Poisoning

The home is loaded with poisons: Cosmetics, Detergents, Bleaches, Cleaning Solutions, Glue, Lye, Paint, Turpentine, Kerosene, Gasoline and other petroleum products, Alcohol, Aspirin and other medications, and on and on.

1. Small children are most often the victims of accidental poisoning. If a child has swallowed or is suspected to have swallowed any substance that might be poisonous, assume the worst—TAKE ACTION.
2. Call your Poison Control Center. If none is in your area, call your emergency medical rescue squad. Bring suspected item and container with you.
3. If the victim is unconscious make sure patient is breathing. If not, tilt head back and perform mouth-to-mouth breathing. Do not give anything by mouth. Do not attempt to stimulate person. Call Emergency Rescue Squad immediately.
4. If the victim is vomiting, roll him or her over onto the left side so that the person will not choke on what is brought up.

5. Be prepared. Determine and verify your Poison Control Center and Fire Department Rescue Squad Numbers and keep them on your telephone.

Drug Overdose

A drug overdose is a poisoning. Alcohol is as much a poison as stimulants, tranquilizers, narcotics, hallucinogens or inhalants. Don't take drunkenness lightly. Too much alcohol can kill.

1. Call for emergency help at once.
2. Check the victim's breathing and pulse. If breathing has stopped or is very weak give Rescue Breathing. Caution: Reviving victims of alcohol poisoning can be violent. Be careful! They can harm themselves and others.
3. While waiting for help:
    A. Watch breathing.
    B. Cover the person with a blanket for warmth.
    C. Do not throw water on the victim's face.
    D. Do not give liquor or a stimulant.

Remember: alcohol in combination with certain other drugs can be deadly!

Burns

1. Minor burns caused by fire, covering only a small area of the body:
    A. Can be treated with cold running water or an ice pack applied for 20 to 30 minutes to relieve swelling and pain.
    B. Do not use grease of any kind. Cold running water is the best first aid.
2. Serious burns:
    A. Require prompt professional care. Call for help immediately.
    B. Wrap the victim in a clean, wet sheet or towel moistened at room temperature.
    C. Burn victims need fluid. Give the victim all the water he or she desires.
    D. Do not attempt to clean the burns or remove clothing or other particles attached to the burnt area.
    E. Keep the victim lying down, calm and reassured.
3. Eye burns:
    A. Should be flushed with large amounts of water.
    B. Then cover the eye with a damp, clean towel and get emergency medical care as soon as possible.
4. Electrical burns:
    A. Are difficult to detect. A person who has received a severe electrical shock may have badly burned underlying tissue, though the surface skin shows little evidence.
    B. Get the victim prompt medical attention. Unattended electrical burns can lead to serious complications.
5. Chemical burns:
    A. Should be washed with plenty of cool, running water. Get the victim into a cool shower, if possible.
    B. After 10 minutes, wrap him or her in a wet, clean sheet and get emergency medical attention without delay.

Quick Reference Handbook Set
BASIC
HEALTH CARE
and Emergency Aid

TITLES AND ASSOCIATIONS ARE AS OF THE TIME OF EACH AUTHOR'S CONTRIBUTION TO THE BOOK

James A. Brussel, M.D.
Assistant Commissioner
Department of Mental Hygiene
State of New York

J. Moore Campbell, M.D.
Clinical Professor of Surgery
School of Medicine
University of Oklahoma

Everett N. Cobb, D.D.S.
Assistant Professor of Operative Dentistry
School of Dentistry
Georgetown University

E. V. Cowdry, Ph.D.
Professor Emeritus of Anatomy
School of Medicine
Washington University

Loren T. DeWind, M.D.
Assistant Clinical Professor of Medicine
School of Medicine
University of Southern California
and California College of Medicine

Mauricio J. Dulfano, M.D.
Assistant Professor of Medicine
School of Medicine
Tufts University

Thomas W. Farmer, M.D.
Head, Division of Neurology
School of Medicine
The University of North Carolina

Ronald N. Grant, M.D.
Director of Professional Education
American Cancer Society

Leonard D. Grayson, M.D.
Clinical Assistant, Allergy Clinic
Medical School
Washington University

Robert A. Hansen, M.D.
Medical Director
Travelers Insurance Company
Los Angeles

Wade B. Irwin Sr., D.D.S.
Assistant Professor of Operative Dentistry
School of Dentistry
Georgetown University

Naomi M. Kanof, M.D.
Chairman, Editorial Board
The Journal of Investigative Dermatology

Jules Kaplan, M.D.
Instructor
Department of Otolaryngology
Medical School
Northwestern University

Mitchell Kory, Ph.D.
Senior Scientist
The Lilly Research Laboratories

Frank W. Newell, M.D.
Professor of Ophthalmology
Eye Research Laboratories
The University of Chicago

Art. H. Panayis, M.D.
Assistant Chief
Department of Obstetrics-Gynecology
Baltimore City Hospitals

Ira A. Roschelle, M.D.
Chief Resident Orthopedic Surgeon
Hospital for Joint Diseases, New York

Isadore Rossman, M.D.
Chief of Professional Services
Home Care Department
Montefiore Hospital, New York

Goodrich C. Schauffler, M.D.
Associate Clinical Professor of
Gynecology and Obstetrics
Medical School
University of Oregon

Lendon H. Smith, M.D.
Assistant Clinical Professor of Pediatrics
Medical School
University of Oregon

Frederick C. Thorne, M.D., Ph.D.
Editor
Journal of Clinical Psychology

James L. Troupin, M.D.
Director of Professional Education
The American Public Health Association

S. O. Waife, M.D.
Assistant Director
Medical Research Division
The Lilly Research Laboratories

Editor

Leroy E. Burney, M.D.
Vice President of Health Sciences
Temple University
Formerly Surgeon General
of the United States

Illustrators

George Geygan
Tom Armstrong
Ellen Zink

UPDATING EDITORS AND CONTRIBUTORS TO THE 1990 EDITION

Updating Editor, 1990 Edition

Isadore Rossman, M.D., Ph.D.
Past President
The American Geriatric Society

Anatomical and Medical Illustrator

Leonard D. Dank

Editorial Coordinator

Cynthia B. Tripp

Contributors

David Altchek, M.D.
Chief Surgeon
Orthopaedic Surgery and
Sports Medicine
The Hospital for Special Surgery
New York

Paul Rossman, M.D.
Staff Psychiatrist
Edgewood Children's Center
San Francisco

Lydia S. Segal, M.D.
Staff Physician, Family Practice
Kaiser Permanente Clinics
Charlotte, NC

C. Al Wood Jr., Pharm.D
Clinical Associate Professor
College of Pharmacy
University of Tennessee

Lisa R. Zablocki, M.D.
Assistant Clinical Professor of Pediatrics
University of Medicine and Dentistry
of New Jersey

THE VARSITY COMPANY
NASHVILLE, TENNESSEE 37214

Published in Nashville, Tennessee, by Thomas Nelson, Inc., Publishers and distributed in Canada by Lawson Falle, Ltd., Cambridge, Ontario.

A compilation of material from earlier editions:
    ©1984, Thomas Nelson Inc., Publishers
    ©1978 Royal Publishers, Inc.
    ©1965, 1972 Stravon Publishers, Inc.

Manufactured in the United States of America

1 2 3 4 5 6 7 8 9 10 — 95 94 93 92 91 90

PREFACE

Like most people in our country, you and your family are more health-conscious today than ever before. At the same time, dramatic progress continues to be made in developing new lifesaving and life-giving medical techniques. Every day doctors learn more about the human body, its chemistry, its physical reactions, and its interrelation with the mind.

This encyclopedia attempts to coordinate this new knowledge and relate it to your own interest in good health in ways that will help you and your family obtain the fullest possible benefits from the major advances of modern medicine. The distinguished physicians and scientists who have written this book present what they consider to be the essential, up-to-date facts on the symptoms, diagnosis, prevention, and treatment of the diseases and disabilities we are likely to encounter today. They tell the facts simply, in language the layman can readily grasp.

As a better informed family—and using this book for ready reference—you will know when to seek medical advice, and will be better able to understand and follow such advice as well as whatever treatment your physician prescribes. Please keep in mind, however, that this is *not* an encyclopedia of home remedies, nor does it replace the need for professional medical care. Importantly, it does outline for you the steps to be taken should an emergency arise, telling you exactly what to do and what not to do until the doctor comes. There are also suggestions on how to care for members of your family at home.

Many changes have occurred in our society within our lifetime which affect the patterns of illness and disability and make it more essential than ever before for you to be well informed. Our population continues to increase—every year adds two or three million more. The two age groups with the greatest proportional gains are the very young and the aging. More than all others, these two groups require medical care. In addition, their health problems are fairly unique: congenital defects, immunization, and infant nutrition are important problems in the very young; cancer, chronic diseases, and mental disorders are most prevalent among the aging.

The number of reported cases of sexually transmitted diseases has soared during the past decade. The numbers continue to rise each month in cases of AIDS, genital herpes, and others. Doctors and research teams have discovered several related complications including pelvic inflammatory disease (PID), recurring infections, and sterility. What can be cured? How does one contract these diseases and how may they be avoided? These and other questions are answered in the section AIDS and Other Sexually Transmitted Diseases.

Our population is highly mobile—about thirty-five million people change residence each year. This increases the family's problems in connection with establishing a relationship with a family doctor or with specialists. On the other hand—and this is an indication of our increased health consciousness—where thirty years ago the average person saw a doctor two or three times a year at best, today the annual average has risen to five visits and even more, especially in the cities. As the cost of medical care continues to rise, more people are turning to nonprescription medications. The FDA has increased the number and variety available to the public without a doctor's prescription. With the help of your pharmacist, you can treat minor symptoms of colds and flus, cuts, burns, and many others. Helpful information appears in the section covering prescription and over-the-counter medications.

In 1930 almost half of all patient visits were made in homes—today very few home calls are made by the physician. Care has been moved from the home to the hospital or other health care institution. This is as it should be, since hospitals are equipped with staffs possessing a broad range of skills; with laboratories to perform the ever-increasing number of tests to aid your own doctor in making a correct diagnosis and instituting proper treatment; with X-ray and other resources, all of which are essential to modern diagnosis and treatment.

Again, many surgical operations are being performed which only ten or fifteen years ago were considered impossible. For example, entire lungs are removed; various types of heart defects are repaired, segments of blood vessels are replaced by synthetic substitutes, and corneas are transplanted from one eye to another to restore sight. Patients are being helped by new heart drugs, improved anesthesia, bone graft banks and blood vessel banks, artificial heart, lung, and kidney machines, and many other lifesaving devices.

Moreover, encouraging and gratifying as medical advances may be, only the well-informed can effectively apply such knowledge, preventing disease before it ever begins, and if it does, preventing irreparable damage by early diagnosis and treatment. To give only one example—it is important for every woman to know at what age—and how often—she should have a cell cytology test, an early-screening technique for detection of cancer of the cervix.

It cannot be emphasized too often that keeping you and your family healthy requires you to be well informed and to accept personal responsibility for initiative and action in this area. The important diseases which strike today are no longer those susceptible to mass prevention and treatment, as was the case a generation ago. In the first part of this century, for instance, the major causes of illness and death in children were the diarrheas and dysenteries and such contagious diseases as diphtheria, whooping cough, and measles. Where once whole communities were incapacitated due to malaria, today state, regional, and local government mosquito-eradication programs have so changed the picture that it is now rare to have a case of malaria reported in the United States. Mass immunization with improved vaccines against diphtheria, whooping cough, poliomyelitis and measles have largely controlled these diseases on a mass basis.

All of this serves to underscore that the average increased life expectancy at birth to seventy years, as well as the lowered mortality rates, are due mainly to our rising educational and economic levels, improved environment, and the development of preventive medicine. Yet the fact remains that the average life expectancy at the age of fifty has increased by only three or four years since 1900. This only emphasizes that the prevention or treatment of heart disease, cancer, arthritis, diabetes, mental illness, and the other chronic diseases are less amenable to public health measures, and hence require vigilance and initiative on your part in recognizing early symptoms and seeking prompt medical advice and care.

This encyclopedia can be invaluable to you in meeting this individual responsibility more intelligently, for it makes accurate information on symptoms, as well as sound advice on when to seek diagnosis and treatment, readily available. Descriptions of diseases and disabling illnesses are followed by the specialists' suggestions as to accepted forms of treatment. It is also explained how and to what extent symptoms may vary in individual cases, and that therapy must therefore be related to individual needs.

The authors have presented their best opinions on the diagnosis and treatment of a broad spectrum of diseases and health problems. But since individual treatment of a specific disease may vary to some extent, you will be wise to follow your own physician's advice carefully, inasmuch as he is the one diagnosing and treating you—or someone in your family—as an individual.

HOW TO USE THIS HEALTH CARE GUIDE

This new edition of Basic Health Care is arranged into twenty-seven medical sections. Each section contains alphabetized entries of terms, conditions and disorders of each medical area. Thus, all the entries on conditions of the eye are in the section EYE AND VISION CONDITIONS, and the entries on nutrition are in the section NUTRITION AND HEALTH. To find an entry the reader can immediately refer to the appropriate section and find a complete listing of topics which are discussed in that section.

The reader should refer to the comprehensive INDEX in the back of the book in order to find entries or discussions that are not immediately located. Frequently, an entry is listed by its medical name, but the index will also list it by its common (popular) name. Occasionally where no separate entry for a disease can be found, a discussion of the particular disease or condition is included in a general discussion covering an entire group of diseases; the index will contain a reference to this specific ailment or condition and, of course, the page number where it can be found.

The first ten sections concern specific bodily systems, arranged in alphabetical order. Listed below is a brief description of each section.

The section CARDIOVASCULAR CONDITIONS identifies the anatomy and physiology of the heart, common disorders (including blood disorders), diagnosis and treatment, and preventive measures of cardiovascular disorders. The section EAR, NOSE, AND THROAT CONDITIONS defines the various physiological structures of the ear, nose, and throat. Perhaps the most common complaints in medical practice today involve conditions of these areas. The section EYE AND VISION CONDITIONS examines the physiology of the eye and discusses how vision is accomplished. Common discomforts and diseases, symptoms and diagnosis, and possible treatments are discussed. The section GASTROINTESTINAL CONDITIONS discusses the physiology and function of the stomach and the intestines. The entries discuss common conditions, diagnostic methods, and possible treatments. The entries in the section GLANDULAR CONDITIONS examine the various glands of the body and how they function, the problems resulting from overproduction or underproduction of the hormones, and possible methods of treatment.

The MUSCULOSKELETAL CONDITIONS section identifies the body's bone and joint structure, defines certain common disorders of the system, and presents possible modes of treatments. The section NERVOUS SYSTEM CONDITIONS examines the physiology of the nervous system and the common neurological disturbances which may be caused by flaws, chemical imbalances, circulatory problems, inflammation, and other disorders of the system. The section RESPIRATORY CONDITIONS examines the process of respiration and the various disorders and conditions that can affect the body's ability to breathe and assimilate oxygen. The section SKIN CONDITIONS presents the physiology of the skin and the symptoms, diagnosis, and possible treatment of common skin disorders. The URINARY CONDITIONS section focuses on the urinary tract and the function of the bladder, ureters, kidneys, and urethra.

The next four sections focus on specific health concerns of different age groups and sexes. There are unique problems experienced by each group, as well as available methods of treatment. For example, a common ailment for a child may pose serious health problems for an adult over sixty-five.

The section AGING: GERIATRICS AND GERONTOLOGY discusses the implications of physical, psychological, and social changes in the elderly, defined as those over sixty-five. References are also given to other health conditions experienced by those in this age group. The section MALE

HEALTH CARE examines the anatomy and physiology of the male, as well as specific medical disorders encountered. The section FEMALE HEALTH CARE discusses the function of the reproductive cycle, as well as basic anatomy and physiology of women. The nature of pregnancy, labor, and delivery are also examined. The INFANT AND CHILD CARE section focuses on the common ailments and concerns of childhood.

Sections Fifteen through Seventeen are concerned with certain vital health care issues. AIDS AND OTHER SEXUALLY TRANSMITTED DISEASES examines the signs, symptoms, and avenues of treatments for these infections. Early diagnosis and treatment is essential, and responsible actions can determine the chances for transmitting or becoming infected with these illnesses. Next, the section INFECTIOUS DISEASES focuses on the symptoms, diagnosis, and sources of treatment for diseases other than sexually transmitted ones. The CANCER section examines the at-risk groups, detection, diagnosis, treatment, and prognosis for cancer patients. Included is a discussion of common cancer sites.

The next sections concern related health fields. The section ALLERGIC CONDITIONS examines the forms of allergies, how they are diagnosed, and how treated. DENTAL HEALTH focuses on the composition and development of teeth, proper dietary and cleaning regimens, and various dental disorders. The section MENTAL HEALTH: PSYCHIATRIC AND PSYCHOLOGICAL CONDITIONS examines certain symptoms of emotionally and mentally disturbed patients and the possible treatments. Then the section MISCELLANEOUS HEALTH CONDITIONS identifies certain disorders, impairments, or departures from good health which do not fit into a neatly categorized system. The section NUTRITION AND HEALTH examines basic dietary concerns, vitamins and minerals, and the new recommended daily allowances. The section SPORTS-RELATED HEALTH CONDITIONS is concerned with the common injuries, symptoms, treatment, and methods of preventing recurrence.

Finally, the last sections concern basic information for home health care. FIRST AID AND EMERGENCIES describe the common first aid and emergency situations and methods of handling them. The section HOME NURSING CARE examines the basic skills required in caring for illness at home and outlines procedures that should be familiar to all adult members of a household. The section QUESTIONS AND ANSWERS ABOUT COMMON SYMPTOMS contains typical patient questions, followed by a clearly outlined physician response. Cross references to other detailed discussions within the text are also given. The questions are grouped with those of a like nature, such as cardiac questions together and so forth. The final section is a GUIDE TO PRESCRIPTIONS AND OVER-THE-COUNTER DRUGS, which outlines certain common medical conditions, the types of medication available, the methods of drug selection, and the possible side effects.

In addition to the twenty-seven sections, there are many black and white illustrations, plus eighty pages of full-color plates designed as ten eight-page color inserts. Each insert may be considered as descriptive of part of the main text or as a complete unit in itself. A comprehensive INDEX is at the end of the volume. The end sheets feature an EMERGENCY SURVIVAL GUIDE.

TABLE OF CONTENTS

COLOR INSERTS

THE CIRCULATORY SYSTEM, Plates B1-B8

THE GLANDS, Plates G1-G8

THE NERVOUS SYSTEM, Plates H1-H8

THE RESPIRATORY AND DIGESTIVE SYSTEMS,
Plates A1-A8

BONE AND SKIN DISORDERS, Plates K1-K8

REPRODUCTION AND FETAL DEVELOPMENT,
Plates J1-J8

CHILD GROWTH AND BEHAVIOR, Plates C1-C8

MUSCULAR AND SKELETAL SYSTEMS, Plates D1-D8

FIRST AID AND LIFE SAVING, Plates F1-F8D

PHYSICAL FITNESS AND REDUCING EXERCISES,
Plates E1-E8D

CARDIOVASCULAR CONDITIONS

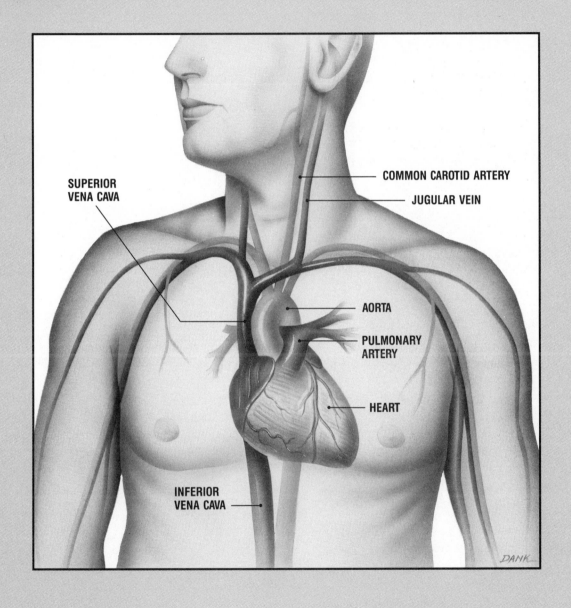

SUPERIOR
VENA CAVA

COMMON CAROTID ARTERY

JUGULAR VEIN

AORTA

PULMONARY
ARTERY

HEART

INFERIOR
VENA CAVA

DANK

Proper functioning of the heart is essential to life. The chief threat the human body faces during its lifetime is a critical decline in the supply of blood to the tissues. When this happens as during a stroke or heart attack, the tissue no longer receives the oxygen and nutrients it requires, and complications and even death can occur quickly. In recent years medical research has advanced in understanding the heart and how to ensure its continued function.

The cardiovascular system is comprised of the organs and vessels that enclose the blood and cause it to move throughout the body. Important components of this system include the heart, the blood vessels, arteries, capillaries, and veins), and their nervous system networks which regulate blood pressure, flow, and distribution of blood as needed by the body's tissues.

This section identifies the anatomy and physiology of the heart, common disorders (including blood disorders), diagnosis and treatment, and preventive measures of cardiovascular disorders. *See also* the questions on anemia (Q-28); on headaches and high blood pressure (Q-33); shortness of breath (Q-46); palpitations of the heart (Q-62); varicose veins (Q-63) in the section QUESTIONS AND ANSWERS ABOUT COMMON SYMPTOMS.

The following is a list of terms identified in this section:

ADAMS-STOKES SYNDROME
ADRENERGIC BLOCKING AGENTS
ANEMIA
ANEURYSM
ANGINA PECTORIS
**ANGIOCARDIOGRAPHY (HEART AND
   BLOOD VESSEL X-RAYS)**
ANGIOGRAPHY, PERCUTANEOUS
ANGIOPLASTY, PERCUTANEOUS
AORTA
AORTA, COARCTATION OF THE
AORTIC ARCH MALDEVELOPMENTS
ARTERIES
ARTERIOSCLEROSIS
ARTERIOSCLEROTIC HEART DISEASE
ARTERIOVENOUS FISTULAS
ATHEROSCLEROSIS
BLOOD CIRCULATION
BLOOD PRESSURE
CAPILLARIES
CARDIAC ARREST
CARDIOMYOPATHY
**CARDIOPULMONARY RESUSCITATION
   (CPR)**
CARDITIS
CHOLESTEROL
COAGULATION

CONGENITAL HEART DISEASE
CONGESTIVE HEART-FAILURE
**CORONARY ARTERY BYPASS GRAFT
   (CABG)**
CORONARY HEART DISEASE
CORONARY INSUFFICIENCY
CORONARY OCCLUSION
CORONARY RISK FACTORS
CORONARY THROMBOSIS
DOPPLER ULTRASOUND
DROPSY
ECHOCARDIAGRAM
EDEMA
EKG
ELECTROCARDIOGRAPHY
EMBOLISM
ESSENTIAL HYPERTENSION
FIBRILLATION
"HEART ATTACK"
HEART CATHETERIZATION
HEART (CARDIAC) DISEASE
HEART DISEASE, EXERCISE AND
HEART-FAILURE
HEART MURMURS
HEART MUSCLE
HEART PAIN (CARDIAC PAIN)
HEART SCANS

ADAMS-STOKES SYNDROME A patient suffering an Adams-Stokes attack loses consciousness and falls into a coma or convulsive attack, perhaps for a minute or more; the catastrophe is caused by temporary but complete cessation of the heartbeat. Its cause may be disease changes, or an inborn defect in the electrical conduction fibers of the heart which can interfere with the intermittent electrical impulse that initiates contraction of the ventricles of the heart.

Symptoms. During an attack of heartblock there is an absence of ventricular contractions, heartbeat, and blood pressure, and circulation of the blood comes to a halt. Spontaneous recovery is, however, the rule, and when the ventricles resume their rhythm, consciousness returns and the symptoms quickly disappear. Attacks occur rarely with some patients, frequently with others. If for any reason the heart fails to resume contractions, death will occur.

Treatment. Drugs can be useful in treating this condition, by speeding up the very slow heart and increasing the ability of the ventricles to resume their own rhythm.

A small electronic device has been developed which can serve as an artificial "pacemaker." Run by a tiny battery, it discharges a very small current at the same tempo as a normal heart. The device is implanted permanently under the skin, and slender wires connect it to the ventricular muscle fibers. The batteries have a life for several years and are replaced in a minor surgical operation under local anesthesia. The presence of the implanted device creates little or no discomfort, and use of the pacemaker has freed thousands of patients from crippling attacks of heartblock and the risk of a fatal seizure.

ADRENERGIC BLOCKING AGENTS Drugs which block the normal response of an organ or tissue to nerve impulses transmitted by the adrenergic nervous system (more or less the same as the sympathetic nervous system). Blocking adrenergic nerves to the heart and blood vessels tends to decrease heart rate and the vigor of heart contraction and to suppress the constriction of blood vessels. Adrenergic blocking agents are often used to treat angina pectoris (since by reducing heart work they reduce its need for oxygen). Some are also used to treat arrhythmias and to control high blood pressure, especially when it is accompanied by a hyperactive heart.

There are two classes of these drugs, alpha- and beta-adrenergic blocking agents. Both

4

can be used in cardiovascular disorders, although beta-adrenergic blocking agents are used more often; of these, propranolol is the most common.

ANEMIA This is a deficiency in the quality or quantity of red blood cells. The red cells may be depleted by loss of blood from the body because of injury, repeated bloody noses, abnormally heavy menstrual flow, bleeding ulcers or fissures, or other conditions leading to blood-loss. Diseases may also produce anemia: cancer, leukemia, tuberculosis, nephritis, rheumatic fever, erythroblastosis of newborn (RH disease) may be responsible. By far the most common type of anemia in children and babies is simple iron deficiency anemia, which is almost always due to inadequate consumption of foods other than milk in the first two years of life.

Treatment. The use of milk should be controlled, iron medication given, and meat and fruit added to the diet. Special blood tests are usually necessary to determine the exact type of anemia and, of course, the specific therapy (which is nearly always iron in some form). Iron supplements should be prescribed by the doctor; unsuitable iron medications or dosages may cause digestive trouble. The distinct form of anemia found in some older persons known as pernicious anemia responds to injections of cyanocobalamin (B_{12}). When rapid treatment of anemia is urgent, whole blood or packed red blood cells are given intravenously.

ANEURYSM If a section of artery wall becomes weakened by disease changes, it tends to thin and bulge out with each beat of the heart. After months or years, a saclike widening finally develops at this weak point along the artery; this bulging, pulsating projection is called an aneurysm. In certain infections (such as syphilis) weakness occurs in the middle, elastic coat of the vessel, the aneurysm wall being made up of remnants from all three layers of the artery.

An arteriosclerotic dissecting aneurysm comes into existence a little differently. First a stony-hard arteriosclerotic patch replaces a section of the innermost (intima) membrane that lines the artery. Since this patch is not firmly united at its sides, pulsations of blood tend to loosen its attachment to the lining membrane, especially when a crack or fissure develops in that line of attachment. As the fissure enlarges, blood is forced under pressure into the potential space between the intima and the middle muscle-coat of the artery. The intima is literally peeled away from its attachment; and the middle coat, now lacking the structural support afforded by its lining membrane, bulges outward with every pulsation of blood. The vessel slowly enlarges and so does the cavity formed between the two blood-vessel layers.

Either type of aneurysm can become quite large over a period of years. Most of them occur in the aorta and adjacent large vessels either because of their size or because of decreased efficiency of circulation, producing symptoms in the vessel system distant from the aneurysm. In quite large aneurysms ruptures can occur, with resulting fatal hemorrhage.

Treatment. Surgery may be indicated if the aneurysm produces symptoms of pain in the chest, abdomen, or wherever it may be present; or if it prevents good circulation to the head, one of the extremities or an important organ of the body. Symptoms of malfunction can come in any of these places. Surgery may also be necessary if the aneurysm is so large that rupture and fatal hemorrhage are a real possibility.

At the time of operation, the aneurysm may be replaced by a section of borrowed vessel or by woven plastic tubing; the aorta in the chest and abdomen lends itself particularly well to this procedure, and it can be life-saving. Replaced segments of artery, whether of natural tissue or made of plastic, can take over blood-vessel function without difficulty for many years. The body usually builds up reinforcing tissue, which surrounds the implanted vessel and strengthens it so that it seems to function as well as a natural arterial conduit.

Sometimes a bypass graft is used and the now-empty original vessel, with its aneurysm, left in place. When this is done, blood flows through the graft that lies beside the diseased vessel. Occasionally the aneurysm can be removed from the artery wall, and the original vessel repaired so that a graft is not needed. (*See also* CORONARY ARTERY BYPASS GRAFT in this section.)

ANGINA PECTORIS   Distinctly a disease of people past middle age and rarely seen earlier, angina pectoris gets its name from the severe chest pain with which it is associated. An attack usually is brought on by physical exertion or emotional stress and generally disappears after a minute or two of adequate rest. The pain occurs because the heart tissue is not receiving as much blood as it needs. Angina pectoris may imply that permanent changes have occurred in the anatomical structure of the coronary arteries. (*See* ARTERIOSCLEROTIC HEART DISEASE in this section.) The individual with angina is at risk of having a heart attack.

The occurrence of angina pectoris in many members of one family and few in another suggests that there may be a hereditary factor involved in its development. Among ethnic groups, too, there is a predisposing influence. For example, the condition is very uncommon in the Bantu tribesmen of South Africa, and rarely is it seen among the Navajo Indians of Arizona, although quite common among other persons in the same area.

Obese individuals have a high rate of coronary artery disease and exhibit a mortality rate from coronary heart disease at least 40 percent higher than among standard-risk persons of average weight. Smoking; a diet excessive in calories, saturated fat, cholesterol, and salt; heavy, regular consumption of alcohol; hypertension; oral contraceptives; family history and sedentary lifestyle are all risk factors. (*See* CORONARY RISK FACTORS in this section.)

Symptoms. If during physical exertion, the heart muscle needs more blood than the width of the coronary arteries can provide, the resulting lack of oxygen (anoxia) and accumulation of metabolic waste products stimulate the sympathetic nerve fibers that surround these arteries. This nerve stimulation can cause pain that is quite severe—a pain usually felt under the breastbone. At the same time, it may spread down the left arm even into the little finger and the one next to it; it sometimes fans out into the neck or jaw, the right arm, or even into the abdomen. The pain usually has a constricting or "squeezing" character.

An attack of angina pectoris is usually brought on by effort, either physical or emotional, and may be relieved in a short time by either sitting or lying down. In some individuals, a large meal can create enough extra heart work to bring on an attack of angina pectoris. Pain may be rather mild and of seconds' duration, or so severe that the person suffering the attack is sure that death itself must be near.

Angina may occur regularly and predictably with a certain amount of physical exertion, so-called "stable angina." When it changes its pattern, becomes much more frequent or occurs at rest, so-called "unstable angina," it may be predictive of a heart attack and hospitalization is advisable.

Sometimes, the pain of angina pectoris is caused by a temporary spasm of one of the heart-artery branches. The spasm causes enough narrowing of the vessel for the flow of blood to heart-muscle fibers served by that particular artery to be restricted, falling short of the constant requirements of muscle tissue for oxygen and nourishment. No permanent damage is done to the heart muscle, since as soon as the spasm passes, normal blood flow to the area is restored and the deficit in tissue requirements can be slowly corrected.

In contrast to a temporary spasm, most angina patients will eventually develop a clot that actually plugs a coronary artery and prevents the flow of blood to the muscle tissue supplied by that vessel. The result is that a segment of heart muscle incurs irreversible injury. Pain that is experienced at the time of vessel blockage may not be very different in character from that experienced during attacks of angina, with one important difference: pain does not disappear after complete rest or even after taking the medication that had always provided relief of pain when vessel spasms alone had caused it.

Treatment. Most patients with uncomplicated angina can, if necessary, carry out light manual work, but any physical activity that increases the frequency of attacks or that causes pain directly must be avoided. A diet is usually advised that does not include rich foods and large meals. Excessive intake of fatty foods should be avoided. Alcohol in moderation does not seem to be harmful.

Drugs in the nitroglycerine group, absorbed from under the tongue, can often avert an impending attack of angina pectoris. Artery dilating medication can be of great value, especially in the period after the acute attack of pain has subsided.

Catheter dilatation or surgical bypasses of the blocking patches within the coronary arteries have restored the ability of those vessels to provide an adequate blood supply to the heart musculature, bringing complete disappearance of the painful attacks in many patients, even after prolonged physical exertion. Operations for the relief of angina pectoris are considered when X-ray studies of the coronary vessels demonstrate significant narrowings. Modern surgical techniques have made these corrective procedures relatively safe, and for that reason many individuals with coronary artery disease now are being studied to determine whether a direct surgical attack can be made on these anatomic changes. (*See also* CORONARY INSUFFICIENCY; CORONARY OCCLUSION; and CORONARY ARTERY BYPASS GRAFT in this section.)

ANGIOCARDIOGRAPHY (HEART AND BLOOD VESSEL X-RAYS) Machines have been designed to take a series of X-ray pictures at intervals of much less than one second; as the heart beats, the changes taking place in its size and shape can be filmed throughout the cycle of contraction (systole) and relaxation (diastole). Study of the precise movements of the heart's outline can lead to important conclusions about its anatomical structure and the efficiency of each chamber in performing the work of pumping the blood.

Angiocardiography is an X-ray study of the movement of blood through the heart and vessels. When a fluid that throws a shadow onto the film (contrast material) is injected into the blood, its passage through the heart, lungs, and blood vessels can be recorded on rapidly-taken X-ray films, or even on motion-picture film that can later be observed in normal or even slow motion. By means of this procedure, the actual pumping can be observed: first the blood enters the receiving chamber of the heart (right atrium) which lies within the right portion of the heart shadow. Next it moves into the pumping chamber (right ventricle) and is then dispersed in the lungs. A moment later, the contrasting material is seen collecting in the left, moving to the left ventricle, then being pumped out of the heart into the aortic system of arteries.

Selective angiocardiograms are usually made during heart catheterization. After pressures have been taken in the heart chambers and samples of blood withdrawn for oxygen saturation percentage, contrast material is then introduced through the same catheter and X-rays taken as it moves through the heart and vessels.

Narrowing of any vessels can be recorded with great accuracy on these X-ray films and the records kept for future reference and comparison. Valve efficiency also is demonstrated well; if any valve happens to be "leaking," the location and quantity of the backward flow can be seen clearly. Any vessel abnormalities, unusual openings between chambers or vessels, can be observed as well.

Angiocardiography can often furnish a good anatomical presentation of the heart in

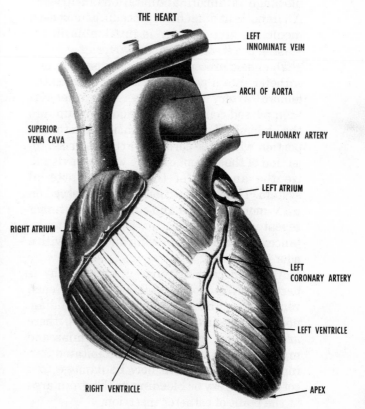

THE HEART

LEFT INNOMINATE VEIN

ARCH OF AORTA

SUPERIOR VENA CAVA

PULMONARY ARTERY

LEFT ATRIUM

RIGHT ATRIUM

LEFT CORONARY ARTERY

LEFT VENTRICLE

RIGHT VENTRICLE

APEX

action when other diagnostic procedures may fail to uncover the precise nature of early disease changes or very small birth defects. In addition, if surgical correction is made, the angiocardiogram can be repeated after operation to demonstrate the improved circulation.

A technique of injecting contrast material into the aorta near the coronary arteries will make the arteries of the heart visible on motion-picture film. Abnormal vessels, narrow points in the coronary artery, and inborn (congenital) defects can be studied by coronary motion-picture angiograms.

From these studies, surgical approaches to diseased coronary vessels can be planned. Each year, more and more patients are having circulation restored to the heart muscle by catheter distention of areas of narrowing or by blood-vessel bypasses which shunt blood to areas past the narrowings.

ANGIOGRAPHY, PERCUTANEOUS
The basic procedure in angiography is the instillation of a dye opaque to X-rays into a blood vessel. The dye produces visualization of the blood vessel, most often an artery, and will reveal areas of narrowing (stenosis), blockage, or abnormal dilatation (aneurysm). An important diagnostic procedure in modern medicine, angiography is invaluable in assessing the state of coronary arteries.

The basic procedure calls for insertion of a catheter into a peripheral artery such as the femoral artery in the groin. The catheter is then passed counter to the blood flow up into the abdominal and then thoracic aorta to that portion where the coronary arteries arise. Injection of the radiopaque dye will then visualize the anatomy of the coronary arterial system. The visualization can be observed on a TV monitor device and captured on film for repeated study thereafter. Of special importance are areas of narrowing and areas with a poor circulation.

Although coronary artery angiography is performed in around 250,000 persons each year and has become almost a routine diagnostic procedure in larger hospitals, there are still some risks to it. Arrhythmias and myocardial infarcts may be precipitated during the process. There may be damage to a coronary artery or bleeding in the groin area at the point of catheter insertion.

ANGIOPLASTY, PERCUTANEOUS
This is a surgical procedure in which an occluded artery is opened up using a catheter that is passed into the artery. Angioplasty is far simpler than bypass grafts, avoids the heart-lung machine, and the painful splitting of the breastbone. The technology that was developed for coronary artery angiography was the base for the procedure of angioplasty. The catheter was modified to incorporate a balloon which could be blown up and thus exert pressure against the arterial wall. (*See* ANGIOGRAPHY, PERCUTANEOUS in this section.)

Indeed it is possible to combine the procedures using the same catheter, first to inject the contrast medium that outlines the arteries and then go on to the procedure.

In the commonly employed balloon dilation method, a segment of the catheter can be blown up so as to exert pressure against the atheromatosis deposit that narrows the artery. The deposit is soft and can be crushed against the wall of the artery. Very often the soft material is dispersed into the arterial wall as the inner lining is fractured by the blown up balloon. When successful, a measurable enlargement of the narrowed area occurs and so a patient may be relieved of the angina.

Originally balloon dilation was limited to a single area of obstruction. More recently reports have appeared of dilation of two but rarely more narrowed segments. In skilled hands and in the absence of complications, patients may go home after no more than a three-day stay in hospital.

In select cases the outcomes are excellent, and the number of patients who have had balloon dilation of their coronary arteries has increased almost rivaling coronary artery bypass grafting. However, there are drawbacks:

- If the narrowed segment is a long one, dilation may not be applicable.
- If there is a good deal of diffuse narrowing throughout the coronary artery system, the balloon method can't be used or will make little contribution.
- There is always the possibility that the fatty material being compressed may move downstream and act as an embolus, thus producing occlusion and myocardial infarction (heart attack). Thus a surgical team able to promptly do bypass surgery

must be available in reserve in such an event.

- Troublesome, even life-threatening arrhythmias may be precipitated by the manipulation—to be contrasted with the non-beating heart in bypass surgery.
- In some persons the dilated coronary segment, more or less, returns to its original state: this is known as restenosis—literally repeat narrowing—and symptoms return. However, the dilation can be repeated.

Despite the aforementioned possibilities balloon dilation has been life-saving especially for patients at high risk for bypass grafting procedures. Various technical advances have made the method safer and more effective. An example is a technique used in a few centers in which the obstructive plaque is neatly destroyed within the arterial lining with a laser. This may well be the method of the future.

It should be noted that balloon dilation is applicable to arteries other than the coronaries. The method has been used for segmental occlusions in the peripheral arteries, most commonly those of the lower extremity. Patients with narrowed femoral or popliteal arteries may be candidates for a balloon angioplasty; when successful these may give relief from intermittent claudication or even the threat of gangrene or loss of limb.

AORTA   The largest artery in the body, the aorta receives all the blood from the left ventricle; it serves as a transport line and reservoir of all newly oxygenated blood. Branching from the aorta are the supply arteries to the head, arms, legs, and—ultimately—every body tissue.

The aorta, like other arteries, has three definite layers in its elastic walls. The intima is the lining membrane—a layer of cells about as thick as heavy wrapping paper. The middle coat is relatively thick, composed of a highly elastic membrane that serves to maintain blood pressure between the heart and the peripheral arteries in between heartbeats. The outer layer (adventitia) is a bed or framework of fibrous tissue, fat, and blood vessels that separates the blood vessel from surrounding tissues, and gives it freedom to expand and contract.

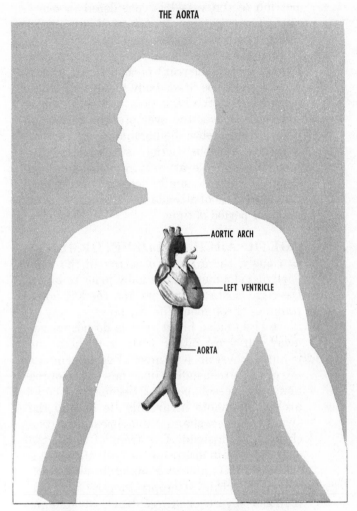

THE AORTA

AORTIC ARCH

LEFT VENTRICLE

AORTA

AORTA, COARCTATION OF THE   A constriction that narrows and may almost completely obstruct the aorta in the upper chest is called a coarctation. A birth defect, it obstructs the flow of blood to the lower half of the body in the usual case. There is circulation to the head and arms because vessels supplying these areas branch from the aorta prior to the point of narrowing.

Symptoms. Although extensive narrowing in the aorta will cause death shortly after birth, most patients with the abnormality survive for many years, often with no symptoms at all. Blood pressure in the arms may be extremely high, but in the legs it can be very low. It is this disparity of blood pressure that often leads to the suspicion of an obstruction within the aorta, and the coarctation can be demonstrated by an X-ray procedure.

Treatment. When the diagnosis has been confirmed, surgical removal of the constricted portion of the vessel is considered in every case. There has been constant strain on the heart which has maintained an abnormally high pressure in the aorta just to squeeze blood through the point of coarctation and to put blood in the lower body vessels. In addition, relief of the high pressure in the head arteries removes the ever present danger of death from cerebral hemorrhage.

In case the obstruction is not severe, the blood pressure elevation is in moderation and surgical relief is usually deferred until about the age of school attendance, sometimes even a longer period of time.

AORTIC ARCH MALDEVELOPMENTS

Curiously, there are two aortas in the very early development of the baby prior to birth; the right aorta disappears and the left aorta remains throughout life. If, however, any of these right-sided blood vessels do not wither away but grow either with or without the usual left system, a number of derangements are possible (depending upon how many of the abnormal vessels persist). Because the right arch components invariably lie behind the swallowing (esophagus) and breathing (trachea) tubes instead of in front of them, the channel within either one or both of these vital conduits is almost completely closed off. When the child attempts to take nourishment, a severe choking attack (dysphagia lusoria) can occur and even cause fatal suffocation.

Treatment. If the choking attacks are severe, or breathing is labored, surgical relief will be required. As soon as the constricting vessel is cut and tied to prevent bleeding, a normal passageway is restored for passage of air to the lungs, or of food to the stomach. Meanwhile, other vessels in the area immediately take over the function of the divided artery.

ARTERIES

The arteries are tubes that carry newly oxygenated blood from the heart, through an elaborate branching system, to all the capillaries and tissues of the body. With every heartbeat, a jet of blood is pressed into the arterial system, which, by its built-in elasticity, insures a constant flow of blood from its smallest branches (the arterioles) into the capillaries, where chemical exchanges are made.

(From the capillaries, blood returns to the heart through a separate system of vessels, the veins.)

ARTERIOSCLEROSIS

More properly now termed atherosclerosis and produced by fatty deposits, this disorder causes more circulatory disease after middle age than any other single cause. Arteriosclerosis is nevertheless occasionally seen in young persons of both sexes and, conversely, many elderly people have little significant manifestation of the condition. It is therefore an oversimplification to say that the condition is the result of stress and wear in the arteries, especially as the result of the aging process. There is, however, one well-recognized form of arteriosclerosis termed Mönckeberg sclerosis associated with advanced aging. In this disorder calcium deposits occur in the middle coat of arteries but with little interference to blood flow.

Although high blood pressure is quite commonly a contributing factor to sclerosis, it may or may not be present in persons with arteriosclerosis. Diabetes can facilitate the development of arteriosclerotic changes; even young patients with diabetes may be severely affected—especially when the diabetes has not been well controlled over a long period of time. The term *arteriolosclerosis* denotes degenerative changes in small arterioles, vessels of small caliber generally within the organs. These are the vessels often damaged by hypertension and diabetes. Small vital units such as the nephrons of the kidney may be damaged or destroyed.

Arteriosclerosis can cause disease changes in specific organs, such as serious kidney disease. Cerebral arteriosclerosis may lead to crippling mental infirmities. Sometimes changes in one or more organs are quite severe, while the rest of the artery system seems to show little significant disease.

Factors contributing to this disease include cigarette smoking, high blood pressure, high blood cholesterols, and diabetes. The male sex, positive family history, and perhaps stress and personality types also seem relevant.

Treatment generally focuses on reducing these risk factors. More specific treatments are available for the disorders that can be caused by arteriosclerosis, such as arteriosclerotic heart disease. Drug therapy may be useful in treating some forms of arteriosclerosis; in others, surgery may be necessary. (*See also* ARTERIOSCLEROTIC HEART DISEASE; ATHEROSCLEROSIS in this section.)

ARTERIOSCLEROTIC HEART DISEASE

Now often referred to as coronary artery disease, this is the most common cause of heart disease in patients beyond middle age and accounts for more deaths in the United States than all other diseases combined. Heart-failure is more frequently caused by arteriosclerosis than any other disease process. The failure may be mild and may persist for many years before death comes as a final manifestation.

Any narrowing of the internal diameter of the arteries of the heart through arteriosclerotic changes can diminish the amount of blood flowing to the heart muscle fibers. In replenishing the vital chemicals constantly needed to energize the heart, blood flow should increase—even if only for a few minutes—every time there is a new demand for intense heart action. (Because of the efficient arrangement of the capillaries in heart muscle, almost no available oxygen remains in the blood after its passage through the heart itself, and therefore additional oxygen can be supplied only by a proportionate increase in blood flow through the coronary arteries of the heart.)

Symptoms. Arteriosclerotic narrowing of the coronary arteries can produce several outcomes. The patient may complain of angina pectoris or the involvement may lead to a clot and damage to a segment of heart muscle which then becomes non-contractile and functionless (myocardial infarction). Degenerative changes in the "heart-triggering" conduction system ("bundle of His") can be the result of arteriosclerotic changes. With these, serious disturbances may occur in the orderly, rhythmic contractions of the heart chambers such as Adams-Stokes attacks and cardiac arrests. This manifestation of arteriosclerotic heart disease is sometimes resolved with a pace-

ARTERIOSCLEROSIS
Arteriosclerosis is a general term for three forms of blood vessel disease.

MEDIAL CALCIFICATION
Medial calcification (Senile Arteriosclerosis) calcifies the middle muscular layer of medium-sized arteries. The artery walls become less flexible, but the blood flow is not impeded.

ARTERIOLAR-SCLEROSIS
Arteriolar-sclerosis is a disease associated with hypertension. The small arterioles can become brittle (A) or the muscle layer may overgrow at the expense of the blood passage (B).

ATHEROSCLEROSIS
Atherosclerosis is a disease of the inner lining in which cholesterol-containing plaques are formed. Eventually the blood flow is impeded by the enlarging plaques.

maker which stimulates cardiac contractions when the need arises.

ARTERIOVENOUS FISTULAS An arteriovenous fistula is an abnormal opening between an artery and a vein. It may be inborn—a defect present at birth—or it may be acquired during life. Usually an acquired arteriovenous fistula is caused by an injury. If a wound should occur in an artery wall, as sometimes results from a knife or bullet injury, the injury may also involve the vein lying next to the artery. These two wounds may then unite the artery and vein walls, tightly fastening them together as the healing proceeds; through this attachment an opening for blood may slowly develop. Blood in the artery, under pressure, can then leak through the opening into the vein by way of the newly formed fistula.

If the opening lies between a large artery and vein, a great quantity of blood may flow out of the artery and return via the vein to the heart without having supplied any of the tissues. This functional leakage can be so large in extent that additional load on the heart may eventually cause heart-failure. On rare occasions, a bacterial infection will develop at the site of the fistula and result in "germs in the blood" (bacteremia).

Treatment. Surgical correction is the only cure for an arteriovenous fistula. In almost every instance, the opening in the artery wall can be closed by fine sutures and the vein moved aside and similarly repaired. A piece of tissue is sometimes placed between the two vessels to prevent a re-forming of the abnormal pathway between the two vessels as they heal.

ATHEROSCLEROSIS The term arteriosclerosis is a general one, used to describe any of the "hardening-of-the-arteries" changes such as calcium deposition while atherosclerosis is a a very specific disease.

The primary tissue-change seen in atherosclerosis is found in the lining membrane (intima) of the arterial tube. While in young, healthy arteries the intimal lining consists of a layer of very smooth and glistening cells loosely adhering to the thicker, medial layer of the artery, in atherosclerosis this lining coat shows deposits of fatty molecules (lipids) as well as variable amounts of scar tissue formation, hemorrhage, and calcification.

Recent studies show that the lipids in circulating blood tend to leak across the lining membrane and be deposited in the space between it and the rather solid (yet elastic) middle layer of the vessel. These lipids are taken into special cells lying in that space (mesenchymal cells). This incorporation of fatty materials into the cells of the blood vessel may represent the earliest form of atherosclerosis. When fat-laden cells leak over into the middle coat of the artery, thickening can result there in addition to formation of intimal-lining deposits. This frequently happens in the larger arteries that supply the brain, the kidneys, and the lower extremities.

As the lipid-filled cells accumulate, fibrous tissue seems to be laid down, the patch of arterial lining membrane then becoming rigid and thickened. As the patch thickens it degenerates, and tiny blood vessels—capillaries—appear within it. These can rupture and produce small puddles of blood within the atherosclerotic deposit itself.

A double process is thus at work: first come the fatty deposits in the cells, together with a heaping-up of these cells in one particular location with degenerative changes that turn the whole mass into a foreign-body deposit; second, there is occurrence of hemorrhage within these accumulations, adding considerably to their bulk. The space inside the vessel still remaining useful for passage of blood becomes smaller and smaller. The vessel itself is sometimes completely blocked by the process, and blood fails to flow through it beyond the affected point. Then too, a clot may form and completely close off a vessel which, while already nearly obstructed to clot-formation, had nevertheless been useful. Calcium may be deposited at any stage of the disease and make the atherosclerotic patch hard and brittle.

Because atherosclerosis is now the most prevalent serious human disease the world over, research about the problems of prevention and control have intensified. In recent years the role of cholesterol has been reaffirmed. Roughly, the higher the blood cholesterol, the greater the degree of atherosclerosis. The total cholesterol can be partitioned into a low density fraction (LDL) which predisposes to the disease ("bad cholesterol") and a high density fraction (HDL) representative of the cholesterol transportable out of the tissues to the liver ("good cholesterol"). It is thought that fats in the diet should be reduced to about 20 or 30 percent of the total caloric consumption. With reduction of lipids and cholesterol circulating in the blood, the precipitation and accumulation of lipids in the intimal lining of the arteries may be reduced to such an extent that the development of atherosclerosis can be held in check.

Reversibility of atherosclerosis changes in animals was clearly demonstrated many years ago. Atherosclerotic deposits in human beings seem to lessen in patients who undergo severe weight loss, or who are on drastic anticholesterol programs. It should be remembered in this connection that there is no cholesterol in the vegetable kingdom and considerably less heart and vessel disease in vegetarians.

Special diets, exercise programs, and careful attention to any metabolic derangements that may be present can sometimes bring about these desirable lower lipid levels in the blood. The degree of reversibility of atherosclerotic deposits is currently under intense study, and opinion is divided. Probably old fixed lesions may not respond. (*See also* ARTERIOSCLEROSIS in this section.)

BLOOD CIRCULATION The design for circulation of blood to all the tissues of the body centers around the pumping action of the heart, through which all blood passes. As the word *circulation* implies, the process is a closed and repetitive cycle.

The heart system. Venous (vein) blood returns to the heart by passing through two major trunks: the superior vena cava, which passively draws blood in from the head, upper arms, and part of the trunk; and the inferior vena cava, which gathers returning blood from the remainder of the body, including all of the abdominal organs.

Through gateways at its upper and lower margins, blood flows into the heart's receiving chamber (right atrium). This chamber serves as a supply depot and also as a contracting chamber which efficiently moves an exact amount of blood into the right ventricular pump chamber for transmission to the lungs.

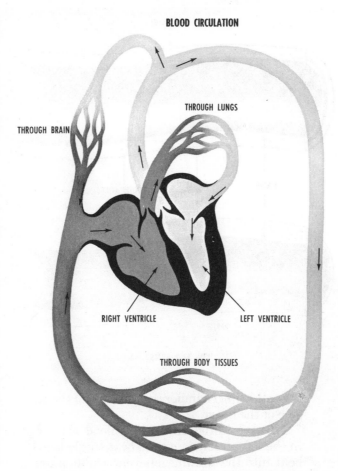

BLOOD CIRCULATION

THROUGH LUNGS

THROUGH BRAIN

RIGHT VENTRICLE   LEFT VENTRICLE

THROUGH BODY TISSUES

With heart contraction, the right ventricle squeezes this measured amount of blood into the pulmonary arteries supplying the lungs. Within the lungs, vessels divide and subdivide hundreds of times, the heartbeat of blood ultimately passing through hundreds of miles of vessels so small that the blood cells must "wiggle" through, almost a single cell at a time. (The diameter of the pulmonary capillaries is scarcely more than the thickness of a single red blood cell.)

The lung capillaries might be said truly to float in the air we breathe, lying as they do against the cells of the terminal air sacs (alveoli) of the lungs. As red blood cells pass through them, carbon dioxide escapes from them into the air about to be exhaled, while oxygen from the air just breathed in passes through the capillary walls and fastens to hemoglobin located within the red blood cells.

Oxygenated, the blood now flows into larger and larger collecting veins and finally arrives, by way of the pulmonary veins, into

VEIN VALVE

OUTER COAT

ARTERY

VEIN AND ARTERY

which has its origin just outside the final valve of the heart, the aortic valve. (This valve prevents arterial blood from slipping back into the heart.)

As the blood reaches the smallest arteries (arterioles), it next flows into the capillaries, whose walls are only single, flattened tissue cells and hence extremely thin; it is through these cell membranes that oxygen and fluid nutrients pass into the tissues. Accumulations of carbon dioxide and fluid waste product are gathered from the tissues after crossing these same capillary walls, and are then swept through the veins to the lungs and excretory organs where they are disposed of.

BLOOD PRESSURE With each heartbeat, freshly oxygenated blood is pumped from the heart and flows under pressure into the largest vessel of the human body, the aorta. At the end of each heart contraction, the valve at the exit of the pumping chamber (left ventricle) snaps closed. It is at this precise moment that pressure in the aorta reaches its highest peak. As the aorta waits for the next burst of blood from the left ventricle, pressure within it gradually drops, because blood is continually filtering out of the arteries into the capillaries.

The large aorta, with its extremely elastic walls, holds a tremendous supply of refreshed blood. It serves as a supply reservoir that, between heartbeats, insures a constant flow of blood into even the smallest vessels, far distant from the heart. Pressure that builds up at the end of ventricular contraction (called systole) is known as the systolic pressure; at rest it should not normally exceed a pressure of 140 to 150 millimeters of mercury.

Between heart contractions, pressure in the aorta falls, reaching its lowest reading while the ventricles are refilling themselves during the diastolic phase of the cardiac cycle. During diastole, the between-beat (diastolic) pressure drops to 90 millimeters of mercury or even less.

Your physician may advise you to buy your own blood pressure measuring device—a sphygmomanometer—and to monitor your blood pressure at home one or more times a day as a means of helping him regulate medication.

the collecting chamber (left atrium) of the left side of the heart.

This measured amount of blood arriving in the left atrium is moved by a single heartbeat into the waiting left ventricular pumping chamber. The ventricle then contracts, and pushes this portion of blood into a large, elastic artery, the aorta, which carries blood away from the heart and supplies the arterial branches which reach into all the tissues.

With each pulsation, the left ventricle ordinarily moves the same quantity of blood from the heart into the body at large as does the right ventricle from the heart into the lungs. Because of this balance, blood is not trapped in the lungs and the volume of blood there remains the same from minute to minute, for each heartbeat empties as much blood from the lungs as is pumped in. If any imbalance does come into existence and the lungs become abnormally engorged with a large quantity of blood, failure of the left side of the heart to evacuate this "stagnating" blood can lead to one type of congestive heart-failure.

The vessel system. Blood circulates from the heart to all the tissues through the arteries of the body. Major vessels to the brain and extremities branch off from the aorta—the main trunk of the body's arterial system—

LIFE-SHORTENING IN UNTREATED HYPERTENSION

Measurement of blood pressure is the most important factor used by insurance companies in predicting life expectancy.

How dangerous is untreated high blood pressure? A study involving 4,000,000 policyholders in 26 large life insurance companies showed that at any given age the higher the blood pressure, the lower the life expectancy.

Age at First Reading	MEN Blood Pressure	Expected Longevity	Loss in Life Expectancy (in years)
35	120/80	76½ years	—
	130/90	72½	4
	140/95	67½	9
	150/100	60	16½
45	120/80	77	—
	130/90	74	3
	140/95	71	6
	150/100	60	17
55	120/80	78½	—
	130/90	77½	1
	140/95	74½	4
	150/100	72½	6
45	WOMEN 120/80	82	—
	130/90	80½	1½
	140/95	77	5
	150/100	73½	8½
55	120/80	82½	—
	130/90	82	½
	140/95	79½	3
	150/100	78½	4

By keeping careful records of your pressure, indicating the date and time of the recording, the name of the drug, the dosage, the time taken, and the nature of your activity before the time the recording has been taken, you can tell him much more than if your pressure were taken only on visits to the office.

Furthermore, blood pressure readings in the physician's office often are higher because of anxiety. In your own home, you become accustomed to it and no longer are tense.

Drugs ordinarily are prescribed on the basis of the blood pressure readings recorded in the doctor's office. Recordings at home permit the doctor to make medication adjustment. When the blood pressure increases, the dosage of drugs can be increased or more potent ones used. When the pressure declines, the dosage can be reduced and the more potent ones discontinued.

You soon learn through home measurements that mental and physical stress will elevate blood pressure and that rest and relaxation will lower it. Thus, you learn to avoid those factors that drive pressure up and promote those factors that bring lower pressure. Regular readings at home also can serve to remind you to take your medication.

In 90 percent of cases of high blood pressure, there is no specific cause. There are, however, certain contributing factors: obesity, high sodium intake, alcohol consumption, oral contraceptives, lack of exercise, and heredity. The disease also tends to develop more frequently in males and in blacks.

CAPILLARIES At the termination of an artery anywhere in the body, a capillary receives fresh blood. A short tube that lies in intimate contact with living cells of the body, the capillary has a wall or membrane made of a layer of thinned-out single cells attached to each other like quiltwork. The cell wall constitutes that semipermeable membrane which permits gas- and fluid-exchange from tissues to the fluids of blood, and vice versa.

The diameter of a capillary will permit the passage of red blood cells lined up in single file. A passive tube with no muscular control of its diameter, it discharges blood into a connecting vein (or venule) for eventual return to the heart by way of the venous system.

CARDIAC ARREST The term cardiac arrest is applied to any sudden and unexpected cessation of heartbeat. It occurs most frequently in older individuals and most often as a manifestation of arteriosclerotic disease.

Circumstances involving any type of stress seem to precipitate an attack. It may occur with severe exertion, during or after a surgical operation, and even without an exciting cause.

Diagnosis is made by noting the absence of pulse or blood pressure and clinched by an electrocardiogram which shows absence of the usual electrical activity. Patients under stress of an accident, an operation, or disease are frequently attached to a cardiac-monitoring device. This electronic machine incorporates a special adaptation of electrocardiographic principles; disturbances in heart rate and rhythm are signaled by a visual or auditory alarm mechanism incorporated in the device.

Treatment. In an acute care facility a cardiac-monitoring device may be arranged to trigger an electrical stimulus to the patient's heart at every prolonged pause in heartbeat, and episodes of cardiac arrest can often be terminated automatically. In very rare instances, however, it may be necessary to open the chest with a surgical incision and massage the heart directly until heartbeat is re-established. This procedure has proven a life-saving measure when promptly employed, no matter what the primary circumstances of arrest.

When an arrest occurs, a special technique of intermittent manual pressure on the breastbone accompanied by blowing air into the lungs—cardiopulmonary resuscitation (CPR)—can often compress the heart artificially and give enough movement of blood through the heart to produce a spontaneous return of heartbeat.

Sometimes electroshock (defibrillation or cardioversion) is needed to break up cardiac standstill or ventricular trembling (fibrillation) before an effective beat of the heart will return. A few drugs are known that will assist and reinforce returning heartbeat. If cardiac arrest is not recognized promptly, permanent brain damage may result after five minutes from lack of continuous flow of oxygenated blood.

CARDIOMYOPATHY Any noninflammatory disease affecting the heart muscle, or myocardium, is known as cardiomyopathy. The cause of primary cardiomyopathy is unknown. Secondary cardiomyopathy can have a wide variety of causes including viral infections, anemia, hypo- or hyperthyroidism, alcoholism, malnutrition, toxic agents, drugs, pregnancy, radiation, bacterial infections, and the aging process. Symptoms are the same as those of heart failure—shortness of breath, coughing, fatigue.

Complete bedrest is required to reduce the heart's workload while the muscle is healing. Treatment is usually directed at controlling arrhythmias and reducing congestion. Primary cardiomyopathy is particularly serious because its cause is unknown.

CARDIOPULMONARY RESUSCITATION (CPR) *See* the section FIRST AID AND EMERGENCIES.

CARDITIS The term carditis applies to any of a number of inflammatory states afflicting the heart. These various inflammatory diseases are ordinarily categorized according to the specific heart tissue involved. A number of such types of carditis are listed below:

Pericarditis. An inflammatory disease of the sac (pericardium) that snugly encloses the contracting heart within fibrous membranes lined with a very smooth surface lubricated by crystal-clear fluid.

Epicarditis. Inflammatory changes in the membrane that covers the heart chambers and envelops the superficial coronary arteries.

Myocarditis. Inflammatory changes in the heart muscle itself.

Endocarditis. Inflammation of the inner membrane of the heart that lies in contact with the blood contained in the cardiac chambers.

Valvulitis. Inflammatory disease that involves the valves of the heart. (The muscle component or the endocardial lining may also be involved.)

Pancarditis. An inflammation of all of the heart components, although usually one may show much more severe changes than the others.

Treatment for myocarditis includes complete bed rest and sedation while managing the underlying infection or other condition that has caused the inflammation. In some cases, corticosteroids may be prescribed. Inflammation caused by bacteria can be treated with a variety of antibiotics, including penicillin, ampicillin, streptomycin, or gentamicin, depending upon the type of bacteria. (*See also* PERICARDITIS in this section.)

CHOLESTEROL   *See* the section NUTRITION AND HEALTH.

COAGULATION   Coagulation or clotting may occur in fluids as diverse as blood and milk. Blood coagulation as a physiologic process is not yet completely understood, but contemporary science believes it is a three-step process, namely: activation of thromboplastin; conversion of prothrombin to thrombin; and formation of fibrin.

Thromboplastin is a substance derived from thrombocytes or platelets which are cells in the circulating blood. Prothrombin is a protein derivative in the blood plasma (serum) from which thrombin (an enzyme) is elaborated when blood is shed. Fibrin is an insoluble protein formed by interaction of thrombin and fibrinogen which results in a meshwork that traps blood cells when blood is shed, hence forming a clot. Fibrinogen is a protein normally present in blood plasma and other tissue fluids in the body.

CONGENITAL HEART DISEASE   Congenital heart disease is present when one or more defects exist in the heart (or vascular system) at the time of birth. Almost one in every hundred live births will show these inborn defects, although discovery and accurate diagnosis may be delayed for months or years.

In its very beginning, many months before birth, the heart is a single tube. Growth causes the tube to enlarge, twist, and divide into chambers, the valves of the heart growing from the walls of these chambers. In final form the human heart has four chambers: two of these, the right atrium and ventricle, collect blood from the tissues by way of the veins and then propel it to the lungs; the other two, left atrium and ventricle, collect blood from the lungs and then move it forward through the arteries to supply every cell in the body with oxygen or nourishment.

In the unfolding process from single tube to highly organized four-chambered organ, thousands of developmental steps take place in orderly sequence prior to birth. Any diversion of effort in an area of growth can slow down or stop a portion of the heart's development and cause a malformation. Contrary to popular belief, fright, tension, nightmares, emotional crises of any sort experienced by the mother during pregnancy have never been proved to cause congenital deformities.

Survival rate. Almost one-fourth of babies with congenital heart abnormalities do not survive the first few weeks of life. Almost another fourth have such severe involvement that they fail to thrive and develop properly, although life is present. At least three-quarters of these latter can be helped or completely relieved by surgical procedures. A little over half do not require surgical correction until school age.

In some defects, the outlook can be grave and surgical risk enormous; but in others, notably patent ductus arteriosus, surgical correction offers no great operative risk.

Congenital heart disease can conveniently be classified into four main groupings:

1. Deformities that obstruct blood-flow (a) at the origin of the pulmonary artery (at or near the pulmonic valve), where blood exits from the heart into the lungs, or (b) at the very beginning of the aorta (at or near the aortic valve), where blood is squeezed from the heart into the large collecting vessel, the aorta.

2. Incompletely developed chamber walls that have resulted in abnormal openings or "windows" between heart chambers. These openings permit blood to leak through, and since pressures are higher in the two chambers on the left side of the heart that squeeze blood into the entire body, that leakage passes from the left heart chambers into their counterparts on the right, which are busy forcing blood into the pulmonary artery and the lungs.

A window between the atrial chambers permits blood that has just passed through the lungs and is in the left atrium to escape into the right atrium; all this leakage must now take a second, purposeless trip through the lungs. If the leak is small, little damage will be done, but the work load of the heart is of course increased somewhat. A large leak may be disastrous and cause heart- and lung-failure early in life.

A window between ventricular chambers produces a leakage of blood with almost the same circulation difficulty as one between the atria: some of the blood is diverted from the aorta and the systemic vessels of the body into the opposite (right) ventricle and must then make a second, unnecessary, trip through the lungs. A small opening between the ventricles can exist from birth to well past the age of seventy, with little or no harm to circulatory efficiency. A large abnormal opening, however, can rob the systemic arteries of much-needed blood volume and as a result produce extreme weakness. At the same time, blood that passes through the lungs repeatedly and without any physiologic advantage may cause early degeneration in the blood vessels of the lungs and thereby lead to complete heart failure quite early in life, unless surgical relief is provided.

3. Ductus arteriosus that persists after birth. Before birth, the lungs are dormant, airless, and are of no use to the unborn child's oxygenation system. A rather large vessel connects the artery leading to the lungs (pulmonary artery) with that leading to the body (aorta). This "shunt" diverts blood which in the normally born infant goes to the lungs, into the entire body; that is, before birth, almost all the output of both the left and right sides of the heart goes into the aorta. Ordinarily, at the time of birth or shortly after, this shunt vessel obliterates itself completely; thereafter, an equal amount of blood flows into the lungs from the right side of the heart, and into the body from the left.

If this close-off process does not occur, blood will flow in a direction through this vessel just opposite to the flow direction prior to birth. Why? Because as soon as the first breath is taken, the lungs expand and pressure in the artery to the lungs falls to a level less than half that in the systemic outflow of the aorta. One-third or more of the blood can escape through the open ductus arteriosus and make another trip through the lungs, for no useful purpose.

4. Double, triple, or more defects (a) in the heart itself and (b) in the blood vessels supplying the entrance and exit of the heart. If there is a window-like defect in the wall of muscle (septum) between either the atria or the ventricles, and in addition there is any obstructive narrowing in the outflow channel to the lungs, blood that should move into the lungs may prefer to move across the abnormal window-defect into a chamber that will pass it to the tissues of the body without its having traveled through the lungs. Blood is rather dark-blue prior to passage through the oxygenating membranes of the lungs. If a sufficient amount moves through the septum defect and is returned to the body without having been oxygenated (and reddened), the patient can show a blueness (cyanosis) of the lips, earlobes, and even of the nail beds and skin over the entire body. Babies suffering from this group of defects have therefore been called "blue babies."

The obstruction from the right side of the heart to the lungs may be caused by an improper development of the valve leaflets separating the right ventricle from the artery to the lungs (pulmonary artery). Furthermore, abnormalities can occur in the veins that supply either the right or the left atrium. Rarely, the aorta and the pulmonary artery have reversed their connections with the ventricles.

As soon as practical, a good anatomic and functional diagnosis must be made in all cases of congenital heart disease. The special techniques of cardiography and X-ray angiocardiography together with heart catheterization will supplement the examiner's diagnosis. These steps will usually give a complete diagnosis of every congenital deformity present in the patient's heart and great vessels.

Treatment. Surgical correction for cure or amelioration is possible in almost every case of congenital heart disease. As soon as a complete diagnosis has been made, the safest and most satisfactory time for surgery can be selected and discussed with the patient, if old enough, and with his family. Delay in diagnosis can be responsible for many unnecessary deaths, because of delay in the optimal time for surgical correction. In the case of patent ductus, especially in the premature infant, there is a medical treatment which may be successful—the administration of the drug indomethacin.

Malformations in the great vessels of the aortic system can be associated with developmental defects in the heart, or can be present even when the heart itself shows no abnormality. The more frequent types of aortic malformations include aortic arch developments and coarctation of the aorta. (*See also* Aortic Arch Maldevelopments; Aorta, Coarctation of the in this section.)

CONGESTIVE HEART-FAILURE When the heart's pumping action and the movement of the blood through one of the divisions of the circulatory system are slowed down and become inadequate, the condition can be called congestive heart-failure. Indeed, a heart that cannot move quite enough blood to and from the lungs and the whole body can be said to suffer from a degree of heart-failure. Inefficiency of the pumping action of the heart is one of the most common of all serious disorders that require medical care. Prolongation of a useful life can come from close cooperation between the patient and his doctor over a period of many years.

Symptoms. Symptoms of congestive heart-failure may occur in the lungs: cough, shortness of breath, or even attacks that can simulate asthmatic disease. On the other hand, the symptoms may be quite distant from the heart itself—the result of sluggishness of the circulation in the more distant parts of the body. There may be swollen ankles, painful legs, numb and cold fingers, or there may be congestive liver enlargement, with loss of appetite, weight loss, and even diarrhea and jaundice.

The same basic circulatory problem affects legs, hands, lungs, liver or intestines—a lack of sufficient fresh blood to provide for tissue oxygenation and nourishment, and an accumulation of waste products of metabolism in the tissues which, because of the impeded circulation, are unable to move on to the proper organs of elimination and excretion.

Congestive failure can occur in any person with heart disease, whenever the disease process—inborn defect, rheumatic valve incompetency, death of heart muscle from coronary occlusion, or some other heart illness—reaches such an acute stage that the heart will no longer move blood through its chambers with sufficient speed and power to refresh all the body tissues and then call back for recircuiting every drop of blood available in the venous return reservoirs.

Inability of blood to move out of tissues and return to the heart causes a pooling of blood in the veins, with swelling (as of the ankles) or enlargement (as noted in the liver). This stagnation of blood leads to an escape of fluid into the tissues, resulting in further swelling. (Medically, such swelling is known as edema.) Most important, however, is the fact that once additional fluid appears in the tissues, it acts as a mechanical impediment to block the free passage of blood back to the heart. For this reason, edema will increase rather than decrease until corrective measures have been taken.

In addition, waste products tend to accumulate in the swollen tissues. In order to make these nontoxic and nonirritating, the body must dilute them with more water, producing additional swelling in the area. Some authorities believe that even the capillary walls themselves are injured in congestive failure, further complicating the fluid- and gas-exchange process at the cellular level.

If the left ventricle is primarily involved, the congestive failure may warrant the specific term left-sided congestive failure; if the ventricle primarily involved is the one supplying the lungs, the condition is referred to as right ventricular failure. After a few hours or days, however, both sides of the heart inevitably become involved in the malfunction.

The natural course of events in congestive failure is slow; sometimes, unless medical help is continuously provided, it progresses rapidly to a fatal conclusion. Conversely, some types of congestive failure may be resolved completely, even permanently, in a matter of hours or days, as for example when failure due to anemia can be corrected by blood transfusions.

Treatment. Congestive heart-failure involves a broad field of medical practice. The heart must be supported, fluid balance restored, and the lungs and kidneys guided into satisfactory physiologic functioning. Diurectics which promote urinary output of excess fluid, "unloading agents" which diminish the work of the heart, drugs which strengthen the heartbeat, and salt restriction are among the common approaches. (*See also* HEART-FAILURE in this section.)

CORONARY ARTERY BYPASS GRAFT (CABG)

One of the more dramatic forms of blood vessel surgery comprises the bypass graft for narrowing of coronary arteries. The extent of narrowing or closing off of coronary arteries can be established by the X-ray procedure known as coronary arteriography and is a necessary preamble to the operation. The arteriography reveals the areas and degree of narrowing in coronary arteries that are the usual cause of angina. CABG is applicable to patients in whom medical treatment is unsuccessful, when angina is severe or produces too great an impairment of a desired life style, or when unstable angina threatens to produce a heart attack. The coronary arteriogram may reveal one, or more often several segments that are narrowed to a greater than 70 percent extent.

The operation has its risks of course, though the operative mortality in the best centers is low. Segments of vein stripped from the lower extremity or from a chest wall artery are used to bypass the narrowed areas. Often several segments are necessary: when three segments are bypassed we speak of a "triple bypass," with four segments and five segments we have "quadruple" and "quintriple" bypasses.

Often the operation brings considerable, even total, relief of angina. Nonetheless precautions are in order post-CABG procedure. One potential threat is clotting with closure within the graft, and a program of aspirin may be useful. Since atherosclerosis tends to be progressive with the years, measures directed against it are still in order. Cholesterol levels should be kept as low as possible. Smoking, of course, is strictly forbidden. A supervised exercise program appears to be of value.

There has been much debate over the years as to whether medical or surgical therapy should be foremost in the approach to the patient with angina. When the angina appears only with considerable effort, and not at all at rest, or when moderate effort angina is eliminated with medications, there may be little drive to undertake an angiogram or contemplate CABG. But when angina becomes frequent and unstable, CABG or an angioplasty may be wise choices.

CORONARY HEART DISEASE

Obstructive disease of the coronary arteries eventually leads to weakness of the heart musculature itself. It is perhaps the leading cause of chronic heart failure and of disturbances in heart rhythm.

In clinical practice, coronary disease is usually discussed in terms of the separate disease processes with which it is associated: angina pectoris (ischemia), coronary thrombosis (infarction), cardiac failure, and arrhythmias of the heartbeat.

CORONARY INSUFFICIENCY

When one or more coronary artery branches are narrowed by a disease, usually arteriosclerosis, circulation to the heart-muscle segment supplied by that artery or arteries can be seriously impaired.

Symptoms. At rest, there may be no symptoms; with exertion, pain in the chest, radiating down the arm or up into the neck, may occur. Severe breathlessness may also be present. Attacks of short-windedness are sometimes the only indication of the disorder. An electrocardiogram will frequently diagnose coronary insufficiency especially after exercise (stress test). An X-ray study of the coronary arteries (a coronary angiogram) may be needed to confirm the diagnosis and show whether surgical techniques may be indicated to remove an arterial obstruction.

Treatment. With proper attention to diet and medication, life may be extended and most useful activities continued for many years.

Bypass grafts or dilation of the blocked points in the heart arteries is sometimes indicated and may restore heart function to relatively normal capacity. In most cases at the present date, however, treatment may remain medical as for example when the angina is "stable" and occurs only on effort. Increasing degrees of angina or its appearance during the night or at rest may be a harbinger of heart attack and needs immediate attention.

Surgery may be indicated. (*See also* ANGINA PECTORIS in this section.)

CORONARY OCCLUSION When a blood clot (thrombus) blocks the passageway (lumen) within one of the major coronary arteries, blood stops flowing through that vessel. Coronary thrombosis or occlusion has occurred, with the closure almost always being permanent. The area of heart muscle supplied by the vessel dies (is infarcted) because it is completely dependent for life upon the blood brought to it by that particular artery.

Although it may occur in both sexes, coronary thrombosis typically attacks the middle-aged man. He may have had a previous heart attack or anginal pain episodes, but this is not very often the case. There is occasionally a warning chest pain and discomfort for several days, or some change in the usual pattern of the angina-pectoris attacks which the patient may have suffered for months or years.

When the coronary occlusion occurs, the patient usually feels an agonizing pain (something like a crushing sensation) beneath the breast bone. This persists for an hour or more, often in spite of the administration of pain-relieving drugs. Rest and nitroglycerine tablets alone cannot relieve the discomfort (although they will in angina pectoris). Collapse of the entire circulation often develops, with profuse sweating, vomiting, and profound shock. Severe breathlessness may complicate the distress.

Collapse, coma, and even death may occur before a satisfactory diagnosis is possible. The blood pressure is low, there is an increase in white-cell count, and blood levels of characteristic chemical substances (enzymes) may be quite high.

Treatment. It has been shown that administering clot-dissolving drugs within the first hours of heart attack may reverse the damage. This can be combined with emergency dilation of the artery in the attempt to salvage heart muscle. Taking aspirin has been found to be of help in preventing spread of the clotting, and long term administration of low dose aspirin is of value in prevention also.

Anticoagulants may be given. These substances prolong the time it takes for blood to form a clot, and for this reason it is thought that additional thromboses can be prevented and enlargement of the already-formed clot adequately curtailed.

If the patient survives the first coronary thrombosis, special attention to diet and general medical care will often result in a relatively normal life-span. Carelessness in health measures and medical attention can often drastically shorten a useful existence, or even result in untimely death.

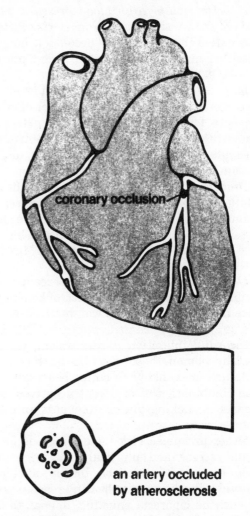

coronary occlusion

an artery occluded by atherosclerosis

CORONARY RISK FACTORS Studies have identified a number of factors that increase the risk of heart disease. Some are unavoidable, such as heredity, gender, and age; others can be changed to lessen the risk.

Children of parents with cardiovascular disease are more likely to suffer the disease. Men in general are at greater risk to suffer cardiovascular disease than women, and black men are at even greater risk because of their tendency to suffer from hypertension. Increasing age is also a factor; fifty-five percent of all heart attack victims are 65 or older.

Major risk factors that can be changed include the following:

Cigarette smoking. This is the number one risk factor for heart disease. Smokers have more than twice the risk of heart attack as nonsmokers. Individuals who stop smoking are able to reduce their risk significantly.

Hypertension or high blood pressure. Second only to smoking as a coronary risk factor, it is called the silent killer because it has no specific symptoms or early warning signals. (*See* HYPERTENSION in this section.)

High cholesterol blood levels. High levels of cholesterol or fat increase the chances of fatty deposits forming on the walls of arteries. Cholesterol levels usually can be controlled through proper diet. (*See* CHOLESTEROL in the section NUTRITION AND HEALTH.)

Diabetes mellitus. Patients with diabetes mellitus have a greater risk of heart disease because of the effect of the disease on the cholesterol and triglyceride levels in the blood. (*See* DIABETES MELLITUS in the section MISCELLANEOUS HEALTH CONDITIONS.)

Obesity. People more than 20 percent overweight have three times the risk of heart disease than those of normal weight.

Use of oral contraceptives. Although myocardial infarction is rare among young, healthy women, those who take birth control pills are more likely to suffer heart attack. The combination of oral contraceptives and cigarette smoking places women at an even greater risk.

Other presumed risk factors include emotional stress and physical inactivity. Although stress cannot be totally avoided, individuals who have unhealthy responses to it, such as cigarette smoking, appear to increase their risk of heart disease. Physical inactivity has not yet been clearly established as a risk factor for heart disease, but it can contribute to other risk factors, such as obesity and hypertension.

CORONARY THROMBOSIS   *See* CORONARY OCCLUSION in this section.

DOPPLER ULTRASOUND   Using high frequency sound waves, a special device called the Doppler probe studies the flow of blood through blood vessels. The study determines whether blood is flowing and at what rate. It is usually painless and is performed while the patient is at rest following light exercise.

DROPSY   Dropsy is one of the traditional terms applied to the body-swellings (edema) of congestive heart-failure or kidney disease (nephritis). The term usually refers to swelling of the feet and ankles often accompanying congestive heart-failure.

ECHOCARDIAGRAM   This diagnostic procedure employs the same sonar principle that ships use to detect submarines. High frequency sound waves are transmitted to the heart through the chest wall to detect changes in structure and motion. The ultrasonic waves are transmitted and received by a hand-held device known as a transducer and are recorded on a strip chart. The sound waves produce "echoes" as they come in contact with various structures and tissues. Movement of a structure intersected by the ultrasonic beam is recorded as a wavy line; a stationary structure produces a straight line.

Echocardiagram is used to diagnose heart murmurs, cardiac tumors, leaking of pericardial fluid, thickening of the heart's wall, dilation of the heart, abnormalities in the motion of the mitral valve, and congenital lesions.

EDEMA   Edema is the presence of excessive amounts of fluid in the tissues, between the cells of the body, or in the various body cavities, and whatever the form it takes, it may cause the symptoms of congestive heart-failure. It may be present in the legs or arms, the pleural cavities, the liver and spleen, the lungs, or the brain. Indeed, accumulations of fluid may appear simultaneously in any combination of the body reservoirs.

No matter what the primary cause of the circulatory weakness happens to be, circulation inefficiency can cause accumulation of edema fluid. Often as much as six quarts can accumulate in the body before edema becomes noticeable to the patient, in the form of swollen ankles or fingers. The condition itself may be a sign of primary congestive heart-failure, but also may be a secondary result of kidney disease, nutritional disorder, or any of a number of other conditions.

In all cases of edema there is usually a rise of pressure in the veins bringing blood back to the heart. For various reasons, fluid has failed to escape from the tissue reservoirs and makes its way into the capillaries which return it, via the veins, to the heart. There is passive venous congestion, with increased venous pressure. This makes for very inefficient pick-up of tissue fluid into the venous circulation.

The edema (or dropsy) of circulatory failure may be due solely to inability of the right side of the heart to move blood efficiently (right heart-failure). Edema in right heart-failure occurs throughout the body, but because there is an inefficient flow of blood from the right ventricle to the lungs, the pulmonary vessels and tissue spaces in the lung itself do not usually show congestion and edema in the early phases of this condition.

More commonly, perhaps, edema is caused by failure of the *left* side of the heart to empty blood efficiently from the lungs. In this case lung edema will be almost immediate. This burden will cause gradual failure of the right side of the heart as well, so that total heart (pancardiac) failure can be present, together with failing circulation to and from the lungs.

As soon as deposits of fluid begin to accumulate abnormally in various tissue spaces, a number of unusual changes in the body's fluid-handling methods begin to appear. For some reason, when circulation is inefficient the kidneys fail to excrete sodium in the usual amount. Excess sodium thereupon accumulates and the body will hold water in an effort to prevent the body fluids from becoming "too salty."

EKG   EKG usually refers to the written record that comes from the electrocardiograph machine. EKG is short for the original German word for the machine. Also known as an ECG.

ELECTROCARDIOGRAPHY   The individual muscle fibers are stimulated to contract by electrical-voltage changes at the junction of the nerve and contracting fiber. To insure rhythmic pumping motion of the heart's chambers, the impulse for contraction begins in healthy subjects at the pacemaker in the wall of the right atrium. The electrical

current (excitation wave) moves along the muscle fibers themselves and is conducted specifically by a system much like a telegraph cable. This special tissue, the bundle of His (beginning at the atrioventricular node) takes the electrical wave from the atria into the ventricles, which ordinarily contract after atrial contracture has concluded. The bundle of His fibers take the wave of excitation to the tip of the ventricles and thence, after dividing into left and right branches, to all the fibers of the ventricular chambers.

Impulse transmission is very rapid along the bundle and its branches but relatively slow as it spreads out in the muscle, gradually passing to all the fibers in the contracting chamber.

In the relaxed, resting state, the heart-muscle fiber is charged positively on the surface. In this state, the muscle cell or fiber is said to be polarized. (The sodium ion at the surface is apparently a major influence in maintaining this positive surface charge.) When the muscle fiber contracts, the sodium ion moves within the cell membrane, and the surface charge turns negative. The muscle fiber is now said to be depolarized.

Experimentally, metal contact-points can be wired to the heart surface and led to a galvanometer, so that the spread of positive-to-negative potential can be traced as the muscle wave of contracture moves from its point of origin to the last heart fiber contracting in that beat. The resulting device is known as an electrocardiograph (EKG or ECG). Abnormal electrocardiogram tracings are present in most of the disease states that affect the heart.

In practice, the wired contacts do not actually touch the heart; the patient's body conducts the current, small though it is, the wires (or leads) being fastened to the arms and legs, and along the wall of the chest over the heart. In these locations they provide a good tracing of the electrical activity within the heart.

Individual waves on the cardiographic tracing are called the P,Q,R,S, and T waves for reference. The P wave is the one which occurs at the beginning of the contraction of the atria. The next wave, the QRS complex, occurs during contraction of the ventricles, and consists of three parts, above and below the zero line. The Q component comes as the impulse produces electrical changes in the fibers of the wall between the ventricles; the R and S components occur as the impulse spreads throughout the ventricles and out onto the heart surface, which is the last to tense. The T wave is recorded as the electrical charge along the conduction system begins to reverse polarity in the recovery, or relaxation, phase of the heartbeat.

In practical use, the electrocardiographic tracing is most useful both in the diagnosis and the observation of clinical progress of most heart patients. The machine is readily available, and little or no discomfort is experienced by the patient as the record is being made.

EMBOLISM Circulatory disease is frequently caused or complicated by embolism, the formation of a foreign body (embolus) such as a blood clot or a cluster of bacteria. After a fracture of bone, a fragment of fatty material may escape from the bone marrow into a vein and form a fat embolus. A laceration of a vein in the neck as made, for example, by a penetrating piece of glass at the time of an automobile accident, will sometimes permit air to enter the circulation and produce an air embolus. Many small gas emboli form in the bloodstream when a deep sea diver is lifted to the surface rapidly; gas that was held in the body fluids by the high underwater pressure suddenly bubbles free (diver's bends).

Within the heart, any diseased area tends to be roughened, and blood may form clots in those surfaces that are not smooth, especially if for any reason there is a slowing of the circulation. In heart disease both roughened intima and slowed circulation are frequently present, especially in association with diseased valve leaflets.

If the embolus forms in the right side of the heart it may fragment and particles of it pass to the pulmonary artery branches: pulmonary embolus. If the clot is formed in and breaks away from the left side of the heart, it can move through the arterial system to any organ of the body: the brain, kidney, or intestine, for example. The embolus can cause serious changes in the organ in which it lodges: even death will result if the vital area of the brain is so involved and deprived of blood supply.

Perhaps most embolization originates in the veins, at points far distant from the heart. Thus, an inflammatory state of the leg veins called thrombophlebitis can produce clots of blood within the veins. Fragments may break away and drift in the moving blood into the right atrium of the heart, skip through the tricuspid valves into the right ventricle, and then push into the pulmonary artery. When the clot reaches a small branch of the pulmonary artery in one of the lungs, it firmly lodges and obstructs blood flow in that particular branch of the vessel. This produces death of the lung tissue supplied by the vessel, the destroyed portion of the lung being a pulmonary infarction.

While a small pulmonary infarct generally produces very little in the way of symptoms (chest pain, blood-tinged sputum), a large pulmonary infarct may even cause the death of a patient.

ESSENTIAL HYPERTENSION Essential hypertension causes a high percentage of all heart disease. It may be found in persons of all social and economic levels.

Most cases of essential hypertension come in middle-aged persons, or those past middle age. Men and women share the disease equally. There seems to be a strong tendency for cases to run in families although what—if any—factor causes the individual to develop this type of blood pressure disability has not yet been discovered.

The physical disability caused by essential hypertension may slowly progress for many years; or it may occasionally advance to complete disability in a few months or years, and even lead to an early death. In spite of widespread research in many directions, little real information has been obtained about the true cause of the disorder and exactly why it leads to progressively destructive changes in the blood supply of the heart vessels and of the heart muscle as well.

There are, of course, many theories. Heredity, emotional stress, hormonal imbalance, and specific substances released abnormally by tissues diseased in a peculiar way are known at times to cause high pressures in the artery system. However, no clear-cut single cause of essential hypertension is yet known.

Even in normally healthy people blood pressure will rise when the individual is under emotional stress. Physical exertion, lifting, and almost any circumstance in which an extra demand for blood is made by the tissues, can also cause an elevation in artery pressures. But as soon as the stress and urgent tissue demands for replenishment of substances or oxygen are over, blood pressure ordinarily falls back to normal in a short period of time. When there is hypertensive heart disease, however, no matter whether the patient is resting or exerting himself, blood pressure stays at levels very much higher than in unaffected persons.

Symptoms. There are few, if any, symptoms directly caused by high blood pressure. Most patients, indeed, feel very well, and typically many of them seem to thrive at a high level of energy and activity at home, in social life, or in business. As a group, these patients seem to be content with themselves and with life. They prefer not to complain about anything, and often the diagnosis comes only after a routine employment or insurance examination.

Headaches and dizzy spells may express circulatory fatigue in persons with essential hypertension. If the structures of the heart or blood vessels, or the lung circulation, have been damaged by excessive pressures over a period of time, shortness of breath, pain in the chest, or cramping legs may be noticeable—especially on severe exertion. These are symptoms of the tissue changes caused by high blood pressure, and can, once they occur, indicate the need for close medical attention.

High blood pressure is never diagnosed as a disease-condition on the basis of a single blood-pressure reading. Repeated examinations must continue to show high readings if essential hypertension is to be diagnosed. As an indication of disease, systolic pressure readings should be consistently above 150 or 160 millimeters of mercury, and the diastolic pressures usually above 90 to 95 millimeters.

Treatment. A large percentage of patients kept under modern drug therapy may expect to lead nearly normal lives, and have a good life expectancy. Neglect of medical care, however, may lead to disaster.

FIBRILLATION An atrium is said to be in fibrillation when its orderly, regular rate is replaced by rapid trembling of heart muscle and ineffective contractions of that chamber. Atrial fibrillation occurs when an irritable focal point causes electrical discharges at a rate of 500 or more per minute, in contrast to the normal and efficient 78 to 80 beats per minute, and produces irregular and ineffective muscular twitching in the atrium instead of a coordinated pulsation. Blood moves into the ventricle without the mechanical assistance of atrial contractions, and only a small portion of the hundreds of electrical impulses are transmitted to the ventricle; in fact, the ventricular rate in untreated atrial fibrillation usually lies between 120 and 200 per minute.

In ventricular fibrillation, the purposeful contraction of the muscular chamber is replaced by chaotic twitching in groups of muscle fibers; the forward flow of blood comes to a halt. Death will occur in a matter of minutes unless artificial maintenance of the circulation is provided until defibrillation can be attempted with the electronic defibrillator.

"HEART ATTACK" The term heart attack has no exact meaning in medical practice. Sudden chest pain, sudden weakness or breathlessness, a sudden blackout, or even sudden death is referred to as a heart attack by many laymen.

Sudden chest pain comes with angina pectoris, coronary insufficiency, aneurysm, and pulmonary infarction, but it may also appear in pleurisy and in disorders completely unrelated to the heart.

Palpitations may indicate heart disease, or on the other hand may be expressions of anxiety.

Sudden unconsciousness may appear in heart disease, but also in cerebrovascular accidents, diabetes, or shock from any cause.

What is often suspected as a heart attack may eventually prove to be an episode completely unrelated to malfunctions of the heart: asthma, epilepsy, gallstone, intercostal neuritis, slipped cervical disc, or even an anxiety state. Until a diagnosis of heart disease is made by the physician, needless anxiety should be held in check, especially by the patient's family and friends.

HEART CATHETERIZATION A catheter is a piece of special tubing that can be introduced into the body to drain out samples of fluid. A rather long section of plastic tubing less than one-sixteenth inch in diameter can be inserted into an arm vein. When this slender tube is pushed inside the vein, it travels with the blood returning to the heart, reaching the right atrium, right ventricle, and then the pulmonary artery and lung vessels. This exploration of the vessels is called right-heart catheterization.

Because the plastic catheter is visible on the X-ray (fluoroscopic) screen, the doctor can observe the path the catheter takes, and serious defects may be studied visually. Thus, the catheter may pass through a defect in the septum that divides the right from the left chambers of the heart, and thereby give pictorial proof of the presence and location of that defect. Then too, any narrow points in the pulmonary valve or vessel may prevent the catheter from passing out of the right ventricle into the pulmonary artery, and may be revealed.

Because the catheter is an open tube, pressure at its tip can be measured. Structural deformities can cause abnormal pressures in the right atrium, right ventricle, and even in the pulmonary circulation; pressure measurements therefore serve a useful purpose in diagnosis and can indicate any unusual strain or work load from which the heart may be suffering.

Defects, or windows between the right and left chambers and vessels, are almost always birth defects. As blood flows through the heart, some of it can move abnormally through these openings, shunting from the high-pressure side of the low-pressure area. The exact position of the catheter tip will indicate the region of the defect; if the pressure changes vary greatly from normal, a serious abnormality may be presumed.

Samples of blood are taken in the right atrium, right ventricle, and pulmonary artery. Oxygen saturation is then measured. Before passing through the lungs, 65 percent saturation may be taken as average, whereas fully saturated blood (97 percent oxygen-laden) circulates in the left heart system. Therefore as the catheter tip passes through the right heart, oxygen saturations higher than usual can indicate an abnormal passageway from one side of the heart to the

other; elevations far above 65 percent will be noted when the catheter tip happens to lie close to the abnormal interchamber connection. The amount of leakage through the defect can be estimated by the amount of saturated blood that moves into the unsaturated portion.

In selective angiocardiograms, contrast material that is visible on X-ray film is injected through the catheter; it will outline the structures in the area of the catheter tip. Repeated small injections can be made and observed on the fluoroscopic screen, so that, for example, exact details of any anatomic changes in that region of the heart can be photographed. Minute variations in the structure and efficiency of valve leaflets can be studied very nicely by this procedure.

Dyes are sometimes injected through the catheter and their concentration in systemic blood can be estimated by photoelectric methods, usually sensed by means of a tiny electronic device attached to the ear. Shunts of blood from right to left can be demonstrated by this method because the time interval between injection and earlobe arrival is shortened when the lung circulation is partially by-passed.

When disease changes are present in the mitral or aortic valves, left-heart catheterization may be helpful. This can be done by passing a catheter inserted in an artery of the body back to the heart and then through the aortic valve leaflets. Pressure and oxygen studies can be done as in right-heart catheterization, and selective angiocardiography carried out. Estimation of rheumatic fever damage to the mitral and aortic valves must be made by left-heart catheterization.

HEART (CARDIAC) DISEASE Heart disease can be the result of tissue changes primarily in the heart itself. Good examples are the congenital heart malformations which, if not correctable by surgery, often lead to death in infancy.

On the other hand, heart disease severe enough to result in a death of cardiac origin can come from disease entirely separate from the heart: failing kidneys can sometimes affect the heart so severely that it develops changes incompatible with life; some tumors of the body may produce severe high blood pressure, with death eventually resulting because of the hypertensive changes produced in the heart.

Some heart diseases show changes in the heart not too different from those found in tissues elsewhere. Thus, changes typical of rheumatic heart disease occur in the lungs, in some of the joints, and in other areas as well. Poisons and drugs that affect the heart will usually also cause disease of the kidneys and liver. High blood pressure is as much an arterial as a heart disorder, and coronary artery disease may be only one manifestation of wide-spread atherosclerosis.

Each variety of heart disease occurs in a characteristic age group, and involves special tissue changes. Symptoms and tissue alterations may be limited to the heart alone or to the entire heart and blood-vessel system, but occasionally other organs, such as the brain, joints, liver, and spleen, are involved in the structural changes brought about by the heart disorder. The patient may even complain bitterly about symptoms in parts of the body completely unrelated to the region of the heart itself.

Important causes of heart disease might include congenital structural defects, rheumatic carditis, syphilitic heart disease, hypertensive (high blood pressure) heart disease, arteriosclerotic heart disease, and bacterial endocarditis. The less common causes of heart disease may include thyroid disease, heart tumors, heart injuries, diphtheria carditis, beriberi and other nutritional heart disorders, and functional heart disease.

Treatment. Diagnosis and management of heart disease must include studies not only of the heart and the efficiency of its functional operation, but also the operational state of the lungs and the demands or requirements of the entire body: whether it requires a higher-than-normal cardiac output and therefore places an abnormal work-load on the heart.

HEART DISEASE, EXERCISE AND

Not long ago, rest was the keystone of treatment in heart disease. The modern trend is to encourage some form of activity or physiotherapy as soon as it is reasonably safe to do so. Recovery from heart disease can be speeded by gradual measures that will include both supervised exercise and occupational rehabilitation. With careful use, the working heart is strengthened and can even facilitate the development of new blood vessels within the heart muscle.

HEART-FAILURE Heart-failure is usually defined as that stage of heart disease at which, even while the patient is resting, the heart can no longer fill the needs of the tissues for oxygenated blood. The symptoms of excessive heart work no longer disappear after rest; fatigue, heart pain, and even attacks of shortness of breath often follow a pattern unique for a particular patient; and the established pattern of their appearance from day to day can rarely be eliminated by enforced rest periods alone.

Symptoms. When the heart is unable to keep up a fresh supply of blood to the tissues, fatigue (muscular weakness) is almost always present. During muscular activity almost all the output of refreshed blood from the heart is diverted from organs to the working muscles. When the output of the heart is unable to increase on demand, as in severe heart disease, even the slightest muscular effort may be hard for the patient to endure.

Often an individual finds himself easily fatigued. This of itself, however, is not often a sign of heart disease. Almost every person will have periods of emotional stress which, even with a healthy heart and blood vessels, will cause useless muscle tension and so deplete the nutritional reserves of muscle fibers. Emotional tension, therefore, and not heart disease is probably the most common cause for the tendency to fatigue.

Everyone may experience breathlessness on effort. As a symptom of heart disease, however, shortness of breath is caused by inability of the heart to move blood through the lungs and into the tissues to keep pace with body demands as these change from minute to minute. Acute distress in breathing, along with a sense of suffocation, may compel the patient to sit down and rest or lie down in a propped-up position.

Fainting is sometimes a symptom of the failing heart, especially when it is produced by either moderate or very little exertion; it is thought to be due to temporary lack of fresh blood circulated to the brain.

Heart-failure of very serious degree causes

very poor kidney function, with a low daily output of urine and accumulation of sodium and fluid in the tissue reservoirs; visible swelling of the feet and ankles may indicate the possibility of this complication. Excessive fluid in the lung tissues may result in a chronic cough, sometimes producing phlegm that is streaked with dark flecks of blood. Abdominal swelling may indicate that excessive fluid has accumulated in the peritoneal reservoir.

Treatment. Satisfactory treatment of heart failure depends upon strict adherence to the doctor's orders. First of all, the cause of failure must be remedied, if possible. A toxic goiter or anemia, for example, can be treated successfully so that heart failure, if caused by either disease, will be completely relieved, if there is a good response to that specific treatment. Structural defects and abnormal vessels may be corrected by surgery and thereby relieve the burdened heart.

If failure occurs during the last months of pregnancy, it may respond well to medical treatment, but when present in the first few months, termination of the pregnancy may need consideration to prevent disaster to both mother and unborn child.

Physical rest is important in treatment, the patient usually being nursed in a half-sitting position. Often an armchair is more convenient than a special bed, for this position itself can relieve congestion in the veins near the heart and reduce heart work to a minimum. Breathing is improved by a somewhat upright position and swelling may drift to the lower legs where it will do the least harm to an overburdened heart.

Drugs in the digitalis group act directly on the failing heart muscle, increasing the strength of its contraction and thereby speeding the evacuation of blood from engorged veins leading to the heart. In addition, medication improves the heart's output so that a greater volume of blood will flow to the kidneys, brain, and other vital organs that have been deprived of an adequate circulation.

A low sodium diet can bring about the removal of excessive body fluid because the sodium already present within the body will "pull water through the kidneys" as it passes through them.

A group of useful drugs that enhance kidney action (diuretics) are very effective as an aid in the removal of fluid trapped in the body by circulatory failure. They may be administered for many weeks without the occurrence of harmful side-effects but the changing salt content of the blood has to be monitored. Once in a while, small skin incisions have been used to provide an escape route for very swollen legs, especially when conservative treatment has not been effective in removal of this "dropsy" (edema) fluid. Drainage, produced through the skin incisions can continue for days with sometimes the fortuitous escape of many quarts of fluid. Fluid that has accumulated in the chest or abdominal cavities may need to be removed by needle puncture. (*See also* CONGESTIVE HEART-FAILURE in this section.)

HEART MURMURS   A heart murmur is an extra heart sound. It sounds like fluid passing an obstruction and is heard between the normal heart sounds. As blood passes through the healthy heart, characteristic sounds are made as the heart valves open by the tensed—and resonating—muscle walls of the heart chamber; and again by the resonant vibrations of the heart valves as they close at the end of muscle contraction (systole).

If there are abnormal surfaces along the valve margins, and especially if these surface changes prevent normal closure of the valve leaflets, murmurs or noises are made by the blood as it rushes past the abnormal surface irregularities or leaks back through misshapen valve leaflets that fail to close completely.

Any defects, inborn or acquired, may be potential causes of murmurs of varying intensity, pitch, and quality. Murmurs recur with each cycle of the heartbeat, and are generally classified as systolic murmurs if they are heard during active contracture of the ventricles, or diastolic if they come during the phase of ventricular relaxation.

Careful study of the murmur, listening to it many times and in a great many areas over the heart, is rewarding to the physician. He can gather an accurate impression of the disorder that causes the murmur, inasmuch as specific changes in the heart chambers or valves tend to produce murmurs that are quite typical. What they sound like, how intense they are, where best heard, and the exact time in the heart cycle when they appear all contribute to the unique character of the various heart murmurs, hence to diagnosis of their underlying causes.

HEART MUSCLE The myocardium, or heart muscle, differs from muscle of the skeletal system in many ways. It has the ability to contract rhythmically both with and without external stimulation, and can do so continuously for long intervals of time with no evidence of fatigue. In the adult, the heart muscle weighs about one pound and provides the pumping pressure to move nearly five hundred gallons of blood through the vascular system every day of a person's life.

HEART PAIN (CARDIAC PAIN) The heart is almost devoid of nerves that carry sensations, so that a great many diseases of the heart are completely painless. There are however two important sources of pain in the heart structures:

Pericardial pain. Some of the sac (pericardium) that encloses the heart chambers is supplied by the same nerve that goes to the diaphragm—the phrenic nerve. Acute inflammation in the pericardium can therefore result in sharp "pleurisy" pains. If the pericardium is irritated by injury or stretched by blood or by fluid trapped within its membranes, a dull, painful ache may be felt over the heart, sometimes spreading to the tip of the shoulderblade.

Coronary-artery pain. Ordinarily, the sympathetic nerves do not carry pain (or even cause it in the conscious mind). There are, however, a number of exceptions to this rule, one of which involves the nerve endings that lace themselves about the arteries of the heart (the coronary arteries). These nerves can be stimulated to produce painful alarm signals when there is deficiency of oxygen for tissue activity in the area supplied by a coronary artery. Painful stimuli travel to the upper sympathetic chain in the left (or at times the right) chest and in some way escape into nearby sensory nerves. The result is real, often excruciating, pain characteristically felt behind the breastbone and down the left arm into one or more fingers. Because the cause of the pain is apparently indirect in its produc-

tion, a great variability in its location, character, and intensity is noticed from one patient to the next.

True heart (or coronary-artery) pain almost always indicates a serious failure of the artery to supply an adequate flow of refreshed blood to the active heart-muscle fibers. This deficit state (myocardial ischemia) can usually be traced to narrowing of the coronary artery's diameter by at least one focal point of partial obstruction.

HEART SCANS Areas of the heart can be scanned using radioactive substances to confirm a diagnosis of coronary artery disease. In one such test, a small amount of radioactive thallium is injected into a vein during exercise while the heart is monitored by electrocardiogram. Thallium is rapidly taken up by contracting heart muscle. Images on a screen reveal areas in the heart where there is no thallium, an indication that coronary circulation is impaired.

A similar test sometimes called a MUGA studies the motion of the heart's wall to determine if there is any impairment of heart contraction.

HEART SOUNDS When listening through the stethoscope, one can ordinarily hear two heart sounds in adults; these are known as the first and second sounds. In children, a soft third sound is often audible, and under unusual conditions a fourth (atrial) sound may occur just before the first.

The first and second sounds are the usual ones to be concerned with. The first is caused by closure of the ventricular (mitral and tricuspid) valves and is audible at the beginning of ventricular contractions (systole). The second sound, in contrast, is due to closure of the aortic and pulmonary valves and is heard just at the beginning of ventricular relaxation (diastole).

HEART TRANSPLANTATION Heart transplantation is performed on patients suffering from end-stage coronary artery disease or cardiomyopathy. The heart is removed from the donor by transecting the great vessels and the atria. It is then transplanted first by suturing the atria to those of the recipient. The great vessels are then connected and air is evacuated from the heart chambers. Heart-lung machines perform the functions of those organs during the surgery.

Following surgery, the patient is kept in protective isolation to prevent infection. Immunosuppressant drugs are used to minimize rejection.

HEART VALVES Four valves control the flow of blood through the heart by opening and closing with each heartbeat. Composed of thin leaflets of fibrous tissue, they permit blood to flow in only one direction. A heart murmur results when a defective valve allows backflow.

The valves include two atrioventricular valves, which separate the atria from the ventricles, and two semilunar valves, which lie between each ventricle and its corresponding artery. The valve between the right atrium and the right ventricle is the tricuspid valve, named for its three cusps. Separating the left atrium and the left ventricle is the mitral or bicuspid valve. The pulmonic valve separates the pulmonary artery and right ventricle and the aortic valve controls the flow of blood between the left ventricle and the aorta. The semilunar valves normally each have three cusps.

HEARTBEAT, IRREGULAR (ARRHYTHMIA) In most persons of all ages, the heart beats at regularly timed intervals, even though the rate can vary from slow to fast. However, if the heart- or pulsebeats are not regular, a disorder—an arrhythmia—of cardiac rhythm may exist.

A disturbance in rhythm can come on and leave quickly, or it can be more or less permanent. The heart may show an occasional irregular beat or a total irregularity (as happens when each beat seems independent of all others, and each interval between beats is of different length). Beats may even come in groups of fast, then slow, pulsations: an "irregular irregularity."

Arrhythmias may have no real significance. Simple ones may be caused by extraordinary stress, strange foods, caffeine, drugs, or even intense excitement. These may be quite a nuisance to the patient, but often cause more embarrassment than real disability.

A serious arrhythmia, however, can cause a profound drop in blood pressure. The patient may become pale, breathless, and weak, or even fall into a state of shock or coma. Occasionally, a patient is quite unaware that he has a heart-rhythm disorder. There may be times, however, when he notices a strange beating in his chest, a "flippity-flop" sensation of fluttering under the ribs somewhere, or a feeling that he is about to "pass out."

Ordinarily, no pain whatever is experienced with a rhythm disorder. If pain is present, it usually means that heart disease may be the primary cause of the irregular heartbeat. All arrhythmias should be called to the attention of a physician, for sometimes a serious crisis may thus be averted.

HEMOPHILIA Years ago any abnormal bleeding in a child was inaccurately called hemophilia. The true hemophiliac is a male who has acquired his bleeding trait through the mother's side of the family. About 1 in 10,000 males in the U.S. have the disease. It can vary from mild to severe, depending on the degree of impairment in the making of the specific blood-clotting factors. Special tests can identify the disorder and its severity (Factors VIII and IX).

Symptoms. The hemophilic boy bruises easily; blood may be passed in his urine from insignificant back injury, or a wrenched knee-joint may fill up with blood and result in a crippling deformity. Dental extraction produces prolonged bleeding.

Treatment. For years, transfusions of fresh blood or plasma were the mainstay of treatment. More recently an essential clotting factor (Factor VIII, AHF-antihemophilic factor) has been isolated. This is now produced by recombinant DNA technology giving a pure product free of potential viruses, such as the AIDS virus. In relatively small amounts it corrects the clotting deficiency of hemophilia. The frequency of administration of the synthetic Factor VIII will vary with the severity of the disease as advised by the doctor. In mild cases it may have to be given prophylactically when surgery or tooth extraction is contemplated. In severer cases it is given at the first sign of any bruising or bleeding or even on a regular basis. The drug is given into the vein and many hemophilics learn to do this for themselves.

HIGH BLOOD PRESSURE (HYPERTENSION) If blood pressure (measured in millimeters of mercury) remains above 150 to 160 in systole, or 90 to 95 millimeters in diastole, even after a period of rest, high blood pressure as a disease entity can be suspected. To prove that a state of high blood pressure exists as an abnormality, the doctor will take a series of pressure readings at various times during the day, after simple exercise tests, or following the administration of certain drugs. If high readings are constantly present, a state of hypertension (high blood pressure) may be said to exist. If present, it may represent a specific disease entity (essential hypertension) or be an indication of a disorder in one of the body organs, such as the kidneys or adrenal glands. (*See also* ESSENTIAL HYPERTENSION and HYPERTENSION in this section.)

HYPERTENSION With each heartbeat, blood is thrust into the elastic artery system under pressure and, propelled by this pressure, is delivered to the capillaries and the tissues. If there is a persistent elevation of the blood pressure, arterial hypertension is present. (When pressure is taken in the arm at the level of, or above the elbow, the upper normal limits for systole and diastole may be as much as 160/90 as measured in millimeters of mercury.) If, after screening for the usual causes of secondary hypertension, the cause of elevated pressure cannot be found, the patient is said to have high blood pressure of unknown cause: essential hypertension. (Secondary hypertension is that which results from a derangement other than that of the heart or blood vessels—as from some of the primary diseases of the kidneys or adrenal glands.)

HYPOTENSION Blood pressure readings that fall considerably below the usual "normal" range are referred to as hypotension. There is no precise range in the sense that some apparently normal individuals consistently have lower than average readings, for example, systolic blood pressures in the 90's and occasionally even in the 80's. These readings are low for an adult and may even warrant some investigation, as for example, for possible adrenal gland insufficiency or a drug effect. The person's usual blood pressure is very relevant in making the diagnosis: in someone known to usually have a blood pressure of 120/80, the finding of 90/70 would warrant a diagnosis of hypotension. Hypotension of disease origin may be found in heart attack, bleeding, salt depletion and various other disorders. It may sometimes only be manifest in the standing position—known as postural hypotension.

Hypotension often is caused by excessive dosages of certain drugs that treat hypertension as well as drugs used in nervous and mental disorders. Hypotension can also be associated with a number of diseases, including diabetes mellitus, pernicious anemia, and Parkinson's disease.

Mild reductions in blood pressure can cause faintness, lightheadedness, visual blurring. More severe episodes can result in loss of consciousness and seizures.

Hypotension can be reduced by stopping the bleeding or treating the disease that may be causing the condition. If drugs are the cause of hypotension, adjustments in the medication can restore normal blood pressure. Milder cases can be treated through the use of ephedrine, increasing salt intake or administering salt-retaining hormones. Nonsteroidal anti-inflammatory agents may also be prescribed. Pooling of blood in the extremities can be reduced through the use of special tightly fitted stockings.

INFARCTION *See* CORONARY OCCLUSION in this section.

INTERMITTENT CLAUDICATION An initial symptom of peripheral vascular disease is intermittent claudication—cramplike pain or weakness in the legs or feet caused by an inadequate amount of oxygen-rich blood during exercise. Sometimes called the "stop and rest syndrome," the discomfort normally subsides once activity stops. The progression of vascular disease can be determined by the amount of exercise that causes the pain. Discomfort while resting indicates a severe degree of arterial or venous obstruction. In addition to pain and weakness, intermittent claudication can cause fatigue, coldness, numbness, and tingling.

The location of the pain can indicate the obstruction site. Reduced blood flow in the superficial femoral artery can cause calf pain, while pain in the thigh may accompany obstruction in the pelvic arteries.

Exercise, usually walking, is recommended for individuals with intermittent claudication. Patients are advised to begin slowly and gradually to increase the distance walked. When discomfort occurs, the patient should stop and resume walking when it subsides. Cigarette smoking should be eliminated because the carbon monoxide produced by cigarette smoking tends to replace the oxygen in smokers' red blood cells and because the nicotine in tobacco decreases blood flow to the legs. A diet low in fat and cholesterol may be advised in order to maintain the proper weight and to slow the atherosclerotic process. A vasodilator, a medication that promotes the dilation of blood vessels, may be prescribed.

Arteriography can be performed to confirm the diagnosis if surgery is being considered. Also, Doppler ultrasonic studies may be used to determine the extent of the obstruction. Tests also might be performed to measure changes in pulse volumes at different levels of the leg and to monitor changes in the pulse and size of the leg with each heartbeat. A lumbar sympathetic block involves the use of a local anesthetic to block sympathetic nerves to the leg. In normal, unobstructed vessels, the block results in a rise in temperature. The temperature stays 'the same or rises only slightly in a leg with atherosclerotic vessels.

ISCHEMIA   Ischemia results from a decrease in the blood supply to a part of the body, thereby denying it oxygen and nutrients. Vascular obstruction—due either to a blood clot, fatty plaque or vascular spasm—is usually the cause. Common locales of ischemia are in the brain, in the heart, and in the legs. The symptoms of ischemia will therefore depend on its site and the tissues involved. In the heart, for example, angina pectoris; in the brain, weakness, confusion; in the legs, pain such as claudication. These conditions require medical intervention as progression of the underlying disease may be potentially fatal.

LEFT-ARM-AND-SHOULDER-PAIN
Left-arm-and-shoulder-pain is a common symptom of coronary artery disease. If the source of the pain is the heart, there is never any spot-tenderness of the shoulder or arm, for the pain only seems to reside in shoulder, arm, or fingers. Movement of the arm or shoulder neither augments, relieves, nor alters heart pain that reflects itself in this area.

When there is an oxygen deficiency at endings of the sympathetic nerves of the coronary arteries, these nerves are aroused to send out pain impulses. The impulses are carried through to collecting stations (ganglia) near the upper five thoracic ribs, a few inches from the spine, and even to ganglia in the neck. From these ganglia, the impulses then escape by pathways near those used by the shoulder and left arm on their way into the spinal cord and hence to the brain.

Apparently this side-by-side position of the sympathetic pathways leading from the arteries of the heart and the peripheral nerve pathways leading from the arm and shoulder may have something to do with the fact that pain originating in the coronary vessels of the heart can appear to originate in the arm and shoulder.

LOW BLOOD PRESSURE   *See* HYPOTENSION in this section.

MYOCARDIAL INFARCTION   *See* CORONARY OCCLUSION in this section.

OPEN-HEART SURGERY   Through the use of a mechanical pump that imitates heart action, and an oxygenating chamber that temporarily assumes the function of lung tissue, the function of both heart and lungs may be suspended for several hours (cardiopulmonary bypass). During this interval, the nearly-bloodless heart can be opened and defects in the muscular or valve structures repaired.

Congenital inborn defects, rheumatic valve damage, aneurysms, and even the coronary arteries lend themselves well to open-heart correction. The procedure of cardiopulmonary by-pass carries little risk when compared to the difficulties caused by the kind of heart damage remedied. (*See also* CORONARY AR-TERY BYPASS GRAFT in this section.)

PACEMAKER   A pacemaker is an electronic device that provides electrical stimuli to the heart muscle to maintain the rhythm of its contractions. A pacemaker may be permanent and may emit a small current at a constant fixed rate or it may discharge only when the heart rate goes below a certain level.

The device, which operates on a tiny battery, is implanted permanently under the skin, and slender wires connect it to the ventricular muscle fibers. The batteries, which can last for several years, are replaced in minor surgery under local anesthesia. The presence of the implanted device creates little or no discomfort.

A pacemaker is used generally when a patient has an arrhythmia or one of several conditions which causes cardiac output to fail, such as heart block or tachycardia.

PERICARDITIS   An acute or long standing inflammation of the external coverings of the heart and the sac in which it lies is called pericarditis. The inflammation and disease may involve only these membranes, or may be a part of disease elsewhere in the heart, particularly the heart muscle or valves. Fluid may accumulate in the sac that encloses the heart; it may be watery fluid (perhaps blood tinged), or it may be rather thick and even purulent.

Accumulation of fluid in the pericardial sac will, of course, make difficult the normal filling of the heart, for the pericardial sac is tough and inelastic, and every ounce of fluid in it can potentially deny space to an ounce of blood entering and passing through the heart with each beat of the cycle.

Acute pericarditis may be a complication of rheumatic heart disease, tuberculosis, or blood poisoning (septicemia). It may also occur in persons with a healthy heart, as in a sudden illness with mild symptoms of vague distress or (at the other extreme) profound prostration.

After the acute phase of the disease is over, a chronic stage may begin. The membranes covering the heart can become thickened and adhere to the heart. The pericardial surfaces lose their lubricating fluid, resulting in a friction rub, a dry, grating sound that can be heard with a stethoscope.

In healing, a fibrous process develops that will tend to shrink and contract the size of the pericardial sac. When this occurs, a constrictive pericarditis is said to be present. The heart is held in a rather rigid envelope of relatively small size. Blood cannot enter the heart chambers in quantities set by tissue demands, but is instead determined by the abnormal anatomic limitations of the constricted sac. Output of the heart, of course, diminishes and blood pressure falls below reasonable levels. Blood that should be readily drawn into the right atrium for passage to the lungs is denied adequate entrance by the constricting pericardium, and the blood dams up in the veins that supply the heart. The liver and spleen become swollen and engorged with blood; neck veins stand out like thick cords, and arm veins are very prominent and fail to empty completely until raised to higher levels than normal.

In the acute phase, aspirin, corticosteroids, meperidine or morphine may be given to relieve the pain. Aspirin also helps to reduce fever and hasten the reabsorption of the inflammatory fluids. Corticosteroids also reduce pain and fever and help prevent the further buildup of fluid. Other medical treatment of pericarditis depends on the cause of the inflammation. Pericarditis caused by bacteria or fungi is treated with specific antimicrobial drugs. Tuberculous pericarditis can be treated with various combinations of the drugs isoniazid, ethambutol, rifampin, and streptomycin.

Treatment. Permanent relief from the very inadequate and disabling circulatory state of chronic pericarditis can only be satisfactorily accomplished by surgical removal of much of the pericardium. This releases the heart, giving it relative freedom to fill properly. Sometimes the surgical relief is so dramatic that it seems as though the patient is rescued from imminent death, and he may be restored to full employment after just a few weeks of postoperative care. The relief is generally permanent since the pericardium does not regrow.

PERIPHERAL VASCULAR DISEASE
When any thickening occurs in the arterial wall, the size of the opening (lumen) within the vessel through which blood passes will become narrowed, even completely closed. Peripheral vascular disease includes all types of change, whatever their causes, that produce these obstructions to adequate blood flow:

Raynaud's disease. In this disorder, the clinical picture is produced by arterial spasm rather than by organic vascular disease, the arteries narrowing as a result of the spasm.

Arteriosclerosis obliterans. This term is used to designate arteriosclerosis which causes complete blockage of the lumen of vessels in the extremities, either because of the arteriosclerotic hardening process itself or because of thrombosis (blood clotting) within the vessel. It is the most common type of occlusive vascular disease in the lower extremities. Sometimes both the intimal (atherosclerosis) and the medial (senile) type of sclerosis are encountered at the same time in affected vessels. The causes of the atherosclerosis have not been made completely clear, although nutritional, endocrine, biochemical, and local vascular phenomena (as well as tissue changes in the intiminal lining substance of the vessels) are known to be implicated in its organization and development.

If vessel blockage completely cuts off the blood supply to an extremity, gangrene will occur in the toes, the foot, and sometimes even at higher levels. Death of the tissue imparts a black, mummified appearance to the skin. If the gangrene is complicated by infection, the affected part appears moist and foul-smelling. There may be considerable sloughing-away of tissue.

Buerger's disease (thromboangiitis obliterans). In this form of blood-vessel disease toxic agents such as nicotine have been implicated, although it is now generally agreed that this drug represents only an aggravating or accelerating influence. Buerger's disease is a condition affecting medium-sized and small arteries, and not infrequently the veins.

In its early stages the affected vessels contract by individual segments, particularly at sites of occlusion. The veins may be similarly involved, and in rare instances may even be the earliest site of involvement. A soft but adherent red-purple clot may be seen within the passageway (lumen) of the affected arteries. Later the clot becomes yellow-gray. Proliferation of vessel-lining may be observed in portions of arteries in which blockage has not occurred. When the lesion is advanced, the lumen is blocked by a thrombus containing vessel-lining cells, clot-related materials, and some red and white blood cells. The musculature of the middle layer of the vessel is well preserved, but the inner lining is thickened by proliferation of connective tissue which in long-standing cases includes adjacent veins. Oxygen-lack changes such as gangrene, softening of the bone, and muscular atrophy may also be present in this disorder.

In addition to the above, there are a number of rare afflictions that may cause arterial obstruction; some of these are attributed to hypersensitivity (allergy) phenomena, others to tissue (collagen) disorders, others still to inflammatory disorders of the arteries. An example of the latter is the arteritis involving the middle-size arteries of the head seen with the rheumatic disorder known as polmyalgia rheumatica.

PERNICIOUS ANEMIA *See* Anemia in this section; Q-28 in the section Questions and Answers about Common Symptoms.

PHLEBITIS *See* Thrombophlebitis in this section.

PHONOCARDIOGRAPHY Heart murmurs can be detected by a specially constructed microphone applied to the chest wall in the same way as a stethoscope. The noise of the murmur can be permanently recorded on moving paper, together with the electrocardiograph (EKG) tracing. This instrument is somewhat greater in sensitivity than the human ear and detects sounds too faint for the ear. Also, it makes possible a permanent record, in case surgery is done or there are changes—as in the case of bacterial endocarditis. Furthermore, a very accurate relationship of murmur to the exact phase of the cardiac cycle is made possible by use of phonocardiograph tracings superimposed on the EKG tracing.

PULMONARY ARTERY The pulmonary artery conducts the blood from the right ventricle of the heart to the lungs. It is separated from the right ventricle by a valve that prevents ejected blood from returning to the ventricular pumping-chamber. A short distance from the heart, the pulmonary artery divides into a right branch that supplies the artery branches in the right lung and a left branch that serves the arteries in the left lung.

Blood pressure in the pulmonary artery is much lower than in the arterial system of the rest of the body. Unless pulmonary-artery disease is present, there is great adaptability to large changes in blood-flow during exercise, with little increase needed in pulmonary artery pressure to insure prompt passage of blood through the capillaries of the lung.

PULMONARY HEART DISEASE

Strictly speaking, pulmonary heart disease is that form of enlargement of the right side of the heart that develops as a result of diseases of the lung, rib cage, pulmonary blood vessels, or from primary pulmonary hypertension. Enlargement of the right side of the heart of lung causation is referred to as "cor pulmonale." Cor pulmonale may also follow mitral stenosis and some types of congenital heart disease.

Development of heart disease following lung involvement depends mainly upon the degree and duration of the resistance to the usual free flow of blood through the lungs at relatively low pressures. Increased resistance to flow through the lung (pulmonary circulation) is usually referred to as pulmonary vascular disease, or pulmonary hypertension.

Cor pulmonale caused by pulmonary vascular disease is seen in such lung diseases as obstructive emphysema and any other structural derangement in lung anatomy that mechanically obstructs the pulmonary blood vessels in such ways that pressure must necessarily rise to force blood through those narrowed vessels. Obstructive emphysema is now recognized as a most common and important cause of cor pulmonale.

Sometimes industrial dusts and chronic infection can affect the lungs and cause cor pulmonale, especially when the disease involves both lungs and produces structural narrowings in the vessel system. Occasionally, multiple blood clots that come into the lungs over a period of weeks and months from

a diseased heart or even from distant veins can gradually block the free flow of blood through the lungs. Pulmonary heart disease will then follow.

RAYNAUD'S SYNDROME This disorder occurs when the small arteries of the fingers (and less frequently the nose and tongue) constrict. Young women are more frequently affected.

Symptoms. The fingers become pale after exposure to cold or during periods of emotional stress and then attain a bluish coloration. Numbness and tingling may also be present.

Treatment. Those with a propensity for Raynaud's disease should wear gloves when reaching into the freezer section of the refrigerator. Avoidance of actions that bring on the disorder is the best treatment. Vasodilator medications are prescribed in some cases. Smokers should quit, as the vasoconstrictive effects of nicotine hasten the onset and frequency of attacks.

RHEUMATIC HEART DISEASE In young adults and children heart disease is usually of rheumatic origin. The antibiotics have so reduced the occurrence of diphtheria and syphilis that rheumatic heart disease is now the only important form of heart disease primarily caused by a specific infection, but it too is becoming much less frequent as time passes.

Acute rheumatic fever is a disease affecting all tissues in some degree. The joints are usually affected and can be swollen and painful for days or weeks. The acute phase of the disease, however, may be so mild that only fatigue is noted, and the young persons so afflicted may even be accused of laziness.

Rheumatic fever is in some way caused by a specific streptococcus (the so-called "Group A beta-hemolytic type"). A sore throat caused by this organism often precedes the rheumatic fever by several weeks. While this group of bacteria does not cause changes in the heart directly, the tissue-reaction and damage related to the organisms are rather characteristic.

Although patients over the age of thirty-five have been known to suffer a first attack of rheumatic fever, it usually comes before the age of twenty. The disease is much more prevalent in the cold, damp areas of the world where upper-respiratory infections and sore throats are common and contagious.

SICKLE CELL ANEMIA Sickle cell anemia is an inherited disorder of the hemoglobin, the substance in blood that carries oxygen. Because of the defective hemoglobin, the red blood cells suffer a deformation and take on a collapsed, sickle-like shape. This structural abnormality, and the loss of oxygen-carrying capacity, may cause or increase the likelihood of extreme fatigue, blood clots, pneumonia, heart failure, and stroke. Many victims die before the age of twenty.

The sickle cell genetic trait occurs predominantly among people of African descent. Just over 10 percent of the American black population have this trait, usually with few or no ill effects. However, when a couple, both possessing the sickle cell trait, produce a child, the child will suffer the full effects of sickle cell anemia.

Many of the manifestations of the disease result from the anemia and the plugging of the blood vessels by clumps of the abnormal red blood cells. The anemia may call for repeated transfusions, especially in the "aplastic crisis" when red blood cell production falls sharply, as with a viral infection. Plugging of blood vessels leads to chronic ulcers of the legs but also to strokes, bleeding from the kidneys, and episodes of severe abdominal pain. There is increased incidence of infections such as pneumococcal pneumonia.

There is no cure for sickle cell anemia. However, treatment that may include drug therapy and blood transfusions has enabled some sufferers to live well into their 40's.

Screening for sickle cell trait is becoming more common. The full-fledged disease could be prevented with premarital genetic counseling which would discourage reproduction by a couple both of whose members have the trait.

STREPTOKINASE This is a protein substance obtained from cultures of a bacterium, a hemolytic streptococcus. Injected into humans, it serves to keep blood clots from forming. It is now produced commercially as an anti-clotting agent for use during or immediately following a heart attack. The substance dissolves clots that may be clogging critical arteries that are nourishing the heart. If instituted within the first several hours of the onset of the attack, it can, in some cases, greatly reduce the amount of damage to heart tissue. (*See also* TISSUE PLASMINOGEN ACTIVATOR in this section.)

STRESS TEST A stress test is a diagnostic method used to determine the body's response to physical exertion (stress). It involves taking an EKG and other physiological measurements (such as breathing rate and blood pressure) while the patient is exercising—usually jogging on a treadmill, walking up and down a short set of stairs, or pedaling on a stationary bicycle.

In individuals with compromised coronary circulation, such as those with angina, the EKG taken during the stress test will often show characteristic changes known to occur when the heart muscle is ischemic. Thus the test is often of value in arriving at a correct diagnosis in the analysis of chest pain. Generally in such cases the individual will complain of the pain with the exercise and there will be abnormalities in the EKG.

A stress test should be monitored by a trained observer since—though rare—untoward events such as arrhythmias may be precipitated.

TACHYCARDIA Tachycardia is unduly rapid heart action. It may be caused by anxiety, excitement, fever, anemia, pericarditis, exercise, and the many varieties of stress that may occur in the human organism. The heart can speed up yet will ordinarily function quite well until it reaches a rate of 160 to 180 beats per minute; any rate beyond this is undesirable, because the heart is unable to fill itself satisfactorily and the beats will become most inefficient.

The heart rate in a resting adult varies, but on the average beats about 80 times per minute. Its pace is set in the sino-atrial node, which is under the influence of both sympathetic nerve fibers which accelerate the rate and vagal impulses from an entirely different set of nerves which tend to slow it. In addition, hormones from the adrenal glands, and even circulating thyroid hormone can alter and even determine the heart rate. In times of emotional stress, the adrenal glands may assist the sympathetic nerves in raising the heart rate. On exercise or exertion, there is an increased return of blood through the veins; this is a factor in increasing the heartbeat to prevent overfilling of the major blood vessels.

A rather serious type of tachycardia is due to disordered function of the heart muscle, the abnormal heart rate being set by a focus in the atrial (or even the ventricular) tissue taking over the normal function of pacemaker. Thus, rapid arrhythmias are classed as supraventricular if the rate of discharge comes from an irritable focus in the atria. In atrial fibrillation, the atria may beat as often as 500 times per minute, while the ventricular rate can remain anywhere between 100 and 200 beats per minute. In a flutter of the atrium the rate of both atrium and ventricle is somewhat slower. Atrial or nodal tachycardia is the usual variety of simple tachycardia. Rapid rhythms produced in an abnormal ventricular area are very rare in patients without heart disease. Ventricular tachycardia may be related to an overdosage of digitalis, but it can easily be aggravated by overexertion or coexisting serious illness. In nodal tachycardia the ventricles beat at the same rate as the abnormal focus—100 to 200 times per minute.

The electrocardiogram can make the exact diagnosis and definitively distinguish whether the increased heart rate has its origin at the ventricular level or above it.

Symptoms. The tachycardias are functional disorders and symptoms are not those of organic disease, unless organic heart changes are present in association with the disorder. Tachycardia is perceived by the patient as extremely rapid heart action, referred to as "fast palpitation." The fluttering behind the breastbone or in the neck is unpleasant and as a rule begins to be felt rather abruptly. Often the tachycardia stops as quickly as it begins. The general rhythm is regular; if it is not, atrial fibrillation is probable rather than a simple tachycardia.

As a rule, attacks of tachycardia rarely last longer than a few hours. They often occur at infrequent intervals over many years, and the patient may learn how to terminate or tolerate them in various ways.

Paroxysmal tachycardia may be considered a rather special type of tachycardia. The awareness of rapid heart action appears without warning, and after a brief period of annoyance, suddenly disappears. It rarely causes any disability except for an awareness of its presence. Characteristically, it repeats itself throughout the lifetime of the patient.

Treatment. If no associated organic heart disease is present, the patient may require no special medication for mild attacks of paroxysmal tachycardia. If severe however, careful clinical or laboratory study will be required to indicate the appropriate measures required for treatment.

THROMBOPHLEBITIS Phlebitis is an inflammatory disease of the vein wall and surrounding tissues. Usually there is an associated thrombosis or clot of blood (thrombophlebitis) that completely blocks the flow of blood through the area of vein holding the clot. Phlebitis can occur in any of the veins of the body, but most commonly occurs in the veins of the legs, thighs, or pelvis.

Symptoms. Acute phlebitis will produce swelling of the extremity involved, together with fever and an elevated pulse rate. Pain may be acute in some patients, especially when motion of the affected part is attempted. Chronic phlebitis is characterized by persistent swelling and physical disability which is caused both by the swelling and the deficient circulation in the extremity.

Treatment. In the acute stage, phlebitis will require rest in bed and careful observation of the changes produced by the blood clot obstructing the large vein. It is customary to institute treatment with drugs that will stop further clotting. Those most commonly used are heparin and warfarin. This is known as anticoagulant therapy. When some of the clot threatens to break away and drift to the lungs (pulmonary embolus), one of the surgical procedures designed to narrow the diameter of the abdominal vena cava and therefore block the passage of the large clot may be indicated.

Often, especially in the leg, an acute phlebitis subsides but a low grade inflammation may occur over the years. This leads to a chronic phlebitis often with some pain, swelling, and redness followed by darkening of the skin. The swelling and deficient circulation can be helped by means of elastic stockings, selective exercise, and diuretics.

THROMBOSIS   *See* CORONARY OCCLUSION in this section.

TISSUE PLASMINOGEN ACTIVATOR (TPA)   Tissue-type plasminogen activator is a naturally occurring enzyme that can break down blood clots. It is now being used to break down clots in coronary arteries that cause heart-muscle damage (myocardial infarctions). Given immediately following the onset of a heart attack (preferably within two hours) TPA, marketed under the trade name Activase®, has been shown to decrease the extent of heart damage and prolong life after the myocardial infarction.

Produced through recombinant DNA techniques, this new clot-destroying substance, despite its high cost, is beginning to replace streptokinase, an earlier but still used substance. TPA is also favored because of its efficacy and ease of application as well as lower incidence of such side effects as massive bleeding and stroke. (*See also* STREPTOKINASE in this section.)

VASCULAR ACCIDENTS   This term refers generally to disease produced by gross circulatory disturbances such as clots or hemorrhages, without overt or identifiable external causation. The term is frequently applied to sudden circulatory events occurring in the central nervous system.

Because of the implied localization to the brain, similar events elsewhere (aorta or other major artery) are referred to as cardiovascular catastrophes. A clot lodged in a lung artery, though a form of vascular accident, would be referred to as a pulmonary embolus.

VEINS   Blood is carried from capillaries to the heart through a network of tubes called veins which course through the body. Composed of three layers of different kinds of tissue, veins have thinner coatings and are less muscular than arteries. These features allow veins to distend and store large volumes of blood. About 75 percent of the body's blood is stored in veins.

Superficial veins near the surface can be seen through the skin. Unlike arteries, some veins have valves that prevent reflux.

EAR, NOSE, AND THROAT CONDITIONS

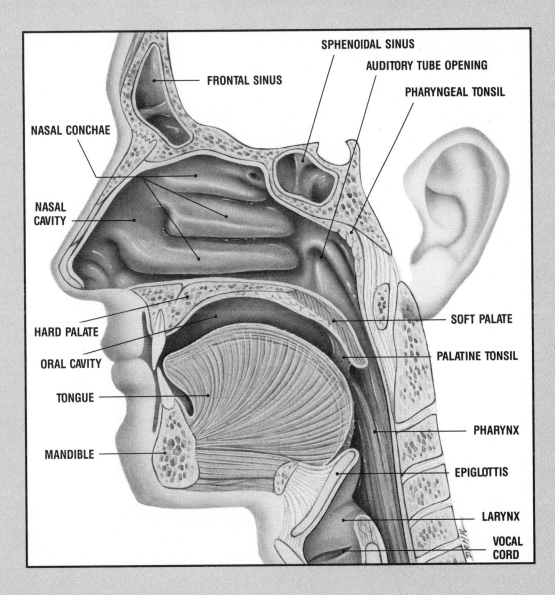

FRONTAL SINUS

SPHENOIDAL SINUS

AUDITORY TUBE OPENING

PHARYNGEAL TONSIL

NASAL CONCHAE

NASAL CAVITY

SOFT PALATE

HARD PALATE

PALATINE TONSIL

ORAL CAVITY

TONGUE

PHARYNX

MANDIBLE

EPIGLOTTIS

LARYNX

VOCAL CORD

The ear, nose, and throat are some of the most important of the body's sense organs. There is interdependence among the elements that need to be identified and understood. The ear is not only concerned with the sense of hearing but also controls our system of balance. The nose, with associated sinus area, and the throat are frequently the sites of irritations and infections associated with allergies, upper respiratory infections, and other conditions. Perhaps the most common complaints in everyday medical practice relate to the ear, nose, and throat (ENT).

This section defines the various physiological structures of the ear, nose, and throat; identifies common inflammatory problems of ear; and discusses some areas of diagnosis and treatment. *See also* the questions on frequent colds (Q-40); sore throat (Q-41); nasal stuffiness (Q-42); sinus infections (Q-43); postnasal drip (Q-44); coughing (Q-45); and poor hearing (Q-38) in the section QUESTIONS AND ANSWERS ABOUT COMMON SYMPTOMS.

The following is a list of terms identified in this section:

ABSCESS, PERITONSILLAR
ABSCESS, RETROPHARYNGEAL
ACOUSTIC TRAUMA
ACUTE EPIGLOTTITIS
ADENOIDS
ANOSMIA
APHONIA
ATROPHIC RHINITIS
AUDITORY CANAL, BLOCKING
   OF THE EXTERNAL
AUDITORY OSSICLES,
   MALFUNCTION OF THE
CERUMEN
CONDUCTIVE HEARING LOSS
DEAFNESS
DEAFNESS, CONDUCTION
EAR
EAR, INFECTION OF THE MIDDLE
EAR, SOME COMMON DISEASES
   OF THE EXTERNAL
EARDRUM, PERFORATION OF THE
EUSTACHIAN TUBE, BLOCKAGE OF THE
HEARING AIDS
HEARING LOSS
HEARING TESTS
HOARSENESS

LINGUAL TONSILLITIS
MÉNIÈRE'S DISEASE
MOTION SICKNESS
NASOPHARYNX
NONCONDUCTIVE (NEUROSENSORY,
   PERCEPTIVE) HEARING LOSS
NOSE AND PARANASAL SINUSES
NOSE, FOREIGN BODIES IN THE
NOSE INJURY
NOSEBLEEDS (EPISTAXIS)
OTITIS MEDIA
OTOLARYNGOLOGY
OTOSCLEROSIS
PERITONSILLAR ABSCESS (QUINSY)
PRESBYCUSIS
RHINITIS
RHINITIS SICCA
RHINOPLASTY
SINUSITIS
SORE THROAT
THROAT
TINNITUS
TONSILS
TUBES IN THE EARS
VERTIGO (DIZZINESS)
VOCAL CORDS, PARALYSIS OF THE

ABSCESS, PERITONSILLAR If infection of the palatine tonsils breaks through the surrounding tissues, an abscess—a localized collection of pus—can occur.

Symptoms. The patient has great difficulty in swallowing, and there is a bad odor to the breath. There is also difficulty in opening the mouth because of inflammation of the jaw muscles.

Treatment. The abscess should be cut into (incised) and drained by the physician. Rapid relief of pain usually occurs when the pressure is relieved.

ABSCESS, RETROPHARYNGEAL An abscess-formation behind the pharyngeal wall and in front of the neck bones or vertebrae (visible in infants and very young children) may be secondary to an infection of the pharynx.

Symptoms. There is difficulty in breathing and sore throat associated with fever.

Treatment. The abscess must be drained in such a way that the infected material is not sucked into the lungs. Antibiotics are used after the drainage.

ACOUSTIC TRAUMA Continued very loud sound or even a single extremely loud blast may lead to noise-induced hearing loss. In reversible cases there may be some ringing in the ears accompanied by the sensation of "listening in a barrel." The hearing may then return. Sometimes, however, the hearing loss is permanent. Therefore, those who are repeatedly exposed to loud sounds (such as rifle or skeet shooters) should wear ear plugs as protection against noise-induced hearing loss.

ACUTE EPIGLOTTITIS When the uppermost part of the larynx (epiglottis) becomes infected, sudden obstruction of the airway may occur. This condition is not common, but is serious, in children. In three or four hours or less the epiglottis of a child can become so swollen that death may occur from inability to breathe. In adults it tends to be more chronic and—taking longer to develop—is not so suddenly devastating.

Treatment. Opening of the windpipe (tracheotomy) is almost always performed when a diagnosis of acute epiglottitis is made, because the obstruction occurs with such rapid-

ity. Antibiotics, humidity, and maintenance of fluid balance are other measures for this respiratory problem. When a young child complains of pain on swallowing and shows difficulty in breathing, he may have epiglottitis and should be seen by a physician at once.

ADENOIDS The adenoids are masses of lymph tissue, closely related to the tonsils in position and function. They are found in the upper back part of the throat, just above and behind the soft palate; thus, they can be seen only with the aid of a special mirror.

Normally the adenoids enlarge during the fourth to the sixth year of life and may, if enlarged or infected, cause obstruction of clear nasal breathing. They may also block the adjacent inner openings of the Eustachian tubes. (These tubes running from the inner ear to the throat equalize the atmospheric pressure on both sides of the eardrums. If the adenoids become enlarged and plug the Eustachian-tube openings, the air from the tubes becomes absorbed and the greater pressure on the outside will push an eardrum in, creating a retracted eardrum and almost always a hearing loss.

Repeated ear infections (*see* OTITIS MEDIA in this section) occurring after colds are often related to enlarged adenoids. If repeated ear infections, mouth-breathing, hearing loss, and swollen, infected tonsils and glands cannot be controlled with conservative management and/or antibiotics, surgical removal of adenoids and tonsils before the age of seven years is a wise decision.

ANOSMIA Anosmia is loss of smell. It may be congenital or acquired. Temporary anosmia is most common in nasal conditions such as the ordinary cold, sinus infection, polyps, and catarrh (inflammation of the mucous membranes). Brain lesions involving the olfactory tract may result in one-sided anosmia which is of diagnostic significance in tumors of the underside of the front of the brain. One- or two-sided anosmia may result from frontal fracture of the skull. Tumors of the temporal portion of the brain may result in olfactory hallucinations. Disturbed sense of smell is not uncommon in psychoses and is sometimes seen as an aura in epilepsy. Treatment for anosmia is that of the underlying cause.

APHONIA   This form of aphasia is marked by loss of speech function. It may be organic in origin but often occurs as a phenomenon of conversion hysteria (a form of psychoneurosis), particularly when the conscious stimulus is a frightening one. In the latter instance, it is assumed that the speechlessness is a reaction to an unconscious emotional conflict.

Treatment. In the absence of organic factors, immediate restoration of speech can be obtained through hypnosis. However, this is not a "cure"; to avoid repetition of hysterical aphonic attacks or equivalent neurotic reactions, psychotherapy must be instituted.

ATROPHIC RHINITIS   When this condition develops, the nasal lining becomes flat with loss of cilia (hairlike processes) and is replaced by skinlike tissue. Without the normal mucosa and its function, the airway is too large and dry, and becomes crusted. Frequently a foul odor emanates from the nose and the patient loses the sense of smell. The direct cause of this uncommon disease is unknown. Removal of the crust and use of oils and hormones have been helpful. Surgery has been used with occasional success.

AUDITORY CANAL, BLOCKING OF THE EXTERNAL   The accumulation of wax (cerumen), bony growth, foreign bodies, or closure of the canal by swelling can all result in significant hearing loss. The canal must be entirely closed before significant hearing loss occurs, for if even a pinhole remains from the sound source to the eardrum, the hearing loss may be negligible. This is why hearing loss tends to result after water enters an ear partially filled with cerumen: the water fills the places between the wax and completely occludes the canal.

It is a very poor idea for a person to try to clean his own ear canal. The old rule that "nothing smaller than your elbow should be put in the ear" is a good one. Wax in the ear is desirable, as it is a special secretion which prevents the thin skin from drying and tends to prevent foreign particles from reaching the eardrum. This function is further aided by the hairs on the outside of the ear canal.

Only if the wax in the ear blocks hearing or becomes hard and painful should it be removed—and then only by a physician. Some-times the services of an ear specialist (otologist) are required. He may irrigate the ear with a special syringe, or use tiny hooked instruments to remove the wax. It may even be necessary to soften the wax prior to cleaning the ear canal. The correct cleaning technique can be selected only by a physician who is able to look into the ear and properly interpret what he sees.

Sometimes young children place small objects in their ear canal. If these objects cannot be easily dislodged at home, they too should be extracted by a physician. Since it is possible for the child to impair his hearing seriously by pushing foreign bodies into the ear, this practice must be strongly discouraged by the parents. Occasionally an object must be removed under general anesthesia, and sometimes an incision must be made in order to remove the offending object. Parents are not in possession of the instruments or skill to remove either wax or foreign objects; this job always belongs to the physician.

External otitis is a common ear disease affecting the skin of the external auditory canal. It ranges from mild irritation (with the sole symptom of itching) to severe purulent infection (with hearing loss and excruciating pain). The cause of external otitis is frequently the fault of the patient. Getting water in the ears, or scratching the ear canal with sharp objects or fingernails, can cause external otitis. Since wax need not be removed from the ear canal except for reasons of pain or hearing loss (and then only by a physician), there is no reason to wash the ears beyond the outermost ear (pinna). Nor is there any need to put bobby pins, hairpins, paper clips, Q-tips®, pencils, safety pins, or washcloths into the ear canal.

If the "elbow rule" is followed and no water is allowed in the ear (particularly when showering, bathing, or washing the hair), most cases of external otitis can be prevented. Cotton plugs in the outside of the ear, shower caps, and ordinary care will prevent water from injuring the ear. Swimming may not be a hazard, although the ears of some people are much more sensitive to the effects of water than others. If the ears are as much as possible cleared of water after swimming, and if diving is not overdone, most people can enjoy the sport without worry. If, however, a person is subject to "swimmer's ear" (which is only external otitis occurring after swimming) the doctor may be able to prescribe drops to use after each day's swimming to serve as a preventive.

Moisture in the ear canal is like water in a narrow-mouthed bottle; it is not easy to get out. The moisture makes the canal skin susceptible to bacterial infection. This, in turn, results in swelling of the skin which adheres very closely to the underlying cartilage and bone. With little room for expansion, the swelling causes severe pain, often requiring narcotics for relief.

Treatment. Treatment is not by home remedy, and a physician (preferably an ear specialist) should treat this condition. Frequently, local medications are enough to combat infections and swelling. A physician may bring the condition under control by cleaning the ear with swab and suction. Long-standing chronic cases with relatively little pain (except for acute flare-ups) require more and longer treatments. After long-standing irritation, the skin actually undergoes changes and long-term therapy is required before the skin reverts to normal.

THE AUDITORY OSSICLES

When sound waves cause the eardrum to vibrate, the chain of bony ossicles also vibrate. Thus, sound waves are transmitted to the fluid-filled inner ear.

AUDITORY OSSICLES, MALFUNCTION OF THE

The three tiny ear bones (ossicles) may be the cause of hearing loss because of noncontinuity, fixation, or absence. Infection, injury, developmental defect, or progressive deafness are the most frequent reasons for these defects.

When the ossicles are not connected and no longer carry the sound vibrations to the ears' fluid system, the eardrums' vibrations are not effective and the patient experiences a moderate to severe hearing loss. Following infection of the middle ear (otitis media), parts of the ossicles may be destroyed. A blow on the head may cause dislocation of the incus and stapes, while developmental defects before birth may result in failure of one or more of the bones to form. Otosclerosis can cause conductive hearing loss by fixation (immobilization) of the stapes (the most common cause of hearing loss in young and middle-aged adults). These are among the more common examples of how difficulties with the auditory ossicles can bring on hearing loss.

Fortunately, if the eardrum is intact and the auditory nerve good, results of surgical repair are highly successful. Ninety percent of these patients can have their hearing restored by current surgical techniques.

CERUMEN

The naturally occurring wax in the outer ear is called cerumen. Wax becomes impacted when excessive amounts are produced. In an attempt to remove excessive wax, the individual may actually push it further into the canal, causing ear pain and a temporary loss of hearing.

Treatment. The wax may be removed by irrigation or by chemical ear wax softeners, and by instrumentation at the doctor's office.

CONDUCTIVE HEARING LOSS

Hearing loss that results from abnormal conditions in the outer or middle ear is said to be conductive. It is very often reparable by use of medication or surgery. (*See* AUDITORY CANAL, BLOCKING OF THE EXTERNAL; EARDRUM, PERFORATION OF THE; AUDITORY OSSICLES, MALFUNCTION OF THE; EUSTACHIAN TUBE, BLOCKAGE OF; EAR, INFECTION OF THE MIDDLE in this section.)

DEAFNESS

Deafness can be either complete or partial. Complete deafness in children is unusual, and modern electronic devices are now helping many who may have thought themselves completely deaf. Congenital (inborn) deafness is usually due to damaged or poorly formed nerves which transmit the sound impulses from the ear to the brain.

It may be difficult to tell if a child is deaf until he is two years old, at which time he should be able to say at least a few words. Since speech is dependent upon hearing, a child who has never been able to hear will be unable to speak.

It is important that deafness be discovered while a child is still young, because current techniques used in educating deaf children are more effective if begun early.

Virus infections of the mother during the first three months of pregnancy are probably the most common cause of congenital deafness. Acquired deafness is usually due to repeated ear infections, persistent fluid behind the eardrum, and/or enlarged adenoids.

Treatment. Ear infections should be treated quickly and adequately. If there are persistent signs of fluid or obstruction, a physician may accomplish drainage by incising the eardrum, with the adenoids and tonsils perhaps being removed later.

DEAFNESS, CONDUCTION

Many causes, known and unknown, are behind conduction deafness. Congenital defects of the ear or parts of the ear or of the Eustachian tube (running from the internal ear to the throat) are not unusual. Major causes of this condition are impacted wax, foreign bodies, tumors, stenosis (narrowing or constriction), perforation, inflammation, or scars of the tympanic membrane, rigidity of the small bones of the inner ear, chronic middle ear disease, otosclerosis (literally, "hardening of the ear") which does not allow the small bones of the inner ear to respond to vibratory stimuli, and blockage of the Eustachian tube.

In children, however, the most common cause is excessive lymphoid tissue in and around the Eustachian tube's opening which so clogs the tube that proper ventilation of the middle ear cannot be achieved. Lymphoid tissue is the same tissue that makes up "enlarged tonsils and adenoids." Otosclerosis is the most frequent cause of conduction deafness in young people, especially girls. It is

most often seen in the eighteen to forty year age bracket. The cause of otosclerosis is unknown, but it seems to run in families.

Treatment. Modern surgical repair includes procedures such as fracturing the small bone known as the stapes with interposition of a vein graft and the making of a window (fenestration) if the stapes-replacement procedure fails. Hearing aids are most useful in conduction deafness, especially when surgery is contraindicated. Hearing aids with transistor tubes are extremely small, to the extent that they can be enclosed in eyeglass frames. Bone conduction aids are worn behind the ear against the skull; air conduction aids are placed in the outer canal of the ear. Specialists perform speech audiometry to ensure that the most suitable instrument is prescribed for the deaf patient. Special classes, such as lip-reading classes, are most useful for deaf children.

EAR

The ear and hearing mechanism is one of the most remarkable sense organs in the animal world. Its complexity is exceeded only by the human brain; its tiny mechanism is as fine and sensitive as the best of our miniscule man-made electrical-mechanical wonders.

There is a natural division of the ear into three parts. The first is the one we see: the outer ear. In some lower animals the outermost ear (pinna or auricle) still has the function of picking up sounds and is even able to turn so as to perform this function more efficiently. The best that man can do is wiggle his ears, and most of us cannot even do that. The outer ear of man serves almost no hearing function. We are concerned about it mostly for cosmetic purposes and for hooking on eyeglasses.

From the outer ear and extending inward is a canal (the external auditory canal) a little over an inch long, which is lined by skin. This canal is supported at its outer third by cartilage and at its inner two-thirds by bone. The outermost skin of the canal has hair follicles and special glands which produce wax (cerumen). The innermost skin of the canal is very thin, tightly bound to the underlying bone, and devoid of hair and glands. The outer ear, then, is composed of the pinna and the external auditory canal.

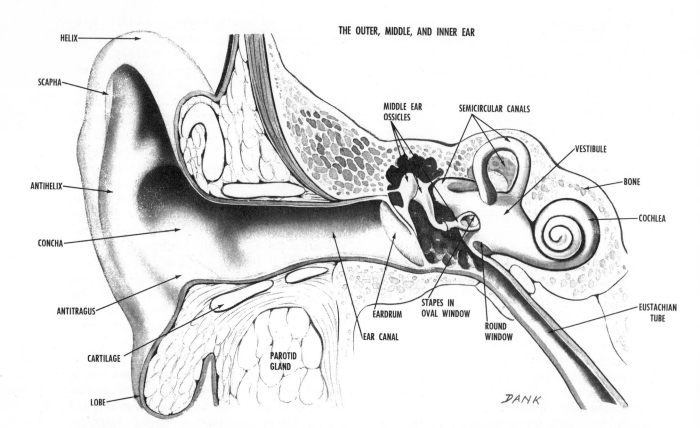

THE OUTER, MIDDLE, AND INNER EAR

HELIX

SCAPHA

ANTIHELIX

CONCHA

ANTITRAGUS

CARTILAGE

LOBE

MIDDLE EAR OSSICLES

SEMICIRCULAR CANALS

VESTIBULE

BONE

COCHLEA

EUSTACHIAN TUBE

STAPES IN OVAL WINDOW

EARDRUM

ROUND WINDOW

EAR CANAL

PAROTID GLAND

DANK

Separating the external from the middle ear is the eardrum (tympanic membrane or drumhead), an exceedingly thin membrane composed of five layers. The eardrum is about three-quarters the size of a dime, with a thickness of 1/250 of an inch.

Embedded in the fibrous layer of the vibrating eardrum is part of the first of the three bones of the middle ear. Shaped roughly like a hammer, this first bone has its handle attached to the eardrum and the head articulated with the second bone, which approximates an anvil in design. The anvil, in turn, has a delicate connection with the smallest bone in the human body, the last of the three bones of the middle ear, which fits into the "oval window" or *fenestra ovalis*. (This smallest bone is shaped very much like a stirrup, so the three bones are sometimes called the hammer, anvil, and stirrup. Their more sophisticated Latin names are the *malleus, incus,* and *stapes,* and it is these which we use in the text.) The stapes is flexibly bound to the oval window by an oval ligament.

The inner ear begins just below the oval window with a two-fluid system and is housed deep in the temporal bone in a special casing

of extremely dense bone. The delicate organs of balance (the semicircular canals) and of hearing (the cochlea) are housed in this special casing and share fluid systems in common. Although they are known by different names, the general mechanical construction of both are similar.

Sound travels through the hearing mechanism as follows: into outer ear—ear canal—tympanic membrane—malleus—incus—stapes—stapes-footplate (which in its vibrations sets the outer fluid in motion)—basilar membrane of the organ of Corti (in the cochlea)—inner fluid—haircells of the organ of Cor cochlear nerve—nuclei of the cochlea—lower brain-centers—higher brain-centers (where sound is recognized, associated, and interpreted).

There is a small tube indirectly associated with hearing which extends from the middle ear to the back of the throat at the level of the nose, called the Eustachian tube. This tube is ordinarily kept closed by muscles at the throat and is opened during yawning and swallowing, thereby keeping the air pressure on the middle ear side of the eardrum equal to that on the outer (atmospheric) side. The ear and hearing mechanisms are enormously complex, and this is a very simplified version; however, sufficient information has been given to understand the more common problems of hearing loss. (*See also* HEARING LOSS; HEARING TESTS; HEARING AIDS in this section.)

EAR, INFECTION OF THE MIDDLE

Infection of the middle ear is called otitis media. This should be not confused with serous otitis media, which (see page 000) does not refer to an *infected* middle ear. Usually the infection results from an upper respiratory infection and affects the middle ear via the Eustachian tube. The symptoms of otitis media are pain in the ear, hearing loss, and fullness in the ear during, or following, an upper respiratory infection.

Treatment. The treatment may be surgical incision of the eardrum with antibiotics or antibiotics alone. (The usual "cold," however, is caused by a virus, not by bacteria. If however, the bacteria *have* gained a foothold, it can be safely assumed that the virus has prepared the way. To put it another way, antibiotics are not in the least effective against the viruses causing colds, and it is only when bacterial invasion has been added that they are indicated. The patient demanding antibiotics for the common cold is therefore foolish and is trying to get the doctor to do something against his better judgment which will not help, and on the other hand may harm, the patient. Only a physician is in a position to decide what medication to use.) In otitis media as in other ear diseases, it is wise to avoid putting any medication in the ear unless prescribed by a physician. If the ear begins to drain, this indicates the drum has broken, providing a natural myringotomy. If this happens, clean cotton may be used in the ear to catch the drainage. The cotton should be very clean and be changed often; washing the hands before and after changing the cotton is a good idea. The doctor should be consulted *as soon as possible*.

Acute extension of a middle ear infection into the air spaces of the mastoid bone (acute mastoiditis) is now relatively uncommon because of the advances in medicine. Chronic mastoiditis is a different condition, however, and is often associated with chronically closed Eustachian tube (or cholesteatoma).

Surgery for this kind of mastoid problem is still relatively frequent.

EAR, SOME COMMON DISEASES OF THE EXTERNAL

The skin of the external ear is subject to the same diseases as skin in other locations of the body. The very thin skin closely bound to the sculptured cartilage of the pinna is most subject to deforming injury. The skin of the ear canal is most subject to chronic inflammation and infections because of the tendency toward retention of moisture.

Frostbite. The pinna is the most frequent site of frostbite. Common signs are loss of skin sensation, color changing from flesh to yellow-white, and hardening of the ear. When these occur, the entire body should be warmed and a physician seen at once. Heat or massage should not be applied to the frostbitten ear. In later stages of frostbite the ear becomes painful and swollen, and blisters (blebs) occur on the skin. Protection against infection and prevention of permanent shut-off of blood vessels may prevent gangrene. Neglect of the condition by the frostbitten patient can result in gangrene and loss of the ear.

Hematoma. Injury to the ear can cause blood to accumulate under the skin, forming a hematoma (literally blood-tumor). The blood should be evacuated and protection against infection secured. Consolidation of the hematoma can produce the "cauliflower ear." Like most ear problems, this is not amenable to home therapy, and a doctor should be seen.

Perichondritis. Perichondritis is an infection of the lining between the skin and the cartilage of the outer ear. It can occur after injury, hematoma, frostbite, burns, or other damage. The ear becomes very thick and dusky red in color. This condition must be vigorously treated with antibiotics. Abscesses must be evacuated. Other modalities such as ultraviolet light may be recommended by the physician.

Sebaceous cyst. The skin behind the lobule of the ear has many sebaceous glands. When obstruction of a gland occurs, a cyst (called a sebaceous cyst) may form. This happens frequently behind the ear or earlobe. Surgical excision is the treatment of choice.

Keloids. Keloids are an accumulation of scar tissue from any damage to the ear. They frequently occur after the earlobe is pierced for earrings. Surgical incision, sometimes followed by small amounts of X-ray, may prevent recurrence.

Furuncles. A localized form of external otitis, furuncles are really just pustules which can cause severe pain and tenderness of the ear. If treatment is started early, the infection can be corrected with local application of medication; later, incision and drainage may be necessary.

Protruding ear. Lop-ear or protruding ear is a condition which can often be corrected by surgery. The purpose of surgery for a protruding ear is purely cosmetic. The ear cartilages are usually too soft to operate upon satisfactorily under the age of four, but after this age results are satisfying. The operation is called otoplasty.

EARDRUM, PERFORATION OF THE

The main mechanism of the middle ear depends upon the relatively large area of the eardrum acting via the three middle-ear bones (ossicles) on the relatively small area of the stapes-footplate. This mechanism is called "the sound-pressure transformer." The eardrum is an extremely important part of the sound-pressure transformer because it provides a seventeen-to-one increase in pressure at the stapes footplate. A perforation of the eardrum lowers this ratio (among other factors), thus causing hearing loss. Keeping water out of a normal ear is a good idea, but keeping water out of an ear with a perforated eardrum is an absolute necessity—and that means no swimming.

Treatment. There are several methods of closing eardrum perforations. If no infection or damage exists other than the hole in the eardrum, any hearing loss caused by the perforation can be remedied if the eardrum is repaired. Because a perforated eardrum more easily allows infection to enter the middle ear, it is wise to see an ear specialist about any eardrum perforation. Home remedies such as oils, peroxide, and water irrigations are definitely to be avoided.

The patient should place a clean piece of cotton in the ear, take an aspirin substitute or other medication for pain, keep the ear dry, and plan to consult a physician soon. From office-treatment to major surgical procedures in the hospital, hearing loss through drum perforation can be repaired in a high percentage of cases. If there are no other defects except the perforated eardrum itself, the chances of successful therapy are over 90 percent.

EUSTACHIAN TUBE, BLOCKAGE OF THE

The function of the Eustachian tube is maintenance of equal pressure on both sides of the eardrum. If the Eustachian tube becomes blocked, this function is unfulfilled. In this case the oxygen in the middle ear is rapidly absorbed; the eardrum is pushed inward by the greater atmospheric pressure outside; and the delicate mucosal lining of the middle ear fills with a watery substance instead of air. The result is hearing loss. This condition is known by several names: serous otitis media, secretory otitis media, tubotympanitis, hydrotympanum, and others.

Treatment. The methods of treatment are directed at relieving the tubal blockage and evacuating the middle ear fluid. This may be accomplished by the procedure called myringotomy, an incision through the eardrum. The myringotomy must be performed carefully by a physician, under adequate lighting, with special instruments in the safe area of the eardrum. Suction may be used to aspirate the middle-ear fluid. The incision heals rapidly, usually in one day. This procedure may be done under general anesthesia for children: local anesthesia or even none will suffice for adults, and probably no anesthesia at all is safest for infants.

The hearing loss is relieved by myringotomy, but in order to avoid recurrence the doctor must also treat the underlying cause: the blocked Eustachian tube. Tubal obstruction may be due to a swelling around the throat (pharyngeal) end of the tube resulting from allergy or from upper respiratory infection (such as a cold). Occlusion may also be due to adenoids, tumor and, rarely, malocclusion of the teeth.

Fluid in the middle ear is the most common cause of hearing loss in children. The factors responsible are usually adenoids and allergy. If allergy is the problem, desensitization and myringotomy may prove successful. If the condition is a long-standing one, with need for long-term allergy management, an indwelling polyethylene tube is sometimes placed through the eardrum to promote drainage and to prevent the eardrum from closing too quickly; this method makes repeated myringotomies unnecessary. When the adenoids are responsible, their removal (and, if indicated, removal of the tonsils) together with the myringotomy should prove successful in relieving the hearing loss.

Medication, alone or in conjunction with opening the eardrum, is often sufficient for treating serous otitis media due to a cold. The danger of a negligent attitude is that after a long period of time the fluid in the middle ear tends to thicken and coalesce, causing possible adhesions. The adhesions then bind the ossicles, preventing their proper vibration and causing hearing loss. This type of hearing loss responds poorly to surgery. Therefore, neglect of the fluid of the middle ear can, in a small percentage of cases, lead to more or less permanent hearing loss. Thus, it is important to care for the ears promptly.

HEARING AIDS The proper way to get a hearing aid is as follows: (1) Go to an ear, nose, and throat specialist. If his diagnosis is a nerve-loss, a hearing aid will perhaps help. (2) Ask the doctor to recommend a place where it is possible to get a "Hearing Aid Evaluation." This is a long series of special hearing tests, which may take several hours, to determine what type of hearing aid will best help. Doctors' offices are usually not equipped to give such tests, but hospital, university, and otology centers are so equipped. For those thinking of a hearing aid, the evaluation test is the best investment which can be made. From the results of these tests the examiners (who are experts in the testing of hearing but usually are not M.D.'s) can tell whether or not a patient will be benefited by an aid, what type he should get, and when and how to use it.

Aids are expensive, and the constant replacement of batteries makes them even more so over the years. It therefore pays to see a doctor to determine whether medication or surgery can help; it pays to get a Hearing Aid Evaluation to find out whether or not a mechanical aid will help, and if so, what type is needed. Merely walking into a store and picking up a hearing aid is a poor way of choosing—even if a thirty-day trial offer goes with it.

HEARING LOSS Hearing loss can result from abnormal conditions affecting any one of the three parts of the ear: outer, middle, or inner. If the outer or middle ear is responsible, the hearing loss is said to be conductive and is very often reparable by the use of medication or surgery. When the inner ear, cochlear nerve, or central connections are at fault, the hearing loss is nonconductive and is called neurosensory or perceptive. Only two kinds of nonconductive hearing loss respond to medical measures: labyrinthine hydrops (Ménière's disease) and psychological hearing loss. (*See also* CONDUCTIVE HEARING LOSS; NONCONDUCTIVE (NEUROSENSORY, PERCEPTIVE) HEARING LOSS in this section.)

HEARING TESTS In order to give the reader a more thorough understanding of procedure in the otologist's office, a brief word about the audiogram is included.

An audiogram is a report plotted on a graph, describing the hearing. There are many special tests which can be performed to give the otologist information about different factors in the hearing mechanism; the basic data recorded by means of the audiometer, however, are the air- and bone-conduction curves.

The audiometer itself is an electronic machine giving off controllable sounds of varying intensity (loudness) and frequency (pitch). These sounds are applied to the outer ear, and the patient indicates when he hears the sound. The audiometrist records this information on a specially prepared graph, this constituting an air-conduction audiogram. When the sounds are channeled to the patient by means of a bone-conductor, most commonly placed on the mastoid bone in back of the pinna, the resulting graph is called a bone-conduction audiogram. The doctor often uses various tuningfork tests to verify the audiogram.

HOARSENESS Hoarseness is a heavy, rough, or harsh quality of the voice, usually lower in pitch than a person's normal voice. It is most common with viral respiratory illnesses and seldom lasts more than a couple of days, then slowly improves. Chronic hoarseness is more likely to be serious. The most frequent causes of hoarseness are inflammation, tumors, trauma, scars, paralysis and foreign bodies. (*See also* VOCAL CORDS, PARALYSIS OF THE in this section; and LARYNGITIS; LARYNX, INJURIES OF THE, AND FOREIGN BODIES IN; LARYNX, TUMORS OF THE in the section RESPIRATORY CONDITIONS.)

LINGUAL TONSILLITIS The part of Waldeyer's ring situated near the base of the tongue can become infected, although less frequently than the larger, deeper-set palatine tonsils. Treatment is similar to that for infections of the palatine tonsils. (*See* TONSILLITIS in the section INFECTIOUS DISEASES.)

MÉNIÈRE'S DISEASE Labyrinthine hydrops or Ménière's disease, is thought to be due to excess fluid in the inner fluid system of the labyrinth. The labyrinth is the term applied to the cochlea and semicircular canals, and their connections and dilatations. The cause of the excess fluid is not definitely known.

Symptoms. Tinnitus (ringing in the ear), hearing loss, episodes of dizziness, distortion of sound, and sensitivity to loud noises are all symptoms. The dizziness is true vertigo and manifests itself by the patient's sensation of his environment whirling around him or the patient whirling around the environment. Incapacitating episodes of vertigo can occur, associated with nausea and vomiting.

Treatment. The usual medical measures are low-salt diet, cessation of smoking, drugs to dilate the blood vessels, and antivertigo and antinausea drugs. Very dilute histamine injections are also used by a few physicians. Medical measures are said to control the symptoms satisfactorily in more than 85 percent of cases, but no one medication is 100 percent effective.

The physician must continue to try different medications until satisfactory control has been achieved. In those cases where the disease is incapacitating and will not respond to medication, surgery is considered. The surgical procedures are divided into two classifications: destructive and nondestructive.

Destructive:
1. Labyrinthectomy. This procedure involves removal of the membranous labyrinth through the oval window or through a window drilled into the hori-

zontal semicircular canal. Both methods destroy the patient's balance mechanism and hearing.
2. Ultrasound. Very high frequency sound is applied to the horizontal semicircular canal via a mastoidectomy approach. This attempts to destroy the balance mechanism while preserving the hearing. Recent analysis of a number of cases has shown a relatively high recurrence rate of vertigo. This procedure offers a good potential but must be further developed.
3. Drugs. Drugs, taken both systemically and by direct injection into the middle ear have been used to destroy the balance mechanism. Streptomycin has been used with some success.

Nondestructive:

Doctors Howard P. and William F. House of Los Angeles, California, world famous ear surgeons, have developed a shunt operation which continuously drains the excess fluid from the inner ear into the fluid system of the brain (the two fluids are very similar). This promising operation is not yet conclusive.

Destructive surgical procedures (and the drug method which sometimes adversely affects the hearing) can clearly be used only if the hearing is already quite poor, and then only in one ear. For patients with intractable Ménière's disease who have useful hearing, the most promising procedure, and the newest, may prove to be the shunt operation.

MOTION SICKNESS *See* VERTIGO in this section.

NASOPHARYNX The nasopharynx, the so-called "back of the throat," can be described as a funnel-shaped cavity with five openings. The posterior nares of the nose are two of the openings; the two Eustachian tubes are two more; and the oropharynx is the fifth opening. The adenoids, when present, sit on the back wall near the roof.

The position of the openings of the Eustachian tubes in children and adults is worth noting. In infants the openings are on a level with the floor of the nose. As the child grows older the relative position rises until in adulthood, the openings of the Eustachian tubes are as high as the lower (inferior) turbinate. The infant and younger child are therefore more prone to middle-ear infections because the wide, horizontal tube, with its opening at the floor of the nose, allows infected nasal secretions to enter the ear easily. The elevated angle of the Eustachian tube of the adult makes the middle ear less susceptible to contamination from nasal secretions.

NONCONDUCTIVE (NEUROSENSORY, PERCEPTIVE) HEARING LOSS Neurosensory hearing loss does *not* respond to surgery; and only Ménière's disease sometimes responds to medication. (Psychological hearing loss, of course, is a separate category and requires the services of a psychiatrist. It responds to psychotherapy and drugs, although the drugs tend only to facilitate psychotherapy rather than act directly on the nerves or blood vessels of the hearing mechanism.) (*See also* MÉNIÈRE'S DISEASE; PRESBYCUSIS; ACOUSTIC TRAUMA in this section.)

NOSE AND PARANASAL SINUSES
The nose is composed of skin-covered cartilage, bone, and an inner lining of delicate tissue—mucous membrane (mucosa). A bony-cartilagenous partition (septum) divides the nose into two nearly equal parts. The nostrils are the front openings of the nose, while the posterior nares are the back openings leading into the highest part of the pharynx (the so-called "back of the throat") called the nasopharynx. The middle part of the pharynx can be seen if one looks into a mirror and says "aahh."

The nasopharynx is just above and behind the soft palate, which may be seen in back and at the top of the mouth by looking at the open mouth in a mirror. The nasal lining (mucosa) covers all the surfaces of the sinuses, mouth, pharynx, larynx, Eustachian tubes, and middle ear, then extends throughout the lower respiratory tract. Although the mucosa varies in structure and thickness in different locations, due to the various roles it plays, essentially it is all the same membrane.

Within the nose, projecting out into the nasal space on either side toward, but not touching, the septum, are three—sometimes four—bony shelves covered by relatively thick

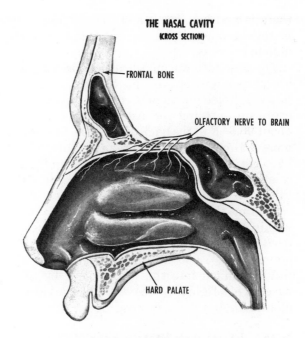

THE NASAL CAVITY
(CROSS SECTION)

FRONTAL BONE

OLFACTORY NERVE TO BRAIN

HARD PALATE

OLFACTORY SENSE
Specialized sensory neurons, capable of being stimulated by airborne odor particles, are located in the roof of the nasal cavity. The neurons collect into numerous small nerves which form the olfactory nerve. The odors most recognized are floral, fruity, herbal or spicy, resinal, and smoky.

mucosa. These shelves are called the turbinates.

The special features of the respiratory-tract mucosa are its cilia and mucus "blanket." The cilia, not visible except under a microscope, are tiny hair-like structures which beat constantly toward the mouth. This ciliary movement carries a blanket of mucus up from deep inside the lungs, as well as from the nose and sinuses downward, into the mouth, where it is swallowed. The function of the mucus blanket and the cilia is to catch foreign material, bacteria, and viruses and to carry them to a place where they will do no harm. This is a remarkable cleansing mechanism and an efficient body defense, since the swallowing allows the body effectively to eliminate unwanted material from the respiratory tract.

When the quantity of mucus becomes excessive, we may cough and spit out some material, but this only occurs in conditions of illness. Some people suddenly become conscious of the great quantity of fluid put out by the mucosa of the respiratory tract and may begin to complain, hack, and spit. However if, after examination, the physician determines there is nothing wrong and the spitting has merely become a habit, the patient is usually able to break it.

The nose also warms the air we breathe to the proper temperature for the bronchi and lungs. Inhaled air, no matter what its temperature on entering the front of the nose, is about 96.8° F. at the back of the nose. Furthermore, almost all the foreign material—bacteria, dust—in the air is gone and the relative humidity of the air is 75 percent. All this is accomplished in about one quarter of a second by the nasal mucosa and turbinates within the four inches of space between the front and back of the nose! Every twenty-four hours about 1,000 milliliters (one quart) of fluid is mixed into the inspired air by the nose. (This figure varies with the environmental air, but it is a fair estimated average.)

NOSE, FOREIGN BODIES IN THE   Just as children sometimes place small objects in the ear, they may also place them in the nose. Easily distracted from one activity to another, children shortly forget the button, bean, or pebble placed there. After a few days, one side of the nose becomes obstructed, and a purulent (pus) discharge which has an unpleasant odor becomes noticeable. These foreign objects should be removed as soon as possible by a physician, and the child strongly cautioned against putting things up the nose. The habit is dangerous because there is always the possibility of suction of the foreign body into the lungs or of serious nasal infection.

NOSE INJURY   The nose is the most prominent and unprotected part of the face and has the highest incidence of all fractures. The most frequent signs of nasal-bone fracture are swelling, black and blue discoloration, nasal bleeding, and movable nasal-bone fragments. X-rays are frequently needed when injury occurs. Ice compresses are helpful until the doctor is seen. A simple, small fracture is not difficult for the physician to set; extensive fractures, however, may require extensive surgery. It is important in either case that fractures not be neglected, either in adults or in children.

Often the septum is displaced during injury, and sometimes a hematoma, which is a localized collection of blood under the septum lining, occurs. If this happens evacuation of the collected blood is necessary. An abscess can form if infection takes hold in an injured septum. This is treated with incision, drainage, and antibiotics. Neglect by the patient of a hematoma or abscess of the septum can result in permanent perforation of the septum.

NOSEBLEEDS (EPISTAXIS)   Epistaxis is simply the medical term for nosebleed. Children seem to have more bloody noses than do adults, probably because they fall on them or pick them more. A nose will also bleed if a fever is high enough to dilate the capillaries within. Since children get many colds and upper-respiratory infections, the mucus secreted will often erode the lining.

Many people have a very red nose lining (nasal septum) with the capillaries very close to the surface. In these people, the slightest jar or sneeze or just dry air will cause this area to split and pour out the blood. Sometimes a respiratory allergy may aggravate this tendency. (*See* Coryza, Allergic in the section Allergic Conditions.)

It is often thought that if a child has many nose bleeds, he has either rheumatic fever or leukemia. This can be so; but there are so many nosebleeds compared to the serious diseases that the latter are last on the list of possibilities.

Treatment. The most important thing to

THE EXTERNAL NOSE

NASAL BONE

LATERAL CARTILAGE

ALAR CARTILAGE

do for nosebleed is to put pressure where the leak is—on the septum (the bony partition that divides the nose into two nearly equal parts). Cold wet rags on the back of the neck, forehead, top of the nose, or under the lip are of little use, since the victim is not bleeding from these areas.

Wet a piece of clean absorbent tissue paper or cotton and press it to the side of the nasal passage. Push it up the canal and squeeze the nose from the outside hard for ten minutes; then leave the pack in place for ten minutes more and slowly withdraw it. This procedure will stop 90 percent of nosebleeds and will leave a clear open passage without a hard, dry clot. If the condition is recurrent, a simple ointment should be applied twice daily for a week (the crack takes this long to heal) to keep the area soft and pliable. If episodes of nosebleed are too frequent, the doctor may need to cauterize the blood vessels of the septum with silver nitrate or a hot needle. (*See also* NOSE-BLEED in the section FIRST AID AND EMERGENCIES.)

OTITIS MEDIA   This common cause of earache is an infection in the middle ear just behind the eardrum, seen most commonly in children following a cold. It is almost always caused by bacteria which seem to build up in the small space behind the eardrum because the cold has closed off the Eustachian tube. (This tube leads out from the middle ear to the back of the throat and allows for proper drainage and equalization of air pressure on the two sides of the eardrum.)

Symptoms. Because the eardrum is very sensitive, even minor inflammation can cause excruciating pain, and the affected child who seemed almost recovered from a cold may suddenly scream out and clutch the ear.

If there is fever the infection has usually progressed to the point of abscess; this may cause the eardrum to bulge and burst, exuding a surprising amount of pus and blood. The fever may then fall and the earache disappear. One may then think that the ear has healed, but the situation remains serious and should be treated. Although not every earache demands treatment, any persistent one accompanied by fever is potentially dangerous, and a doctor should be consulted.

Treatment. The common feelings of "full-ness" in the ear experienced during a respiratory infection are often helped by decongestant pills (many of which are sold over the counter), nose drops, and aspirin. When pain and diminished hearing are complained of, home treatment is treading on dangerous ground. The doctor should be consulted, and it is customary to rely on the use of an appropriate antibiotic. Otitis media and its sequel, the "running ear," have become rare with the advent of antibiotics. Only occasionally will a physician find it necessary to puncture the drum to permit drainage of fluid in the middle ear.

OTOLARYNGOLOGY   The term otolaryngology refers to the surgical specialty devoted to diagnosis and treatment of diseases of the ear, nose, and throat. (The name is actually a shortened version of the full name, otorhinolaryngology, oto-referring to the ear, -rhino- to the nose and sinuses, and -laryng- to the larynx.) This field also includes the pharynx and almost all the structures of the neck.

OTOSCLEROSIS   *See* DEAFNESS, CONDUCTION in this section.

PERITONSILLAR ABSCESS (QUINSY)   *See* ABSCESS, PERITONSILLAR in this section.

PRESBYCUSIS   Presbycusis, which may begin as early as age thirty-five and as late as sixty-five, is the most common cause of hearing loss in the older age group. A neurosensory type of hearing loss, it is sometimes complicated by an inability to discriminate correctly between similar sounds. When discriminative faculty of the hearing mechanism is functioning poorly, merely increasing the loudness of the voice is ineffective in helping the hard-of-hearing person. The problem is one of insufficient signals leading to understanding. Speaking slowly and clearly, and letting the hearing-impaired person watch the speaker's lips, will aid materially in achieving understanding of speech. This problem—of not understanding speech even if it is made loud—can occur in many types of neurosensory hearing loss and is not restricted to presbycusis. This phenomenon does not occur in purely conductive loss.

RHINITIS   *See* ATROPHIC RHINITIS; RHINITIS SICCA in this section.

RHINITIS SICCA   Chronic rhinitis sicca (literally dry rhinitis) is not common in young healthy adults or children. It occurs more frequently in women at the time of the menopause, or in persons with chronic debilitating diseases such as diabetes or chronic kidney problems. The symptoms are dryness of the nose and annoying crusting with a heavy odor. With rhinitis sicca there is no atrophy of the nasal lining or bone, thus distinguishing it from the more severe atrophic rhinitis. Treatment consists of local medication which promotes secretion of the nasal mucosa and restoration of general health as much as possible.

RHINOPLASTY   Reconstruction of the nose may be indicated either because of injury or for reasons of developmental deformity. Sometimes it is intended to aid breathing and other times is done for purely cosmetic purposes. This operation, called a rhinoplasty, is performed by the ear-nose-and-throat surgeon, who may, if necessary, straighten the nasal septum at the same time.

Rhinoplastic surgery may make the nose look more attractive, and it may make breathing easier; but it will not change life situations, open the door to romance and adventure, or solve personal problems. Given the proper motivation, this is a useful operation even when done solely for cosmetic purposes; with poor and erroneous motivation, even a beautiful surgical result may prove unsatisfying to the patient.

SINUSITIS   The air-containing sinuses of the head, situated around and emptying into the nose, are called the paranasal sinuses. They are lined by mucosa similar to that of the nose itself, but modified and much thinner.

Whenever there is an infection of the nose (such as a cold) the sinus membranes, being continuous with that of the nose, are also affected. This does not mean that every time one has a cold one has sinusitis, for sinusitis refers to retained secretions in the sinuses.

Symptoms. The most common symptom of sinus disease is discharge; head pain is much overrated as a symptom. An acute sinus infection will often give a feeling of weakness and fever.

Treatment. Treatment should be by the physician, who may use antibiotics, nosedrops, and/or drainage of the sinuses.

SORE THROAT   Sore throat has many causes, the most common of which is acute pharyngitis (without membrane-formation). This may be caused by viral diseases such as the common cold or influenza, or by noninfectious inflammations resulting from inhalation of irritant substances, excessive dryness, or ingestion of very hot foods or liquids. All of these are self-limited conditions, disappearing when the offending mechanism no longer causes pharyngeal infection or irritation. Infections of any part of Waldeyer's ring can also cause sore throat. (It should be noted that sore throat can also cause ear pain because of a common nerve supply.)

The organisms causing syphilis and tuberculosis, as well as certain fungi, can also produce throat infections. These are not common and require special diagnostic procedures. Pharyngitis and tonsillitis can also become chronic and manifest themselves by persistent sore throat—as can certain blood diseases. Cancer frequently first shows itself as a chronic sore throat and/or a lump in the neck.

Treatment. A sore throat should not be neglected. *If lasting more than a few days, it should be seen by a physician.* Bed rest and fluids are helpful for a sore throat. Hot salt water gargles are soothing. Further details for treatment are given under the specific ailment.

THROAT   The throat is a general term applied to the pharynx, the larynx, and the associated muscles, blood vessels, and other tissues of the neck.

TINNITUS   Tinnitus refers to a ringing in the ears. Subjective tinnitus is noise only the patient can hear and is the most common type. Objective tinnitus is noise an examiner can hear as well. There are countless reasons for tinnitus and it is usually associated with a hearing loss. Occasionally, after the hearing loss is corrected, the tinnitus disappears.

Tinnitus is not a cause of hearing loss as

many people think; it is only associated with it. Some people are sure that if they can get rid of their tinnitus, they will hear better. This is not true. If they get rid of their hearing loss, however, the tinnitus may disappear. This is particularly true of otosclerosis. The noise may be high- or low-pitched, constant or intermittent, and usually seems worse at night.

Treatment. Tinnitus is very difficult to treat. Many people simply become accustomed to it; this may be the best answer when there is a noncorrectable hearing loss. A careful examination should be made by the physician to rule out any dangerous causes of tinnitus. If the doctor's examination reveals no danger, then learning to live with tinnitus is the most effective way of handling the problem.

TONSILS   The lymphoid tissue at the back of the nasopharynx is really the pharyngeal tonsil; when it becomes enlarged, it is called (in the plural number) the adenoids. These can cause obstruction of the Eustachian tubes and are removed surgically when the obstruction causes hearing problems or ear infections. This lymphoid-tissue mass is part of a ring of lymphoid tissue which, unless allergy or infection is frequent, tends to grow smaller and becomes functionless as adulthood is approached. The other components of the ring (Waldeyer's ring) are the lingual tonsil, the lateral pharyngeal bands, and the palatine (faucial) tonsils. (When the term tonsils is used without qualification, it refers to the palatine tonsils, the ones we can easily see through the open mouth.)

Any of the tonsils may become infected, and any and all may have to be removed. The most common troublemakers, however, are the palatine tonsils and adenoids. It is when these tissues cause more trouble than their protective benefits are worth, that the physician recommends removal. Indications for tonsillectomy are recurrent tonsillitis and abscess in the tonsillar area. Indications for adenoidectomy are blockage of the Eustachian tube leading to hearing loss; recurrent middle-ear infection; fluid in the ear; and nasal obstruction that causes mouth-breathing.

The above described indications comprise about 90 percent of the reasons for tonsillec-tomy and adenoidectomy. Frequently the tonsils and adenoids are removed at the same time, when both are enlarged and diseased, and when there are indications for surgical removal of both organs. On occasion, however, the tonsils or adenoids alone may be at fault and either one—but not both—is removed. This decision must be left to the physician.

Not all children need tonsillectomies and adenoidectomies (T-A's), and this, like any other operation, has specific indications. It is a safe procedure, but in children it is performed under general anesthesia, and any general anesthesia carries with it a small risk. The danger from T-A itself is very small, the major complication being bleeding. Bleeding can occur immediately after surgery, in the hospital, where the doctor can control it; or it can occur when the healing membrane sloughs off, about a week after surgery. Sometimes the child must be brought back to the hospital. True, bleeding of this kind does not occur often, but it will happen on occasion even to the most cooperative patient with the best doctor in the finest hospital. (*See also* ADENOIDS in this section.)

TUBES IN THE EARS   *See* EUSTACHIAN TUBE, BLOCKAGE OF THE in this section.

VERTIGO (DIZZINESS)   Dizziness involving faintness or lightheadedness should be distinguished from true vertigo, which involves sensations of whirling in space or of seeing the surroundings rotating. A common symptom of vertigo is nystagmus, a rhythmic horizontal or vertical oscillation of the eyeballs which is exaggerated by turning the eyes in different directions. (Many older people experience a transient dizziness on getting out of bed or coming suddenly to an upright position. This is caused by a delay in the body's adjustment of blood pressure to accommodate for a change in posture. It has no particular significance and is relieved simply by moving more slowly, or by resting a moment after standing up, to allow blood pressure to adjust.)

Ordinary dizziness usually involves transient interruption of blood circulation to the brain. True vertigo, in contrast, involves a disturbance of the balancing mechanism of the middle ear.

Treatment. The most common types of vertigo caused by car and motion sickness are relieved symptomatically by use of Dramamine®. In more complex organic conditions, treatment depends on exact diagnosis and removal of the underlying causes. Ordinary dizziness is far more easily overcome, usually by putting the head between the legs or by lying down until normal blood pressure returns.

VOCAL CORDS, PARALYSIS OF THE

Paralysis of one or both vocal cords as the cause of hoarseness is surprisingly common. In about 20 percent of cases it is not possible to determine the cause.

Symptoms. When one vocal cord is paralyzed there is mild hoarseness at the onset of paralysis, but the larynx compensates and a normal-sounding voice may be the eventual outcome. When both vocal cords (bilateral) are paralyzed and cannot be moved apart from their midline position, the voice usually remains of good quality but the airway is often inadequate under physical stress.

Treatment. The treatment of paralysis is therapy of the causative factors. In addition, in cases of bilateral paralysis, operations are possible which return the vocal cords to a more normal position and thereby enlarge the airway.

EYE AND VISION CONDITIONS

ACUTE IRITIS

CONJUNCTIVITIS

CATARACT

GLAUCOMA

The eye has been called the window of the soul. What we see and how we see it determines to a large sense the manner in which we function in the world. Many people consider vision to be one of the most important of our sense organs. The mechanism for sight is a complex one, one which involves degrees of depth and light perception. Over the lifetime of an individual, the eye may be subject to certain stress and deterioration, primarily as a result of the aging process.

This section examines the physiology of the eye and how vision is accomplished. Discussion is also given of common discomforts and disorders, symptoms and diagnosis, and possible treatment. Depending of the level of eye care needed, professional examination can be provided by an ophthalmologist, a physician who specializes in the treatment of diseases of the eye; an optometrist, one who is certified in the treatment of certain visual defects by the use of corrective lens and other measures; or an optician, one who makes and sells eyeglasses and other optical instruments. *See also* the question on poor vision (Q-39) in the section QUESTIONS AND ANSWERS ABOUT COMMON SYMPTOMS.

The following is a list of terms identified in this section:

ACCOMMODATION
AMBLYOPIA
APHAKIA
ASTIGMATISM
BLEPHARITIS
BLINDNESS
BLINKING
CATARACT
CATARACT, CONGENITAL
CHALAZION
CHOROID, DISEASES OF
CILIARY BODY, DISEASES OF
CONJUNCTIVITIS ("PINKEYE")
CONTACT LENSES
CORNEA AND SCLERA
CORNEA, INFLAMMATION OF
CORNEAL TRANSPLANT
CROSS-EYE (SQUINT OR STRABISMUS)
DARK-ADAPTATION
EYE, ARTIFICIAL
EYE, BLOWS TO THE
EYE, BURNS OF THE
EYE, CHAMBERS OF THE
EYE, DRY
EYE, FOREIGN BODIES IN THE
EYE, HYGIENE OF THE
EYE, INJURIES OF THE
EYE, OPTICAL DEFECTS OF THE

EYE, PARTS AND FUNCTIONS OF THE
EYE, SCRATCHES OF THE
EYE, TUMORS OF THE
EYELIDS
EYELIDS, DROOPING (BLEPHAROPTOSIS)
EYELIDS, FUSED
EYELIDS, INFLAMMATION OF THE
EYELIDS, TURNED-IN (ENTROPION)
EYELIDS, TURNED-OUT (ECTROPION)
EYELIDS, TWITCHING OF THE
FARSIGHTEDNESS (HYPEROPIA)
GLARE
GLAUCOMA
GLAUCOMA, ANGLE-CLOSURE
GLAUCOMA, CONGENITAL
GLAUCOMA, SECONDARY
GLAUCOMA, SIMPLE
INTRAOCULAR PRESSURE
IRIS, DISORDERS OF
IRITIS
KERATITIS
LACRIMAL GLAND
LENS
NEARSIGHTEDNESS (MYOPIA)
NIGHT BLINDNESS (NYCTALOPIA)
OCULAR MUSCLES
OPTIC NERVE

ACCOMMODATION Accommodation refers to any change in the focusing power of the lens; thus the eye is able to focus on both near and far objects. The crystalline lens of the eye is changed in shape by the action of the ciliary muscle so that objects are clearly focused on the back of the eye. Thus the normal individual is able to see objects clearly both at near and far distances. With increasing age the lens thickens and loses its elasticity, and after the age of forty to forty-five, glasses are usually necessary for clear vision at near distance. An exception would be in the case of myopia, "nearsightedness." Persons with nearsightedness may find that the accommodative changes produced by aging enables them to read somewhat better in their middle years and even perhaps dispense with their glasses. A majority of the population however will need "reading glasses."

The muscles that alter the lens, like muscles anywhere, may tire and impair accommodation. Their action may also be impaired by some medications so that one of their side-effects may be blurring of vision.

AMBLYOPIA Amblyopia is dimness of vision not corrected with glasses and not arising from disease of the eye. It may occur if the patient failed to use an eye in the early childhood years, because of poisons to which the eye is sensitive or because of hysteria.

Symptoms. There is poor vision in one or both otherwise healthy eyes. There is no pain, and the individual may not even be aware of the visual defect until the eyes are tested separately. When an eye crosses before the age of five years, the eye is not being used and the development of vision in the crossing eye is arrested. Vision is usually developed before the age of five and crossing after this time does not affect visual acuity. Poisons and hysteria cause a dimness of vision in both eyes. The classic example of the latter is the "sharp shooter's blindness" described during World War I. Usually of sudden origin, a rifleman would complain of severe visual loss. The eyes were normal to examination and vision would be "restored" when the soldier was removed from the front lines. Diagnosis may be extremely difficult.

In years past, tobacco was considered to be a cause of amblyopia, but this has been disproved. Amblyopia occurring in alcoholics is due to a vitamin B deficiency and is not a direct effect of the alcohol.

Treatment. This must be directed to the cause. Amblyopia due to a crossed eye must be treated before the age of seven. Usually the better eye is covered with a patch so as to force use of the poorer eye. This method is continued until there is no further improvement in vision.

Toxic amblyopia must be corrected by iden-

60

tification and removal of the causative poison. Vitamin B is frequently administered.

Hysteria as a cause of visual loss occurs in an individual who has a personality deficiency in facing emotional conflicts. Such an individual may require removal from a stressful situation and skilled psychiatric care.

APHAKIA This is the optical condition which follows removal of the lens in cataract surgery. A powerful convex lens is required, and inasmuch as accommodation for near vision is not possible, increased power for close work is usually provided for by a bifocal lens. There is increasing resort to an intraocular lens as the best replacement. (*See also* CATARACT in this section.)

ASTIGMATISM If rays of light entering the eye are bent unevenly, they do not all come to focus at the same point. In astigmatism the focusing is such that the rays of light entering the eye form a line instead of a point. Astigmatism may be farsighted, nearsighted, or mixed (in which one line is focused in front of the retina and another would be focused behind if it did not strike the retina first). Minor degrees of astigmatism are practically universal, presumably as a result of the weight of the upper lid resting upon the eye.

Symptoms. Marked astigmatism causes reduction in either near or far vision, sometimes in both. Intermediate amounts of astigmatism are considered to be a particularly likely cause of eyestrain, inasmuch as a slightly blurred image is seen which cannot be put in more distinct focus by accommodation.

Treatment. Astigmatism is neutralized by cylindrical lenses which refract in one plane and not in the plane at right angles. Considerable judgment is required in prescribing lenses to correct small degrees of astigmatism.

BLEPHARITIS *See* EYELIDS, INFLAMMATION OF THE, in this section.

BLINDNESS This term includes not only absence of all sight but may be applied to conditions in which vision is so reduced as not to be useful. As defined by industry and the Internal Revenue Service, blindness is considered to be vision of less than 20/200 (*see*

VISION, MEASUREMENT OF in this section) in both eyes with the best possible glasses, or contraction of the visual field within twenty degrees of the point of fixation. There are about 350,000 blind persons in the United States, and approximately 35,000 are blinded annually.

Information concerning the blind may be obtained from the American Foundation for the Blind, Inc., 15 West 16th Street, New York, New York 10011, or from the local state agency for the blind.

The causes of blindness vary markedly in different parts of the world, with trachoma, a viral inflammation of the eye, the most common one. However, this disease can be cured by use of sulfonamide medications and is no longer a serious problem in the United States. The chief causes of blindness in the United States are glaucoma and senile cataract. Systemic diseases such as diabetes and disorders of the blood vessels which cause destruction of the retina are the second most common cause. The third most common cause are birth defects arising from failure of the eye to develop normally during the period of growth in the womb. Inflammations of the eye, injuries, poisoning, tumors, and unknown causes account for the remaining cases.

BLINKING Spontaneous blinking occurs in each person because of a number of factors relating to moisture of the eyes, external lighting, fatigue, and the like. Frequent blinking, particularly in children, is seldom serious and many times appears to be an attempt on the child's part to attract attention.

Frequent forcible closure of the eyelids occurs as a result of eye or nervous disease and may be extremely disabling. The condition is referred to as blepharospasm. Muscle relaxants by mouth or local injections into the lids may be of value for the spasm.

CATARACT The crystalline lens of the eye is located directly behind the colored iris that surrounds the pupil, the central circular opening of the eye. Ordinarily, the lens of the eye is wholly transparent. The term cataract is applied to any loss of this transparency, whether slight or marked. A cataract is not a growth, but solely a loss of transparency of the lens. An entirely opaque lens is "ripe," while one that retains some transparency is "immature."

The most common cause of cataract is aging (senile cataract). Cataracts present at birth are called congenital, and may occur because of a hereditary tendency, or because of illness of the mother during the first three months of pregnancy. Other causes include injury from a blunt or penetrating blow to the eye, exposure to heat or X-rays, inflammation of the interior of the eye, and diabetes mellitus. Markedly lowered blood calcium and rare skin and muscle diseases may also be associated with cataract.

Symptoms. The chief symptom of cataract is a gradual dimming of vision that is not associated with pain or redness of the eye. In the early stages, there may be double vision in one eye only, but this disappears with further decrease in vision. Vision is frequently better in a dim light which permits dilation of the pupil. When one looks at a bright background such as the sky, there may be spots that do not dart about but remain in one position.

The diagnosis of cataract is based upon direct observation of the loss of transparency of the eye lens. When the cataract is very far advanced, the pupillary area is gray or white rather than black. Less advanced cataracts are diagnosed by special instruments.

Treatment. Nothing can restore the original transparency of the crystalline lens. During the period of dimming vision, wearing accurately prescribed spectacles will often maintain vision at a functional level.

Physical examination should be made with careful attention to the possibility of diabetes mellitus or reduced parathyroid gland activity. Examination of the eyes will usually indicate if the cataract is due to injury or inflammation.

Surgical removal of a cataract is indicated when the cataract itself causes glaucoma or an inflammation of the eye or when the defect in vision interferes with one's daily activities. As long as there is good vision in one eye, cataract removal may not be recommended solely for the purpose of improving the poorer eye. Because of the improvement in contact lenses, however, many surgeons have been recommending removal of a cataract even though the other eye is good. If one is unable to wear a contact lens, then the procedure may initially produce annoying double vision.

Cataract surgery is seldom indicated when there is a disease of the front or back of the eye affecting vision, making it unlikely that removal of the cataract will improve vision.

The surgical removal of cataracts is an operation usually performed with local anesthesia. The surgeon may use extreme cold to freeze the lens to a surgical probe, thereby permitting the removal of the cataract. Another technique makes use of high frequency sound waves that "dissolve" the clouded lens, which then can be drained away.

Because the lens is one of the main focusing parts of the eye, eyeglasses or special contact lenses are required after lens removal. Some cataract patients require a bifocal lens that is much thicker and heavier than an ordinary lens. When contact lenses are worn, magnification and optical defects are reduced. If such a lens is used, an additional lens for reading may be required. Perhaps the best solution may be the implantation within the eye of a new lens: the intraocular lens. A majority of cataract extractions are currently being followed by implantation of the lens.

The decision to operate on the second eye, if a cataract is present, is based on much the same factors as those governing the initial removal. If cataracts are present in both eyes, the surgeon may recommend operating on both eyes in one procedure. "Ripe" or swollen cataracts usually require removal. In other instances surgery is based upon the activity and visual needs of the individual. A sedentary person may see adequately with one eye, while a more active individual may determine he or she must have the use of both eyes.

CATARACT, CONGENITAL Any loss of transparency of the ocular lens which is present from birth is a congenital cataract. It may be familial, due to the occurrence of German measles in the mother during the first three months of pregnancy or due to inflammation in the eye of the infant before birth.

Symptoms. These are the same as those occurring with other types of cataracts. There may be additional eye defects which require careful examination to discover. Many types of congenital cataract do not interfere with vision, do not progress, and are discovered only in the course of an eye examination.

Treatment. The degree of interference with vision governs the selection of treatment.

When congenital cataracts are associated with other eye defects, even skillful surgical removal may not improve vision. Generally, if the cataract is present in one eye and the other eye is normal or nearly so, surgery is not indicated. If cataracts are present in both eyes but vision is as good as 20/70 with eyeglasses, normal schooling is possible and surgery is not recommended. If the cataract is marked in each eye, surgery is indicated and this is usually carried out in about the second or third year of age. In borderline conditions, surgery is delayed until vision can be evaluated carefully, usually about the fifth year.

Following surgery, correcting lenses must be worn to compensate for the loss of focusing power.

CONGENITAL CATARACT
(Lids are pulled away from eye.)

CHALAZION This cyst-like nodule results from an inflammation in one of the glands in the fibrous plate (tarsus) of the eyelid. The resultant closing of the duct of the gland and its enlargement may leave an ongoing swelling in the lid often thought initially to be an ordinary sty.

Symptoms. There is an area of redness on the inside of the lid and an associated tenderness. The attacks tend to repeat, and between infections there is a hard pebble-like nodule in the lid which may cause a lump in the skin.

Treatment. When infected, hot compresses and a local antibiotic ointment are indicated. Repeated infections may make it necessary to remove the infected gland.

CHOROID, DISEASES OF The choroid is the blood-vessel layer of the back of the eye. It lines the sclera and provides nourishment for that portion of the retina adjacent to it. It extends from the optic nerve behind, to the ciliary body (with which it is continuous) in front.

An inflammation of this tissue, choroiditis, arises from a variety of causes: tuberculosis, syphilis, sarcoidosis, and viral diseases. It may follow injury. Many cases are probably the result of an allergy to bacteria, viruses, yeasts, or other small organisms.

The choroid is also the site of the most common malignant tumor of the eye, malignant melanoma.

Symptoms. Decreased vision, without pain, is the most common symptom of choroidal disease. It arises from two causes: interference with the function of the adjacent nerve tissue, the retina; or an outpouring of inflammatory cells into the vitreous cavity. Long-continued disease of the choroid may cause a cataract with even further loss of vision.

Treatment. This must be directed to identification and elimination of the cause of the inflammation. It depends upon careful examination, a number of skin tests, and laboratory examinations. Some infectious diseases may be corrected by means of specific drugs. In some instances, steroid compounds are given to reduce inflammation.

CILIARY BODY, DISEASES OF The ciliary body is located inside the eye, directly behind the outer margin of the iris. It is continuous with the iris in front and the choroid behind, and is held in position by an attachment to the outer covering of the eye, the sclera. In addition to blood vessels, it also contains the muscles responsible for the change in focusing power of the lens (accommodation).

Inflammation of the ciliary body (cyclitis) arises from the same causes as inflammation of the iris or choroid, both of which are usually secondarily involved in a ciliary-body inflammation. The disorder is often referred to as a uveitis. Paralysis of the muscles of the ciliary body is sometimes deliberately induced by the instillation of medicine in the eye, or may follow interference with the nerve supply.

Paralysis of the ciliary-body muscles is without pain, but it is impossible to change the focus of the eye. Thus, near work is blurred, although distance vision may be unchanged. The pupil is usually dilated.

Symptoms. Inflammation of the ciliary body causes a dull aching pain deep within one eye, associated with redness of the eye. If there are a large number of inflammatory cells released into the interior of the eye, vision may be reduced.

Treatment. This is directed toward identification and elimination of the cause of the inflammation. Frequently medicines are used which dilate the pupil and paralyze the ciliary muscle. This promotes healing as do eyedrops which also reduce inflammation. Many of the conditions causing inflammation are self-limiting and heal spontaneously, but tend to reoccur. Among the systemic illnesses which are the background to cyclitis and uveitis are several forms of rheumatoid arthritis, some parasitic and viral infections, TB, and sarcoidosis.

CONJUNCTIVITIS ("PINKEYE") This is an inflammation of the thin, nearly transparent tissue (conjunctiva) which covers the white of the eye (sclera) and lines the inside of the eyelids. Because of its exposed position, it is liable to a variety of infections by bacteria or viruses, allergies, and irritation.

Symptoms. The eyes burn and the lids feel heavy, and there may be rapid fatigue with any task requiring intensive use of the eyes. A discharge may be present, varying in consistency from that of tears to thick, heavy pus. There may be dried pus on the eyelids, and the lids may be stuck together upon awakening. Blood vessels on the surface of the eye may be prominent. Vision is usually not affected.

Treatment. This is directed to the cause. Many types of conjunctivitis are contagious, and in order to protect others, affected persons should use separate towels and practice meticulous cleanliness. The eyes should not be bandaged. The use of dark glasses may afford some comfort, and either hot or cold compresses may provide relief from burning and/or itching. Pus should be removed from the eyelashes by means of moistened cotton applicators. If only one eye is involved, care should be taken not to spread the infection to the other eye with the fingers.

In conjunctivitis due to bacteria and some viruses, main reliance is placed upon frequent instillation of drugs to which the causative organism is sensitive. A medicine dropper and not an eyecup should be used. Conjunctivitis due to irritation from smog, smoke, chemical fumes, and the like requires elimination (frequently difficult) of the cause.

There are a number of special types of conjunctivitis. Ophthalmia neonatorum is any inflammation of the conjunctiva occurring within two weeks of birth. The most serious type is that due to the bacteria causing gonorrhea (gonococcus). The practice of instilling silver nitrate in the eyes immediately after birth has nearly eliminated blindness from this source. Other causes include various bacteria, particularly staphylococci, and the virus which causes a mucus-discharge (inclusion blennorrhea). Gonorrheal inflammation occurs within a period from a few hours to a few days after birth, while the others do not cause symptoms until five or more days after birth. In all cases there is profuse discharge of pus, and medical care is indicated.

Trachoma is a chronic conjunctivitis caused by a virus. Although it is the chief cause of blindness in the world, it is rare in the United States except among Indians in the Southwest. The disease produces scarring of the conjunctiva and cornea, with distortion of the lids and reduction of vision. Trachoma is treated with various antibiotics and sulfonamides. Currently a vaccine is being developed to immunize infants at birth.

Vernal (or spring) conjunctivitis (catarrh) is an allergic disease associated with severe itching and marked thickening of the conjunctiva. It occurs principally in the tropics and is relieved by removal to a climate free from heat and dust. There is no specific therapy.

CONTACT LENSES Contact lenses are thin, usually plastic, discs worn over the cornea and beneath the lids to correct errors of refraction. There are two main types: corneal and scleral. The corneal is a thin wafer which floats on a surface of tears covering the cornea. The scleral type overlies both the cornea and sclera and is worn with a layer of fluid between the lens and the cornea. The chief medical indication for contact lenses is irregular astigmatism caused by a corneal abnormality such as cone-shaped cornea or scarring. They should not be worn in glaucoma, nor when the cornea has been the site of a virus infection or a recent infection. They should also be avoided by individuals who have no corneal pain sensation, due to involvement of nerves going to the eye, since injury may occur without suitable warning.

The risk of corneal injury is higher if the lens is not kept scrupulously clean or if it is worn for longer periods than recommended by the manufacturer. Of the two forms of contact lenses available, hard and soft, the latter has become more popular since they are permeable to oxygen and little adaptation time is required. In one recent version, the "throwaway" type, the wearer replaces the old with the new lens at approximately weekly intervals, thus doing away with the need for cleaning procedures, sterilization, etc.

In 1989 the FDA cautioned users of extended-wear and disposable contact lenses not to wear the lenses longer than seven days before replacing them. The FDA's warning was designed to forestall the formation of a bacterial infection (ulcerative keratitis) that can cause blindness. The FDA also advised contact-lens manufacturers to change their label instructions from thirty days continuous wear to seven days and to emphasize to the public the importance of thorough cleaning for the extended-wear type lenses before using them again.

CORNEA AND SCLERA

The outer coat of the eye, the cornea and sclera, is fairly tough tissue approximately one-twenty-fifth of an inch thick. Five-sixths of the eye, the white (sclera), is opaque while the remaining portion, the cornea, is transparent. The cornea is the front portion of the eye through which the colored iris and black pupil can be seen. It is the main focusing portion of the eye, and the quarter-inch at its center is most important to clear vision.

CORNEA, INFLAMMATION OF

The cornea is the transparent tissue of the eye which lies in front of the iris and pupil. It is prone to injury and infection because of its exposed position. Inflammation of the cornea, called ulcer or keratitis, may be superficial or deep.

Superficial keratitis includes catarrhal keratitis, due to secondary infection of the cornea by the agent causing conjunctivitis (staphylo-coccus is the usual cause); serpiginous keratitis, an acute corneal infection caused by bacteria or other infectious agent which enters through mechanical injury; dendritic keratitis, a virus inflammation of the cornea caused by the same virus that causes cold sores (herpes) of the lip; like cold sores, it tends to be recurrent, and it is triggered by injury, fever, menstruation, and so on; lagophthalmic keratitis, an inflammation which may follow exposure when the lids do not cover the eye (lagophthalmos), associated with a lack of pain sensation in the cornea.

Deep or interstitial keratitis is usually due to congenital syphilis. It occurs between ten and fifteen years after birth and is associated with many new blood vessels growing into the cornea, with subsequent reduction of vision. Effective treatment of syphilis has made the condition rare in the United States.

Symptoms. Inflammation of the cornea usually causes a marked sensation of a foreign body in the eye. The eye waters and is markedly uncomfortable. The eye becomes markedly reddened. If the ulcer involves the line of sight, vision is reduced. The involved area may appear as grayish-white, or it may be necessary to stain the area with a special dye and observe it with a microscope.

Treatment. An eye bandage may be applied to make the eye more comfortable, and hot compresses may give some relief. Eyedrops to combat infection and to dilate the pupil may be used. Skilled diagnosis is required, as drugs which aid in some conditions may cause damage in others. If the cornea has no sensation, or the lids do not cover the eye, lid surgery may be necessary to protect the globe.

SCLERA

CORNEA

CORNEAL TRANSPLANT

An entire eye cannot be transplanted. However, replacement of a diseased with a healthy cornea can be carried out by transplanting either the full thickness of the cornea (penetrating) or the front two-thirds (lamellar). The operation is indicated either to improve vision or to remove infected or injured tissue. The donor-eye is usually secured by prompt removal after death. (Healthy eyes of living individuals are never used. Arrangements to donate one's eyes after death can be made with a local eye bank; information may be obtained from the local Lions' Club.) The graft always "takes," but visual results vary with the disease for which the operation is performed.

CROSS-EYE (SQUINT OR STRABISMUS)

Crossed eyes may be divided into those in which there is a paralyzed muscle and those in which the ocular muscles are normal. If the eyes turn in toward the nose, the condition is called esotropia; if the eyes turn outward, it is called exotropia.

Nonparalytic (comitant squint) cross-eye is the most common type. The degree of crossing is the same in all directions of gaze. It may occur because of some disease preventing clear image-formation on the back of the eye; because of disturbances in the ratio between focusing and converging for near work; or because of disturbances in the perception of images by the brain.

Paralytic crossing of the eyes arises from a disease or injury involving the ocular muscles or their nerve supply. The amount of crossing is more marked when the eyes move toward the field of the paralyzed muscle. A common example may be seen in diabetics who are subject to neuropathies, disturbances in various nerves which may be those going to ocular muscles. When this occurs the person may develop a paralysis of an eye muscle and strabismus, with diplopia (double vision). The condition usually resolves in six to eight weeks, and there is no specific treatment.

Symptoms. In nonparalytic cross-eye, the turning of the eye inward or outward is usually the only sign. In the early stages the eyes cross alternately, but eventually one eye is usually turned at all times. If double vision is present, the child is usually too young to describe it and soon ignores the image from the poorer eye. If an eye remains turned in or out constantly before the age of five, there is arrest of visual development in the deviating eye (amblyopia).

A paralytic crossing, if acquired after the development of binocular vision, causes the individual to see double. This, in turn, may lead to tilting of the head.

Treatment. Treatment of nonparalytic cross-eye is initially directed to tests and examination to learn whether or not there is any disease preventing normal image-formation on the retina. Farsightedness or myopia must be fully corrected; most eye physicians believe that this can be done only after instillation of medications in the eye to paralyze the focusing mechanism. Drops which make the pupil small may be helpful in eliminating abnormal focusing mechanisms. The most important step is to prevent poor vision in the crossing eye. Usually this is carried out by covering the better eye in order to force use of the poorer. Prior to the age of seven years, patching should be carried out for at least two months before it is concluded that vision in the deviating eye cannot be improved. If there

CROSS-EYE (STRABISMUS)

Strabismus is a squint deviation of one eye from its proper direction so that the visual axes cannot both be directed simultaneously at the same objective point.

is improvement, patching should be carried out until there is no further improvement. Generally after the age of seven there is no more improvement in vision with patching.

There is a sharp division of opinion as to the value of eye exercises in crossing. Most doctors agree that the exercises do not have any effect on the eye muscles or the development of fusion (stereoscopic vision).

To bring about a parallel orientation of the eyes, surgery is carried out. This has no effect on ability to see, although it may align the eyes in such a way that fusion is possible. Usually it has no effect upon the need for correcting lenses. The surgeon's aim is to do the minimal operation that will correct the crossing. If there is any danger of overcorrection, it is preferable to do a series of operations rather than attempt full correction in one operation. Usually six months should elapse between operations to permit stabilization and evaluation of the procedure.

The management of paralytic crossing depends upon the cause. When present at birth, it may be impossible to distinguish the paralytic from the nonparalytic type.

DARK-ADAPTATION

An increased sensitivity of part of the eye occurs when there is an extremely low level of illumination. The process involves the rods of the retina, which are so arranged that although form and color vision are poorer than in bright illumination, there is a marked increase in side vision and in the ability to detect movement. Sensitivity is further increased by dilation of the pupil which permits more light to enter the eye. Dark-adaptation is decreased in vitamin A deficiency, glaucoma, retinal degenerations, and many other conditions.

EYE, ARTIFICIAL

After injury or disease it is sometimes necessary to remove the eyeball. A sling remains within the socket which consists of connective tissue and the eye muscles, known as Tenon's capsule. The artificial eye is placed within this capsule of tissue and can, to a variable degree, be pushed by the contraction of the unattached muscles. Artificial eyes do not have the range of movement of the normal eye, and those wearing one should move their head rather than the eye to look to the side. Infection may be introduced into the socket by the fingers; the hands must therefore be scrupulously clean before touching the artificial eye to clean it. If one eye has been lost, it is wise to wear shatterproof lenses to protect the remaining one.

EYE, BLOWS TO THE

The eyes are well protected by the bony structure surrounding them, and large blunt objects usually damage only the eyelids. A "black eye" consists of blood beneath the thin skin of the eyelids and is usually associated with swelling. If vision is normal, it is usually of minor import. During the first twenty-four hours, cold or iced compresses applied for ten minutes every hour will limit swelling. After twenty-four hours, hot compresses may be used. (*See* EYE, HYGIENE OF THE in this section.)

A blow to the eyeball itself may cause severe injury. If the vision is decreased, if the pupil is not round, or if there is blood in front of the colored iris, immediate medical attention is indicated.

EYE, BURNS OF THE

Chemical burns of the conjunctiva and cornea are best treated by immediate irrigation with water. No time should be wasted in seeking the appropriate neutralizing solution, but rather the eye should be copiously irrigated as soon as possible with clear water. The most effective method is to plunge the entire face into a container of water and then open the eyes under water.

Acid burns are quickly neutralized by the tissues and the immediate injury is usually the full extent of the damage; alkali burns, however, become worse as time goes by. Medical care should be sought as soon as possible after a chemical burn has been irrigated thoroughly.

Heat burns of the eye usually involve only the eyelids because the eyeball is fairly well protected from injuries by quick closure of the lids. Burns from cigarettes or matches require medical care. Washing the eye as described under chemical burns may remove foreign particles. Bandaging or closing both eyes will then prevent the eyeball from moving and will minimize pain.

Burns of the eyelid may be extremely serious and if severe enough to cause blisters (second degree) must have medical care. Salves and lotions should not be applied except under medical direction.

Ultraviolet rays from arc welding, from reflections of sunlight off sand or snow, or from a sun lamp may cause extreme eye irritation. Like sunburn, the effect adds up and, usually during the night following exposure, the eyes burn and water and feel filled with sand. The irritation is so extreme that it may be nearly impossible to open the eyes. If the individual recalls exposure to ultraviolet rays, the diagnosis is usually simple, since there are few conditions which cause such discomfort in both eyes. The condition persists for from twelve to twenty-four hours. Bandaging of both eyes; rest in a quiet, darkened room; and sedation are usually all that is required. Medicines which anesthetize the eyeballs give comfort but delay healing and should be used only under medical direction.

1 CORNEA
2 CONJUNCTIVA
3 IRIS
4 PUPIL
5 LENS
6 SCLERA
7 RETINA
8 OPTIC NERVE

THE EYE
(CROSS SECTION)

EYE, CHAMBERS OF THE   The eye contains three chambers which interconnect with one another. The front chamber is in front of the iris and behind the cornea. It contains a clear, slightly salty fluid called the aqueous humor, which continually drains out of the eye through a channel at the junction of the cornea and sclera. Obstruction of this channel causes increase in pressure in the eye known as glaucoma.

A very small chamber, the posterior chamber, is located behind the iris and in front of the supporting fibers of the lens. It is important because this is where the ciliary body secretes the nutrient material for the lens, which has no blood supply of its own to feed it.

The fluid secreted by the ciliary body flows through the pupil into the anterior chamber.

The largest chamber of the eye is the vitreous cavity containing a clear, gelatin-like material in which are suspended very few cells but much water. This is the vitreous humor.

EYE, DRY   This occurs because of decreased tear secretion which may follow scarring of the lining of the lids, or occurs as part of a disease complex which includes decreased salivary secretion and rheumatoid arthritis. This combination of disorders is known as Sjögren's syndrome. The eyes are dry and feel sandy, and are constantly irritated. Diagnosis is made by measuring tear-formation. Treatment is by instillation of artificial tears.

Milder forms of dry eye are complained of in old age. The eyes may burn and the irritation may, paradoxically, lead to tearing. Artificial tears may be quite soothing. These generally have a methylcellulose base and act as a lubricant.

EYE, FOREIGN BODIES IN THE   Dirt and cinders may be blown into the eye and cause a typical foreign-body sensation. Nearly always it feels as though the material is beneath the outer portion of the upper lid. There is watering of the eye but no disturbance of vision. The foreign body is usually lodged on the transparent tissue of the cornea or on the inside surface of the upper lid. If the foreign body is on the cornea, it may sometimes be washed out of the eye by placing the face in a basin of clean water and opening the eye under water. If this is not effective, the foreign particle may have to be gently lifted off the eyeball by a physician. Rubbing the eyelids is not helpful.

Foreign bodies on the lid are removed after first turning back the lid. A cotton-tipped applicator or the corner of a clean handkerchief should be available before doing this, and a good light should be used. (The individual must look downward or the upper lid cannot be turned.) The lashes are grasped and the lid drawn gently away from the eyeball to break the suction. With a match or cotton-tipped applicator held against the lid at the level of the fold in the skin about one-quarter of an inch above the margin, the lid may be folded back on itself. A cinder will frequently be at about the middle of the reddish exposed surface. The lower lid may be turned by placing the thumb against the skin surface and pressing gently inward.

Foreign bodies within the eye are extremely serious inasmuch as they damage the eye upon entering, may introduce infection, and may dissolve within the eye, causing further injury. Large objects are likely to destroy the eye. Most objects retained within the eye are small. Usually, but not always, the pupil is no longer round after the injury.

If the foreign object is wood or similar material, it may carry bacteria and cause an abscess to form in the eye. Small metallic foreign bodies frequently are sterilized by heat and are less likely to cause infection. Vision is frequently much reduced, and a cataract may form.

X-rays indicate metallic objects within the eye but frequently fail to show wood, plastics, and glass. Iron and nickel foreign bodies may be removed by a surgeon with a magnet, but other metals and materials are not magnetic. Some materials such as glass and some plastics are well tolerated by the tissues and need not be removed, while others are quickly covered by scar tissue and cause no harm. Some metals such as copper cause much damage; hence every effort must be made to remove them. In household accidents, the tool that may have been the source of the injury should be made available to the surgeon so he can learn its composition.

EYE, HYGIENE OF THE   The eyes are remarkably organized to provide vision with a minimum of care. They arise as an outgrowth of the brain and, like the brain, are designed for—and cannot be injured by—use.

Every individual should assure himself from time to time that his vision is unchanged, by testing each eye separately for both near and distant vision, and then checking side vision (see VISION, MEASUREMENT OF in this section). Eye examinations are particularly important during the third year of life; in the first, fourth, and ninth grades; and at about age eighteen. After the age of forty to forty-five, examination every one or two years is desirable.

Poor lighting, excessive use of the eyes for close work, the wrong prescription glasses, or the need for glasses may give rise to burning and discomfort of the eyes, sometimes associated with headaches. The headaches are never severe and are always relieved by discontinuing the task at hand. If not relieved, the headaches are not caused by the eyes. The factors cited cause no permanent change but only discomfort. Excessive blinking, which occurs particularly in children, is seldom serious and usually disappears if attention is not directed to it.

It should not be necessary to use eyewashes at any time, unless prescribed for a definite disease. If an eyecup is used, it should be sterilized in boiling water and allowed to cool immediately prior to use. If one feels an eyewash is necessary, a satisfactory one can be made by dissolving a teaspoon of table salt in a pint of water, boiling for ten minutes, and then storing in a sterilized bottle. Old medications should be discarded. Inasmuch as the symptoms of many different eye diseases are the same, medicines should not be used by other family members.

The wearing of tinted and colored glasses is a personal preference and is rarely indicated for eye disease. The colored lenses provided by industry for protection in certain occupations should not be used outside of work as they frequently reduce vision excessively or interfere with the color vision necessary to recognizing traffic signals. A neutral gray or a greenish tint is the preferred color for sunglasses. Reddish tints may interfere with recognizing the red of traffic lights. All colored and tinted lenses interfere with night vision and should never be used at night. Individuals with normal eyes do not require colored lenses indoors. Protection against the harmful effects of sunlight on the lens and retina can be obtained by using glasses which have been treated with an ultraviolet B filter. This can be superimposed on prescription glasses. The filter is particularly needed for sunglasses, as many ultraviolet rays will still pass this portion of the light spectrum. Neighborhood drugstores may have such non-prescription sunglasses.

The use of safety lenses made of plastic or hardened glass is preferable not only in industry and home workshops, but for general use. They should be worn even by those with normal vision in school laboratories and when working at home. Tools should be discarded if there is any danger of metal breaking off.

Hot or cold compresses may relieve tired eyes and swollen eyelids. A washcloth wrung out in running hot or cold water, and then applied to the lids for ten minutes, relieves many nonspecific conditions. It is not necessary to add any medicine to the water.

EYE, INJURIES OF THE   Prompt and appropriate care of injuries of the eye may prevent much disability and may even be instrumental in making major corrective surgery unnecessary. If vision is to be saved prompt evaluation by an ophthalmologist should be sought. (*See also* EYE, BLOWS TO THE; EYE, BURNS OF THE; EYE, FOREIGN BODIES IN THE; EYE, SCRATCHES OF THE in this section.)

EYE, OPTICAL DEFECTS OF THE Rays of light entering the eye are bent by the transparent cornea, next to the lens; they then come to a focus. If the length of the eye is proportionate to the bending, the rays come to a focus at the back of the eye on the retina and a clear image is formed. If the degree of bending is not proportionate to the length of the eye, the focus is either in front of the retina or would be behind it if it were not stopped by the retina. Such a disproportion causes an error of refraction. Minor errors arise as a variation in growth and cannot be modified by such external influences as eyedrops, diet, lenses, exercises, or use of the eyes. (*See also* APHAKIA; ASTIGMATISM; FARSIGHTEDNESS (HYPEROPIA); NEARSIGHTEDNESS (MYOPIA); PRESBYOPIA in this section.)

EYE, PARTS AND FUNCTION OF THE The eye is a hollow organ about one inch in diameter. It contains light-sensitive tissue, the retina, which is connected to the brain by nerve fibers in the optic nerve. It is protected by bone on all sides except at the front, and rests in a tissue hammock, surrounded by fat. Its movements arise from the action of six muscles.

In front, the eyelids keep the eye moist and protect it from external irritants and excessive light. The optical portions of the eye are transparent to permit transmission of light. The cornea and the crystalline lens both form images of external objects upon the retina.

The pupil acts as a diaphragm to control the amount of light entering the eye and to reduce such blurring of the image as would be created by stray light entering a large opening.

EYE, SCRATCHES OF THE   Scratches of the eyelid are generally not serious and require only cleanliness and treatment similar to that given for such injuries elsewhere in the body. Scratches of the surface of the eyeball are extremely painful. Inasmuch as they may become infected, prompt medical care is advisable. Some comfort may be obtained by closing or bandaging both eyes.

Cuts or lacerations of the eyelids vary in severity, but even apparently minor injuries may produce concealed damage. Cuts that parallel the lid margin may bleed profusely but, if there is no deeper damage, usually heal well, with the scar concealed in skin folds. Cuts at right angles to the lid margins usually gape widely and require skilled repair to avoid notching the lid.

Cuts of the eyeball are always extremely serious and require prompt and expert medical care. They are recognized by the protrusion of the iris through the surface of the eye (so that the pupil is not round) or by the brownish tissue gaping through the cut. Both eyes should be bandaged and the individual should be moved on a stretcher. Examination of the eye should be avoided until surgical facilities are available. Even with expert care the damage may be so severe that vision cannot be saved.

Sympathetic ophthalmia is an inflammation of both eyes that follows a deep laceration of one. It requires at least fourteen days after the injury for this condition to develop and will not happen if the injured eye is removed before that time. After the disease has been established, removal of the injured eye is not helpful, and it is probably best to retain it, since it may still be the better eye after the inflammation clears. The disease is now uncommon and responds fairly well to cortisone-like drugs.

EYE, TUMORS OF THE   Because of the ease with which they can invade the deeper structures of the head, if neglected, skin tumors are somewhat more serious in the eyelids than those elsewhere in the body. The most common new growth of the lid is a basal-cell cancer which usually occurs in the aged among those who are exposed to sun and wind. It is generally about one-fourth of an inch in diameter and has heaped-up sides with a depression in the center. It is treated either with surgery or by X-ray.

The most common malignant tumor in infants and young children is the retino-blastoma. It arises in the retina and in 40 percent of the patients who survive is transmitted as a dominant hereditary characteristic to the children of survivors. It may occur in either one or both eyes, usually before the age of one year. It is usually first noticed when there is a white mass visible through the pupil or in the evaluation of strabismus. Such an eye must be removed as quickly as possible. Exact examination is required to detect early tumors in the remaining eye, which occur in about 25 percent of cases. If a tumor is present, the second eye is treated with X-rays, anti-cancer medicines, and sometimes by an intense light directed through the pupil to coagulate the tumor. If the tumor continues to progress, it is necessary to remove the eye. Otherwise the tumor spreads by direct continuation into the brain and through the body via the bloodstream. It may also invade the nose and throat.

The most common eye tumor in adults is malignant melanoma, which arises in the blood-vessel coat of the eye—the choroid. The first symptoms arise because of loss of function in the adjacent retina with a resultant "island" of blindness. As the tumor grows, the island increases in size; later the eye becomes hard (secondary glaucoma), inflamed, red, and painful. The tumor spreads via the bloodstream to other parts of the body. Treatment for malignant melanoma is removal of the eye; if this is done while the tumor is relatively small, there is a good likelihood that malignancy has not spread to other parts of the body, hence that lasting cure can be achieved.

EYELIDS The front surface of the eye is covered by the eyelids—upper and lower curtains of skin, muscle, glands, mucous membrane, and a cartilage-like material. The eyelids serve to distribute fluid over the surface of the globe by periodic blinking and to protect the eye from external irritants and excessive light.

The skin covering the eyelids is extremely thin and is thrown into numerous folds to permit lid movements. It can stretch enormously following injury or when inflamed. Because of the thinness of the lids, blood vessels beneath the skin may be seen, sometimes as a dark blue line and at other times as a diffuse bluish discoloration of the entire lid. The conjunctiva is the mucous membrane lining the lid; it is continuous from the lid margin to the junction of the white (sclera) and the transparent portion (cornea) of the eye.

The lids contain voluntary and involuntary muscles which function in opening and closing. The muscle mainly responsible for closing is the orbicularis oculi, a circular muscle in the upper and lower lid; this muscle holds the lids in close contact with the eyeball. The upper lid opens by means of the levator muscle which arises from the area surrounding the stem, or apex, of the orbit. Involuntary muscles in the lid elevate the upper and lower eyelid and give "tone" to the tissue.

Stability is provided in the lid by a modified plate of dense tissue, the tarsus, which extends along the lid margin and deep into the lid. It contains glands producing an oily secretion which prevents the tears from overflowing.

The lid margins meet tightly to prevent fluids and irritating material from entering the eye. These margins each contain two layers of eyelashes and oil and sweat glands which may become infected to cause stys.

EYELIDS, DROOPING (BLEPHAROPTOSIS) If the upper lids are too heavy because of scarring or tumors, or if there is weakness in the muscles which elevate them, they will droop. In old persons because of muscle laxness and sagging of the tissues, noticeable ptosis (drooping) can develop. If marked enough, the lids cover the pupil and interfere with vision.

Symptoms. These arise only because of mechanical interference with vision and are a cosmetic defect.

Treatment. This depends upon the cause. If slight, no treatment is recommended; if severe, the condition must be corrected surgically. Occasionally a "crutch" can be attached to a spectacle lens and support the lid.

In children ptosis (drooping) usually occurs as a birth-defect and may involve one or both eyes. Later in life it occurs primarily because of disease of the nerves, particularly strokes, myasthenia gravis, and muscular dystrophies.

EYELIDS, FUSED

Fusing of eyelids may occur as two clinical entities: ankyloblepharon and symblepharon. In ankyloblepharon the borders of the eyelids have grown together, partially or completely. In symblepharon the eyelid partially or completely adheres to the eyeball. Both conditions result from old inflammatory disorders, injury, or burn. Sometimes infants are born with either defect. Plastic-lid surgery is necessary to correct the condition.

EYELIDS, INFLAMMATION OF THE

The exposed position of the skin of the eyelids makes them particularly subject to irritations and infection. Marked swelling may occur after insect bites and is best treated by cold compresses. Skin allergies from nail polish, perfumes, colored or scented soaps, medicines, and the like may particularly affect the lids, sometimes only on one side when the irritant is carried to the lids by the fingers. The condition recurs until the offending agent is removed.

Inflammations of the lid margin (blepharitis) causes an unsightly redness with fine, powdery scales on the lashes. The condition is frequently associated with dandruff of the scalp. There may be chronic irritation from bacterial infection, smoke, chemical fumes, or repeated rubbing. Treatment must be directed toward eliminating the cause.

EYELIDS, TURNED-IN (ENTROPION)

This condition, a turning-in of the lid margin, is most often caused by scarring of the inside associated with chronic inflammation.

Symptoms. The turned-in lashes irritate the eyeball and cause redness and discomfort.

Treatment. Relief can sometimes be obtained by drawing the outer portion of the lid downward by means of adhesive tape; but if severe and persistent, surgery is required.

EYELIDS, TURNED-OUT (ECTROPION)

Turning-out of the lid margin is caused by scarring of the skin of the lids, by paralysis of the muscle closing the lids, or excessive laxness of the tissue.

Symptoms. Irritation and tearing are produced by exposure of the inner lining of the lid.

Treatment. Surgical correction is indicated.

EYELIDS, TWITCHING OF THE

The delicate muscles of the lid may spontaneously contract. The condition is annoying but usually not serious, and is due to fatigue. Adequate rest is then an effective treatment.

In some older persons not previously subject to such twitching, it is thought that hyperactivity of certain brain cells may be involved. Muscle-relaxing drugs by mouth or injection into the eyelid muscles (botulinus toxin) may be helpful.

FARSIGHTEDNESS (HYPEROPIA)

In this condition light rays from a distant object strike the retina before coming to a focus so that a blurred image is formed. The condition arises because there is either too little bending of light rays or too short an eyeball. It is extremely common and is usually compensated for by a change in the shape of the lens (accommodation) which increases its focusing power.

Symptoms. Minor degrees of farsightedness cause no symptoms, and both near and far vision are good because of the adjustment by accommodation. If there is a marked degree of farsightedness, accommodation may adjust the eye so that distant objects are seen clearly but the additional accommodation required for close work causes eyestrain or blurring of vision. Inasmuch as accommodation occurs less with age, an older eye cannot compensate as well for farsightedness as a youthful eye.

Treatment. Farsightedness is corrected by means of convex (magnifying) lenses. Considerable medical judgment is required to learn if symptoms arise because of the farsightedness, what should be the power of the lens required, and whether glasses should be worn constantly or only occasionally.

GLARE   Any brightness within the field of vision that causes an unpleasant sensation or temporary blurring of vision is defined as glare. It cannot be measured scientifically and symptoms vary considerably in different persons. Particular sources of glare are reflections: from bright surfaces such as desk tops, automobile windshields and hoods, sand, and sky. Unshielded light sources may cause discomfort. Colored lenses may minimize symptoms, but a change in lighting conditions is more effective. In some older persons with early cataract, bright light may produce complaints of glare.

GLAUCOMA   This is an eye disease in which the pressure within the eye is so increased as to cause interference with vision. The severity of the increased pressure is not the same in every eye, and some individuals may tolerate for long periods a pressure which would rapidly blind another. A pressure of 24 mm. of mercury, as measured with a special instrument, is usually considered the maximum pressure compatible with continued health of the eye. In some persons glaucoma may be found in one eye and borderline or even normal pressure in the other. Frequently however, the condition is bilateral so that both eyes are treated.

Glaucoma is divided into primary and secondary types. Primary glaucoma is in turn further divided into two sub-types: simple glaucoma and angle-closure glaucoma.

GLAUCOMA, ANGLE-CLOSURE   This is an uncommon type (5 percent of all primary glaucoma) in which the iris is too close to the cornea. The pressure in the eye is normal, but conditions which cause dilation of the pupil, (such as looking at movies, being in prolonged darkness, emotional disturbances, and the like) result in the iris touching the cornea and closing the area through which fluid exits from the eye.

Symptoms. An acute attack is ushered in with a dull, aching pain in one or both eyes, which gradually becomes more severe. There is marked loss of vision, sensitivity to light, watering of the eye, and extreme redness of the affected eye. The pupil is dilated, the eye is sensitive to the touch, the iris pattern appears muddy, and the individual appears severely ill.

Treatment. This is directed initially to lowering the pressure within the eye by means of local eye drops, injections behind the eye, and systemic medication. If the acute attack cannot be interrupted immediately, surgery must be performed. If the acute attack is stopped, surgery is indicated in the interval between attacks.

Most individuals with angle-closure glaucoma have mild transient attacks that do not damage the eye. The chief symptoms are mild dimness of vision and halos around lights. The attack is frequently corrected by sleep, during which the pupil is small and constricted. The predisposition to attacks of angle-closure glaucoma can be detected by careful examination of the position of the iris in respect to the cornea, sometimes by controlled dilation of the pupil.

Once diagnosed, angle-closure glaucoma should be corrected by surgical means. Even faithful use of medications designed to prevent acute attacks may be useless, while the disease *can* be cured with surgery. Treatment with laser beams is often more successful and is gradually replacing older surgical approaches.

GLAUCOMA, CONGENITAL   This is a secondary type of glaucoma which arises because of a developmental abnormality involving the outflow channels of the eye. Males are affected about twice as frequently as females.

Symptoms. Signs may be evident at birth or up to one year of age. The earliest sign is marked tearing of the eye with an associated sensitivity to light. The normally transparent cornea becomes hazy, and the pattern of the colored iris is seen with difficulty. The eye then enlarges and there is loss of vision.

Treatment. Surgical correction should be carried out as soon as the diagnosis is made.

GLAUCOMA, SECONDARY   Increased pressure of the eye occurs as a complication of a number of eye diseases. The main signs and symptoms are those of the primary disease. Treatment is usually directed toward the cause of the glaucoma rather than toward the increased pressure itself.

GLAUCOMA, SIMPLE This is the most common type of primary glaucoma and frequently causes severe visual damage without prominent symptoms. It arises because of an obstruction to the exit of fluid from the eye.

Symptoms. The eye has a normal appearance. There may be loss of focusing power for near objects and a development of farsightedness. Night vision may be poor. If there is a sudden increase in eye pressure, there may be blurring of vision and the appearance of halos around lights. This last symptom, however, is not as common in simple glaucoma as in the angle-closure type.

As the increased pressure continues, the optic nerve is injured and there is loss of side vision. Vision directly ahead (central vision) is usually preserved until a late stage. If the disease is detected and treated in time, optic-nerve changes are not likely to occur.

The condition is diagnosed by discovering increased pressure in the eye by means of an instrument applied directly to the eye (tonometer). If optic-nerve damage is present, it may be evaluated by means of an instrument directing light through the pupil (ophthalmoscope). Measurement of side vision will indicate the degree of damage present.

Treatment. This is directed to maintaining the pressure within the eye at a normal level by means of drops in the eyes and sometimes tablets taken by mouth. Coffee is usually limited to no more than two cups daily, and drinking excessive amounts of fluid is discouraged. Usually the drops are used at regular intervals, and before and after a person has been in prolonged darkness, such as at the movies, which tends to dilate the pupil.

Medical treatment is preferred in simple glaucoma; but if the disease progresses despite adequate care, surgery is indicated. A variety of surgical procedures is used, to lower eye pressure either by establishment of drainage valves, or reduction of the flow of fluid through the eye.

INTRAOCULAR PRESSURE The eyeball is hollow and in order for it not to collapse it must have an internal pressure in excess of the surrounding atmospheric pressure. Usually the pressure inside the eye is only slightly (10–20 mm. of mercury) above the atmospheric pressure. The pressure inside the eye arises from secretion of fluid, blood pressure, and a delicate control of the flow of fluid into and away from the eye.

IRIS, DISORDERS OF Diseases, injuries, and abnormalities of the iris give rise to variations in its color, a loss of tissue substance, a distortion in shape of the pupil, and failure of the pupil to become smaller when bright light shines in the eye.

Absence of the whole iris (aniridia), usually of congenital origin, gives the eye a black appearance. It is associated with poor vision and frequently with treatment-resistant glaucoma.

The iris may change in color. Change of a brown iris to blue may occur because of an inflammation of unknown cause (heterochromic iritis) frequently associated with secondary glaucoma and cataract. A blue iris may become brown when a piece of metal containing iron is retained in the eye.

Blunt blows to the eye may tear the iris from its root and cause the appearance of two-pupils—the normal central one and another at the edge. There is frequently blood in the anterior chamber between the iris behind and the cornea in front. If small, the rip in the iris is frequently not corrected.

Finally, in diabetes (and following closure of a retinal vein) new blood vessels may form on the iris surface and cause a glaucoma which is nearly impossible to control either medically or surgically. The disease usually involves only one eye and requires a microscope to diagnose accurately. (*See also* IRITIS in this section.)

IRITIS Inflammation of the iris may occur because of the same conditions that cause choroiditis and cyclitis.

Symptoms. The eye frequently becomes red and it aches. Vision is reduced and the iris pattern appears cloudy. The pupil at first is semidilated; later it adheres to the lens behind it and is irregular in shape.

Treatment. This is directed to dilation of the pupil by medication and treatment of the specific cause. Frequently cortisone-like eyedrops are used to minimize inflammation. Attacks tend to recur.

KERATITIS *See* CORNEA, INFLAMMATION OF in this section.

LACRIMAL GLAND Tears are mainly formed by the lacrimal gland located in a depression in the front, upper, and outer portion of the bony orbit. Tears flow over the surface of the eyeball to the inner portion, where tiny openings are located in both the upper and lower lid. These openings lead to a duct which carries tears to the nose.

LENS The lens of the eye is located behind the pupil and is held in position by fine fibers (the zonule) which are inserted into the ciliary body. The lens is transparent and, because of varying tension exerted by the zonule through connections with the ciliary body, varies in focusing power so that the normal eye forms clear images for objects located both near to and far from it (accommodation). The lens is formed by enclosure of a tissue which forms skin elsewhere in the body and is secondarily involved in some skin diseases. Like skin, it forms new layers throughout life, but unlike skin, it does not cast off the old ones; rather, these become concentrated in the center of the lens. These older fibers lose elasticity and their accumulation results in a gradual loss of focusing power (presbyopia), so that in about the forty-fifth year of life glasses may be necessary for clear close vision.

Sometimes, in cataracts, the loss of clearness of the hard fibers in the center of the lens results in a marked increase in total focusing ability, so that the eye becomes nearsighted and it is possible to read without glasses late in life. This "second sight" of the aged, however, is associated with decrease of vision for distance and is frequently not permanent.

NEARSIGHTEDNESS (MYOPIA) In this condition light rays from a distant object come to focus in front of the retina. It occurs because the ratio between the bending of light rays and length of the eye is not proportionate, either because of too much bending or too long an eyeball. An object which is located close to a nearsighted eye is focused on the retina so that one can see objects clearly from this point.

Symptoms. Nearsightedness causes an inability to see clearly at a distance. Objects

THE LACRIMAL APPARATUS

The lacrimal gland secretes tears which are poured over the eyes through small ducts. The tears collect in the inner corner of the eye and pass through two small openings into the lacrimal ducts and into the lacrimal sac. The sac empties into the nose.

may be brought close enough to the eye to be in focus, but they may be so close that eyestrain occurs.

Treatment. The condition is neutralized by concave lenses. Most individuals are farsighted at birth and become nearsighted between the tenth and twentieth year. Thereafter, there may be minor changes, but the condition is stabilized.

Temporary nearsightedness may occur in diabetes or be associated with excessive use of the eyes which remain focused for near vision (spasm of accommodation). The condition disappears when the underlying cause is removed. In some types of cataract in the aged, nearsightedness occurs so that vision is clear for close work without lenses. However, there is a parallel reduction of vision for distance, and if the cataract progresses, near vision is also disturbed.

NIGHT BLINDNESS (NYCTALOPIA) Night blindness is a condition in which sight is deficient in reduced illumination or in the dark of night, although it is normal in good illumination. It sometimes occurs in atrophy of the optic nerve, abnormality of the retina (in anemia, scurvy, etc.), and in vitamin A deficiency.

OCULAR MUSCLES Movement of the eye is provided by six ocular muscles responsible for fine adjustment. Generally the eyes remain directed approximately straight ahead and the head rather than the eyes moves when objects are located far to one side. Four of the muscles, the rectus muscles, arise deep in the orbit from a tendon surrounding the opening through which nerves and blood vessels enter and leave the orbit. They attach to the outer covering of the eye, the sclera. Two other muscles, the oblique muscles, arise from the roof and the floor of the orbit. Except for the two muscles which move the eye inward and outward, the others function in elevating and lowering the eyes, holding the eyeball steady when it is turned in or out, and rotating the eye when the head is tilted toward either shoulder.

OPTIC NERVE The retina is connected to the brain by the optic nerve. This is about one-fifth of an inch in diameter and consists of numerous fine fibers from all portions of the retina. Shortly after leaving the bony orbit and entering the brain cavity, the inner half of the optic nerve from each eye crosses to the opposite side and joins optic-nerve fibers from the outer half of the eye on that side. Each eye is thus connected with each side of the brain. In side vision, objects on the nose-side of the eye's field of vision are perceived by the half of the brain on that eye's side; while objects towards the outer (temple) part are perceived by the portion of the brain on the opposite side of the head.

OPTIC NERVE, DEGENERATION (ATROPHY) OF Fibers of the optic nerve may die or deteriorate because of retinal disease, glaucoma, infection, inflammation, loss of blood supply, injury, poisons, or brain tumors.

Symptoms. The outstanding symptom is visual loss which may involve only side vision, central vision, or both. The optic nerve can be seen by means of an instrument (the ophthalmoscope) and appears white. A large number of serious conditions must be differentiated in making the diagnosis.

Treatment. This is directed to the cause. Frequently it is not possible to restore vision, but correction of the disease causing it will prevent further loss. Diseases which must be considered in the diagnosis of optic atrophy include syphilis, vitamin B (particularly thiamine) deficiency, multiple sclerosis, methyl (wood) alcohol poisoning, blood-vessel disease, meningitis, and encephalitis.

OPTIC NERVE, DISORDERS OF The optic nerves convey signals stimulated by light from the eye to the brain. Just after entering the skull, the inner half of each optic nerve crosses to the opposite side, and from this point each optic nerve carries fibers from the nasal half of the retina of the eye on the opposite side and from the temple (temporal) half of the eye on the same side. Thus, diseases of the optic nerve back of this crossing cause a loss of half of the vision in each eye. Diseases in front of the crossing affect only one eye. Abnormalities in the optic nerve may arise because of brain tumors, inflammation of the central nervous system, infections, and diseases of the eyes.

OPTIC NERVE, INFLAMMATION OF THE (OPTIC NEURITIS) The optic nerve may become inflamed anywhere in its course, from back of the eye to deep in the brain. Usually inflammation can be diagnosed only if it occurs in front of the crossing of the nerves in the brain. When the inflammation occurs on the surface of the nerve within the eye, it is called papillitis. If it occurs in the course of the optic nerve, it is called retrobulbar neuritis.

Symptoms. In each case, the chief symptom is loss of central vision with retention of side-vision. Retrobulbar neuritis may also cause pain upon movement of the eye. The disease usually occurs suddenly, with rapid loss of vision in one eye. The visual loss may range from slight dimness to complete blindness. The condition arises from a variety of diseases: multiple sclerosis, virus infection, malnutrition, syphilis, and others. Frequently a cause cannot be found or cannot be diagnosed until long after the attack.

Treatment. There is a marked tendency for recovery with or without treatment. Steroid drugs taken by mouth are commonly used. There is a tendency for recurrence, and as each attack causes some damage to the optic nerve, there may be permanent change.

OPTIC NERVE, SWELLING OF THE (PAPILLOEDEMA)

The optic nerve may become swollen in inflammations (papillitis) and secondarily to interference with drainage of blood in its veins. Papilloedema occurs in conditions in which the pressure within the brain is elevated and also in local conditions within the orbit which disturb venous drainage from the eye.

Symptoms. Vision is good until late in the disease. Frequently it is a sign of brain tumor or other serious intracranial disease. There are associated symptoms of the primary disease.

Treatment. This must be directed to the cause. If not relieved, the papilloedema causes optic atrophy. If corrected, it recedes and leaves no signs.

ORBIT

The orbit is the bony cavity which contains the eye. It is approximately pear-shaped, with a central expansion in the middle to contain the eye, the stem being the apex of the orbit where nerves and blood vessels enter and leave. The front margin of the orbit is composed of heavy bone which surrounds the eye except on the outer side, where it is deficient so as to permit side vision. The orbit is recessed deeply within the head. Above and on the outside, it is adjacent to the brain; inside and below, it is adjacent to the nasal sinuses. The lacrimal gland, which forms tears, is located in the upper and outer portion of the orbit.

ORBIT, ABNORMALITIES OF

The bony orbit which contains the eye is slightly more than a fluid ounce in capacity. In addition to the eye, it contains muscles, blood vessels, nerves, and fat. Most diseases and abnormalities of the orbit cause mainly a bulging forward of the eye or eyes, called exophthalmos or proptosis. This appearance can be caused by retraction of the upper lid, which makes the eyes appear more prominent, or by an unusually enlarged eye. The symptoms of proptosis (drooping) arise from exposure of the eye to irritation and sometimes from infection. Treatment must be directed to the cause.

A wide variety of congenital defects cause orbits which are too shallow or too far apart.

Generally the cosmetic defect cannot be corrected.

Both eyes or one eye may become prominent in thyroid overactivity. Correction of the thyroid disease may sometimes be followed by bulging forward, so that surgery is required. Tumors may impinge on or grow within the orbit, and many inflammations also cause prominence of an eye. Hemorrhages and blood-vessel defects also cause proptosis.

PRESBYOPIA

The power of accommodation (focusing for close work), is gradually lost, and at about the age of forty-five it is no longer possible to do close work comfortably. This is called presbyopia, a visual change that is part of normal aging except in pre-existing nearsightedness (myopia).

Symptoms. The chief symptom of presbyopia is gradual increase in the distance from the eye at which close work can be seen clearly. There may be difficulty in seeing small print or seeing clearly in poor light.

Treatment. The condition is neutralized by convex lenses which must be made stronger as the condition progresses.

The lenses used to correct presbyopia cause blurring for distance, so that bifocals are frequently used for clear vision both near and far. If glasses must be worn at all times, bifocals are preferable to single-vision lenses. If a lens is required only for close work, a reading-glass may be preferred. Presbyopia occurs in all eyes, but the nearsighted individual may achieve clear near vision by removing his glasses. Selection of single-vision or bifocal lenses is a personal preference only; but usually, if it becomes evident that glasses are required at all times, it is best to adjust to bifocals as early as they are required.

PUPIL, ABNORMALITIES OF

The central black opening in the colored iris is the pupil. It controls the amount of light entering the eye by becoming small in bright illumination and large in dim. Usually the pupils are large in youth and become smaller with the passing years. They are small in sleep, following medicines used in glaucoma treatment, following the use of morphine, and when adherent to the iris after iritis. The pupils markedly enlarge in dim light, when the eye is blind, following medicines used in the treatment of certain eye inflammations, and in death. Most medical attention is directed to whether the pupils constrict with light directed into the eye and dilate when it is discontinued. Failure of the pupils to react may occur with many serious diseases of the eye and the nervous system and is a signal for careful study.

RETINA   The innermost layer of the eye, the retina, is a complicated and highly organized nerve network which converts light impulses to nerve impulses by means of a chemical reaction not yet entirely understood. There are two main layers in the retina: an outer pigment layer which supports nutrition of the cells receiving light impulses; and an inner nerve layer. The nerve layer contains cells—the rods and cones—which undergo changes in chemistry in response to light impulses, giving rise to a nerve impulse. Each such impulse is magnified in the retina and conducted to the brain through nerve fibers which combine to form the optic nerve.

RETINA, BLOOD VESSEL CHANGES IN   The blood vessels which nourish the retina may be seen by means of an ophthalmoscope. Changes occurring in hardening of the arteries, diabetes, kidney disease, blood cancers, and many other conditions can be detected by changes in the retina. Frequently, however, these diseases are not reflected in the eyes, and the presence of normal eyes is no assurance that systemic disease is not present.

RETINA, CLOSURE OF CENTRAL ARTERY OF   In high blood pressure, hardening of the arteries, heart disease with scarring of the valves, certain obscure inflammation of arteries, migraine, and some other conditions, the blood supply to the retina through its main artery may stop.

Symptoms. There is a sudden loss of all vision in the eye, unless only a branch is involved—in which instance only the area of the vessel is injured. Examination with an ophthalmoscope indicates a spasm of the artery, with the retina milky white.

Treatment. This must be carried out immediately. Blood vessel dilating pills used for heart pain (angina), such as nitroglycerin,

may be useful for this eye emergency. Breathing into a small paper bag may dilate the involved vessel. Rubbing the closed eye with the fist through the lids for fifteen seconds, followed by ten seconds' rest, over a total of five minutes may be helpful. Early medical care is urgent if vision is to improve.

RETINA, CLOSURE OF CENTRAL VEIN OF   This is most likely to occur in hardening of the arteries, glaucoma, conditions in which blood flow is slowed, and conditions favoring clotting of the blood.

Symptoms. Vision is lost over a period of several minutes. Inspection with an ophthalmoscope shows the vein to be dilated and sausage-like, with intermittent narrowing and a large number of hemorrhages.

Treatment. Massage as described for retinal arterial closure is of questionable value. Treatment is directed towards lowering pressure in the eye and reducing the coagulability of blood, both obviously under close medical supervision. There may be gradual improvement over many months, but the condition may be complicated by the development of glaucoma.

RETINA, DETACHMENT OF   The retina may become separated from its underlying layer of pigment in primary detachment, or it may become elevated because of hemorrhage or new growth in the underlying choroid. Primary retinal detachment (serous) occurs because of the formation of a hole in the nerve layer. The hole occurs because of degeneration or injury.

Symptoms. The first symptom is commonly a localized area of bright lights flashing in the eye, followed by a sudden appearance of minute "floaters"; the detachment causes a progressive loss of side (peripheral) vision. The condition is diagnosed by examination with an instrument which illuminates the interior of the eye (ophthalmoscope) and must be differentiated particularly from a tumor of the choroid, which causes a secondary detachment.

Treatment. The treatment is nearly always surgical; medical attention should be sought immediately. The hole in the retina is closed by creating scar tissue in the choroid adjacent to it. Sometimes the outer wall of the eye is indented by means of a plastic rod to push the wall in slightly and bring the choroid toward the retina.

RETINA DISORDERS The retina is a complex nervous structure for converting light to nerve impulses which are then carried to the brain. Because of the delicacy of structure of the retina, even minor disturbances reflect themselves in changes in vision. The change involved may be in recognition of letters or objects (form), in color, in side vision (peripheral), or in dark-adaptation. Retinal disorders themselves never cause pain or redness of the eye, although these may accompany complications or involvement of other structures.

RETINA HEMORRHAGE Bleeding into the retina may occur because of injury, congenital abnormalities of blood vessels, diseases involving a bleeding tendency, inflammations within the eye, or from rupture of newly formed blood vessels. Symptoms depend upon the area of retina involved. Treatment is directed to the cause of the disease.

RETINA MACULAR DISEASE The area of the retina at the very back of the eye contains cones responsible for clear central vision and color vision. Disturbances in this area (macula) cause dimness of vision, with an island of blindness surrounded by an area of vision. The macular area may be affected in a large variety of diseases, including congenital disorders which may occur with mental retardation and muscle paralysis.

In aging, the blood supply in the choroid which supplies the macular area may gradually fail, causing gradual loss of clear central vision. There is never complete loss of vision. Treatment may not be effective. Some macular degenerations occur because of an inherited tendency and become evident only late in life.

RETINA, OXYGEN DAMAGE TO (RETROLENTAL FIBROPLASIA) Premature infants with a birth-weight of less than three pounds may, in order to survive, require oxygen in addition to that in the surrounding atmosphere. In some infants the oxygen interferes with the orderly growth of blood vessels in the retina, and the retina is converted to scar tissue. There are varying degrees of severity, and in the worst forms all vision is lost. The possibility of the disease developing is minimized by using oxygen as rarely as possible, and never in a concentration exceeding 50 percent. However, some cases do occur in infants who have not received any oxygen, and other unknown factors are involved.

RETINA, PIGMENTED DEGENERATION OF (RETINITIS PIGMENTOSA) This is a hereditary disorder beginning in adolescence in which there is gradual loss of side vision and decreased night vision. In severe instances vision is entirely lost by about age fifty. The condition is diagnosed by measurement of side vision, recognition of characteristic changes in the back of the eye, and a number of special tests. There is no effective treatment.

SCLERITIS Inflammation of the sclera of the eye may be superficial (episcleritis) or deep (scleritis). Causes include irritation, inflammatory infections, injury, rheumatism, gout, syphilis, and tuberculosis.

Episcleritis is usually harmless and is marked by slight discomfort, tearing, and pain. Occasionally there are more severe manifestations. There may be a slightly raised patch, red or purple in color, which causes congestion of the conjunctiva and the sclera. After a few weeks this lesion disappears, but recurrences, one after the other, are not uncommon. The condition may resemble certain types of conjunctivitis; it may become a frank scleritis.

Therapy is chiefly sedative, such as warm compresses using boric acid solution. If the cornea or iris is involved, atropine is administered to dilate the pupil and as an anesthetic and antispasmodic. Anesthetic drops relieve discomfort and pain. Antibiotics (by mouth or in drops) are also employed. Treatment is also of the underlying condition, as mentioned above.

The symptoms of scleritis are acute, the course of the affliction is protracted, and consequences may be serious. Involvement of both eyes is fairly common and relapses are usual.

Severe pain, tenderness to the examining finger, tearing, and marked sensitivity to light are the major indications. The doctor finds that the tension of the eyeball is often increased; there may be secondary glaucoma. Other elements of the eye may be involved leading to markedly impaired vision, even blindness.

Therapy is that as given above, except that it is vigorously pursued, and energetic treatment of the underlying cause, if it can be determined, is followed as soon as possible. Sulfa medication and antibiotics have been of great help in bacterial infections.

STY   A boil (sty) on the lid margin arises because of an infection in one of the glands of the lashes. There is a tendency for the infection to involve successive glands so that the sites occur in "crops."

Symptoms. The eyelid is tender and red until the sty ruptures.

Treatment. Hot compresses applied for ten minutes every hour give comfort. It may be necessary to open the sty surgically when it comes to a head; however, this decision should only be made by a physician and *never* attempted by a layman. Generally it is unnecessary to administer antibiotics either locally or systemically.

TEAR DUCT, PLUGGED   Stoppage of the tear duct is a common affliction during the newborn period; there is a congenital blockage of the tiny canal that allows the tears to flow from the inner corner of the eye into the nose.

Symptoms. Since tears are formed at a constant rate, if dammed back they will cause a watery eye and will flow over the lid and down the cheek. There is nothing wrong with the eye itself, but because the fluid is a good culture medium for germs, babies with blocked tear duct are frequent sufferers from conjunctivitis.

Treatment. Nine out of ten babies with this problem will outgrow it by the age of ten months; a mucus plug is expelled and/or the canal simply opens up. If the stoppage persists, an eye specialist (ophthalmologist) should be seen for treatment. Mere passage of a probe may be all the medical treatment required.

TEARS   The tears are secreted by an almond-shaped gland located in the upper, outer portion of the orbit. Additional tears are secreted by glands on the inside of the lids. Relatively few tears are normally formed, but they are evenly spread over the eyeball and keep the eye moist, preventing growth of bacteria.

TEARS, EXCESSIVE   These are formed when crying, or when the eye is irritated by cold, a superficial injury, a foreign body, or infection. Blocking of the drainage ducts for tears may cause overflow of a normal amount of tears. With aging, the lids become relaxed and tears may no longer be guided to the drainage ducts and overflow. Excess tears may be merely a nuisance, or they may be a sign of serious disease. Tearing in an infant's eye should alert one to infantile glaucoma which requires immediate surgical treatment. However, an infant's eye may also water because of failure of the tear duct to open during the early weeks of life. Glaucoma may be recognized by the loss of clearness of the cornea and difficulty in seeing the iris and pupil clearly.

UVEA   The middle coat of the eye, the uvea, consists of the iris, ciliary body, and choroid. The iris, the colored portion of the eye visible through the cornea, surrounds a central opening, the pupil, which controls the amount of light entering the eye.

The iris contains two muscles, one for dilating the pupil and the other for making it smaller. Structurally, it is a thin tissue consisting of two layers. The front layer is composed of thin filaments, while the back layer is dark brown. The color of the iris depends upon the number of filaments in the front layer. If many are present, the eye is blue; if fewer, the eye is hazel or green-gray; if very sparse, the eye is brown.

The size of the pupil is mainly governed by the amount of light entering the eye, but varies first of all with the individual; also with instillation of some ophthalmic medicines or certain drugs taken by mouth; with anger, fear or similar emotions; and with optical defects of the eye.

The ciliary body is continuous with the iris and is located behind it, so that it is not visible from without. This body provides nutrition to the interior of the eye and tends to maintain intraocular pressure. Fine fibers attached to the lens and ciliary body (the zonule) support the lens in position. A muscle in the ciliary body gives rise by contracting and relaxing to changes in shape of the lens, with focusing through the zonular fibers. (Focusing for near objects is known as accommodation.)

The choroid is the blood-vessel layer of the eye and provides nutrition for the portion of the retina adjacent to it. It is continuous with the ciliary body in front and ends at the optic nerve behind. It consists mainly of blood vessels with pigment interspersed between them.

VISION, MEASUREMENT OF   The function of the eyes involves several different types of vision.

Central vision is measured by the reading of a chart with different-sized letters, numbers or pictures. The measurement numbers usually used, such as 20/20, 6/6, are not a fraction and do not indicate the percentage of vision present. The first number indicates the distance from the eye to the test material, in either feet or meters; the second number indicates the distance at which a normal eye can read the test matter—more accurately, the distance at which the objects subtend a 5 foot angle. "Near tests" are frequently carried out to learn the smallest object or print that can be seen without respect to distance from the eye. In general most attention is given to testing with the best possible correcting lens rather than to vision without lenses.

The most important visual function for moving about is the ability to see to the side (peripheral vision). One may have entirely normal central vision; but if side vision is lost, one is blind for practical purposes. Side vision can be measured accurately by a variety of tests. A rough measurement is made by closing one eye and having someone else signal with fingers from a given side until one can recognize the number of fingers used.

There may be a loss of color vision with loss of central vision, but many individuals are born with a decreased color sense. This loss may be very marked and easily evident by the inability to see color. In others, it may be very slightly depressed and require elaborate test-ing to demonstrate. There is no treatment for hereditary color blindness.

The ability of the eye to increase in sensitivity in dim illumination is dark-adaptation. Testing is fairly complex and seldom done. Much of the same information may be obtained by testing the electrical response of the nerve network (retina) at the back of the eye.

Eye examinations are particularly important during the third year of life; in the first, fourth, and ninth grades; at age eighteen; and yearly after age forty to forty-five.

VISUAL AIDS   A number of aids to vision are used, ranging from partially closing the eyes to make the lids act as a pinhole, to looking through a small opening in the closed fingers. (A pinhole admits only parallel rays of light to the eye. These do not have to be bent by the lens or cornea to come to a clear focus at the retina.) A number of pinholes in a piece of paper may also be used.

Spectacles consist of either concave or convex lenses, frequently with different powers at right angles to each other to correct astigmatism. Lenses of additional strength may be fused to them by heat to make bifocals or trifocals.

Spectacles are frequently made of safety glass or plastic, so as not to shatter if struck by a hard object. Plastic lenses have the disadvantage of scratching more easily than glass, but they are lighter in weight. Most safety-glass lenses are manufactured by "case-hardening," in which the lens is heated and then cooled suddenly, thus making the outside surface very hard. Rarely, safety lenses are made by laminating an unbreakable plastic between two layers of glass, as is done with automobile windshields.

A number of different types of lenses are provided for those whose vision is defective even with ordinary lenses. The most popular is a magnifying lens held over reading material. An arrangement of lighting so that a bright light is directed on reading material is frequently useful. (Generally the light should be in front of the eyes and strike the reading material at an angle.) Most lenses for improving near vision cause magnification, and the reading material must be held close to the eye. The lens sometimes permits only one or two letters to be seen at a time, and great patience is required to read. Most devices for visual aid are designed only for close work. A small collapsible telescope can be used for distance; this is mainly useful in viewing street signs, bus routes, and the like.

Those with legal blindness (vision with correction less than 20/200, or a visual field contracted within a 20 degree radius) are eligible for "talking books" from the Library of Congress (books recorded on phonograph records, together with a phonograph) and many other aids. (Write to American Foundation for the Blind, 15 West 16 Street, New York, New York 10011, for information.) (*See also* EYE, ARTIFICIAL in this section.)

VITREOUS, DISORDERS OF   The vitreous is a clear, gel-like structure which fills the eyeball between the lens and the retina. It has very few cells and does not partake actively in any disease process.

Normally the vitreous contains small strands of protein fibers which are opaque and can be seen as dark lines when viewing against a bright background such as the blue sky. They are of no significance.

In injury and disease, white or red blood cells may enter the vitreous from adjacent structures. Treatment is directed against the cause.

GASTROINTESTINAL CONDITIONS

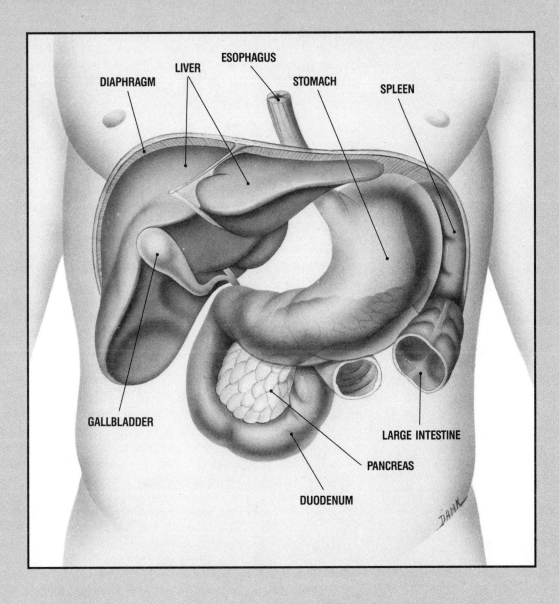

The gastrointestinal tract is comprised of the stomach and intestines and is basic for nourishment and elimination. The gastrointestinal system functions through a complex system of self regulating and fail-safe features throughout the life of an individual. By its very nature, this system will be subject to many stresses and outside elements which will cause aging and deterioration.

This section discusses the physiology and function of the various elements of the gastrointestinal tract, some common disorders and other conditions, and diagnostic methods and possible treatments. *See also* the questions on burning in the stomach (Q-6), bloating, gaseousness, and other minor digestive disorders (Q-8, Q-9), bowel irregularities (Q-11, Q-12), and hemorrhoids (Q-13) in the section QUESTIONS AND ANSWERS ABOUT COMMON SYMPTOMS.

The following is a list of terms identified in this section:

ABDOMINAL PAIN
ACHLORHYDRIA
ACIDOSIS
ACID STOMACH
ANUS
APPENDICITIS
BILE
BILIARY COLIC
BILIOUSNESS
BOWEL OBSTRUCTION
CECUM
CELIAC DISEASE
CHOLECYSTITIS (GALLBLADDER
　INFECTION)
CIRRHOSIS
COLITIS
COLOSTOMY
CONSTIPATION
DIARRHEA
DIGESTIVE DISORDERS
DIGESTIVE TRACT
DISTENTIONS
DIVERTICULOSIS AND DIVERTICULITIS
DUMPING SYNDROME
DUODENUM
DYSPEPSIA
ENTERITIS
ESOPHAGUS AND ESOPHAGITIS
FLATULENCE (GAS)
GALLBLADDER
GALLSTONES

GASTRIC JUICES
GASTRITIS
GASTRITIS, CHRONIC
GASTROINTESTINAL SYSTEM
HEARTBURN
HEMORRHOIDS (PILES)
HERNIA
HIATAL HERNIA
HIGH-RESIDUE DIET
HUNGER, UNUSUAL
HYPERACIDITY
ILEITIS, REGIONAL (TERMINAL ILEITIS)
ILEOSTOMY AND COLOSTOMY
ILEUM AND ILEITIS
INDIGESTION
IRRITABLE BOWEL DISEASE (IBD)
LACTOSE INTOLERANCE
LARGE INTESTINE
LIVER
MEGACOLON
NAUSEA AND VOMITING
OMENTUM
PANCREAS
PEPTIC ULCER
PERITONITIS
PORTAL VEIN
PROCTITIS
PYLORIC STENOSIS
RECTUM
SMALL INTESTINE
SPHINCTER MUSCLE

ABDOMINAL PAIN   Pain in the abdominal region is a symptom of many diseases which may either be of no consequence at all or extremely serious. Pain may arise from structures within the abdomen, or it may be referred from an extra-abdominal site.

Common abdominal disorders which cause pain include appendicitis, gastroenteritis, peptic ulcer, colitis, hernias, intestinal obstructions, tumors, regional ileitis, diverticulitis, and colic. Many genito-urinary disorders, such as kidney stones, urinary-tract infections, tumors, pregnancy and its complications, inflammation of the pelvis, menstrual cramps, and ovarian cysts can cause abdominal pain. Diseases of associated organs (gallbladder, liver, pancreas, and peritoneum) are other sources.

Conditions that arise in other locations but may cause abdominal pain include pneumonia, heart disease, neuritis, disorders of the blood, blood clots, systemic infections, spinal arthritis, and poisons such as lead and arsenic.

Symptoms. The description of the pain is most important in helping the physician in determining the cause. Such characteristics as onset, location, severity, and the methods that the patient uses to obtain relief are important. Certain types of pain are more or less characteristic of a specific condition. Thus, pain which occurs after eating a fatty meal and which tends to radiate under the right shoulder blade is often seen in cholecystitis. Peptic ulcer pain often occurs one or two hours after eating and is sharply localized in the upper mid-abdomen. Acute intestinal obstruction will often cause increasingly severe colicky pain with relief between spasms. Flank pain which is associated with bloody urine and which radiates into the genitalia or inner thigh is commonly seen with kidney stones. Tubal (ectopic) pregnancy can cause severe abdominal pain and a history of a missed period with sudden shock and vaginal

bleeding should alert one to this possibility. A coronary thrombosis may cause abdominal pain. Shingles (herpes zoster), which is a viral infection of the nerve root, can cause severe burning abdominal pain which is difficult to differentiate from other conditions until the characteristic blisters appear.

ACHLORHYDRIA   This term refers to the complete absence of acid-production by the stomach. It has been estimated that this condition is present in between 10 and 20 percent of all individuals over the age of fifty and is therefore usually not associated with any particular disease or symptom. The importance of the condition lies in the' fact that several serious disorders may be associated with absence of acid: pernicious anemia, gastric polyps, cancer of the stomach, and (sometimes) certain vitamin deficiency diseases. Less commonly, it may accompany certain chronic diseases such as nephritis, diabetes, chronic alcoholism, chronic cholecystitis, and colitis.

Symptoms. Few if any symptoms can be specifically ascribed to achlorhydria. Complete digestion of proteins and fats will still occur due to pancreatic and intestinal enzymes. Rarely, some cases of diarrhea may be associated with achlorhydria and respond to administration of dilute hydrochloric acid by mouth. Achlorhydria may be produced by X-irradiation of the stomach, a treatment sometimes resorted to for chronic peptic ulcer.

Treatment. Usually little or no treatment is required, but it is desirable to have reasonably frequent medical check-ups because of the possibility of the existence of certain conditions which may be associated with it. The diet should be balanced and easily digestible.

ACIDOSIS   The body has a superb mechanism for maintaining the proper acidity-alkalinity of its tissues. This delicate and sensitive system involves buffering substances in the blood, sensing areas in the central nervous system, and careful control of carbon dioxide-oxygen transfer in the lungs.

A state of excess acidity not compensated for by bodily means is known as acidosis. (In reality, the term is used when there is depletion of alkali.) This condition occurs in connection with several disorders, among them, uncontrolled diabetes, kidney disease, and severe diarrhea.

The body normally produces an excess quantity of acidic substances. Most are neutralized by the free alkaline (basic) elements, particularly the sodium in plasma. (This sodium comes from sodium bicarbonate. When sodium combines with an acid, the remaining bicarbonate is converted into carbon dioxide which is breathed out.) Other acid-eliminating reactions also occur.

Symptoms. Weakness, nausea, and vomiting are common in acidosis. The breath may have a sweetish fruity odor. Drowsiness may proceed to coma.

Treatment. Treatment requires hospitalization for proper chemical determinations which are guides for fluid and (electrolyte) alkali replacement. In diabetic acidosis and coma, insulin, fluids, sodium, potassium, and other substances must be given promptly.

ACID STOMACH   The term acid stomach is misleading. The stomach (gastric) juice should be—and normally is—acidic. The acidity is actually an aid to digestion; indeed, lack of gastric acidity can lead to definite health problems.

The phrase, as used in everyday speech, is applied to a sense of burning, irritation, or distress felt at the lower edge of the "breastbone" (sternum); this minor gastrointestinal sensation may be due to regurgitation of stomach contents up into the lower segment of the esophagus. True gastric hyperacidity is another matter and is discussed in the entry GASTRITIS in this section.

ANUS   The anal canal is the final portion of the rectum and large intestine (colon). The anus is guarded by the anal sphincter, a circular muscle which surrounds the canal. Piles (hemorrhoids), fissures, proctitis, and other common disorders of the region are discussed under their appropriate headings.

APPENDICITIS   Surgical removal of the appendix (appendectomy) because of an infection (appendicitis) is one of the more common abdominal operations. Appendicitis is most often seen in the ten-to-thirty age group, although it may strike at any age. Its incidence has been decreasing rather dramatically in recent years, a decline ascribed to the more liberal use of antibiotics. The causes of acute inflammation of this organ are not entirely clear; however, since it is a dead-end tube, substances which enter the appendix may find difficulty in leaving; obstructions are thus thought to occur, with subsequent swelling, inflammation, and finally bacterial invasion. Hardened pieces of intestinal contents lodged in the appendix for long periods of time are a common cause of obstruction. Occasionally, intestinal worms may also cause obstruction.

Symptoms. The usual combination of symptoms is classical, hence, diagnosis is not particularly difficult; there are, however, enough variations to make proper diagnosis extremely challenging. Normally, the typical attack is characterized at an early stage by intermittent or colicky pain, either throughout the abdomen or around the naval (umbilicus). The pain gradually becomes localized in the right-lower abdomen. Onset of pain is often followed by nausea and vomiting, and loss of appetite is common. After the pain has settled in the right-lower abdomen, it tends to become constant rather than cramping, and is increasingly severe. Occasionally the pain becomes extremely severe, then suddenly ceases. This is the "calm before the storm," as it often means that the appendix has ruptured and that peritonitis will ensue. The fever ordinarily does not exceed 101° F. Constipation is often a symptom. It is extremely important not to give cathartics or enemas to anyone suspected of having appendicitis.

While the above-mentioned are the usual symptoms, there are many variations; also, because of the mobility of the intestine, the appendix may be found in the *left*-lower abdomen, and if it is far to the rear of the cavity it may mimic the pain usually associated with kidney stones. Other conditions which must be differentiated from appendicitis include intestinal obstructions, femoral hernia, and—in the female—inflammation of the pelvic organs. In fact, almost any disease that may affect the abdominal cavity has been mistaken for appendicitis, and vice versa.

Particularly today, with modern techniques and treatment readily available, it is probably the wisest course to have an exploratory operation if appendicitis is at all suspected, since the mortality after delay is great. In addition to peritonitis, complications of acute appendicitis may include abscess-formation, intestinal obstruction, and (occasionally) a fistula or infected opening into a surrounding structure such as the bladder. It must be remembered that in the very young, the elderly, or in people who are chronically ill from other conditions, the classical signs of appendicitis may not be present, and in these instances the doctor must very carefully evaluate abdominal pain.

Treatment. The treatment is surgical removal as soon as the diagnosis is firmly established or cannot be ruled out. There may be rare instances in which for one reason or another surgery is not feasible. In these cases, massive doses of antibiotics and careful observation may suffice; but the instances are few where this course of action is considered prudent.

BILE   Bile, a secretion of the liver, is a thick greenish-yellow fluid; its chief components are salts, pigments resulting from the metabolism of broken-down red blood cells, cholesterol, and fat. Bile is primarily a collection of materials to be excreted into the intestinal tract and discarded, except for the bile salts which aid in the splitting and digestion of fats. Bile is collected in liver tubules which lead to the bile ducts which in turn carry the bile to the gallbladder. There it is stored and concentrated until the presence of food in the small intestine causes it to be discharged. In cases of severe vomiting, bile may be regurgitated into the stomach and subsequently found in the vomitus.

BILIARY COLIC   *See* GALLSTONES in this section.

BILIOUSNESS   This is a rather imprecise term which pertains to a feeling of nausea or uneasiness, usually after meals. There may be heartburn or vague pain in the right-upper abdominal region. The symptoms may be early signs of infection of the gallbladder, but ordinarily subside spontaneously and do not recur with any regularity. Avoiding overindulgence and highly seasoned foods, eating meals in a pleasant unhurried atmosphere, and chewing food well are often all that is required to relieve these symptoms.

BOWEL OBSTRUCTION   Obstruction to the passage of the intestinal contents may result from a variety of causes. The obstruction may be partial or complete and may occur anywhere along the course of the small or large intestine. Common mechanical causes include a kinking (or volvulus) of the bowel, adhesions as a result of previous abdominal operations, pressure from a tumor of neighboring tissue, strangulated hernia, impacted stool or foreign bodies, or strictures or tumors of the bowel wall. Inability of the musculature of the bowel to contract may simulate a mechanical obstruction, with abdominal swelling and pain. An example would be an impairment of the blood supply to a part of the bowel which may impair its motility. A particularly serious type of obstruction follows the plugging of a large blood vessel supplying a segment of intestine, and the resulting death of that portion of the bowel. Often after surgery or during the course of peritonitis the bowel may become temporarily paralyzed, a condition termed ileus.

Symptoms. Symptoms of bowel blockage vary according to the cause, duration, location, and completeness of the obstruction; but usually include intermittent crampy pain, vomiting, and abdominal distention. If the obstruction is in the large intestine, the pain is usually less severe. Vomiting may not be prominent and there may instead be occasional passage of bloody stools. In the paralytic type distention is prominent and the pain steady rather than colicky. X-rays of the abdomen will usually reveal the diagnosis.

Treatment. The treatment is directed at relieving the cause of the obstruction and often requires surgery.

CECUM   The cecum is the pouch-like portion of the large intestine at its juncture with the small intestine; the appendix is attached at the apex of this pouch. Rarely, the cecum may be involved in an inguinal hernia on the right side, and conditions which affect the large intestine will also involve this portion.

CELIAC DISEASE

Celiac disease is a chronic intestinal disorder of infants and young children characterized by fat in the stools (steatorrhea), loss of appetite, decreased growth rate, and symptoms of impaired nutritional absorption. The cause is unknown, but most patients seem to be unable to tolerate wheat gluten, a form of wheat protein. There are disturbances in the activity of intestinal enzymes. The disease is usually seen between the ages of six months and six years.

Symptoms. A characteristic finding is a prominent abdomen. The stool is large in size, loose, foul smelling, and often frothy. Alternating diarrhea and constipation may occur occasionally. The disease has an irregular course, improvement and relapse alternating in cycles.

Certain laboratory tests are helpful in making the diagnosis. These include laboratory examination of the stool to detect increased fat and carbohydrate. A test dose of vitamin A taken by mouth can be shown to be poorly absorbed. Anemia may be present.

Treatment. With adequate treatment, recovery occurs in most cases after a prolonged period of as much as several years.

Gluten-free diets, from which all products containing wheat and rye are eliminated, have been successful. Skimmed milk and the gradual addition of ground lean meat, cottage cheese, egg white, and pureed vegetables are the basis of diet therapy. Vitamin supplements may be needed. Because they may produce a relapse, starchy foods are added last.

CHOLECYSTITIS (GALLBLADDER INFECTION)

Infections of the gallbladder are generally caused by bacteria. They are frequently associated with gallstones, although it is now well established that stones may be present for many years without any symptoms or complications.

Symptoms. The symptoms are usually moderate to severe attacks of pain (often perceived under the right shoulder blade), indigestion after a fatty meal, fever, nausea, and vomiting. A large percentage of cases of gallstones are accompanied by some degree of infection. In prolonged cases, the infection may pass upward into the ducts leading to the gallbladder and thus cause obstruction and jaundice. In severe cases the gallbladder may perforate, spilling its contents into the abdominal cavity and thus producing severe peritonitis. Occasionally the pain is difficult to distinguish from appendicitis. Many acute cases subside spontaneously with the help of antibiotics; in such cases, surgical intervention is not required. Should the symptoms increase, however, with rupture or peritonitis, surgical removal becomes necessary. Patients with frequent recurrences of acute cholecystitis, particularly when gallstones are demonstrable, should be considered logical candidates for surgical treatment. This is the removal of the gallbladder, an operation called a cholecystostomy. Most cases of chronic cholecystitis are associated with gallstones. In patients who have recurrent indigestion or "biliousness," where function is otherwise normal and no stones are demonstrable by X-rays, the diagnosis should be questioned.

CIRRHOSIS

A chronic disease of the liver, cirrhosis produces an increased amount of connective tissue and destruction of the functioning cells. This results in hardening of the organ and eventually a marked obstruction to the normal flow of blood. Although many cases are due to chronic alcoholism, this is by no means the only cause. Cirrhosis may occur after a severe case of hepatitis (infectious jaundice), long-standing malnutrition (the probable cause of alcoholic cirrhosis), untreated malaria, chronic congestion due to heart-failure, and obstruction of the normal flow of bile caused by gallstones or infection of the bile ducts. Cirrhosis may also be caused by a rare disorder, hemochromatosis (bronze diabetes).

Symptoms. Initially the liver is usually enlarged because of an infiltration of fat. Later it becomes scarred, nodular, and shrunken. The symptoms are ill-defined at first and consist of loss of appetite, nausea and vomiting, weight loss, and vague abdominal pain. In advanced cases jaundice, foul breath, red palms, abdominal swelling due to fluid in the abdomen, and gastrointestinal hemorrhages are common. Because of the many functions of the liver, the effects of cirrhosis can be profoundly serious. Abdominal fluid (called ascites) collects as a result of obstruction to the flow of blood from the intestines to the liver (through the portal vein) as well as because of a decreased amount of proteins in the blood. When severe, this portal obstruction may also cause formation of varicose veins in the esophagus and rectum (the routes by which the blood must flow when the normal channels through the liver are obstructed). Rupture of the veins in the esophagus can cause a massive and often fatal blood loss.

Treatment. The treatment of far-advanced cirrhosis is usually unsatisfactory; in early cases, however, it can be halted or reversed by proper nutrition, strict abstinence from alcohol, supplemental vitamins, and rest. Occasionally, surgical procedures designed to relieve the pressure in the portal vein are successful in preventing hemorrhages, but careful treatment of the underlying condition is mandatory.

COLITIS Mucous colitis, or irritable colon, is a common functional disorder of the large intestine which should be clearly differentiated from the much more serious ulcerative colitis.

Symptoms. In mucous colitis, a benign but often distressing condition, the irritable colon exhibits uncoordinated, irregular contractions of its lower portion, with excessive mucous production. Constipation may occur and gas can then be trapped, causing sensations of bloating and fullness. Occasionally the spasm will cause frequent loose stools with much intermixed mucus.

Treatment. The causes are poorly understood, but successful treatment often requires relief of emotional tensions and reassurance that the condition is not serious, does not predispose to cancer, and that simple constipation does not result in the absorption of "bowel toxins," headaches, or various other diverse and unrelated symptoms. Regular meals, avoidance of straining at the stool, and general measures are of great benefit. (*See also* CONSTIPATION in this section).

COLOSTOMY *See* ILEOSTOMY and COLOSTOMY in this section.

CONSTIPATION Healthy persons may have normal bowel movements as often as two or three times a day, or as seldom as once every four or five days. Much needless worry and consternation could be avoided by the realization that it is not essential for good health to have at least one movement a day. Ideally, perhaps, the bowels should move at least every other day, but the frequency is not so important a matter as is the difficult passage of hard, dry stools. In these times, with dieting so prevalent, it must also be remembered that a scanty diet will inevitably result in scanty stools. The habitual passage of hard, dry stools may lead to such constant use of laxatives that spontaneous movements eventually become impossible. Chronic constipation may predispose to secondary rectal trouble such as hemorrhoids, fissures, and proctitis. Injudicious use of strong laxatives and frequent "cleansing enemas" may result in loss of muscular power in the rectum and is to be avoided. Failure to respond to the urge to move the bowels, lack of exercise, improper diet, and inadequate fluid intake can all be important in causing constipation. Rectal pain due to spasm of the anal sphincter, or other rectal diseases, may reduce the urge to defecate and further amplify the problem. Emotional disturbances likewise are a common predisposing factor.

Treatment. Treatment should be directed to clearing up any underlying cause and then to reeducation, which mainly consists of setting aside a specified time of day, usually after a meal, for defecation. Avoidance of straining at the stool, responding promptly to the urge to defecate, proper exercise, diet, and adequate fluid intake are usually helpful measures. Stool softeners and bulk forming agents made from psyllium seeds, bran, and other fiber may also be beneficial in treating constipation. Habitual use of laxatives and enemas is to be avoided. (*See also* the section HOME NURSING CARE.)

DIARRHEA This term refers to abnormally frequent bowel movements of fluid-like fecal matter. Diarrhea is frequently caused by minor infections of the intestinal tract and is commonly referred to as acute enteritis or intestinal flu (no relation to influenza).

Many disorders of the alimentary canal are accompanied by diarrhea of varying severity. Colitis, regional enteritis, some liver disorders, and emotional disturbances may have diarrhea as the cardinal symptom. The term dysentery usually refers to a condition of greater severity, in which blood and mucus make up a prominent portion of the stool. (*See also* the section HOME NURSING CARE.)

DIGESTIVE DISORDERS A broad definition of digestive disorders would include any condition or disease that interferes with the breakdown and absorption of ingested foodstuff. Impaired digestion may result from mechanical problems such as ill-fitting dentures or poor dental repair. Extensive surgery on the gastrointestinal tract may leave a shortage of absorptive surfaces. An obstruction due to tumors, scar tissue, kinking of the bowel, or a foreign body will impede the passage of food and hamper the digestive process.

Generalized infections may cause a temporary decline in the efficiency of the digestive apparatus such as is seen in the vomiting which accompanies many illnesses. Localized infections of the stomach, liver, gallbladder, pancreas, and intestine can cause disturbances in the secretion of the necessary digestive ferments or enzymes, and interference with absorption may likewise result from infections of specific portions of the intestine. In cases of diarrhea, ingested food passes through too quickly to be utilized, and in chronic cases severe malnutrition may result. Certain diseases such as sprue (lack of vitamin B_6) and celiac disease are characterized by poor absorption of fats. Voluminous, greasy, foul-smelling stools may result. The treatment of these various disorders depends upon their cause.

DIGESTIVE TRACT The digestive (alimentary) tract comprises the mouth or oral cavity, the gullet or pharynx, the esophagus, stomach, small intestine (considered to have three areas—duodenum, jejunum, and ileum), large intestine or colon, rectum, and anus. In addition to this irregular tubular structure, the digestive tract involves such food-processing organs as the salivary glands, liver, gallbladder, and pancreas.

The digestive tract consists basically of a cavity (lumen), through which nutrients pass. This is lined by mucous membrane (mucosa), behind which there is a muscular layer. Behind the muscle, in turn, there is an outer layer of connective tissue. The mucosa is lined with various cells: some produce mucus, a thick lubricating fluid, whereas others secrete digestive enzymes. Folds of mucosa (villi) enable an enormous surface area to be exposed to the substances in the digestive canal for the purpose of absorption.

DISTENTIONS Abnormal collections of food or gas as intestinal contents may cause localized swelling and distress. Most cases are temporary and subside spontaneously. A temporary "paralysis" of the gastrointestinal tract is often present after abdominal surgery and acute stomach distention can be particularly troublesome. To prevent this it is customary to keep a nasogastric tube (a tube placed through the nose down into the stomach) hooked up to a drainage bottle for several days after the surgery. This tube drains off gases and fluids and keeps the abdomen decompressed. When bowel sounds return—"gas pains"—the drainage can be discontinued.

DIVERTICULOSIS AND DIVERTICULITIS Diverticulosis is the presence of diverticula, which are small pea-sized out-pouchings, usually of the lining of part of the large intestine (sigmoid colon). (These may occur elsewhere in the alimentary canal, but they are the most common in this location.) Causes for their formation are not known; ordinarily they cause no symptoms and do no harm. Inflammation or diverticulitis occurs when the opening into the sac becomes obstructed, favoring bacterial invasion of local tissue; abscess formation and subsequent perforation and peritonitis may follow. Fortunately, such severe complications are rare; the usual case of diverticulitis will subside with conservative treatment.

Symptoms. The symptoms are constant pain in the lower left abdomen, slight fever, abdominal distension, and perhaps an inability to pass gas.

Treatment. Treatment with antibiotics, rest, and cleansing enemas (after being cer-

THE INTESTINAL TRACT
(ALSO CALLED ALIMENTARY CANAL OR DIGESTIVE TRACT)

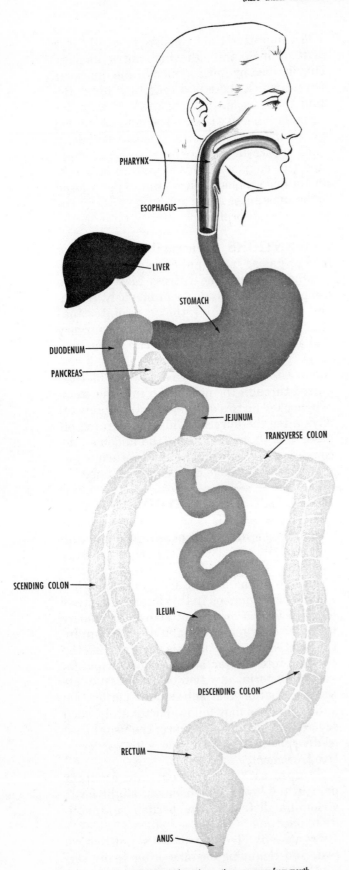

PHARYNX

ESOPHAGUS

LIVER

STOMACH

DUODENUM

PANCREAS

JEJUNUM

TRANSVERSE COLON

SCENDING COLON

ILEUM

DESCENDING COLON

RECTUM

ANUS

PANCREAS

SCHEMATIC CROSS SECTION

The schematic cross section illustrates the general plan
of any part of the digestive system.

1 OUTER COVERING
2 OUTER MUSCLE LAYER
3 INNER MUSCLE LAYER
4 SUBMUCOSA
5 MUSCULARIS MUCOSA
6 LAMINA PROPRIA WITH GLANDS
7 VILLUS
8 GLAND IN SUBMUCOSA
9 EXTERNAL GLAND DUCT

The intestinal tract is a continuous passage from mouth
to anus. The liver and pancreas empty into the tract.

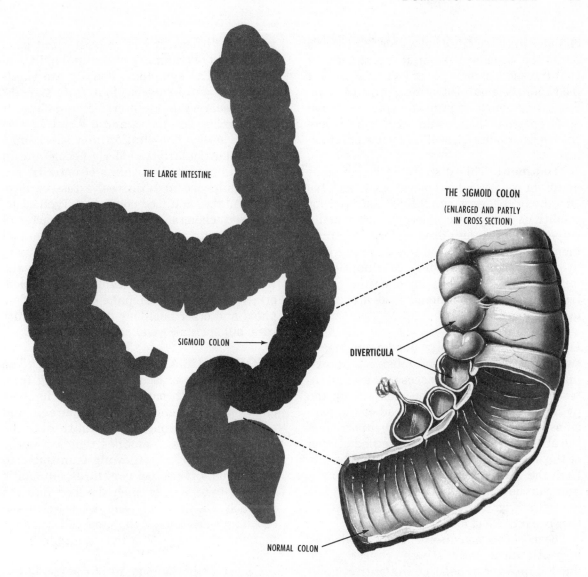

THE LARGE INTESTINE

THE SIGMOID COLON
(ENLARGED AND PARTLY
IN CROSS SECTION)

SIGMOID COLON →

DIVERTICULA

NORMAL COLON

DIVERTICULOSIS AND DIVERTICULITIS

tain that no complications are present) usually suffice. In the long-term treatment of diverticulosis, bulking agents which produce large stools are favored. Examples are the various products containing psyllium (e.g., Metamucil®), and stool softeners. Bran and other high-fiber items may also be added to the diet.

DUMPING SYNDROME   After the surgical removal for any reason of all or part of the stomach, a group of symptoms known as the dumping syndrome sometimes occur. The symptoms occur from two different mechanisms. In the first or immediate dumping syndrome the patient is aware of pain, distention, and sometimes nausea and vomiting immedi-

ately after eating. These symptoms occur as a result of the decrease in storage space due to the removal of a portion of the stomach; the ingested food then distends the first part of the intestine, causing the pain and vomiting.

In the second and more serious type of dumping syndrome, the symptoms occur usually about one-half hour to an hour after eating; therefore its name, the delayed dumping syndrome. In both cases, the symptoms are abdominal pain, palpitation, occasionally nausea and vomiting, and (in severe cases) actual loss of consciousness. The cause of these distressing symptoms is not entirely known or understood, but the presumption is that there are large fluid-shifts from the bloodstream into the small intestine, causing changes in the delicate balance of fluid in and out of the vascular system. It is also thought that the sudden entrance of large amounts of food into the small intestine causes the pancreas to secrete larger amounts of insulin and other enzymes than would occur if food were released periodically, as it is in a normal stomach.

Treatment. This distressing condition is one of the reasons why removal of stomach tissue should be very carefully considered for conditions like peptic ulcers, which usually respond to other, less drastic, forms of treatment. The treatment for the dumping syndrome consists of avoiding consumption of large amounts of food at any one time. Small frequent feedings of bland food are consequently recommended.

DUODENUM   Literally duodenum means twelve fingerbreadths and refers to approximately the first twelve inches of the small intestine. It is joined at the stomach by the pylorus, curves around the head of the pancreas, and extends to the left upper portion of the abdomen where it joins the second portion of the small intestine (the jejunum). The bile from the gallbladder empties into the duodenum via the common bile duct. The pancreatic juices likewise empty into it to aid in the further breakdown of food.

The most common disorder of the duodenum is peptic ulcer. Interestingly, cancer of the duodenum—and indeed of the entire small intestine—is an extremely rare condition. Because of the constant irritation of the surface cells, this is an unexpected finding. Inflammation, perhaps with spasm in this area, is referred to as duodenitis. It may or may not be associated with a duodenal ulcer, but the condition may produce much the same symptomatology and require similar treatment.

DYSPEPSIA   *See* INDIGESTION *in this section.*

ENTERITIS   Enteritis is an inflammation of the lining of any portion of the small intestine. The most common form of enteritis encountered is that which is referred to as intestinal flu. (The influenza virus has nothing to do with the cause of this disorder.) This condition is often caused by several different types of viruses and is characterized by a rapid onset of cramping, abdominal pain, and diarrhea. The symptoms usually are short-lived and within twenty-four to forty-eight hours recovery is more or less complete. If the diarrhea is intense, and if vomiting also occurs, severe dehydration and shock may ensue—particularly in elderly people and in young infants. Other causes of enteritis are overindulgence in laxatives, excessive alcoholic intake, and food-poisoning. Typhoid fever and cholera produce severe bacterial forms of acute enteritis. It has been estimated that until modern times, enteritis or dysentery probably killed more soldiers than the wounds of battle. In the United States, modern, sanitary facilities make outbreaks of typhoid and other bacillary dysenteries rather rare, but sporadic cases continue to occur.

ESOPHAGUS AND ESOPHAGITIS   The esophagus is a muscular tube leading from the back of the throat down through the chest cavity and an opening in the diaphragm and ending in the stomach. The first third of the esophagus contains muscles that are under voluntary control; swallowing is initiated in this region. In the other two-thirds, automatic reflexes take over to push the food into the stomach. The lining of the lower portion of the esophagus has some of the same cells that are found in the stomach, secreting enzymes and acid.

Occasionally the muscles of the esophagus will go into spasm, and it is thought that this is one cause of the familiar symptoms of heartburn. Often a case of esophagitis causes pain and discomfort that resembles other health problems. Caustic poisons such as lye or commercial acids, when swallowed, can cause severe inflammation and scarring of the esophagus so that surgery may be necessary to widen the passage. Diverticula (balloon-like projections from the wall of the esophagus) are sometimes seen and can cause burning pain and difficulty in swallowing.

FLATULENCE (GAS)   Excessive gas may accumulate in either the stomach or the intestine. An excess in the stomach may be expelled by belching, while collections of intestinal gas are relieved by the passage of flatus rectally.

Gas in the stomach is the result of swallowing air, usually while eating or drinking; the ingestion of large quantities of carbonated beverages will likewise cause stomach gas. If excessive, the swallowed air can cause symptoms of pressure, fullness, and occasionally heartburn. Some individuals attempting to relieve this pressure by belching can cause further discomfort by swallowing more air.

Intestinal gas also results mostly from swallowed air, forced through the tract by peristalsis. Putrefaction of intestinal contents by bacterial action produces the rest. As is well known, certain foods such as beans, tomatoes, and other raw vegetables tend to cause excessive amounts of intestinal gas. Flatulence in this region can cause the same symptoms of fullness, abdominal cramping, and general distress as stomach gas. Gas-pains after abdominal surgery can be extremely distressing and must often be relieved by the use of a rectal tube. (This accumulation of gas is caused by a temporary paralysis of the intestinal tract so that the patient is unable to pass flatus voluntarily.)

GALLBLADDER This sack-like structure is primarily a reservoir for bile, which is produced by the liver. It is situated under the right lobe of the liver in the right-upper portion of the abdominal cavity. Bile helps in the digestion of fatty substances and is a thick liquid containing many salts. It is released from the gallbladder into the duodenum via the common bile duct. Removal of the gallbladder (cholecystectomy) does not seem to be harmful in any way and digestion continues as before. Infections of the gallbladder (cholecystitis) are relatively common, as is stone formation (cholelithiasis). (*See also* CHOLECYSTITIS in this section.)

GALLSTONES Many individuals may have a gallbladder loaded with stones and yet never have symptoms. By contrast, others may have only a single gallstone which can cause agonizing pain and serious difficulties requiring extensive surgery. Acute attacks of biliary colic often occur in overweight, middle-aged women of light complexion. The causes of gallstones are not entirely known. Faulty metabolism of cholesterol (one of the substances in bile), chronic infection of the lin-

THE GALLBLADDER AND LIVER

ing of the gallbladder, and partial obstruction of the bile duct are all thought to play a part.

Symptoms. Typically, a gallbladder attack will start as a cramping pain in the upper right portion of the abdomen, usually after a heavy meal. The pain then becomes more severe and often radiates into the back under the right shoulder blade. (This type of radiating pain is characteristic of gallbladder disease.) Nausea and vomiting are common, and the pain can become extremely severe.

Occasionally a stone will travel into the common bile duct and obstruct the flow of bile. If the obstruction continues, bile will back up through the liver and eventually stain the skin, causing jaundice; the characteristic color of this condition is due to certain pigments that are found in bile. If the obstruction is severe, the stools may become very light since the normal brown color of feces is due to bile pigment. An attack of biliary colic usually subsides spontaneously in a few hours, only to make its presence felt at some later time.

Treatment. Surgical removal of the gallbladder and its stones is by far the most effective cure. Pulverization of stones by shock waves (lithotripsy) and dissolution through taking certain drugs by mouth are alternate approaches. Other useful measures are reduction in weight and the avoidance of fats in the diet. Surgery is seldom indicated in patients whose gallbladders contain a single large stone where there is no danger of passage into the bile ducts and no associated infection. However, acute and chronic infections of the gallbladder are commonly associated with gallstones. These conditions are discussed under CHOLECYSTITIS in this section.

GASTRIC JUICES The lining of the stomach secretes a variable mixture of powerful digestive juices including hydrochloric acid; the enzymes pepsin, rennin, and lipase; and a thick, protective mucus. The secreting cells respond to stimuli initiated by the sight, smell, or thought of food, as well as by reacting to the presence of food in the alimentary canal.

GASTRITIS Gastritis is an acute inflammation of the lining of the stomach. Usually of brief duration, it is sometimes sudden and violent. Several types of gastritis exist. One form may be caused by the ingestion of single substances, such as alcohol, creosote, sulfa drugs, antibiotics, iodine or bromine compounds, very hot foods, an allergy-producing food (such as milk, eggs, or fish when taken by hypersensitive individuals), and so forth. Another type may be caused by swallowing strong acids or caustics (iodine, arsenic, zinc, lead, etc.). Still a third type of gastritis is produced by infectious or toxic material and may be seen in patients with influenza, measles, scarlet fever, pneumonia, or diphtheria. A recently recognized bacterium campylobacter has been found to cause acute gastritis and also gastric ulcers.

Symptoms. In gastritis the lining of the stomach is often congested with small areas of hemorrhage, and there may actually be ulceration. Symptoms include loss of appetite, pain or pressure sensation in the stomach area, headache, vomiting, and exhaustion. In milder cases these symptoms may subside within twenty-four to forty-eight hours. If the gastritis is due to a corrosive poison, there will be collapse, severe pain, and a rigid abdomen, and chills and fever will occur if the cause is toxic or infectious.

Treatment. In the more common form of gastritis, complete bed rest is necessary. Drugs that reduce the tendency to nausea are indicated, and analgesics or narcotics may be given for severe pain. (Morphine, however, is not to be given in the presence of nausea or vomiting.) No solid or semi-solid food should be given for the first day or two. Water, bouillon with salt, hot tea and sugar, and thin soups may be given orally, although in some cases nourishment must be given intravenously. Later, bland foods may be taken. These include buttered toast, soft-boiled eggs, cooked cereals, mashed potatoes, milk and cream, gelatin desserts, and so forth. This type of diet may be necessary for several weeks.

GASTRITIS, CHRONIC Chronic gastritis is a continual inflammation of the wall of the stomach. The cause is unknown, although some instances may be psychosomatic. The organism campylobacter may be involved in some cases. Patients have a sensation of heartburn or fullness in the upper part of their abdomen, especially after the ingestion of food. Loss of appetite, nausea and vomiting, or hemorrhages occur infrequently. An ulcerlike pain is present in many patients and loss of weight is common.

Treatment. When chronic gastritis is suspected, all stomach irritants such as alcohol, nicotine, spices, aspirin-related or iodine compounds, or harsh laxatives, should be avoided. A bland diet, such as is used for peptic ulcer, is recommended. Because of the nutritional limitation of foods in this diet, vitamins may be added. In view of the fact that the disease is hard to distinguish from peptic ulcer or other more serious conditions of the gastrointestinal tract, the patient should be placed under a physician's care. The campylobacter organism responds to some antibiotics and to bismuth subnitrate.

GASTROINTESTINAL   SYSTEM The gastrointestinal system (or alimentary canal) can properly be considered a hollow tube with various bulges and attached glands, extending from mouth to anus. Its purpose is to prepare and extract fluid and nourishment from foodstuffs, to provide energy and building material for the body, and then to reject resulting waste at the convenience of the host. This tube is lined with various types of cells which, in addition to other specific functions, protect the body in much the same way as does the skin. The canal should be considered not as an inner part of the body, but merely as another surface in contact with the outside environment.

The alimentary canal includes the mouth, the esophagus (or tube from throat to stomach), and stomach, the small intestine with its associated organs—the liver, gallbladder, and pancreas—the large intestine, the rectum, and the anus. This complicated apparatus is subject to many diseases and malfunctions, both of its components individually and of the system as a whole. Disturbances of function may arise from infections, ingested food or poisons, injuries, tumors, lack of essential foods, and in many instances from so-called psychosomatic or "functional" difficulties.

In our society a vast amount of attention is given to conditions of the alimentary canal. The infant is urged to eat; the adult is urged not to eat after the previous lessons have been too well learned; the teenager fears halitosis (a term coined by an advertising man for the promotion of a certain mouthwash); and nearly everyone is at least occasionally preoccupied with "regularity" or lack of it. It is no wonder that an estimated 30 percent of patients with gastrointestinal complaints are found to have no demonstrable disease to account for their symptoms. Conversely, very real and often serious disorders such as peptic ulcers, ulcerative colitis, and even cirrhosis of the liver may have at least partial psychologic origins.

HEARTBURN This commonly used term describes a sensation of burning and pressure under the lower portion of the breastbone. It results from distension of the lower portion of the esophagus or from the presence of regurgitated stomach-contents in that area. Heartburn does not necessarily result from the presence of stomach acid, as persons with no acid-production may experience this symptom. Simple measures, such as change in position or the drinking of a small amount of milk or antacid mixture, will most often relieve this condition.

HEMORRHOIDS (PILES) Hemorrhoids are swellings of the veins in the lower rectum and anus. If they protrude through the anal opening (sphincter) they are external. If they are confined to the anal canal they are internal. Hemorrhoids are seldom painful unless the blood becomes clotted in these swollen areas. Hemorrhoids have been called "a disease of upright posture," as they are seldom noted in four-footed creatures. They may result from constipation, pregnancy, rectal infections, an enlarged prostate gland, severe obesity, or lack of exercise. Rarely, the appearance of hemorrhoids may signify an obstruction of the normal blood flow from the intestinal tract to the liver via the portal vein, such as seen in cirrhosis of the liver.

Symptoms. Internal hemorrhoids may cause itching, a feeling of fullness in the rectum, and pain if they become filled with clotted blood. Frequently the first sign of internal hemorrhoids will be bright-red blood from the rectum coating the stool. Bleeding is often not associated with pain. External hemorrhoids can be felt as small grape-like protrusions from the anus. They often contain clotted blood and can be extremely painful. Because of the pain associated with the passage of a bowel movement, the patient is likely to neglect his normal bowel habits, causing further hardening of the stool and thus making passage even more difficult. It cannot be assumed that all bright-red painless bleeding from the rectum is due to hemorrhoids, because painless tumors or polyps may also bleed even though hemorrhoids are known to be present. Examination is essential in these cases.

Treatment. The treatment of hemorrhoids may be very satisfactorily accomplished by such simple measures as sitz baths and anesthetic ointments. The avoidance of constipation and of the consequent straining at stool is most important in eradicating this condition. Severe pain and bleeding or chronic recurrence are indications for surgical removal.

HERNIA A hernia or rupture is defined as the abnormal protrusion of a loop of the intestine or of some part of an internal organ through an abnormal opening of the cavity which contains it. In the gastrointestinal system, the commonly seen hernias include hiatus hernia—protrusion of a portion of the stomach through the hole in the diaphragm through which the esophagus passes; ventral hernia—protrusion of intestinal loops through a defect in the midline of the abdominal wall; and inguinal and femoral hernia—loops of intestine which pass through the inguinal canal into the scrotum or (in females) through the femoral canal into the upper thigh.

A hiatus (diaphragmatic) hernia is usually the result of a congenitally large hole (or hiatus) in the diaphragmatic muscle which allows a portion of the stomach actually to protrude into the chest cavity; rarely, severe injury to the abdomen may force a portion of the stomach up through the hiatus.

A ventral hernia may occur in the midline of the abdomen, particularly after repeated pregnancies. This is due to the relaxation and separation of the muscles of the abdomen and can be quite distressing. Occasionally a ventral hernia may protrude through the site of a former incision in the abdomen. This is known as an incisional hernia.

Inguinal hernias are of two major types: indirect and direct. The indirect type refers to the protrusion of a loop of intestine through the inguinal canal which leads from the abdominal cavity into the scrotum. (Normally the entrance to this canal closes over shortly after birth.) A direct inguinal hernia, on the other hand, does not travel through the length of the inguinal canal, but pushes into it at some distance beyond its origin. If the loop of intestine which herniates through the abnormal opening becomes kinked (strangulated), serious consequences may follow unless the hernia is quickly reduced. This procedure may require skill and experience, though some patients learn how to do this on themselves: gentle pressure is applied on the hernia near its exit point and the hernia is gradually tucked back in. If, because of blockage to intestinal flow, a bowel obstruction is present, the flow of blood becomes impaired, and there is actual tissue-destruction. This type of strangulated hernia is a surgical emergency. In many instances, however, the defect is relatively large so that the loop of intestine is easily pushed back up into place, either manually (without surgery) or by a truss (a supportive device which is worn to prevent enlargement of the hernia). Inguinal hernias may result from excessive straining or lifting, but a preexisting weakened inguinal canal is usually necessary for producing a hernia in this manner.

A femoral hernia is the protrusion of a loop of intestine (usually in women) into the femoral canal—the potential space through which the large blood vessels and nerves leave the pelvis and go into the upper leg. This type of hernia may likewise be relatively benign, producing no symptoms, but occasionally surgery is required.

In a certain percentage of newborn babies there is protrusion of a loop of intestine at the naval, causing an umbilical hernia. This may be rather frightening to the parents, but such hernias almost always disappear after one or two years and seldom require surgical repair. However, if surgery is required for a large hernia, the baby will take only about two to four weeks to recover.

HIATAL HERNIA   *See* HERNIA in this section.

HIGH-RESIDUE DIET   This type of diet is indicated in constipation due to lack of muscle tone (atonic constipation) and for conditions such as diverticulosis. The intestinal muscles are stimulated by bulky foods that are high in cellulose content—basically fruits and vegetables. Bran products and plant extracts such as psyllium (e.g., Metamucil®) will also increase the bulk and weight of the stool. This approach has been derived from observations which indicate that in societies where people consume high bulk diets there appear to be fewer cases of such common disorders as constipation, diverticulosis, and colon cancer.

HUNGER, UNUSUAL   Hunger is a complicated sensation that has physiological as well as psychological origins. True hunger should not be confused with appetite, as appetite may continue long after hunger pangs have been satisfied by the first few mouthfuls of food. Hunger pangs result from actual contractions of the stomach, causing disagreeable sensations in the upper abdomen when expected food is not forthcoming.

The level of circulating blood-sugar (controlled by insulin from the pancreas) is thought to be important in the regulation of hunger sensations. Thus, pancreatic disturbances may cause unusual hunger if excessive amounts of insulin are being secreted. Where the food that is actually digested and absorbed is inadequate, continued hunger may result. At times of increased need for foods, such as during the heavy growth periods of teenagers, hunger is also prominent. Because of the intimate psychological relationships between hunger and appetite, however, there are many instances of chronic disease when hunger is strangely not present. Persistent unusual hunger in an individual who is consuming adequate amounts of food should lead one to suspect the possibility of hyperthyroidism, an insulin-secreting tumor, food malabsorption, intestinal parasitism, and other systemic disorders.

HYPERACIDITY   The overproduction of gastric acid by the specialized glands in the lining of the stomach results in hyperacidity. The term refers to gastric acid only and has nothing to do with the delicate acid-base balance of the blood and other body fluids. The consumption of acid-containing foods and liquids contributes very little to gastric acidity, as the acids contained in fruits and vegetables are extremely weak when compared with the hydrochloric acid manufactured by the stomach. Acid secretion is initiated by the ingestion of food, as well as by nervous impulses from the brain. This latter mechanism is the usual cause of hyperacidity and emotional stress is therefore a powerful contributing factor. Prolonged hyperacidity may cause gastritis and in many cases is a direct cause of a peptic (gastric or duodenal) ulcer.

ILEITIS, REGIONAL (TERMINAL ILE-ITIS)   The cause of this inflammatory condition which usually affects the final eight to twelve inches of the ileum (final portion of the small intestine) is not known. It is most frequently seen in young males but may affect all ages of both sexes. In the commonly seen form of the disease there is diarrhea, cramping, abdominal pain, loss of weight, and a continued low fever. Occasionally the onset may be abrupt, with localized pain in the right lower abdomen, and differentiation from acute appendicitis may be determined only at surgery. Many cases subside spontaneously; chronic cases, however, usually progress steadily and surgery may eventually be necessary. Because of the extensive involvement of the lining of the intestine, there is interference with the absorption of certain foods—particularly fats and certain vitamins.

Diagnosis can usually be made in chronic cases on the basis of the patient's history and X-ray examination of the intestinal tract. This condition must be differentiated from functional gastrointestinal disorders, ulcerative colitis, sprue, and tumors. Rarely, tuberculosis of the intestines may cause similar symptoms.

ILEOSTOMY AND COLOSTOMY   In cases where extensive portions of the large intestine or rectum have been surgically removed, the construction of an artificial anus may be necessary. This is accomplished by suturing the cut end of the bowel to an opening in the abdominal wall. The resulting opening is called an ileostomy or colostomy, depending upon whether the ileum or the colon has been brought up to the abdominal wall. An ileostomy, because of the fluid nature of the contents of the small intestine, is likely to require somewhat more care and the use of a bag held in place by various mechanical devices is often required; however, after training and experience, the individual with an ileostomy can carry on a completely normal life without fear of embarrassment. Most patients with a colostomy, because of the more normal consistency of the contained stool, are usually able to train themselves to have relatively normal bowel movements at predictable intervals and do not require any particular attachments to cover their abdominal opening.

There are thousands of patients with ileostomies and colostomies who lead perfectly normal lives. There are, in fact, formal societies (ostomy clubs) of patients who have had procedures in most large cities throughout the country. Regular meetings are scheduled to which patients with recently acquired ileostomies or colostomies are invited. Much self-confidence is obtained through such organizations and the care and use of altered eliminatory apparatus becomes much less formidable.

ILEUM AND ILEITIS   *See* SMALL INTESTINE in this section.

INDIGESTION   Indigestion (also known as dyspepsia) is an indefinite term that is used differently by various writers. Because the term is so nonspecific, it is really not useful.

The most common interpretation of the term is as a group of symptoms, including nausea, heartburn, upper abdominal pain, belching, passage of gas, a sense of fullness, and a feeling of distention.

Symptoms. Although the symptoms may be caused by organic disease of the digestive tract, they are more commonly produced by eating too much or too rapidly, inadequate chewing of the food (sometimes due to poor dentures), eating during emotional upsets or mental strain, and the swallowing of large amounts of air. Indigestion may also be produced by poorly cooked foods; those with high fat content; and—for some people—by specific items of diet, such as cucumbers, radishes, gas-forming vegetables (beans, cabbage, etc.), and highly seasoned foods. Chronic gallbladder disease and allergies to specific foods can also cause symptoms.

The symptoms seem to be due to an alteration in the activeness (motility) of the digestive tract. Instead of a normal, smooth, rhythmic wave of contraction down the tract pushing the food material onward, under conditions of nervousness, anxiety, fear, depression, or pain, the muscles may be inhibited or may go into spasm and not relax. Because similar symptoms may be associated with significant organic disease, any patient who has frequently recurring episodes of indigestion should see a physician.

Treatment. The patient should eat a balanced diet. Food should be thoroughly chewed without haste, and meals should be eaten, whenever possible, in a pleasant, quiet, relaxed environment. Foods should be properly cooked, prepared in an appetizing way, and eaten in moderate amounts. Smoking immediately before meals should be prohibited. Excitement should be avoided after a meal. A number of drugs are used for indigestion; most of these act on the psychological aspects of the digestive process, but others are used to relieve spasm, reduce gastric acidity, improve bowel function, and so forth.

IRRITABLE BOWEL DISEASE (IBD)

Also known as spastic colon and irritable colon syndrome, IBD most commonly affects the young to middle-aged, and more often women. IBD is a malfunction of the colon's propulsive activity and appears to be made worse by emotional stress. No underlying specific disease of the bowel has ever been found.

Symptoms. Alternating cycles of diarrhea and constipation are accompanied by abdominal pain. The pain is achy rather than cramping and is often relieved by a bowel movement. The majority of patients with IBD have prolonged periods of waxing and waning of their symptoms. Attacks often follow emotional stress, depression, and anxiety.

Treatment. There is no single therapy that works for the majority of symptoms. Dietary changes to include high-fiber foods, bulking agents, and avoidance of foods that appear to initiate attacks have been partially successful. There are a variety of medications, including anti-depressants, anti-diarrheal and anti-constipating agents that have been used but all with limited success. Often a thorough medical examination and the physician's assurance that no underlying serious illness exists may alleviate many of the symptoms and prolong the patient's symptom-free periods.

LACTOSE INTOLERANCE

Lactose intolerance is the inability to digest milk and milk products. It is caused by a deficiency or absence in the gut of the enzyme lactase. This enzyme breaks down complex sugars into small digestible fragments. This condition often occurs in infants and children.

Symptoms. Common symptoms include bloating, flatus, abdominal cramping and diarrhea.

Treatment. The obvious treatment is to avoid the offending foods. Generally, processed cheese and yogurt are well tolerated, because the milk sugar in these products is already partially broken down. Recently introduced enzyme tablets are designed to make troublesome milk foods more digestible.

LARGE INTESTINE

The large intestine, or colon, is joined to the ileum (the final portion of the small intestine) at the cecum, a blind pouch to which the appendix is affixed. The colon is composed of four parts. The first portion, or ascending colon, originates in the lower right abdomen and rises along the right flank to just under the liver. The transverse colon crosses the upper part of the abdomen and makes a sharp turn downward, becoming the descending colon. Along the left flank, the descending colon dips into the pelvis and is then called the sigmoid (S-shaped) colon and ends at the rectum.

The main functions of the large intestine are storage of fecal material and the absorption of water. In this context it should be noted that the concept of intoxication due to poisons being absorbed through the wall of the colon has been amply disproved. Cleansing enemas are accordingly seldom required in the normal, healthy individual, and may in fact be harmful if resorted to frequently. The lining of the colon contains many mucus-secreting cells which aid in lubricating the fecal material and protecting the lining from excess roughage.

A condition called megacolon (large colon) is occasionally seen, in which the large intestine may attain a huge size due to a congenital defect in the nerve supply (see MEGACOLON in this section). Unlike the small intestine, the colon is relatively prone to tumors often

arising from small polyps which may extend from the wall of the organ. Most authorities agree that polyps, whenever discovered, should be removed for this reason. Mucous colitis, or irritable colon, is a fairly common, annoying, but not serious condition. Diverticulitis is another relatively common affliction of the colon and is described under a separate heading. Ulcerative colitis, a much more serious disease, requires early recognition and careful treatment. (*See also* COLITIS; ULCERATIVE COLITIS in this section.)

LIVER   The largest organ in the body, the liver is situated mainly in the right-upper portion of the abdominal cavity, but it does extend into the left upper quadrant as well. Because of the dome-like shape of the diaphragm (the muscular partition between the chest and the abdomen), the liver is normally protected by the lower ribs; in healthy individuals it is seldom felt on abdominal examination. The liver has many functions and is

THE COLON

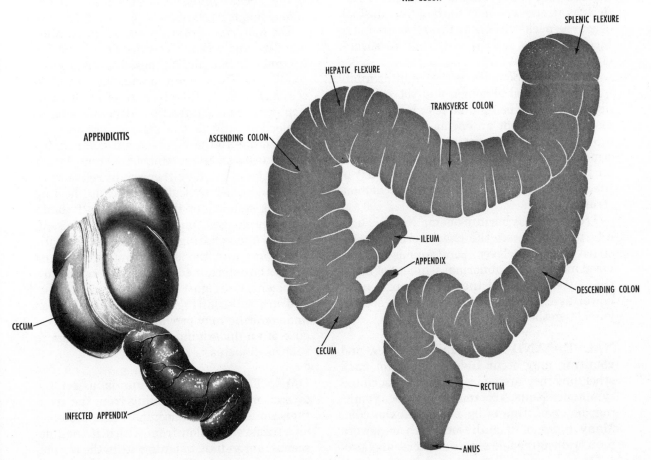

APPENDICITIS

CECUM

INFECTED APPENDIX

SPLENIC FLEXURE

HEPATIC FLEXURE

TRANSVERSE COLON

ASCENDING COLON

ILEUM

APPENDIX

DESCENDING COLON

CECUM

RECTUM

ANUS

indispensible for life. Fortunately it has a great capacity of regeneration, and liver failure occurs only after an overwhelming infection or repeated injury. Among its more important functions are storage of digested food-products and energy; the manufacture of proteins; the storage of certain vitamins (the normal liver can store more than a year's supply of vitamin B_{12}); the production of bile from the breakdown products of the red blood cells; the manufacture of antibodies; and the detoxification of many harmful substances which may occasionally be present in the bloodstream. Its major functions are therefore storage, synthesis, and detoxification. The more common disorders of the liver include hepatitis, cirrhosis, and subsequent jaundice. (*See also* CIRRHOSIS in this section; HEPATITIS in the section INFECTIOUS DISEASES; JAUNDICE in the section MISCELLANEOUS HEALTH CONDITIONS.)

MEGACOLON   In the congenital condition megacolon (literally, huge intestine), there is a narrowing of the rectum due to a nerve deficiency in one section of the bowel-wall: stool, of course, packs up behind this stricture in the large intestine (colon) and leads to severe, chronic constipation.

Symptoms. Sometimes the infant exhibits a very distended abdomen and there is usually a history of being unable to have a bowel movement without an enema, a suppository, or a finger. Psychosomatic (psychogenic) constipation can be distinguished from megacolon in that the former does not start so early in life, and no rectal stricture can be demonstrated.

Treatment. A barium-enema X-ray is usually used to detect the characteristic rectal structure, and a clever operation has been devised in which the abnormal segment of intestine is removed and the normal portions of bowel at each end of the nerveless section joined together.

NAUSEA AND VOMITING   Nausea and vomiting may occur independently of each other, but they are usually closely associated symptoms. Nausea commonly precedes vomiting; however, this is by no means the rule. Many types of stimulation, such as severe pain or disagreeable sights or odors, may pro-

voke nausea and subsequent vomiting. Stimulation from the organs of balance in the middle ear may cause nausea, as in seasickness. The actual act of vomiting requires a center of the brain for coordination and is therefore rather complex.

A type of vomiting not preceded by nausea, in which the stomach contents are ejected forcibly, sometimes occurs after severe head injuries, and is thus a valuable diagnostic sign. Acute infectious diseases, too—particularly in children—very often have vomiting as one of the preliminary symptoms. Practically all diseases and conditions affecting the upper digestive tract may also cause nausea and vomiting. The vomiting of early pregnancy is little understood but widely experienced. Certain types of heart or endocrine disease can be associated with nausea and vomiting. In sensitive individuals, mere stimulation of the rear portion of the throat may cause gagging and vomiting. In some persons nausea and vomiting seem to be psychogenic or emotional in origin; these patients rarely suffer malnutrition because of it, since the actual amount of food lost is negligible.

The material actually vomited up is called vomitus, and its characteristics can be of importance in diagnosing possible underlying conditions. Thus, vomitus with the odor of feces may indicate the presence of an obstruction in the small intestine. Although streaks of blood usually have no significance (mere irritation due to the vigorous muscular action may cause a small amount of bleeding), larger quantities of blood—either bright red or dark brown—usually indicate significant bleeding into the stomach or the esophagus. If vomiting is prolonged, bile is commonly present. Nausea and vomiting are usually nonspecific symptoms and the underlying cause must always be determined. Most cases are due to a transient viral gastritis or gastroenteritis, and are self-limiting. Occasionally, nausea and vomiting may provide a clue to the presence of an underlying metabolic disturbance such as diabetes.

OMENTUM   The omentum is a double-layered membrane extending from the liver, then separating to encompass the stomach and transverse colon from which it then descends, apron-like, to hang within the abdominal cavity and cover the coils of the small intestine. The main function of the omentum is fat storage. A membranous structure, the omentum can be involved in any generalized peritonitis in the abdominal cavity. (*See also* PERITONITIS in this section.)

PANCREAS The pancreas, a long slender organ, lies on the rear wall of the abdominal cavity behind the stomach and has two major functions. The first is secretion of pancreatic juice, which aids in the digestion of the intestinal contents; this is carried to the first part of the intestine (the duodenum) by way of the pancreatic duct. The second pancreatic secretion is insulin, which is concerned with the metabolism of sugar. When insulin is insufficient or is altogether lacking, the result is diabetes.

Because of the inaccessibility of this organ, a tumor of the pancreas is very difficult to diagnose until it has progressed to dangerous proportions. Inflammation of the pancreas (pancreatitis) can be quite severe and is often caused by reflux of bile or by stone blockage of the pancreatic duct. Acute pancreatitis is a dire abdominal emergency, requiring hospitalization, intravenous fluids, and possibly surgical procedures. Occasionally, pancreatitis becomes chronic, and because of the diminished amounts of pancreatic juice formed, the patient is likely to have severe digestive difficulties and intermittent bouts of abdominal pain. Pancreatitis may also be caused by acute or chronic alcoholism.

The pancreas is also involved in cystic fibrosis, a childhood condition due to abnormal function of various glands throughout the body. Malnutrition, retarded growth, thick mucus, and lung infections are common and are particularly difficult to treat.

Occasionally, fluid-filled cysts are formed in the pancreas, and these may reach rather large proportions. Symptoms of cysts are pain in the abdomen, nausea, weight-loss, vomiting, and jaundice. Treatment is surgical removal.

PEPTIC ULCER Peptic ulcers are erosions of one or more layers of the stomach or duodenum (the first portion of the small intestine). Depending on their location, they are therefore classified as either gastric or duodenal. These lesions result from an inability of the mucous-membrane lining of these organs to withstand the powerful digestive action of the enzyme pepsin and an increased amount of hydrochloric acid; these overabundant secretions from the stomach are uniformly found in peptic ulcers. Occasionally, if the ulcer is found in the stomach, it becomes important in the older-age group to determine if acid is being produced at all. In its absence other diagnoses must be considered.

In times of particular emotional turmoil, acid secretion tends to become excessive—hence the common belief that the hard-driving executive type is especially prone to develop an ulcer. Recent studies have shown, however, that persons in all walks of life are susceptible. Moreover, many cases have been seen in newborns and very young infants.

Symptoms. Ulcer pain is usually very characteristic. It tends to be sharply localized in an area just below the tip of the breastbone and is often described as feeling like a red-hot poker. The pain is noteworthy for its predictable appearance at specific times of

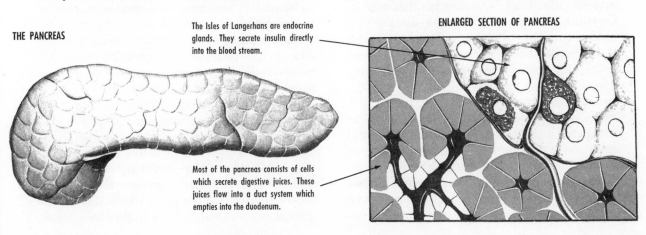

THE PANCREAS

The Isles of Langerhans are endocrine glands. They secrete insulin directly into the blood stream.

Most of the pancreas consists of cells which secrete digestive juices. These juices flow into a duct system which empties into the duodenum.

ENLARGED SECTION OF PANCREAS

the day or night. Typically it comes on an hour or so before lunch and dinner and often around 2:00 A.M. In uncomplicated cases the burning discomfort is usually relieved promptly by food or antacids such as bicarbonate of soda. This "pain-food-relief-pain" cycle is so characteristic that a diagnosis can be strongly suspected from this history alone. Confirmatory X-rays are desirable to make sure that other conditions requiring different treatment are not present.

PEPTIC ULCER

A peptic ulcer is a benign crater in the mucous membrane of the stomach or duodenum, caused by the action of the acid gastric juice.

Rarely, an ulcer can attain a large size without pain. The first indication that there is anything wrong in these instances may be a sudden vomiting of blood or other indications of internal bleeding, such as severe weakness or fainting and the passage of black, tarry stools. Bleeding as a complication of an ulcer results from the actual destruction of a blood-vessel wall in the ulcer crater. This should be considered an emergency, and prompt medical attention is mandatory. If the crater becomes too deep, the wall of the stomach or duodenum may actually perforate. The spillage of gastrointestinal contents into the abdomen can cause severe peritonitis. If a perforation oc-

curs in the rear wall of the duodenum, the pancreas—which is adjacent at this point—may become involved. The ensuing pancreatitis, while uncommon, can be a very serious complication. In long-standing chronic cases of duodenal ulcer, the passageway may become so scarred and/or swollen with inflammation as to be completely obstructed. The resulting constant vomiting, pain, and dehydration point to another grave complication of peptic ulcer.

Treatment. The vast majority of peptic ulcers can be treated by diet and medication. The nature itself of the disease-process suggests the proper treatment, namely: neutralization of stomach acid; a bland diet to prevent irritation of the injured tissue; and attainment of a measure of tranquillity and freedom from emotional stress. One old program consists of hourly feedings of milk or food, alternating with one of the many available antacid preparations. Medications designed to reduce the secretion of acid—ranitidine, cimetadine (H_2 blockers)—are very effective. This regime is rapidly successful in relieving the pain, and in a few days the diet can be gradually made more liberal. Some studies indicate that many ulcers may heal quite well on a regular diet. All spicy and heavily seasoned foods must be avoided. Alcohol in any form is contraindicated, as it is known to be one of the most powerful stimulants to the acid-producing cells. The use of tobacco should likewise be greatly curtailed.

The length of time necessary to heal an ulcer in certain locations in the stomach may vary from a few weeks to several months. Since recurrences are notoriously common, certain dietary restrictions may be required indefinitely. Sometimes it becomes necessary to recommend a change of employment or some other alteration of a hostile environment so as to aid the healing process. The management of the previously discussed complications may require surgical intervention. Prompt diagnosis and judicious surgery may be lifesaving. In middle-aged or older patients, an ulcer may require direct visualization with an instrument (endoscope) and biopsy, because of the possibility of cancer. In a small percentage of chronic and recurrent ulcers surgery for the ulcer itself may be required; but most authorities agree that medical management must be given a fair and adequate trial before resorting to these more drastic procedures.

Two procedures currently have their advocates, and both are designed to cut down on the secretion of acid. The more direct approach consists of the removal of a portion of the stomach—a partial gastric resection. There are certain complications which occasionally result from this procedure (*see* DUMPING SYNDROME in this section). A vagotomy and pyloroplasty, the other commonly performed operation, consists of interrupting the fibers of the vagus nerve (which controls the secretion of acid in the stomach) and widening the pyloric canal, the narrow band of tissue that separates the stomach from the duodenum. Ulcers have gained a certain amount of respectability in our society as the mark of the successful man. Most patients would agree that the price is exorbitant.

PERITONITIS Peritonitis is a widespread inflammation of the membranous lining of the abdominal cavity (peritoneum). This condition—while still extremely serious and requiring prompt and early medical attention—is fortunately much less common and dreaded than in the days before the sulfas and antibiotics. Because of the extensive surface-area involved, it is a very generalized infection and causes profound symptoms.

Peritonitis is caused by infectious agents or foreign material within the abdominal cavity. Practically any type of bacteria gaining entrance will multiply rapidly, since the peritoneum and its lubricating secretions make an ideal growth-medium. Bacteria may gain access by perforation of the intestinal tract resulting from appendicitis, peptic ulcer, diverticulitis, severe gallbladder disease, typhoid fever, bowel obstructions, or dysentery. (Occasionally bacteria may gain access through the female genital tract.) A chemical peritonitis may result if bile or pancreatic juices are spilled into the abdominal cavity. Occasionally the infection is not generalized and a local abscess will form.

Clinical features are quite variable, since they depend upon the cause of the infection. A localized peritonitis is common with appendicitis, and in this instance pain is confined to the inflamed area. If the appendix then ruptures, the peritonitis may spread rapidly.

Symptoms. The inflammatory process usually causes a rising temperature, chills, an increase in the number of white blood cells, vomiting, and severe pain. Because of the discomfort, the abdominal muscles are usually very rigid—this being a valuable sign to the physician. Peritonitis is most often a complication of an underlying condition in the abdomen, and signs of appendicitis, gallbladder disease, intestinal obstruction or other such conditions are also present.

Treatment. A localized peritonitis may result in spontaneous recovery, but a generalized condition requires prompt and vigorous treatment. Appropriate therapy depends upon the underlying condition and may require surgical intervention. Vigorous and prompt administration of appropriate antibiotics has reduced the incidence and gravity of the disease immeasurably, but prompt recognition and treatment are essential.

PORTAL VEIN The portal vein is a large vessel which collects blood from the gastrointestinal tract and transports it to the liver, where absorbed foodstuffs can be extracted and stored until needed. Harmful substances which may have been absorbed into the bloodstream are rendered harmless in the liver before entering the general circulation. Obstruction to the flow of blood in the portal vein may occur from cirrhosis or hardening of the liver, cancer of the pancreas-head, and rarely by a clot (thrombosis-formation). If the flow through the portal vein is completely obstructed, the blood must find other routes to gain access to the general circulation; swollen or varicose veins of the esophagus, the rectum, and the anus (hemorrhoids) may result.

PROCTITIS Proctitis is an inflammatory disease of the rectum which may be due to various agents. Frequent enemas or cathartics, heavy pinworm-infestation, and chronic constipation may be causes. Irritating discharges from diseases higher up in the intestinal tract can cause a secondary proctitis. Sometimes the inflammatory process that leads to ulcerative colitis is prominent in the rectum and is referred to as a proctocolitis.

Symptoms. Symptoms vary, depending

upon the cause. In general, diarrhea, occasionally mixed with blood and pus, rectal discomfort, and pain are the common manifestations. Chronic proctitis may occasionally lead to the development of inflammatory polyps which have a tendency to become malignant.

Treatment. The diagnosis depends on inspection of the area and treatment is directed towards the underlying cause.

PYLORIC STENOSIS Between the stomach and the duodenum (the first part of the small intestine) there is a slightly narrowed segment called the pylorus. In its wall are a large number of muscle fibers which run in circular (sphincter) fashion around this area. It is assumed that the chief function of the pylorus is to keep food in the stomach until its digestive activity is complete. A few newborn babies develop an enlargement of these muscle fibers, so that the passageway from the stomach is narrowed (becomes stenotic) to such an extent that little or no milk or food will move into the duodenum.

Symptoms. The condition occurs almost exclusively in first-born males in the first six weeks of life. Sometime in the first two or three weeks the infant begins spitting up; this is assumed to be a feeding problem and the child may go through several milk-changes, always with the same result. The spitting becomes vomiting and the vomited material may be shot out two to four feet (projectile vomiting). Stools become hard and infrequent and the urine scanty. The child loses weight and may become severely dehydrated. If proper care is not given early he may die. The diagnosis is made on the basis of these symptoms and confirmed by the doctor, who can feel the tumor-like swollen muscle and also observes the abdominal waves moving across the upper abdomen.

Treatment. After fluids have been restored by injections and the baby is in better general physical condition, the surgeon treats pyloric stenosis by making an amazingly small incision to find the pylorus; he then partially cuts the fibers. Within just a few hours the baby is eating normally. There seem to be no residual effects. Recurrences of pyloric stenosis are practically unknown.

RECTUM The rectum is the final portion of the large intestine, which leads to the anus. Its function is primarily the storage of feces until evacuation is convenient. As the rectum becomes distended with feces, the urge to move the bowels is created. Disregarding this urge repeatedly may lead to chronic constipation. Bleeding from the rectum may be the first sign of rectal cancer and demands investigation. It can be a dangerous mistake to ignore such a sign by assuming the source of the blood to be piles or hemorrhoids. Fissures and abscesses in the rectal area can be the source of much discomfort, as can internal and external hemorrhoids. Irritability and irritation of the rectal area in children should raise the possibility of pinworm infestation. This diagnosis is simple to make and the treatment, while occasionally tedious, is effective and well worth the trouble.

SMALL INTESTINE The small intestine is a thin-walled muscular tube about one inch in diameter and approximately twenty feet in length. It is divided into three parts, the duodenum, the jejunum, and ileum.

SPHINCTER MUSCLE The anal sphincter is a well-developed circular muscle in the anal canal that closes the passage until such time as defecation is to take place; conscious effort causes the muscle to relax and allows the stool to pass. Inflammatory conditions of the mucous-membrane lining of the canal may cause a spasm of the sphincter and make passage difficult. Conditions such as hemorrhoids, fissures, and rectal abscesses are common causes. Chronic rectal conditions may give rise to excessive scar tissue in the area and cause permanent narrowing of the anal canal. The ensuing straining necessary to force the stool past the region may then cause additional irritation, worsening the condition, and causing further constipation. Surgery is sometimes necessary under these circumstances.

SWALLOWING DIFFICULTIES Most cases of swallowing difficulty are due to obstructions in the esophagus (the tube from the throat to the stomach). Hiatus hernia may cause similar symptoms. In patients over fifty years of age a gradually progressive difficulty in swallowing should be given prompt attention, as cancer of the esophagus is a common cause. Pain is usually absent, and the diagnosis is easily confirmed or rejected. Another common cause of this distressing symptom is spasm at the entrance to the stomach. The cause is not known, but the symptoms are usually transitory. Pain and vomiting are commonly associated with the swallowing difficulty. Treatment with medications is usually satisfactory. Narrowings or strictures as a result of lye or other corrosive substances on the lining of the esophagus are a common cause of swallowing difficulty in children. Swallowing a foreign body (such as bridgework or too large a bite of meat) may cause difficulty, but the cause is usually readily apparent. Occasionally, the complex nerve-control of the act of swallowing will become impaired by such diseases as poliomyelitis, diptheria, or strokes. Rare causes can be myasthenia gravis—a poorly understood disorder of nerve-impulse transmission—or an opening (fistula) between the esophagus and windpipe. A common complaint in nervous individuals of a lump or sense of constriction in the throat is usually easily diagnosed because there is no actual demonstrable difficulty in swallowing.

TAPEWORM Tapeworms are a common cause of human parasitic disease. These long, flat, thin worms (which *do* look like "tape") live in the human intestine. The species that most commonly infest man are the beef *(Taenia saginata),* pork *(Taenia solium),* fish *Diphyllobothrium latum),* and dwarf tapeworm *(Hymenolepsis nana).*

Man becomes the host by consuming raw or improperly cooked flesh-food or food or water contaminated with droppings from infected dogs, rats, etc. Thorough cooking will destroy the larvae stages.

The adult tapeworm has a head (scolex) with little hooks or sucking disks attaching it to the bowel lining. This head is followed by a long ribbon-like string of segments (proglottids), each capable of reproducing additional segments or producing eggs. The number of segments range from three to several thousand. Segments and eggs are passed in the stool, and the diagnosis is made by finding them on microscopic examination.

Symptoms. Symptoms of tapeworm are quite variable and depend on both the type and number of worms present and the general health and nutrition of the host. In fully developed cases, there is diarrhea, weakness, anemia, and weight loss despite a surprisingly good appetite.

Treatment. A number of drugs, called vermifuges, are used in an attempt to dislodge the tapeworm. Unless the head is removed, however, new segments and eggs will continue to be produced.

TONGUE The tongue is a muscular organ with a rich blood- and nerve-supply. Its functions include the manipulation and perception of materials placed in the mouth, the initiation of the act of swallowing, and—aided by the nose—the appreciation of taste. This latter function is important in digestion, as the sensation of taste evokes reflexes necessary for the secretion of the indispensable gastric juices. Because of its rich blood-supply, minor injuries are rapidly healed; bacterial infections are rare for the same reason. Vitamin deficiencies resulting in pellagra can cause a severe inflammation of the tongue, but this is now a relatively rare disorder in the United States. The disappearance of the taste buds (papillae) may signal the onset of pernicious anemia, a condition caused by the individual's inability to absorb vitamin B_{12}. An interesting, but benign, condition known as geographic tongue is so named because of the peculiar map-like appearance produced.

ULCER AND ULCERS An ulcer is an erosion of the surface lining of a tissue, usually accompanied by varying degrees of inflammation. Ulcers may occur in any area and can have various causes. Viral or bacterial infections, burns due to heat or caustic chemicals, increased secretion of pepsin and acid by the stomach are common causes of ulcers in the digestive tract. (*See also* in this section PEPTIC ULCERS; ULCER DIET; ULCERATIVE COLITIS.)

ULCER DIET Patients with ulcers of the stomach or duodenum (the first few inches of intestine following the stomach) are usually placed on a bland diet. The principle of the diet is to dilute the acid gastric juice frequently by providing several meals daily of easily digested, palatable, nonirritating foods. Milk is the basic food in a bland ulcer diet; other foods are gradually added as tolerated.

The following types of food neutralize the acid already in the stomach and are therefore included in an ulcer-diet:

- Protein foods such as milk and milk products
- Cereals, chicken, fish
- Foods that are soft and smooth (no raw fruits or vegetables)
- Salt and lemon juice, for seasoning

Meals should be frequent and small in amount so as to take up the acid; three snacks in addition to the regular three meals are usual.

Certain other habits of eating are also recommended:

- Rest before meals if tired or nervous.
- Allow plenty of time for meals and eat slowly.
- Rest fifteen minutes after meals if possible.
- While on the diet, the bowel functions should be kept normal by using orange juice as a natural laxative. Use the juice of one orange in one glass of warm water before breakfast and, if still constipated, repeat this at the noon meal.

Foods which must definitely be omitted from the diet of the ulcer patient are the following:

- Foods highly seasoned with mustard, pepper, vinegar, or other spices
- Meat broths, gravies, nuts, pickles, and hot sauces
- Foods that are ice-cold (ice cream should be partially melted)
- Coffee, carbonated beverages (cola drinks, soda pop, etc.) and alcohol

Below is a sample ulcer-diet menu:

Breakfast:
  Enriched refined cereal with milk and
    sugar
  Egg
  White bread and butter
  Milk or cocoa
  Strained fruit or juice at meal's end

Lunch:
  Cream soup
  Lean meat
  Potato, rice, or spaghetti
  Bread and butter
  Milk
  Strained fruit juice
Dinner:
  Lean meat, fish, or fowl
  Potato
  2 strained cooked vegetables
  Bread and butter
  Bland dessert (custard)
  Milk

Milk, in one form or another, is often recommended between meals and at bedtime. The physician can modify the general principles described here for the individual patient.

However, many physicians believe that a regular diet may be taken in the presence of an ulcer, especially in conjunction with the newer gastric acid suppressants.

ULCERATIVE COLITIS This serious chronic disorder of the colon should not be confused with mucous colitis, a relatively benign functional disorder. Ulcerative colitis is characterized by repeated episodes of severe inflammation and ulceration of the large intestine. The exact causes are not well understood, but emotional factors are thought to play a significant role.

Symptoms. Symptoms of ulcerative colitis include abdominal cramping; as many as ten to twenty bowel movements a day; the passage of blood and mucus from the rectum; and fever, weight loss, and prostration. The attacks may be mild at first, but with repeated episodes of increasing severity the potential seriousness of the illness becomes evident. The ulceration may become so severe that the stool contains little else but blood. With vigorous treatment the disease may become dormant for long periods of time, but then may begin anew. Stools may be relatively normal, depending upon the region of intestine involved. However, between bowel movements there are discharges of blood and pus, and generalized symptoms of fever, nausea, vomiting, and gradual weight loss are seen. The diagnosis can usually be confirmed by direct examination and X-rays.

Treatment. Conditions such as amoebic dysentery (*see* DIARRHEA in this section) must first be ruled out as the treatment is quite dissimilar. The maintenance of adequate nutrition, replacement of blood, control of infection, and a recognition of the emotional aspects of the disease are the foundations of successful therapy. Often the surgical removal of the offending portion of the colon is mandatory.

VOLVULUS A volvulus is an obstruction of the intestine due to the twisting or kinking of a segment of the bowel. This not only prevents passage of the intestinal contents but usually shuts off the blood vessels as well. A volvulus most often occurs in the sigmoid portion of the large intestine because of the peculiar anatomic attachments at this point. The most common predisposing cause is the presence of adhesive bands of scar tissue, often as a result of previous abdominal surgery. Interestingly, a high percentage of volvulus is seen in patients who are vegetarians. It is presumed that this more bulky diet is in some way responsible.

Twisting may occur in other portions of the large intestine but is rare in the small intestine. Because of the disruption of the blood supply to the involved section, gangrene and perforation of the bowel are common if early surgery is not performed. The symptoms are similar to those in any intestinal obstruction. In occasional instances, the twist will right itself, but surgical treatment is usually necessary.

WORMS (ASCARIASIS) Worms are estimated to inhabit 80 percent of the intestines of the two-to-ten year olds at one time or another. The most common worm is the pinworm. This white worm is only about three-eighths of an inch long and is as thick as a piece of thick thread. The adult female comes out of the rectum at night to lay her hundreds of eggs about the anus; this sets up an intense itch, the victim scratches, and gets many eggs on his hands and under the nails. During the day he then transmits these eggs to his toys and clothes, his friends, and of course, to his own mouth. Once the eggs reach the intestines, they hatch and mature, male

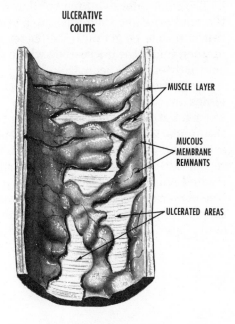

ULCERATIVE COLITIS

MUSCLE LAYER

MUCOUS MEMBRANE REMNANTS

ULCERATED AREAS

Colitis is an inflammation of the mucous membrane and walls of the large intestine, in the pathologic picture of which ulceration predominates. Ulceration generally begins in the rectum and spreads upward, eventually involving the entire colon. The symptoms are fever, malaise, prostration, persistent diarrhea, and the passage of blood, mucus, and pus.

meets female, the female is fertilized, and the cycle is repeated.

Some children are much more susceptible because they suck their thumbs, pick their noses, or for some reason or other have their hands frequently in contact with their faces. Pinworm infestation is not caused by eating candy or sitting on cold cement; furthermore, pinworms come from other humans and not from animals.

Symptoms. Worms will not cause convulsions. The usual symptoms are an itchy anal area, wakefulness at night, stomachaches, and a grouchy disposition. The best method of diagnosing the condition is to inspect the anal region about an hour after the child has retired at night. A strong light is used and the worms may be seen coiling and twisting about, and in a girl even crawling into the vagina, where they may occasionally carry infection, such as vaginitis.

Worm eggs are microscopic and cannot be seen by the naked eye. For accurate diagnosis it is recommended that the sticky side of transparent adhesive tape be placed against the anal area and then taped to a glass slide; this can then be given to the doctor to be examined under the microscope where the characteristic eggs are seen.

Treatment. Newer and more effective medicines are now on the market to kill pinworms, but physical cleanliness (especially of the hands) is a vital part of the treatment; otherwise the worms will soon be back. It is also recommended that whole neighborhoods be treated simultaneously, for even if a child is free of worms he will soon get them from his untreated playmates. It is no longer considered a sign of unclean living to be afflicted with worms; it is merely a sign that a child has friends who may have worms.

ZOLLINGER-ELLISON   SYNDROME
This is a disorder comprising an increased gastric acid level, peptic ulcer disease, and a non-insulin producing pancreatic tumor.

Symptoms. Peptic ulcers, diarrhea, fatty stools, and abdominal cramping are the most common symptoms.

Treatment. High dose anti-ulcer drugs are now the preferred initial treatment. Surgery, reserved for severe non-remitting cases, may involve removal of portions of the pancreas and stomach.

GLANDULAR CONDITIONS

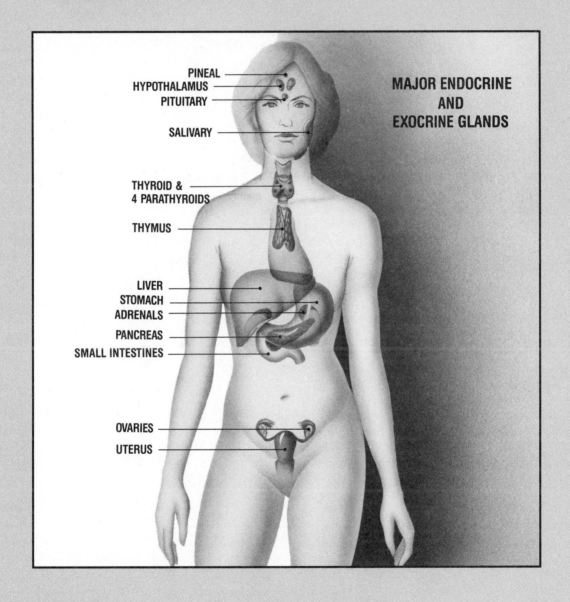

PINEAL
HYPOTHALAMUS
PITUITARY

SALIVARY

THYROID &
4 PARATHYROIDS

THYMUS

LIVER
STOMACH
ADRENALS
PANCREAS
SMALL INTESTINES

OVARIES
UTERUS

MAJOR ENDOCRINE
AND
EXOCRINE GLANDS

The glandular system provides for the normal functioning of the body and for the interrelationship of the various organs in the body. The internal secretion glands comprise a network of tissues that manufacture chemical messengers called hormones. These hormones may travel to distant sites through the bloodstream to stimulate activity in a target tissue.

There are two main types of glands: those that secrete substances directly into the digestive tract or the skin (exocrine or duct glands) and those that secrete directly into the bloodstream (endocrine or ductless). This section examines the various glands of the body and how they function, the disorders resulting from overproduction or underproduction of hormones and possible avenues for treatment. *See also* the questions on glandular trouble (Q-29, Q-30) in the section QUESTIONS AND ANSWERS ABOUT COMMON SYMPTOMS.

The following is a list of terms identified in this section:

ACROMEGALY
ACTH
ADDISON'S DISEASE
ADRENAL GLANDS
ADRENALIN (EPINEPHRINE)
ADRENOGENITAL SYNDROME
ANDROGENS
CORTISONE
CRETINISM
CUSHING'S SYNDROME
DIABETES INSIPIDUS
DUCTLESS GLANDS
DWARFISM, PITUITARY
ENDOCRINE ADENOMATOSIS
ENDOCRINE SYSTEM
ESTROGENS
GIGANTISM
GOITER
GRAVES' DISEASE
GROWTH HORMONE
HERMAPHRODITISM
HORMONES
HYPERPARATHYROIDISM
HYPERGLYCEMIA

HYPERINSULISM (OVERPRODUCTION
   OF INSULIN)
HYPOGLYCEMIA
HYPOPARATHYROIDISM
HYPOPITUITARISM
HYPOTHYROIDISM
MYXEDEMA
OVERACTIVE THYROID
   (HYPERTHYROIDISM)
PARATHYROID GLANDS
PAROTID GLANDS
PITUITARY GLAND, ANTERIOR
PITUITARY GLAND, POSTERIOR
PITUITARY TUMORS
PUBERTY
SIMMONDS' DISEASE
STEROID HORMONES
THYMUS GLAND
THYROID GLAND
THYROIDITIS
UNDERACTIVE THYROID
   (HYPOTHYROIDISM)
VASOPRESSIN

ACROMEGALY   In this condition there is enlargement of the hands and feet, with marked prominence of the jaw, thickness of the lips and tongue, and unusual enlargement of internal organs. The disease develops gradually and is usually accompanied by se- vere headaches. It is caused by a tumor of the anterior pituitary gland. As the tumor grows pressure develops against the optic nerves, producing defects in vision. Effects on the other endocrine glands ensue when the tumor grows to such a size that it destroys by pres-

113

sure the remainder of the anterior pituitary gland. Activity of the thyroid, adrenals, and sex glands is depressed.

Treatment. Treatment is by surgical removal or by X-ray irradiation of the tumor. The latter form of treatment is usually preferred and is very satisfactory—particularly where the radiation dose can be accurately delivered to the pituitary gland by modern techniques.

ACTH   ACTH is the abbreviation for *adrenocorticotrophic hormone*. It was first made available for clinical testing in 1946. This hormone is secreted by the anterior pituitary gland and stimulates the adrenal glands to secrete cortisone and other substances. It is the normal regulator of adrenal gland function in healthy people. It has been extracted from pituitary glands and in purified form is used in the treatment of some forms of arthritis, lupus erythematosus, and severe skin disorders. The beneficial effects of injected ACTH result from its stimulation of the adrenal gland cortex, which releases large quantities of naturally formed cortisone.

ADDISON'S DISEASE   This condition occurs when the adrenal glands are absent or completely inactive. In former years tuberculosis of the adrenal glands was a common condition and often responsible for their inactivity; recently, however, it is more common to find atrophy of the glands without demonstrable cause or inactivated after prolonged use of steroid drugs and in some acute septic states. Thus persons with diseases that require cortisone-type drugs for months or longer will experience atrophy of their adrenal glands. If they stop taking these drugs suddenly, without tapering off, they may have a sudden onset of an Addisonian-like state. A sudden acute adrenal insufficiency has been observed in overwhelming bacteremias in which there may be hemorrhage into the adrenal glands. The glands are also removed surgically in some cases of Cushing's disease.

Patients with Addison's disease are constantly in a precarious state of health. If untreated, they may go into shock and collapse at any time and even die suddenly. Usually they are subject to repeated attacks of vomiting and weakness with severe drop in blood pressure. The discovery of cortisone has been life-saving to such persons. Fortunately, cortisone can be easily administered by mouth and is effective in relatively small doses. Sometimes, however, patients with Addison's disease will need to take an additional substance to promote retention of salt, which in this disease characteristically leaves the body excessively via the kidneys.

ADRENAL GLANDS   The two adrenal glands rest atop the two kidneys in "cocked hat" fashion. The glands are composed of an outer layer (cortex) and an inner zone (medulla). The adrenal cortex secretes cortisone, as well as hormones which have some masculinizing properties. In excessive doses some of these diminish muscle, redistribute fat, and raise the blood sugar (Cushing's syndrome). Still another substance (aldosterone) secreted by the adrenal cortex regulates the body content of salt and water. The adrenal medulla is closely related to the sympathetic nervous system and secretes adrenalin (epinephrine).

ADRENALIN (EPINEPHRINE)   The secretion of the inner portion of the adrenal glands (medulla) is known as adrenalin (epinephrine). It is responsible for producing contraction of smooth muscle and is therefore capable of elevating the blood pressure by constricting the small arteries. It may also produce an increase in pulse rate, perspiration, and a general feeling of fright. Its secretion helps the individual to cope with stressful experiences.

Secretion of adrenalin is increased in the body when a rare type of tumor (a pheochromocytoma) is present in one of the adrenal glands. This produces a very serious condition, responsible for episodes of rapid pulse and high blood pressure, and is treated by a delicate surgical operation.

Injected adrenalin is useful in the treatment of asthma, hives, and other allergic reactions and is always to be found in any list of emergency drugs.

ADRENOGENITAL SYNDROME   This very serious condition occurs when the adrenal glands overproduce androgen (male hormone).

In adults it may be due to benign hyperplasia (overgrowth) of adrenal cortex tissue or to an actual adrenal tumor (which may be benign or malignant).

Symptoms. Women afflicted with this adrenal disturbance develop increased body hair growth, a beard, thinning of scalp hair, loss of feminine body configuration, increased muscle strength, and deepening of the voice. Sexual interest may be increased but no homosexual (lesbian) tendencies are noted if they were not present before.

Treatment. Treatment is by surgical removal of a tumor if one can be found, or by long continued administration of cortisone if benign hyperplasia is diagnosed by appropriate testing, which consists of measuring the adrenal secretions in a urine sample.

In children, the disorder is spoken of as congenital (prenatal) androgenic adrenal hyperplasia. It is due to a biochemical block in the manufacture of cortisone by the adrenal cortex. The hormones produced in place of cortisone are masculinizing in their effects. If they are present in prenatal life in males, they produce increased growth of the normal male genitalia, which is obvious at birth. In female babies, prenatal stimulation with androgens (male hormone) affects differentiation of urogenital structures, so that at birth casual inspection may cause confusion about the child's sexual identity. Sometimes the genitalia appear so much like normal male structures that the male sex is erroneously assigned. Once many such individuals were considered to be true intersexes (*see* HERMAPHRODITISM in this section) and were raised as boy or girl depending largely on the appearance of the genital structures. Cases are known of girls with large clitorises and scrotal-appearing labia, raised as boys, and accepting the male role, until puberty when menstruation, breast development, or other evidences of femininity assert themselves. This occurrence can be a psychological catastrophe, and careful consideration must be given to the future of the individual when the true sex is made known. Some adolescents are mature enough to decide intelligently whether they wish to undergo an apparent "transformation" to their true sex (feminine), in which case appropriate plastic surgery and hormone therapy will usually permit a completely successful assumption of the feminine role. If continuation of the sex of rearing (male) is elected, the individual must be told that extensive plastic surgery including removal of ovaries and breasts must be performed, and that reproduction will not be possible, although a moderately satisfactory sex life may be pursued.

In view of the tremendous psychologic impact of a change in sex, most authorities agree that the sex in which a child is reared should not be changed unless this change can be made before the age of two and one half years, or when the individual is sufficiently mature to understand and adapt to the transformation.

Treatment. Even though adrenogenital syndrome is serious and frightening to the parents, treatment is easy and satisfactory consisting of administration of cortisone by mouth. This must usually be continued throughout life in order to prevent return of the abnormal adrenal secretions.

ANDROGENS The characteristic hormonal secretions of the testes are known as androgens. These are steroid chemical substances, secreted into the bloodstream, which stimulate the muscles, bones, and skin to produce the characteristic changes associated with masculinity. Smaller amounts of androgens are also found in adrenal and ovarian secretions. Preparations of androgen are available for injection and oral use in therapy.

CORTISONE The most important secretion of the adrenal cortex is cortisone, which belongs to the family of substances known as steroid hormones or corticosteroids. They are lacking in patients with Addison's disease and in those who have had their adrenal glands removed; their secretion is low in patients with Simmond's disease and other forms of hypopituitarism.

Cortisone is obviously the treatment of choice in patients whose adrenal cortex activity is either low or nonexistent. It is also used—in much larger dosage—to treat rheumatoid arthritis, lupus erythematosus, and other diseases of connective tissue, as well as asthma and allergies.

CRETINISM   A dwarfed individual who also lacks a functioning thyroid gland is known as a cretin. Children with this disease may be readily recognized by a trained observer: even in early infancy, a cretin has a dull facial expression, lack-luster eyes, a runny nose, and a thick protruding tongue; the hair is dry and there is an excess of it on the skin of the body. When the child begins to walk—at a rather late age—there is a swaybacked and potbellied appearance. All reactions are slowed, and development of speaking, walking, bowel- and bladder-training, and self-feeding are delayed. In some iodine-poor areas of the world this condition is common, and is known as endemic cretinism. Cretinism also appears sporadically and may be due to destruction of the thyroid before birth by antibodies developed in response to material from the mother's thyroid which enters the fetal circulation. It may also be due to other unknown toxic substances.

Diagnosis of this condition is quite easy for a physician with some experience in treating children. When there is doubt about the exact diagnosis, however, blood tests may be helpful. The thyroid usually registers low in cretinism. Also helpful is an X-ray taken to reveal several centers of bone growth: these appear spotty and fragmented in cretinism. When even after all available tests there still is doubt about the diagnosis, thyroid hormone is usually administered for several weeks. If the child is not a cretin, no response will be evident. In the cretinoid child, on the other hand, dramatic changes occur after administration of thyroid hormone. In the event that the diagnosis is still in doubt, further administration of thyroid substances can do no harm, and may be of great value in the long run.

Treatment. A number of thyroid hormone preparations are on the market which are inexpensive, effective, and readily available everywhere. The hormone is administered by mouth, and may be given dissolved in milk in very young infants, or on a spoon with soft foods. It is important that the medication be given regularly and in the prescribed amounts. If doses are omitted, the child may fail to develop a normal mentality. One of the most tragic sights encountered by the physician is the child or adolescent who appears normal in all respects except for mental development, and who has a history of cretinism which remained untreated until the age of three or four. Once mental deficiency exists, it may be accurately diagnosed; but nothing can be done to accelerate the mental development of youngsters afflicted with it.

CUSHING'S SYNDROME   Cushing's syndrome is a hormonal disorder in which excessive amounts of cortisone are secreted by the adrenal glands. It may arise because the pituitary gland drives the adrenal gland to oversecrete, or as a primary disorder of the adrenal itself.

Symptoms. Symptoms may include obesity, hypertension, hirsutism, fatigue, and edema. The face is characteristically rounded, appearing "moon face," and plethoric. Patients with Cushing's frequently have diabetes.

Treatment. One treatment consists of the surgical removal of the tissue producing the excessive hormone. Other treatments involve medications and irradiation.

DIABETES INSIPIDUS   In this rare disorder, which is unrelated to diabetes mellitus, damage to the posterior portion of the pituitary gland causes the passage of large volumes of water in the urine due to the disruption of the secretion of antidiuretic hormone. In some cases as much as twenty-five quarts of urine per day may be excreted, compared to the normal amount of about one quart per day.

Symptoms. There is excessive thirst with affected individuals perhaps consuming as much as fifteen quarts of water daily. Diagnosis of this condition is sometimes difficult because people with certain nervous disorders are also inclined to drink large amounts of water.

Treatment. Treatment of diabetes insipidus is with a posterior pituitary hormone that restores the body's antidiuretic ability. This hormone may be taken by injection, in tablet form, or by blowing a powder into the nose. Treatment is usually lifelong, although some cases have improved spontaneously.

DUCTLESS GLANDS   Glands which secrete their products directly into the bloodstream, instead of through ducts into the other organs or to the exterior of the body, are known as ductless or endocrine glands. (*See also* Endocrine System in this section.)

DWARFISM, PITUITARY Failure of the peanut-sized pituitary gland at the base of the skull to secrete growth hormone before the age of maturity results in dwarfism. Pituitary dwarfs retain their childlike body proportions and do not undergo the normal prepuberal growth spurt. Because sexual maturation is absent or incomplete, older pituitary dwarfs may be considered by untrained individuals to be simply small children. Growth retardation is often apparent in early childhood: on the other hand, slow growth may continue into the mid-twenties, with eventual heights of four to four and one-half feet.

When failure to develop into adulthood becomes evident, the pituitary origin of the problem is suspected. If the entire pituitary gland is nonfunctional, as may occur with certain congenital anomalies and tumors, the child will also have signs of deficiency of thyroid and adrenal secretion. In about half the cases of pituitary dwarfism, the cause cannot be found. Intelligence is usually normal unless there is an associated thyroid deficiency or abnormality of the brain, either of which by itself would produce lack of mental development. Emotional immaturity is often present because dwarfed children continue to be treated by adults as though they were younger.

Because our knowledge of growth hormone is still incomplete, it is often not possible to make an accurate diagnosis of pituitary dwarfism at an early age. Until the age of one or two years, the child may appear to be as fully developed as other children. When concern about growth is brought to the attention of the physician, he must consider such things as family background, nutrition, and the presence of other congenital or hereditary diseases which limit growth and the function of other glands—particularly the thyroid. One of the specific laboratory tests for diagnosing pituitary dwarfism consists of measuring growth hormone (GH) in the blood after injection of insulin or the substance arginine.

Treatment. The treatment of pituitary dwarfism will undoubtedly undergo revolu-

GLANDS

Exocrine glands (with ducts) empty into intestines or onto the skin.

Endocrine glands (ductless) empty directly into the blood stream.

tionary changes in the next few years. Use of the new gene technology in cells in modern laboratory techniques has made growth hormone much more available and should make dwarfism a treatable disease. For those individuals who have associated deficiencies in other endocrine glands, it is possible to obtain maturation and some degree of growth by treatment with thyroid substance, adrenal hormones, and—at the proper age—with male or female sex hormones. It is very important that persons having daily contact with those afflicted with pituitary dwarfism should be aware of the nature of their problem so they may be handled in accord with their age, and not with their height. This applies especially to parents and other relatives, teachers, social workers, schoolmates, and playmates. With proper care dwarfed individuals will have a normal life expectancy.

ENDOCRINE ADENOMATOSIS This condition exists when benign secreting tumors arise simultaneously in several endocrine organs. Although rare, it is important for the physician to recognize. Tumors may be seen at one and the same time in the parathyroid, the pancreas, and the pituitary, each of which produces its own characteristic effects which mingle with the effects of the tumors in the other glands. This complexity makes the entire disease picture exceedingly difficult to diagnose. Surgery for the tumors is the basic approach.

ENDOCRINE SYSTEM The group of glands which secrete their products directly into the bloodstream are known collectively as the endocrine (ductless glands) system. The glands are to a great extent interrelated, the thyroid, adrenal glands, and sex glands being dependent for their normal functioning on secretion of the pituitary gland. It is for this reason that the pituitary is known as the "master" or controlling gland. The function of the pituitary gland is in turn regulated by a "feedback" mechanism which permits the pituitary to turn off its supply of hormones when they are not needed. Thus we may speak of a pituitary-thyroid or pituitary-adrenal axis which keeps the glandular secretions in balance.

ESTROGENS Hormones produced by the ovaries, the estrogens are responsible for the

GOITER

A goiter is an enlargement of the thyroid body, causing a swelling in the front part of the neck.

development of female sex characteristics (development of breasts, general female contour of the body), and the preparation of the uterus for the monthly menstrual flow. Cessation of estrogen-production results in the female climacteric or "change of life." Natural and synthetic estrogens are commercially available and are used for the treatment of various abnormalities caused by estrogen deficiencies.

GIGANTISM When a pituitary tumor of the eosinophil type develops before maturity, it stimulates overgrowth in all body tissues. Because the growth of bone is not complete, such afflicted individuals grow to an excessive height. In addition, there occur some of the features described under ACROMEGALY in this section, and the treatment approach is similar.

GOITER When the thyroid gland becomes enlarged for any reason, it is spoken of as a goiter. Various forms of goiter occur: the toxic goiter with hyperthyroidism; the nontoxic goiter present with iodine deficiency or due to congenital or hereditary disturbances; and swelling of the thyroid in various forms of thyroiditis. The treatment of goiter depends upon its cause. A toxic goiter is treated by surgery or by administration of radioactive iodine or antithyroid drugs. Simple goiter, if due to iodine deficiency, is treatable by administration of iodine in the form of drops or iodized salt. Goiter which is due to congenital disorders is usually best treated by the administration of thyroid hormone.

GRAVES' DISEASE When the thyroid gland becomes overactive and diffusely enlarged, the increased amounts of circulating thyroid hormone produce changes throughout the body. These changes, especially noticeable in the heart and circulatory system, are known as thyrotoxicosis, or Graves' disease (named after the man who described the changes many years ago). Chiefly affected are women between the ages of twenty and forty.

Symptoms. Characteristically, patients with Graves' disease appear highly nervous and overactive. They are quite apt to be emotional and excitable and often complain of intolerance to heat. Weight loss is common; there is excessive perspiration, and a tremor

THE ENDOCRINE GLANDS

THE PITUITARY
The pituitary is a small reddish gland attached to the base of the brain.

THE THYROID
The thyroid is a large reddish gland located in front of, and on the sides of the trachea.

THE PARATHYROIDS
The parathyroids are four small nodes located on the back of the thyroid.

THE ADRENALS
The adrenals are paired yellowish glands located above the kidneys.

THE PANCREAS
The pancreas is a large gland located below and behind the stomach. Only the Isles of Langerhans are endocrine in function.

THE TESTES
The testes, the male reproductive glands, are located in the scrotum. They correspond to the female ovaries.

is often noticeable. The eyes usually present a staring appearance and often bulge noticeably; indeed, eye symptoms may be the most prominent and serious feature of Graves' disease. Diagnosis is made by measuring the circulating thyroid hormones and in more recent years by the use of the radioactive iodine-uptake test. (For many years the basal metabolic rate was a standard test; this is usually elevated by 30 or 40 percent when Graves' disease is present.)

Treatment. A number of so-called "antithyroid drugs" are available for temporary alleviation of this condition; however, they are rarely capable of producing a lasting cure. The two definitive forms of therapy are surgery and administration of radioactive iodine. Before surgery can be performed, it is necessary to bring thyroid overactivity under control by means of antithyroid drugs and iodine; radioactive iodine, on the other hand, is usually administered without prior preparation.

Because of the unpredictable nature of Graves' disease, it may be expected that a good number of the patients treated either by surgery or radioactive iodine will develop permanent underactivity of the gland— hypothyroidism. This is easily treated by administration of thyroid hormone, however, and is a much less dangerous and formidable condition than is Graves' disease itself. In a few individuals the eye protrusion becomes worse after treatment of the thyroid condition. If the eyes become too irritated or swollen, surgical removal of a portion of the bony orbit may become necessary. Often, however, the protrusion will stabilize after several months and slowly recede.

GROWTH HORMONE

This product of the pituitary has been actively investigated in recent years and is now available in a few clinical centers for experimental administration to human beings. Its availability up until recently was limited by the availability of human pituitary glands at autopsy. The recent development of new genetic techniques has made it possible to harvest the hormone from specially treated cells in tissue culture. It will greatly increase the availability of growth hormone treatment. (*See also* DWARFISM, PITUITARY; GIGANTISM in this section.)

HERMAPHRODITISM

This rare condition is named after the Greek god Hermes and the Greek goddess Aphrodite. In mythology, their child Hermaphroditos possessed the traits of both sexes, and the name has been applied to conditions which represent male and female features in the same individual. True hermaphrodites have one or more testicles and one or more ovaries. The individual may have the physical appearance of a male or female, depending on the predominance of the ovary or the testis. Often the true hermaphrodite will appear to be a completely normal female who is found at surgery to have testes in the groin region. (*See also* ADRENOGENITAL SYNDROME in this section.)

HORMONES

A hormone is a substance of complex chemical composition secreted by an endocrine gland directly into the bloodstream, traveling to organs and tissues where it stimulates chemical reactions. Glands which secrete hormones are the pituitary, thyroid, adrenals, male and female sex glands, and the parathyroid. (Hormones are also secreted by the stomach, liver, and kidney, but these are not as well understood.) Hormones are used in the treatment of deficiencies of the glands which normally manufacture them. Certain hormones have been synthesized in the laboratory; most important of these are cortisone, thyroxine, and sex hormones. Thyroid, cortisone, and sex hormones may be given by mouth. Insulin and ACTH are examples of hormones which must be given by injection.

HYPERPARATHYROIDISM

Excessive parathyroid secretion (hyperparathyroidism) may be produced by generalized enlargement of the parathyroid glands or by a growth in one of them.

Symptoms. The most indicative finding in hyperparathyroidism is an elevated level of calcium in the bloodstream. It is this hypercalcemia which is the cause of the other symptoms of the condition. The increased level of calcium in the blood produces a high level of calcium in the urine. When the calcium becomes too concentrated in the urine, it precipitates in the small tubules of the kidney or in the larger collecting ducts. Stones form and may cause severe pain or destruction of kidney tissue. When there is widespread calcification of the kidneys, much of their function is lost and the patient develops kidney failure (uremia) often resulting in death. In hyperparathyroidism it is also common to experience abdominal pain due to ulcers of the stomach and duodenum.

Treatment. The only known treatment for hyperparathyroidism is surgical removal of the enlarged glands. The operation is delicate but carries little risk in the hands of a skilled surgeon.

HYPERGLYCEMIA *See* the section MISCELLANEOUS HEALTH CONDITIONS.

HYPERINSULISM   (OVERPRODUCTION OF INSULIN) This very rare condition is due to a tumor of the Isles of Langerhans in the pancreas. Fortunately, it is usually amenable to surgical treatment by removal of the isle-cell tumor.

Some persons often secrete excessive amounts of insulin, so that their blood-sugar is kept low (hypoglycemia) when they are not eating, and the result is an almost constant state of nervous irritability, chronic headache, and fatigue. It is important to distinguish this condition from psychoneurotic states, which will not respond nearly as satisfactorily to the diet therapy discussed under HYPOGLYCEMIA in this section.

HYPOGLYCEMIA Hypoglycemia, which occurs when blood sugar level falls too low, is caused by too much insulin in the system. In diabetics this may be due to an overdose of insulin, too little to eat, strenuous activity, or not eating after insulin has been administered. Sugar or glucose should be given by mouth immediately if the affected individual is conscious and capable of swallowing. If the individual is unconscious, immediate medical attention is required.

Many people who are not diabetic suffer from mild to severe forms of hypoglycemia. Symptoms can include trembling, cold sweating, headache, feeling of fainting, fatigue, and anxiety. A glucose-tolerance test can measure the extent of the condition; a prescribed amount of glucose is taken by the patient on an empty stomach followed by analysis of blood sugar levels at stated intervals.

The prudent hypoglycemic strives to maintain a steady blood sugar level through a high protein diet. He or she eats a "good" breakfast immediately upon rising, does not skip meals or go too long between meals, if necessary having supplemental snacks such as nuts, cheese, or milk during the day and at bedtime. Discreet use of sweets may possibly be included in the diet if taken in conjunction with the necessary protein.

HYPOPARATHYROIDISM When the parathyroid glands are absent or inactive, blood calcium levels fall and a condition ensues known as tetany. This is characterized by spasms of the muscles in various parts of the body, numbness of the fingers, and (sometimes) convulsions.

Although this condition may occur spontaneously, it is more frequently seen in patients who inadvertently have had their parathyroids removed in an operation for removal of the thyroid gland.

Diagnosis is made by measurement of calcium and phosphorus levels in the blood, and by the presence of clinical signs of irritability of the muscles.

Treatment. This condition does not yield to treatment by replacement of the absent hormone (parathormone). In fact, no effective preparation is available for long-term use. It is fortunate, however, that the symptoms may be well controlled by administration of calcium and vitamin D.

HYPOPITUITARISM *See* SIMMONDS' DISEASE in this section.

HYPOTHYROIDISM *See* UNDERACTIVE THYROID in this section.

MYXEDEMA When thyroid activity is very low or absent, the skin becomes thickened and the tissues under the skin become filled with a mucinous thick substance. This condition is spoken of as myxedema. The same term is also often used to refer to the entire symptom complex of hypothyroidism. (*See also* UNDERACTIVE THYROID in this section.)

OVERACTIVE THYROID (HYPERTHY-ROIDISM) Excess secretion of thyroid hormone is characterized by intolerance to heat, increased sweating, loss of weight with increased appetite, shakiness, muscle weakness, and—in some patients—diarrhea, staring eyes, and enlargement of the thyroid gland. The most common cause of hyperthyroidism is the release of excessive amounts of thyroid hormone into the circulation by a diffusely enlarged gland. (*See* GRAVES' DISEASE in this section.) When excess hormone is secreted by a portion of the gland, usually felt as a nodule, the condition is called Plummer's disease.

Diagnosis is made by discovery of a high blood thyroxine level, elevation of the amount of radioactive iodine taken up by the gland during a six or twenty-four hour period, and elevation of the basal metabolic rate. In Plummer's disease (nodular hyperthyroidism) a special scan of the gland after administration of radioactive iodine helps to outline the nodules.

Treatment. (For treatment of diffuse hyperthyroidism *see* GRAVES' DISEASE in this section.) Nodular hyperthyroidism is usually best treated by surgical removal of a solitary nodule or subtotal removal of a multi-nodular gland.

After treatment of hyperthyroidism, it is necessary to observe for signs of low or absent thyroid activity (*see also* UNDERACTIVE THYROID in this section), which is treated by administration of thyroid hormone.

PARATHYROID GLANDS These glands are usually four in number and lie just behind the thyroid gland in the lower neck. Their function is quite well understood: they secrete a substance known as parathormone which regulates the level of calcium in the blood. This activity is accomplished by the hormone's effects on the kidneys and on bone. The parathyroid glands may become completely inactive or may be removed surgically, producing a state of hypoparathyroidism, characterized by painful muscle spasms and convulsions.

PAROTID GLANDS Located in the cheek at the angle of the jaw, the parotids are the largest of the salivary glands. The saliva which they secrete is transported by a duct which opens into the mouth opposite the second upper molar on each side. The parotid glands are affected in mumps, and the swelling is characteristic. In elderly people, acute infections of the parotid glands may result from inadequate fluid intake. Because of the heavy concentration of various salts in the saliva, it is not uncommon for stones to form in the duct, giving rise to rather severe pain and inflammation, termed parotitis. This may subside with administration of local heat, antibiotics, and fluid intake by mouth. Occasionally probing the duct for the obstruction is necessary.

PITUITARY GLAND, ANTERIOR The pituitary gland at the base of the skull is divided into two portions, the posterior and the anterior. It is the anterior or forward portion which is responsible for secreting the hormones regulating the function of the thyroid gland, the adrenals, and the sex glands; in addition, it secretes growth hormone. The anterior pituitary is made of several cell-types, some of which have a secretory function. It may be the site of tumor, hemorrhage, or atrophy, all of these causing it to lose its characteristic function, thus also depressing the function of the glands which it controls.

PITUITARY GLAND, POSTERIOR The rear part of the pituitary gland is a direct extension downward of the brain and is richly supplied with nerves. It is responsible for secreting hormones with powerful effects on the uterus and the smooth muscle of blood vessels. It is also the site of secretion of the antidiuretic (anti-urination) hormone which acts to keep the body from losing too much water through the kidneys. Destruction of the posterior portion of the pituitary gland produces a tremendous increase in the output of urine (diabetes insipidus) together with thirst.

PITUITARY TUMORS Tumors of the pituitary gland are classified according to the type of cell which predominates. Most common is the chromophobe (color-fearing) tumor, so called because the cells do not take up the high color stain which is usually used in the laboratory.

Inasmuch as these cells do not secrete any

of the known hormones, this tumor does not affect the other endocrine glands except by destruction of normal pituitary cells when the tumor becomes large. Treatment is by radiation or surgical removal.

Other types of pituitary tumor do have endocrine effects. Eosinophile tumors of the pituitary produce gigantism or acromegaly. Basophile tumors are thought to produce Cushing's syndrome, but they may not appear until a patient with Cushing's has been treated by surgical removal of the adrenal.

PUBERTY   Puberty is that stage of growth and development when the generative organs achieve the capability of functioning reproductively. In the boy, this is accompanied by the discharge of semen (physiologically observed usually by nocturnal emission—the so-called "wet dream"), deepening of the voice, and development of pubic and facial hair.

In the girl, it is marked by the menarche (onset of menstruation), development of the breasts, and an interest in feminine attractiveness (dress, hair, cosmetics, etc.).

In psychiatry, puberty is the physiological milestone on the road to psychosexual development heralding the advent of heterosexuality. (*See* specific entries in the sections FEMALE HEALTH CARE and MALE HEALTH CARE.)

SIMMONDS' DISEASE   This term is used to describe the condition resulting from the destruction of the anterior pituitary gland either by disease or injury. It is accompanied by wasting of the body musculature, emaciation, generalized weakness, loss of body hair, thinning of the skin with accompanying yellow coloration, low sex drive, and manifestations of deficiency in the other endocrine organs. It is treated by administration of hormones to replace the deficiencies found in all endocrine organs governed by the pituitary—thus, cortisone, thyroxine, and sex hormones.

STEROID HORMONES   These chemical substances consist of four rings of carbon atoms with attachments of hydrogen and oxygen. Carbon-containing side chains are present in some compounds. Metabolic reactions in the adrenal glands and the sex glands are responsible for the manufacture of steroid hormones; their configurations are character-

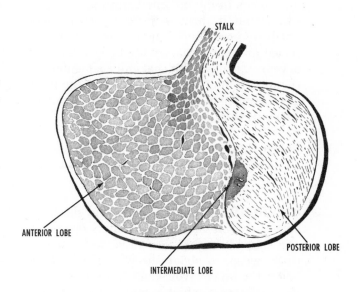

THE PITUITARY GLAND
(THE MASTER ENDOCRINE GLAND)

STALK

ANTERIOR LOBE

POSTERIOR LOBE

INTERMEDIATE LOBE

The anterior lobe produces at least six chemicals (hormones). These exert control over the other endocrine glands and the body in general. The posterior lobe secretes two hormones which control urine output and uterine muscular contractions. The function of the intermediate lobe is not certain.

istic of the particular gland, and each substance is able to perform a distinctive function within the body.

The chief steroid hormone groupings are the androgens (male hormones), and estrogens (female hormones); the progestins, which are responsible for maintaining pregnancy; and the products of the adrenal cortex (including cortisone). Steroid hormones are available for use in therapy by injection and by mouth. Combinations of progestins and estrogens are used as birth control pills, and some of the adrenal-cortex hormones are used to treat inflammations and diseases of connective tissue.

THYMUS GLAND   This gland is set in the anterior part of the chest known as the mediastinum, just above the heart and great blood vessels. In childhood it is quite large, but decreases markedly in size at adolescence. Until recently its function was not well understood, although it was known to be implicated in the rare disease known as myasthenia gravis in which the muscles fatigue very rapidly with use. During the past several years, however, it has been discovered that the thymus gland is important in the production of antibodies in infants and children; it is very likely that it shrinks in adulthood because antibody-producing function is well established in other tissues of the body. A number of years ago it was felt that enlargement of the thymus in infants was a dangerous condition often responsible for sudden death. In many patients this led to treatment of the gland by means of radiation therapy. It is now believed that such treatment is unnecessary and that the gland would reduce in size without it.

THYROID GLAND The thyroid gland is a structure weighing approximately one ounce and shaped roughly like an H, which is partially wrapped about the windpipe directly below the larynx (voicebox). It secretes a hormone (thyroxin) which is responsible for regulating the rate of metabolic activity in all organs and tissues. For proper functioning of this gland iodine is a necessity, and in regions poor in this element this may be easily supplied in the diet through use of iodized salt.

THE THYROID GLAND

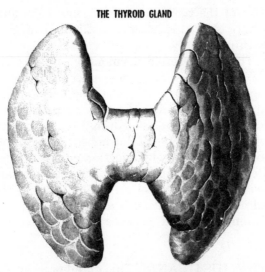

The thyroid is a large reddish, endocrine (ductless) gland located in front of, and on either side of, the trachea. It consists of two lateral lobes and a connecting isthmus.

The thyroid gland is composed of clusters of cells arranged to form pockets filled with a gelatinous substance known as colloid, which contains stored thyroid hormone. When the gland is extremely active, the colloid disappears and the cells become tall and more numerous.

The thyroid is controlled by the pituitary gland through the secretion of thyrotropic hormone. There is also a "feedback" mechanism, whereby depletion of thyroid hormone stimulates secretion of thyrotropic hormone by the pituitary. Should the amount of thyroid circulating in the body be too high, the secretion of thyrotropic hormone by the pituitary is immediately inhibited. Thus, under normal conditions, the secretion of thyroid hormone is kept within a rather narrow range.

The blood thyroxine (T_4) level measures the amount of circulating thyroid hormone. The function of the thyroid gland is also assessed by measuring the uptake of radioactive iodine and by the basal metabolic rate. In an overactive thyroid, one of the standard treatments is its partial removal by surgery (thyroidectomy). Thyroid substance used as medication is prepared from dried thyroid glands of domestic animals. It is prescribed by physicians when either the thyroid or the pituitary is underactive, and also in some cases of obesity and menstrual disturbance.

THYROIDITIS In addition to the other well-known conditions which afflict the thyroid gland, it is frequently the seat of inflammation which is usually nonspecific in origin. (It may be that the gland becomes sensitive to some of its own hormone, thus setting up an inflammatory response which temporarily or permanently inhibits the secretion of thyroid hormone.) This condition is accompanied by pain in the anterior region of the neck, fever, and symptoms and signs of thyroid overactivity. If untreated, this condition slowly subsides, but the individual may be left in a hypothyroid state. Treatment is usually by means of thyroid substance, cortisone, and medication to relieve pain. It is important to distinguish this condition from hyperthyroidism or other afflictions of the gland, as inappropriate treatment may result in permanent damage. Chronic forms of thyroiditis do exist and are called Hashimoto's disease and Riedel's struma. The gland becomes enlarged, firm to the point of simulating a tumor and infiltrated with lymphocytic cells, a finding associated with immunologic disturbance.

The gland is thereby destroyed with resulting hypothyroidism.

UNDERACTIVE THYROID (HYPOTHYROIDISM)

In this condition the amount of circulating thyroid hormone is low. In extreme form, it appears as myxedema or, in children, as cretinism. Not many patients, however, are afflicted with this severe form.

Symptoms. Mild cases of hypothyroidism show easy fatigability, dry skin and hair, increase in body weight, decreased tolerance for cold, and increased nervous irritability. The incidence of hypothyroidism is quite high, as has been demonstrated in several studies in which blood iodine measurements have been taken in the general population. It is often present in people with goiter and in patients previously treated for overactive thyroid conditions. Diagnosis is not always easy because the condition can be confused with anemia, underactive pituitary (hypopituitarism), nervous conditions, and general fatigue states. The basal metabolic rate was once the most useful test in diagnosing this condition. In recent years, however, thyroidologists have developed direct testing for the thyroid hormone in the blood (thyroxine) which measures the functional action in the gland itself and the radioactive iodine-uptake test.

Treatment. Treatment of hypothyroidism is usually quite easy and may be effected with oral administration of a variety of thyroid preparations. Thyroxine itself is available as well as the metabolic product active at the cellular level, triiodothyronine. Treatment must usually be continued for a long period of time, sometimes indefinitely. Usually the individual thus treated will show remarkable improvement in energy, strength, general vigor, and ability to accomplish daily activities.

VASOPRESSIN

Vasopressin (anti-diuretic hormone) is secreted by the posterior pituitary gland and is responsible for stimulating contraction of smooth muscle, especially of blood vessels. It also promotes the absorption of water by the kidney tubule, thus producing a urine-reducing (antidiuretic) action. Lack of vasopressin is responsible for a condition known as diabetes insipidus.

Musculoskeletal Conditions

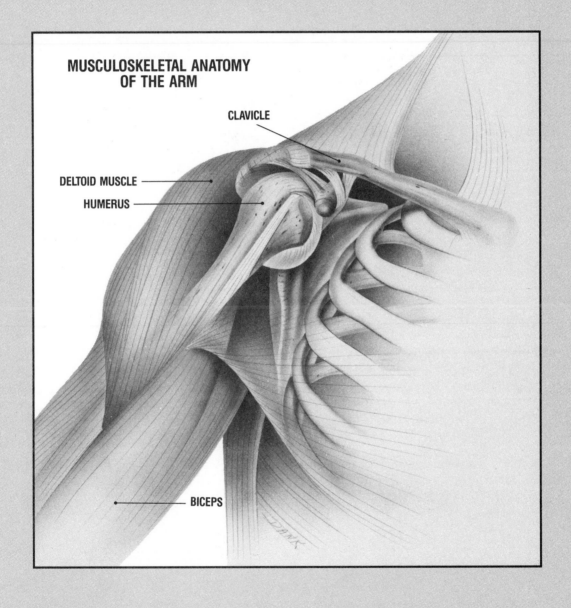

MUSCULOSKELETAL ANATOMY
OF THE ARM

CLAVICLE

DELTOID MUSCLE

HUMERUS

BICEPS

The musculoskeletal system provides the framework for the body and makes possible its range of movement. Bones, muscles, ligaments, tendons and joints are involved in all motions from writing or playing an instrument to throwing a ball and walking.

This section identifies the body's bone and joint structure, defines certain common disorders of the musculoskeletal system, and presents possible mode of treatments. Physicians who specialize in the field of orthopedics are best qualified to determine the source of these complaints. *See also* the questions on lower back pain (Q-50, Q-51, Q-52); thickening in the finger joints (Q-53); and neck pain (Q-54) in the section QUESTIONS AND ANSWERS ABOUT COMMON SYMPTOMS.

The following is a list of terms identified in this section:

ADHESIVE CAPSULITIS
ARTHRITIS
ARTHRITIS, DEGENERATIVE, OR
  OSTEOARTHRITIS
ARTHRITIS, GOUTY
ARTHRITIS, INFECTIOUS
ARTHRITIS, RHEUMATOID
BONES AND JOINTS
BURSITIS
CLAWFOOT (PES CAVUS)
DISLOCATION OF THE KNEECAP
  (PATELLA)
DISLOCATIONS
FLATFOOT
FOOT PROBLEMS, ADULT
GOUT
HERNIATED DISK
KNOCK-KNEES
LEG CRAMPS

LIGAMENTS AND SPRAINS
LOW-BACK PAIN
MEDIAL TIBIAL TORSION
METATARSUS VARUS
MUSCULAR DYSTROPHY
ORTHOPEDIC CONDITIONS, CHILDHOOD
ORTHOPEDICS
OSTEITIS
PERTHES' DISEASE
PHYSICAL THERAPY AND EXERCISE
RECTUS MUSCLE
REHABILITATION
RHEUMATISM AND ARTHRITIS
SCIATICA
SCOLIOSIS
SHOULDER, PAINFUL
SLIPPED CAPITAL FEMORAL EPIPHYSIS
TENDINITIS

ADHESIVE CAPSULITIS A syndrome in which the shoulder is limited in its motion by pain and also by fibrous capsular adhesions, adhesive capsulitis is frequently the result of bursitis in which inadequate exercise was performed and adhesions formed. It may also result from inactivity of the shoulder, as, for example, when the wrist is immobilized by a cast for a fracture and the shoulder is not adequately exercised; thus, this condition often occurs in bedridden patients who are not receiving adequate shoulder exercises. These various causes are mentioned in detail so as to stress the importance of preventing this painful, disabling syndrome.

Treatment. Treatment of this syndrome is not always completely successful. Physiotherapy, traction, and manipulation play a role in the successful management of the patient.

ARTHRITIS The term arthritis as used by the orthopedist refers to conditions of the joints characterized by varying degrees of pain, swelling, stiffness, and loss of motion. There are innumerable causes of such conditions. (*See also* RHEUMATISM AND ARTHRITIS in this section.)

ARTHRITIS, DEGENERATIVE, OR OSTEOARTHRITIS Degenerative arthritis is the most common form of arthritis in the United States. It is due to the wear and tear of ill-matching (incongruous) joint surfaces rather than to a specific inflammatory disease, as rheumatoid or gouty arthritis. When generalized, osteoarthritis is a manifestation of the aging process; when localized in one joint, it is usually the result of previous deformation of the joint. For example, osteoarthritic involvement of one hip may be due to old Perthes' disease, while osteoarthritis of a knee may be the result of a severe knock-knee deformity.

Symptoms. Osteoarthritis is usually manifested in the weight-bearing joints of the body, since these joints are subject to far more wear and tear than the joints of an upper extremity. However, it is common in the finger joints especially in women and for some reason seldom affects the ankle. The osteoarthritic patient complains of joint pain which is worse on awakening in the morning than later in the day. If he has pain in the hips or knee, he will experience great difficulty in getting out of low or soft chairs. When loose bodies are present within the joint, the patient will note crackling sounds and locking of the joint.

Treatment. Treatment includes rest of the acutely painful joint and pain-reducing (analgesic) medication. There are no specific drugs now available to treat this mechanical condition. Treatment today is preventive in the early stage, protective during acute flareups, and reconstructive in the advanced degenerative stage.

Any patient with a tendency toward osteoarthritis should keep his weight under control, since obesity places added strain on the already-taxed joints. A cane is very helpful in taking stress off involved limbs. With hip pain, the cane should be used on the opposite side, but it may be more comfortable on the same side in cases of knee pain.

ARTHRITIS, GOUTY This condition presents essentially the same symptoms as infectious arthritis, but it is due to increased uric acid in the bloodstream, not to an offending bacterial organism.

Symptoms. Gout is far more common in men than in women and most commonly involves the big toe; however, all other joints may also be involved. In many cases there are extensive, easily palpable, soft-tissue deposits of uric-acid salts (urates) which are called tophi.

Treatment. Treatment is carried out along several lines: anti-inflammatory drugs are used in acute flare-ups, and in the quiescent periods specific drugs such as allopurinol are used to lower the circulating uric-acid level. Dietary control is also of great help during the quiescent periods. Gouty patients should restrict their intake of fish, meat, and alcoholic beverages, since these contain large amounts of uric acid precursors.

ARTHRITIS, INFECTIOUS This type of arthritis is due to bacterial involvement of a joint. The joint is acutely hot, swollen, and painful. If not rapidly treated, the offending organism will destroy it and lead to ankylosis.

Treatment. Treatment includes antibiotics, joint immobilization, and either suction (aspiration) or drainage. Before the antibiotic era, the result of infectious arthritis was always catastrophic, but now there is a fair chance of healing with preservation of normal joint function.

ARTHRITIS, RHEUMATOID An inflammatory condition of unknown cause, like the other collagen diseases, rheumatoid arthritis appears to be related to the body's immune mechanisms. The blood of rheumatoid arthritis patients contains abnormal amounts of certain proteins, among them a fairly specific substance known as "rheumatoid factor."

Symptoms. In classical rheumatoid arthritis, joint involvement tends to be symmetrical and intermittent. The patient may complain of painful swelling of both wrists or pain in both ankles which begins at much the same time. The symptoms will then abate, only to recur in the future either in the same or in other joints; in severe cases most of the joints of the body will be involved to some degree. Along with the joint swelling, fibrous scarring of the joint capsule and overgrowth (hypertrophy) of the joint's lining wall (synovium) takes place. If untreated, the joint becomes markedly deformed with time.

Treatment. Aspirin has traditionally been used to treat rheumatoid arthritis and even

There are three main types of arthritis:

1 Osteoarthritis
2 Rheumatoid Arthritis
3 Gouty Arthritis

OSTEOARTHRITIS

The most common form of arthritis, occurring most frequently in elderly people, is due to the wear and tear on bones. Thickening of the bones can cause deformity. The joints nearest the finger tips are favorite sites.

RHEUMATOID

This is a chronic, severely disabling inflammatory disease marked by deformity and union of bones.

GOUTY

Gouty arthritis is caused by excess uric acid in the blood. Uric acid deposits in the joints interfere with movement and form enlarged, painful tophi (deposits of sodium urate) around the joints.

NECK

SHOULDER

ELBOWS

SPINE

HIP

WRIST

FINGERS

KNEE

ANKLE

TOE

now provides the mainstay of treatment. It acts to relieve pain and to minimize the inflammatory response around the involved joints. A large number of non-steroidal anti-inflammatory drugs have been developed, referred to as the NSAIDS, of which ibuprofen (Motrin®) is best known. These may be more effective than aspirin and usually are more convenient. Like aspirin all tend to produce stomach irritation and occasionally gastro or duodenal bleeding. In the past decade cortisone and the other steroids have been less widely prescribed for their anti-inflammatory effect. There is some evidence now that the steroids do not affect the progress of the disease, but rather only control the acute symptoms.

An acutely painful joint should be splinted. As soon as the pain and swelling abate, the joint should be vigorously exercised to regain strength and mobility. Physical therapy plays an important role in the overall management of the arthritic patient. Heat in various forms is used to relieve pain and spasm, and gentle manipulation is prescribed to overcome early contractures. Paraffin baths are very helpful in increasing the mobility of rheumatoid hands and may be self-administered by the patient in the home.

Various surgical operations are being developed to reconstruct involved joints and restore motion to stiffened arthritic limbs. Surgery now has much to offer the severely incapacitated arthritic patient and will presumably play an important role in the total care of such patients in the future.

BONES AND JOINTS   Bone provides the rigid supporting structure for the human body. It consists of an abundant calcified "scaffolding" (matrix) which encloses the true bone cells (osteocytes). The long bones consist of an outer shell of dense cortical bone surrounding and enclosing the spongy cancellous bone which, together with the marrow, fills the interior. Surrounding the bone is the periosteum, a fibrous sheath responsible in part for nutrition of the bone and in part for appositional bone growth. Even though bones appear superficially to be rocklike, they are actively live organs and even in their most dense areas have an excellent blood supply.

There are 206 bones in the human skeleton, and they are classified according to shape—flat, irregular, long, and short. (An example of a flat bone would be a rib.) With increasing age bones tend to become more brittle, and scientists are currently discovering some new reasons for this occurrence.

Although bones serve primarily as a support structure, they protect some vital organs, such as the skull's covering the brain. Bones also provide points of attachment for muscles; acting as levers, they make movement possible.

Joints are the articulations between bones. The contour of the joint determines the function it performs. For example, the shoulder joint is a ball-and-socket and therefore allows motion in all directions, while the finger joints are hinged and allow only flexion and extension. The joint surfaces of the bones are capped with cartilage, a slippery, smooth tissue magnificently able to bear weight and allow gliding motion. The joints contain a small amount of lubricating fluid which is secreted by the synovium, the lining wall of the joint. Surrounding the joints and binding them in place are the joint capsules and ligaments.

BURSITIS   This condition is due to inflammation of the gliding surfaces (bursae) which are placed around the joint. Occasionally an acute calcium deposit is also present. Common sites are the shoulder, arm, elbow, and hip.

Symptoms. The patient awakens with acute throbbing pain localized at the shoulder and radiating down to the elbow. The shoulder may be slightly warm to the touch and swelling may be present. All motion of the shoulder is painful, and the patient cannot lift the arm from the side. If X-rays reveal a calcium deposit as the cause of the difficulty, needle suction of this material may completely relieve the pain. Rest in a sling is usually prescribed while the pain is acute; as the pain subsides, vigorous pendulum and figure-eight exercises are useful in restoring motion to the inflamed shoulder: the patient bends forward and toward the painful side, swinging the arm through ever-increasing pendulum arcs for two minutes; then, after a period of rest, the arm is swung through figure-eights for a few minutes. This exercise is repeated three times

BONE AND BONES

Bone is composed of mineral crystals deposited around collagen fibers. These components make it a hard but flexible material.

HEAD

NECK

SHAFT

CANALICULI

LACUNA

MARROW CAVITY

COMPACT BONE

ENLARGED SECTION OF BONE SHAFT

The hollow construction reduces weight and frees the marrow for blood-cell production.

ENLARGED SECTION OF COMPACT BONE SHOWING PART OF A HAVERSIAN SYSTEM

Concentric layers of bone are applied around a center containing a capillary.

ENLARGED SECTION OF THE HAVERSIAN SYSTEM

Bone cells live in the lacunae. The connecting canaliculi transport nutrients from capillary to the cells.

BASIC BONE SHAPES

LONG BONE (HUMERUS)

FLAT BONE (SCAPULA)

IRREGULAR (VERTEBRA)

SHORT BONE (CUNEIFORM)

THE CLASSIFICATION OF JOINTS

IMMOVABLE

Bones are united by a thin layer of fibrous tissue. The sutures of the skull are typical.

SLIGHTLY MOVABLE

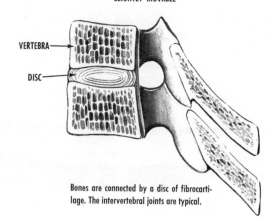

VERTEBRA

DISC

Bones are connected by a disc of fibrocartilage. The intervertebral joints are typical.

FREELY MOVABLE

Gliding joints (the carpal bone joints are typical) permit gliding movement only.

FREELY MOVABLE

HUMERUS

SYNOVIAL MEMBRANE AND CAVITY

BONES COVERED WITH ARTICULAR CARTILAGE

ULNA

Hinge joints (the elbow or humero-ulnar joint is shown) permit only forward and backward movement.

FREELY MOVABLE

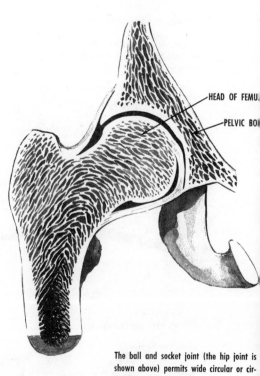

HEAD OF FEMUR

PELVIC BONE

The ball and socket joint (the hip joint is shown above) permits wide circular or circumduction movement.

a day. Aspirin and related groups of drugs are useful in reducing pain and discomfort brought on by bursitis.

CLAWFOOT (PES CAVUS)

Pes cavus, or clawfoot, or high-arched foot is a foot disorder in which the longitudinal arch is abnormally high. It is very often seen with a clawlike contraction of the joints between the toes and the bones behind them. Pain is due to pressure on the foot which is exerted on the heads of these small bones, over which calluses form. Usually there is shortening of the Achilles tendon (the tendon above the heel) which results in further weight being thrown on the front part of the foot.

Treatment. A sponge rubber bar placed across the fore part of the sole or a leather bar similarly placed toward the outer side of the sole of the shoe afford marked relief.

DISLOCATION OF THE KNEECAP (PATELLA)

Dislocation of the kneecap (patella) is a condition in which the kneecap slips out of its groove in the knee joint. The patient usually states that the knee went out of place and then immediately jumped back in place. This may be due to a number of causes, including abnormally shaped kneecaps (patellae), knock-knee, and misshaped knee joints. In most cases the condition is recurrent, and some patients affected with it are afraid to straighten their knees for fear that dislocation will occur. Each fresh episode may inflict damage on the joint surfaces, and this in turn may lead to degenerative arthritis. Treatment of this condition is surgical.

DISLOCATIONS

Dislocations are the result of sprains of such a degree that the normally opposing bones are no longer in place. Dislocations involve greater force than sprains, since the tear is of sufficient magnitude to separate the joint surfaces and to force one or both of the bones out of the joint through a tear in the joint capsule.

Treatment. The object of treatment is gentle, non-damaging reduction of the dislocation and immobilization of the part to allow healing of the tear in the capsule. Failure to recognize a dislocation early may make manipulative reduction impossible, and an open operation may be required.

Perhaps the most common complication of a dislocation is recurrent dislocation of the same part. Recurrences are due to inadequate healing of the capsular tear after the first dislocation and as a rule require surgical repair of the deficient capsular and ligamentous structures.

FLATFOOT

Flatfoot is a layman's term used to describe a loss of height in the longitudinal arch of the foot. In rare cases it may be due to abnormality of the bone, but is usually due to ligament or muscular weakness. Flatfeet are rarely painful in childhood, and most adults with flatfeet are able to lead active lives without any pain or discomfort. If foot discomfort develops, it may be relieved by appropriate shoe modifications such as heel wedges and pads and, if the foot is mobile, by an arch-support.

Some orthopedists feel that children with painless flatfeet should nevertheless be treated by means of shoe modifications and exercises in an attempt to strengthen their weak feet. The patient is taught consciously to try to flex his toes as he walks and to walk with his feet pointing directly forward, vigorously resisting the tendency of his feet to turn outward.

FOOT PROBLEMS, ADULT

Most commonplace adult foot complaints are either due to, or aggravated by, poorly fitting shoes; painful bunions and hammertoes are almost exclusively related to pressure from tight shoes. Improper length is rarely a problem in shoe fit. Improper width and abnormal tapering of the toe box cause most of the difficulties. It is impossible to fit an ellipsoid foot into pointed shoes. Either the foot will deform the shoe or the shoe will deform the foot. Properly fitting shoes should be firm about the heel and amply wide in the toe area.

The fit of a shoe is best checked with the body in the upright position. There should be half an inch of room in front of the big toe, and enough room at the level of the bases of the toes for the foot to be able to move ever so slightly inside the shoe. Any shoe that causes pain is improper and should not be worn.

Shoe modifications (such as arches, insoles, metatarsal pads, and wedges) are helpful in the relief of pain due to static orthopedic deformities. To achieve best results, professional examination by an orthopedist or podiatrist and prescription is advised. If improperly selected, commercially available appliances may increase rather than relieve the painful symptoms.

**FALLEN ARCH
(FLAT FOOT)**

GOUT Gout is a body-chemistry disturbance with recurrent attacks of acute arthritis which may become chronic and deforming. The disease has been known since ancient times and occurs predominantly in middle-aged males. The cause is unknown. It is obviously a disturbance in the processing of vital chemicals known as urate and purine. The protein materials found in the nuclei of cells (nucleoproteins) are the principal source of the body's uric acid; certain foods, such as organ meats (liver, kidney, and sweetbread) and sardines, are the source of purine in the diet. In gout, the serum uric acid level is elevated. Urate deposits, which eventually form small nodules called tophi, are a distinguishing feature. These nodules may be found in cartilage, certain parts of the bone, ligaments, and tendons.

Symptoms. In acute gout there is a sudden, sharp, severe pain, often at night, and not infrequently in the joint of the great toe. The joint becomes swollen and extremely tender. The skin is red, hot, and shiny. There may be fever and chills. Attacks may last for a few days or may persist, with intermissions, for several weeks.

Only after numerous attacks over a period of years in inadequately treated patients will there be permanent deformity. This can take the form of limited motion in many joints of the hands or feet, and sometimes in other joints.

A frequent and sometimes serious complication is kidney disease. This is usually related to urate stones that develop in the kidney.

Treatment. A patient with acute gout responds rapidly to large doses of colchicine. Other forms of arthritis do not respond to this drug. Cortisone derivatives and the nonsteroidal anti-inflammatory drugs (NSAIDS) are also useful.

In recent years a new form of therapy appeared with the development of the drug allopurinol (Zyloprim®). Allopurinol reduces the body's manufacture of uric acid and thus acts on the fundamental mechanism behind the disease. It has to be taken several times per day on an indefinite basis in most patients.

HERNIATED DISK *See* SLIPPED DISK in the section NERVOUS SYSTEM CONDITIONS.

KNOCK-KNEES These disorders in leg growth and development are rarely present at

45°   45°

OUTLINE OF FEET
SHOWING NORMAL
ANGLE IN STANDING

NORMAL RANGE OF FOOT

20° FLEXION

45° EXTENSION

birth and usually are not manifest until the child walks. When either condition is mild, the child may be expected to outgrow it. If it is progressive, however, orthopedic attention is required. The child's diet should meanwhile be checked to make sure that he is receiving adequate milk and vitamin D, since these deformities are commonly seen in rickets, a disease due to vitamin D deficiency. Since these conditions are rarely painful in childhood, treatment is directed toward prevention of disability in adult life. Shoe wedges, manipulation and massage, and occasionally braces may be necessary to treat these deformities.

LEG CRAMPS   One type of painful muscle contraction in the legs (leg cramps) occurs during physical exercise, such as running, jogging, and other sport activities. Usually there is a sudden onset of painful cramping. This type generally subsides within one to two minutes of rest. A second type occurs during rest, often while the person is asleep and affects the calf and foot. Some types of cramping are due to a form of arteriosclerosis or hardening of the arteries.

Treatment. Treatment includes exercise modification for those with activity-related cramping. Certain medications may also be helpful. Weight reduction and smoking cessation are beneficial. Some patients find that the frequency of rest-related cramps are reduced if the diet is supplemented with vitamin E or quinine.

LIGAMENTS AND SPRAINS   The ligaments are bundles of tensile connective tissue specifically placed between adjacent bones. At the joints the ligaments are part of the joint capsule. The ligaments maintain the proper anatomical arrangement between the bones, acting in some instances as protective struts to limit unwanted motion and in others as guy-ropes transmitting force from one bony part to another.

A sprain is an injury to a limb in which ligaments and other soft tissues are torn. Marked pain and swelling are usually associated with it.

Treatment. The object of sprain-treatment is to control the distressing pain and swelling and to allow the torn structures to heal precisely. The sprained limb should be put to rest, and an icebag applied locally in an attempt to prevent further swelling; an elastic compressive dressing may be applied to provide temporary support and to control the pain.

These home measures will in most cases be adequate treatment for minor sprains, but medical attention should be sought if pain and swelling persist for more than a few hours. A severe sprain may require taping, compression dressings, or plaster immobilization to allow adequate healing. Occasionally the tear of the ligaments may be sufficient to warrant surgical repair. Untreated sprains lead to unstable and weak joints, which are then subject to repeated sprains from minor damage which would not be capable of injuring intact joints.

LOW-BACK PAIN   Low-back pain is one of the most common complaints of mankind. It is probably related to man's erect posture since the four-legged animals rarely develop spinal difficulties. The terms lumbago and sciatica are commonly used to describe the clinical syndrome. Lumbago denotes pain localized to the low-back area and is increased by motion of the back; sciatica refers to acute pain in the back, radiating down the back of the leg along the distribution of the sciatic nerve.

Symptoms. A low-back syndrome may develop spontaneously or may follow an injury. The patient may state that his back "gave out" after he bent down to pick up a heavy object. Sciatic pain may or may not be present acutely. The patient describes difficulty in standing erect; his trunk is tilted forward and to the side; and he walks with a halting, painful gait. For many years this syndrome was labeled sacroiliac disease because of the pain localized over the sacroiliac joint, but there is now general agreement that the sacroiliac joint itself is rarely implicated.

Treatment. Mild acute low-back syndromes may be due to muscle sprain and will be relieved by a period of bed rest and a back support. The more severe cases are usually due to herniation of intervertebral disks, the disks sandwiched between adjacent spinal bones (vertebrae). In a severe injury, the retaining ligaments are disrupted and the disk material drops (prolapses) backward, pressing against a spinal nerve root.

Several days to weeks of bed rest on a firm mattress, with or without bed boards, is the usual treatment. When symptoms subside, the patient is slowly allowed to move, and a back brace or corset is prescribed to limit motion and provide some support to the weakened back. Certain rules are helpful for avoiding recurrence of back pain:

- Never lift anything by bending forward at the hips only. Always bend the knees and lift from a squatting position.
- Never sit up in bed with the legs fully extended. Always get out of bed by rolling out sideways.
- Never twist the trunk. Rather, maintain the trunk as a column and turn about at the hips.

The patient should lie down and rest whenever his back "gives out." Even when free of back symptoms, the low-back patient should sleep on a firm mattress and actively protect his back. Most low-back syndromes will be resolved under this regime. With massive disk protrusion and unabating neurological signs, surgery is occasionally required to relieve nerve-root pressure.

MEDIAL TIBIAL TORSION This is a common cause of "in-toeing" in childhood. When this condition exists, the ankle joint and the foot face further inward than the rest of the leg. Tibial torsion is frequently self-correcting with growth, but severe cases may require brace or cast correction. Its cause is unknown, but in some cases at least there is good evidence that it is due to some degree of immobilization of the developing fetus in the uterus. This occurs because there is relatively less amniotic fluid in the last months of pregnancy, and the fetus is more likely to be wedged into place with less room for movement.

METATARSUS VARUS This is a congenital deformity of the foot in which the inner part of the fore region of the foot is elevated, the heel remaining in a normal or slightly turned-in position. Treatment consists of corrective plaster casts which, as they are changed, gradually return the foot to normalcy. The sooner this therapy is instituted, the better the prognosis.

MUSCULAR DYSTROPHY This is a genetic disease with a hereditary characteristic. The disease is marked by a primary progressive atrophy of the muscles. As the weakening and wasting progresses the patient becomes confined to a wheelchair and ultimately to bed. As yet no cure is known. There are a number of distinct forms which involve different groupings of muscles. In the most common, Duchenne muscular dystrophy which appears in boys age three to seven, weakness first occurs in the pelvic and lower extremity musculature. This leads to general weakness, repeated falls, and to the use of a wheelchair by age ten to twelve. The muscles of the shoulder are never involved. Milder combinations of regional dystrophies have been described. Unfortunately no basic treatment is available for any of the hereditary dystrophies.

ORTHOPEDIC CONDITIONS, CHILDHOOD Congenital and acquired childhood musculoskeletal deformities are fairly common. Some of these may be relatively minor and may be self-correcting through normal growth and development. Others (for example, clubfeet) require vigorous therapy and all the ingenuity of the orthopedic surgeon to achieve good results.

ORTHOPEDICS Orthopedics is the surgical specialty concerned with the care of the musculoskeletal system. The word orthopedics is derived from the Greek words meaning straight child, and from the time of Hippocrates to the end of the nineteenth century orthopedists were concerned with the care of children afflicted with congenital or acquired crippling deformities. More recently, orthopedists have also assumed the care of fractures and other injuries to the limbs and spine in adults as well, and presently orthopedic surgeons are making major advances in the surgical management of patients with arthritic conditions. For example, a prosthetic hip can abolish the pain and limitation of an osteoarthritic hip, and knee replacement is similarly available.

OSTEITIS Osteitis is a general term describing inflammatory changes in the bones. A common form of osteitis called osteitis deformans is also known as Paget's disease, and produces characteristic bending and bowing of the extremities with irregular thickening of the skull, visible by X-rays. In osteitis fibrosa cystica the bone has areas of spongy tissue which under X-ray look like holes. This condition is still seen in patients with hyperparathyroidism, but it is not as common as in former years, probably because of the greater availability of calcium in the diet. Surgical removal of the parathyroid tumor of three out of four of overfunctioning glands may lower the blood calcium and the outward flow of calcium from the bones.

PERTHES' DISEASE This is the most common hip malady in the two-to-six-year-old age group. The head of the femur bone, set in the hip, temporarily loses its blood supply and the bone softens, crumbles, and deforms.

Symptoms. The usual symptom is the gradual onset of a painless limp. At the same time, the child may complain of inability to spread his legs as far as usual and of mild pain in the knee. (This knee-pain originates in—is "referred" from—the hip and is not a sign of knee involvement. Many children have had only knee X-rays by mistake when the true seat of disease was in the hips.)

In mild cases, Perthes' disease is a transient problem and may even go unnoticed. In severe cases, however, it requires several years to resolve. If untreated, it results in destruction of the hip joint and in incapacitating degenerative arthritis in adulthood.

Treatment. Since the bone is softened while the deforming force itself is the weight of normal walking, treatment of the disease involves putting the child to bed for several months in order to remove the weight-stress and to allow the femoral head to re-form under the stimulus of its new blood supply. A gradual increase of weight bearing is then allowed, using crutches and an ischial weight-bearing brace, a Sam Browne sling, or an abduction device.

PHYSICAL THERAPY AND EXERCISE
Physical therapy is the technique by which physical means such as light, heat, electricity, and exercise are utilized to help patients overcome pain and increase the strength and mo-

bility of the involved parts. Heat is widely used to relieve tension, relax tense muscles, and increase joint mobility. It may be applied superficially, with a hot-water bottle, heat lamp or hydrocalator packs (warm moist applications) or deeply, with shortwave diathermy or ultrasound. Massage, as applied by a trained therapist, may be very helpful in reducing muscle spasm and in freeing tightened structures. Well-performed massage should be vigorous enough to achieve its goal without being so violent as to inflict damage.

Exercises are planned muscular activities designed to increase limb strength, joint control, and motion. Active exercises are those in which all muscular effort is expended by the patient, while passive exercises are those in which the joint is put through a range of motion by the therapist. Active exercises are superior because the patient, limited by his pain, is unlikely to damage the limb. Passive exercise is hard to control, and the patient is dependent on the therapist's experience.

Walking is considered an excellent exercise for persons in the older age group. In recent years, jogging has been heralded as an important exercise, especially for its tonic effects on the heart and the increment in cardiac capacity that results. A hoped for, although still unproven, effect might be a decrease in coronary artery disease. Progressive jogging should not be undertaken by sedentary or middle-aged persons without prior medical clearance. A general rule is that one should consult his physician when considering any significant change in exercise regime.

Sedentary people may benefit from conditioning exercises, such as those illustrated in "Physical Fitness and Reducing Exercises" (color plates E1 through E8) and Isometrics.

RECTUS MUSCLE This is a long, flat muscle which arises from the pubic bone and is inserted into the cartilage of the lower ribs. It affords protection and aids in bending the trunk. The rectus muscle is divided in its midportion by fibrous tissue. After repeated pregnancies, this tissue occasionally separates allowing the abdominal contents to protrude, and thus causing a ventral (belly) hernia. A binder may help keep the abdominal contents in place, but surgical repair is often required.

REHABILITATION One of the most important public health and educational problems is rehabilitation of those suffering from physical or mental disorders so that they may resume working and supporting themselves. It is now recognized that most handicapped people have both physical and psychological problems and require psychiatric as well as physical rehabilitation.

Among the more important methods of rehabilitation are retraining of the blind; provision of hearing aids and of artificial limbs; muscular retraining for the physically crippled; special job situations for those with physical handicaps; and psychotherapy for those among them who are too emotionally disturbed to be able to work. Perhaps most important in rehabilitation is improvement of self-confidence and morale to such an extent that one wishes to become self-supporting and independent again.

RHEUMATISM AND ARTHRITIS The terms arthritis and rheumatism are used synonymously for afflictions of joints or supporting structures.

Arthritis is inflammation of a joint. However, because arthritis seldom occurs without pain, arthralgia (joint pain) must be linked with it.

Physicians have been trying to establish a classification for arthritic and rheumatic disorders. To date there has been no success. The following classification, based chiefly on causes or alleged causes, is the one generally used.

Due to Specific Agents
(the more common ones)
    Gonorrhea
    Tuberculosis
    Staphylococcus (osteomyelitis)
    Brucellosis

NORMAL AND ABNORMAL POSTURE

The normal vertebral column has three curves — a forward cervical, a forward lumbar, and a backward thoracic. Lordosis is an excessive forward curvature of the ce ' or lumbar curves; kyphosis is an excessive backward thoracic curve.

NORMAL   RELAXED FAULTY POSTURE   KYPHOSIS AND LORDOSIS   LORDOSIS (SWAYBACK)   FLAT BACK

Syphilitic arthritis
Undulant fever
Rheumatoid arthritis
Paget's disease
Osteoarthritis
Rheumatoid spondylitis
Backache (lumbago and sciatica)
  Sprains, strains, and poor posture
  Spondylitis and spondylolisthesis
  Osteoporosis
  Slipped disk
Gout
Lupus erythematosus
Polyarteritis nodosa
Scleroderma
Schönlein-Henoch purpura
Hemophilia
Bursitis

SCIATICA   *See* LOW-BACK PAIN in this section; and SCIATIC NERVE and SLIPPED DISK in the section NERVOUS SYSTEM CONDITIONS.

SCOLIOSIS   Scoliosis is lateral curvature of the spine which may be congenital in origin or due to faulty posture, organic causes such as rickets or spinal paralytic disease, or a series of vertebrae which are constantly deviated from the normal spinal axis. Depending on cause and severity, treatment is special exercises, orthopedic braces, surgery, or a combination of all three.

A common form of scoliosis comes on in adolescence and is attributed to asymmetrical growth in vertebral bodies and may have a hereditary aspect. The condition is more common in girls. It may lead to loss of height and later in life may contribute to impaired respiration and displacement of the heart.

SHOULDER, PAINFUL   Pain in the shoulder may be due to a multitude of causes: it may be a manifestation of generalized arthritic disease, and in some cases represents pain "referred" from internal organs; heart disease, pleurisy, and gallbladder disease may all present symptoms of shoulder pain. Adults with pain in the shoulder not accompanied by tenderness on palpation of the shoulder and not accompanied by limitation of motion should suspect the possibility of internal disease and undergo careful medical evaluation. Bursitis and adhesive capsulitis are the most common local shoulder conditions.

SLIPPED CAPITAL FEMORAL EPIPHYSIS   This disease is an adolescent hip malady showing much the same symptoms as Perthes' disease. What happens is that the growth-center (or epiphysis) of the bone becomes loosened from its attachment to the shaft of the femur and slowly slips into an abnormal position. Since this malady develops in children during puberty, it is thought to be related in some manner to the sex hormones, but no definitive cause has been established. Slipping of the femoral head occurs very gradually, and the child can rarely recall an injury to the hip. If untreated, this condition also leads to degenerative arthritis of the hip. Hip-nailing is usually required to hold the femoral head and neck aligned so that no further slipping occurs.

TENDINITIS   Tendinitis is the inflammatory reaction that occurs when a tendon, the tissue that binds a muscle to a bone, undergoes some form of stress, injury, excessive exercise, or arthritis. Common sites are around the shoulder, hip, and elbow. "Tennis elbow" is a well-known example of tendinitis.

Symptoms. Pain and swelling along the length of the tendon are the typical symptoms.

Treatment. Application of heat or cold, pain relievers, and non-steroidal anti-inflammatory drugs are the customary treatments. In serious cases, steroids are injected directly at the site of the inflammatory reaction. Special exercise may be helpful.

Nervous System Conditions

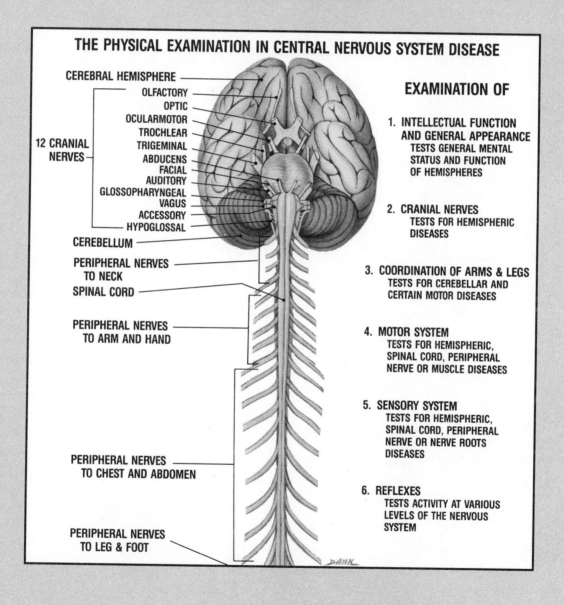

THE PHYSICAL EXAMINATION IN CENTRAL NERVOUS SYSTEM DISEASE

CEREBRAL HEMISPHERE

12 CRANIAL NERVES
- OLFACTORY
- OPTIC
- OCULARMOTOR
- TROCHLEAR
- TRIGEMINAL
- ABDUCENS
- FACIAL
- AUDITORY
- GLOSSOPHARYNGEAL
- VAGUS
- ACCESSORY
- HYPOGLOSSAL

CEREBELLUM

PERIPHERAL NERVES TO NECK

SPINAL CORD

PERIPHERAL NERVES TO ARM AND HAND

PERIPHERAL NERVES TO CHEST AND ABDOMEN

PERIPHERAL NERVES TO LEG & FOOT

DANK

EXAMINATION OF

1. **INTELLECTUAL FUNCTION AND GENERAL APPEARANCE** TESTS GENERAL MENTAL STATUS AND FUNCTION OF HEMISPHERES

2. **CRANIAL NERVES** TESTS FOR HEMISPHERIC DISEASES

3. **COORDINATION OF ARMS & LEGS** TESTS FOR CEREBELLAR AND CERTAIN MOTOR DISEASES

4. **MOTOR SYSTEM** TESTS FOR HEMISPHERIC, SPINAL CORD, PERIPHERAL NERVE OR MUSCLE DISEASES

5. **SENSORY SYSTEM** TESTS FOR HEMISPHERIC, SPINAL CORD, PERIPHERAL NERVE OR NERVE ROOTS DISEASES

6. **REFLEXES** TESTS ACTIVITY AT VARIOUS LEVELS OF THE NERVOUS SYSTEM

The central nervous system is the command center of the body. From the brain and through the spinal cord, commands and directions are sent to the peripheral muscles, the heart and blood vessels. All data collected by the sense organs are also transmitted within the system to the brain.

This section examines the physiology of the nervous system and the common neurological disturbances which may be caused by flaws, chemical imbalances, circulatory problems, inflammation, and other disorders of the system. Physicians in the field of neurology are concerned with examination and treatment of nervous system disorders. *See also* the questions on headaches (Q-34, Q-35) in the section QUESTIONS AND ANSWERS ABOUT COMMON SYMPTOMS.

The following is a list of terms identified in this section:

ACUPUNCTURE	HYPOGLOSSAL NERVES
APOPLEXY	MEDIAN NERVE
ATAXIA	MENINGES
AUTONOMIC NERVOUS SYSTEM	MULTIPLE SCLEROSIS
BERIBERI	MYASTHENIA GRAVIS
BRAIN	NARCOLEPSY
BRAINSTEM	NERVE CELL (NEURON)
BRAIN TUMORS	NERVE FIBERS
CAUSALGIA	NERVOUS SYSTEM
CENTRAL NERVOUS SYSTEM	NEURALGIA
CEREBELLUM	NEURITIS
CEREBRAL EMBOLUS	NEUROLOGIST
CEREBRAL HEMORRHAGE	NORMAL PRESSURE HYDROCEPHALUS
CEREBRAL THROMBOSIS	(NPH)
CEREBROSPINAL FLUID	NYSTAGMUS
CEREBROVASCULAR ACCIDENTS	ORGANIC BRAIN SYNDROME
CEREBRUM	PARESIS, GENERAL
COMA	PARKINSON'S DISEASE
CONCUSSION, BRAIN	PERIPHERAL NERVES
CONTUSION, BRAIN	RADIAL NERVE
CONVULSIONS	REFLEX ARC
CRANIAL NERVES	SCIATIC NERVE
ELECTROENCEPHALOGRAM (EEG)	SENSORY NERVE CELL (NEURON)
EPILEPSY	SHAKING PALSY
EXTRADURAL HEMATOMA	SLIPPED DISK
FACIAL NERVES	SPASTICITY
FACIAL PARALYSIS (BELL'S PALSY)	SPINAL ACCESSORY NERVES
GLOSSOPHARYNGEAL NERVES	SPINAL CORD
HEADACHE	STROKE
HEADACHES, MIGRAINE	SUBDURAL HEMATOMA
HEMORRHAGE, SUBARACHNOID	SYNAPSE
HUNTINGTON'S CHOREA	TRIGEMINAL NERVES

TRIGEMINAL NEURALGIA
ULNAR NERVE
UNCONSCIOUSNESS

VAGUS NERVES
VOLUNTARY NERVOUS SYSTEM
WATER ON THE BRAIN (HYDROCEPHALY)

ACUPUNCTURE More than 2000 years ago the Chinese developed a system of medical treatment called acupuncture. This treatment involves the insertion of needles at specifically designated points on the body, which will then have a beneficial effect on the part of the body that corresponds with the insertion point. Some acupuncture practitioners identify up to 1000 distinctive points on the body that can be used as needle placement sites.

In the West medical authorities are most interested in applying acupuncture techniques as an element in anesthesiology and in the treatment of chronic pain. Acupuncture used as an anesthesia (frequently the needles carry a very slight electrical current) has advantages over conventional methods during surgery. Patients are conscious during the operation, and they rarely experience nausea during recuperation. However, the method has not made any significant inroads into U.S. anesthetic practice. It is not as reliable as our usual methods and critics have pointed out that even in China "supplements" of local or other kinds of anesthesia may have to be used for major surgery.

How acupuncture works is not yet clearly understood. Traditional explanation maintains that the body possesses various energies that often become imbalanced. The proper placement of an acupuncture needle allows these energies to either drain or build up, thus returning the body to a normal, healthy condition. Modern explanations concerning the anesthetic capabilities of acupuncture involve the idea that stimulation of nerve fibers at specific points with acupuncture needles may block the nerve fibers' ability to send impulses of pain or discomfort to the brain.

Further research into the way acupuncture works may yield new applications for its use, such as in the treatment of obesity and narcotic addiction. In the United States acupuncture treatment is restricted to physicians who have been trained in acupuncture procedures.

APOPLEXY Apoplexy is a sudden decrease or loss of consciousness, sensation, and voluntary motor power caused by rupture or obstruction of an artery of the brain. The outstanding finding is usually paralysis of one arm and leg. Occasionally only one extremity, or all four extremities, may be weak or paralyzed. The patient may be drowsy, confused, or completely unconscious. Associated findings include speech disorders, partial blindness, double vision, facial paralysis, or difficulty in swallowing. (*See also* CEREBROVASCULAR ACCIDENTS in this section.)

ATAXIA Ataxia refers to unsteadiness of the arms, trunk, or legs. In the hand and arm it is manifested by difficulty in eating, writing, sewing, and performing other coordinated movements. If the arm is at rest, there is no tremor. However, a rhythmical tremor does develop with purposeful movements. Ataxia of the trunk or legs results in difficulty in walking. The individual walks with his feet apart and has difficulty with balance. He may fall due to difficulty in coordinating leg movements properly.

Cerebellar ataxia is due to failure of development, degeneration, intoxication with alcohol or drugs such as Dilantin® (dimenhydrinate), or abscess or tumors of the cerebellum. When there is involvement of the central portion of the cerebellum, unsteadiness of the trunk is a prominent symptom. A tumor or abscess involving one lateral cerebellar hemisphere will produce unsteadiness in the arm and leg on the same side.

Sensory ataxia is due to destruction of sensory pathways, chiefly those for determining the sense of position in space. The sensory fibers may be destroyed in the brainstem, spinal cord, or peripheral nerves. If the destructive process is in the brainstem or cervical spinal cord, ataxia is present either in the arms alone or in both the arms and the legs. Involvement of the lower spinal cord results in ataxia in the legs. If the damage occurs in the peripheral nerves, it may involve the legs, the arms, or both.

AUTONOMIC NERVOUS SYSTEM The autonomic nervous system is that part of the nervous system which supplies those motor structures which are primarily not under voluntary control. These structures include smooth muscle (for example, the intestines), heart muscle, and glands. Fibers of the autonomic nervous system are distributed to the smooth muscles of all parts of the body.

The autonomic nervous system is subdivided into the sympathetic and parasympathetic divisions. Anatomically, the sympathetic outflow is from the middle (thoracic and lumbar) parts of the spinal cord, whereas the outflow of the parasympathetic division is from the top and bottom (cranial and sacral) portions.

The autonomic nervous system serves as a balance-adjusting (homeostatic) mechanism to preserve the internal stability of the body. Control over peripheral autonomic mechanisms is maintained by centers located in the cerebral hemispheres, hypothalamus, and brainstem.

The autonomic nervous system controls the muscular tone of blood vessels and regulates the activity of the viscera. A large part of the control of bladder and bowel function is a function of the autonomic nervous system. The control of respiration, heart rate, and body temperature are also under autonomic control.

BERIBERI Beriberi is the name given to the clinical state produced by deficiency of thiamine (vitamin B_1). The disease takes two forms—the type called dry beriberi, in which there is primarily a disturbance in the nerves of the arms and legs (peripheral neuritis), and wet beriberi, a form of heart disease with accumulation of fluid (edema). Early symptoms of thiamine deficiency include loss of appetite, fatigue, nausea and vomiting, irritability, vague fears, and depression.

Symptoms. Early signs of nerve disorder are burning of the soles of the feet and numbness and tingling of the feet and legs. This may be followed by hypersensitivity and, later, loss of sensitivity in the toes. Shooting pains in the legs, muscle cramps, tenderness of the calves, weakness of the muscle, and abnormalities in the reflexes may also be observed, and the heart itself is enlarged.

In wet beriberi, the heart rate is rapid. There may be pain and shortness of breath on exertion, and the lips and nail beds may be somewhat bluish. Certain heart murmurs and disturbances in rhythm may be detected; the electrocardiogram shows characteristic findings. There is enlargement of the liver, and local accumulation of fluid—particularly around the ankles—is frequently observed.

Infantile beriberi occurs in breast-fed infants of mothers who have thiamine deficiency. Although this has not been seen frequently in the United States, it is quite prevalent in Japan and other Far Eastern countries. There is loss of appetite and vomiting, rapid pulse and respiration.

Treatment. In these forms of beriberi, the response to large doses of vitamin B_1 (usually by injection, occasionally by mouth) is often dramatic.

Other clinical forms of thiamine deficiency may also be found. One of these, known as Wernicke's syndrome, is characterized by weakness or paralysis of the muscles moving the eyeball. Lack of muscular coordination and mental disturbances are occasionally seen. Severe alcoholics often have complex vitamin deficiencies. Thus thiamine and other members of the vitamin B complex have been valuable in the treatment of delirium tremens and other acute psychotic diseases associated with alcoholism. The susceptibility of the nervous system to a deficiency of this vitamin is explained by the central nervous system's dependence on glucose (carbohydrate) metabolism and by thiamine's role in this metabolism.

BRAIN The brain is the portion of the central nervous system which is contained within the skull. It includes the cerebrum, the brainstem (medulla oblongata), and the cerebellum, and is the central organ which directs voluntary and involuntary bodily functions. It is the seat of memory, consciousness, emotional expression, and learning. The brain enables the individual to control voluntary musculature. Nearly all of the brain substance is composed of nerve cells and nerve fibers, which have specific functions. Therefore, damage to any segment of the brain results in disorder of function. The site of damage determines the type of resultant disability.

THE BRAIN
(CROSS SECTION)

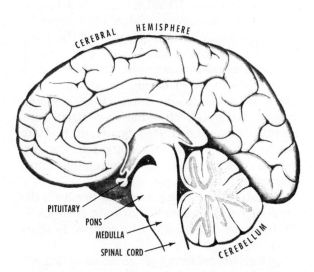

BRAINSTEM The brainstem is that narrower portion of the brain located underneath the cerebral hemispheres and cerebellum. It is located inside the lower part of the skull. Through it pass all of the sensory and motor tracts connecting the cerebrum and cerebellum with the spinal cord, and most of the cranial nerves arise from nuclei in the brainstem. Certain pathways in the upper portion of the brainstem are related to consciousness. Vital functions of heart rate and respiration are also controlled by mechanisms located in the brainstem. The term "brain-dead" refers to a state in which there is an absence of electrical activity in the cerebral hemispheres, but brainstem activities go on, sometimes referred to as a persistent vegetative state.

Damage to a relatively small portion of the brainstem results in pronounced deficits in neurologic function. Extensive damage to the brainstem is often fatal.

BRAIN TUMORS Brain tumors may develop in the cerebral hemispheres, cerebellum, or brainstem, and occur both in children and in adults. Such tumors may spread to the brain from tumors elsewhere in the body, or they may be primary in the brain itself. Some tumors are encapsulated, while other (cancerous) ones invade nervous tissue. The cause of tumor cell growth is not known.

Symptoms. Tumors of the brain may produce symptoms due to local compression or due to invasion of nervous tissue. Other symptoms are due to generalized increase in pressure within the skull. If a tumor arises from the optic nerves, early loss of vision may occur; similarly, a tumor may compress the acoustic nerve and produce deafness. Convulsions occur as a first symptom in many tumors arising in a cerebral hemisphere. These convulsions may be associated with progressive weakness, numbness, or language difficulty. With involvement of the cerebellum, the gait becomes unsteady. Headache, nausea, and vomiting occur with increased intracranial pressure.

Treatment. Diagnostic procedures developed over recent years (the CAT scan and the MRI, magnetic resonance imaging) are used to locate brain tumors. The primary treatment is surgical. Encapsulated tumors are removed. If the tumor is invading nervous tissue (that is, is cancerous), the neurosurgeon removes as much of it as is deemed advisable; subsequently, invasive tumors may be treated with X-ray therapy.

If an encapsulated tumor is successfully removed, permanent cure is usually accomplished, although regrowth of tumor may occur. The treatment of invasive tumors by operation and X-ray therapy is usually followed by recurrence of tumors after a period of months or years. Surgical therapy for tumors which have spread to the brain from elsewhere in the body is usually effective only for periods of months.

CAUSALGIA Causalgia is a constant burning pain, secondary to injury of sensory or mixed peripheral nerves. It is often associated with incomplete damage to the particular nerve. A rare complication of nerve injury, it may occur immediately after the injury or after an interval of several weeks.

Symptoms. After a nerve injury (frequently of the median nerve) the patient may become aware of a constant burning sensation in the distribution of the nerve involved. Any stimulation of the skin in the area of distribution of this nerve increases the pain.

Treatment. Mild pain may disappear spontaneously after a few weeks or months; with severe causalgia, burning pain persists. Surgical treatment with sympathetic nerve block or sympathectomy may be successful.

CENTRAL NERVOUS SYSTEM The development of human higher mental functions is directly related to the complexity of the central nervous system—CNS—both in the history of the human race and in the development of each individual. The CNS is a marvelously complex communication system which receives, transmits, associates, retains, integrates, and sends out electrical messages from all its parts, much like a telephonic communication system. It includes the brain and the spinal cord. It provides the direction and control of the activities of skeletal and smooth muscles, as well as of glands of secretion. It also controls the secretion of endocrine glands. Much reflex integration of bodily functions is carried out at the spinal cord level.

The basic unit of the nervous system consists of the nerve cell (neuron), which picks up and transmits different kinds of messages from different parts of the brain in the form of very slight electrical potentials. In general, all bodily function is controlled by a delicate balance of excitatory and inhibitory nervous control; for example, all movements are controlled by a delicate balance of excitation of one set of muscles and inhibition of opposing muscles.

The hindbrain (medulla oblongata) contains the vital centers for integrating the vegetative functions of the body—making possible swallowing, digestion, respiration, circulation, and elimination. The midbrain (thalamus and cerebellum) contains centers regulating consciousness, feelings and emotions, sleep, muscle tone, and postural coordination. The forebrain (cerebrum) controls the highest mental functions—coordinating sensations, voluntary motor actions, and associative thought processes.

The ways in which currents in nerve cells are translated into conscious mental activity are still unknown, though much progress has been made in mapping out the functions of the different brain centers and recording the small electrical discharges (brain waves) underlying brain functioning.

The action of different parts of the nervous system can be tested medically by neurological examinations which check the functioning of the different nerves and brain centers; the functioning of sensory nerves is tested by studying the normality of the senses. Motor functions are studied by checking muscular movements. The functioning of the cerebellum is tested by studying postural coordination. Cerebral functions are tested by giving complex psychological tests which measure all factors of ability.

The nervous system is subject to all the kinds of disease and injury which can attack other systems of the body. In general, damage to sensory nerves or centers produces loss of sensation; damage to motor cells and centers, loss of muscular functions; and damage to the cortex, loss of higher mental functions. The exact cause and nature of lesions (damage) to the nervous system can be determined only by neurological examination.

The functions of the nervous system can be just as easily disturbed by emotional disorders as any other organ systems. Before diagnosing disease of the nervous system, therefore, it is always necessary to rule out emotional upsets.

CEREBELLUM The cerebellum is the lower part of the brain which lies below the cerebrum and back of the brainstem. It consists of two lateral lobes and a middle lobe. A large number of pathways connect it with the cerebrum, brainstem, and spinal cord. The cerebellum receives stimuli relating to the position of the body and parts of the body in space and regulates the coordinated control of those muscular activities which permit walking, running, sewing, and similar activities.

Disorders involving the central portion of the cerebellum produce unsteadiness in walking. If one lateral cerebellar hemisphere is involved, the arm and leg on the affected side reveal incoordination and tremor.

CEREBRAL EMBOLUS Cerebral embolus is a bit of matter, usually a blood clot, which is carried by the bloodstream until it lodges in a cerebral artery and obstructs it.

Most emboli come from clots within the heart chamber and are associated with the arrhythmia known as a trial fibrillation; others come from the heart valves and are associated with bacterial infection (endocarditis); they may, however, come from the lungs or elsewhere. On rare occasions, fat droplets entering the circulation at the site of a bone fracture, air, tumor cells, bacteria, and foreign bodies may also produce cerebral emboli.

Symptoms. The obstruction of a cerebral artery by an embolus produces an area of tissue destruction or infarction. (For discussion of cerebral infarction, *see* CEREBRAL THROMBOSIS in this section.) This results in the sudden onset of neurologic symptoms which are frequently those of weakness, paralysis, loss of sensation, or similar deficits. Partial or complete recovery usually occurs, although emboli to large vessels may be fatal. Cerebral embolus may be a fatal complication of coronary thrombosis with infarction.

Treatment. If cerebral embolus is secondary to endocarditis, drug therapy may be successful in treating the cause of the embolus and in preventing recurrence. In persons who have a trial fibrillation, anticoagulant therapy may be prescribed. Physical and occupational therapy and speech retraining may be of symptomatic value during the convalescent period after a cerebral embolus.

CEREBRAL HEMORRHAGE Cerebral hemorrhage represents bleeding into the substance of the brain from a ruptured cerebral vessel. In a patient with high blood pressure, a cerebral artery may occasionally rupture without any external head injury. Also, in patients with aneurysms or vascular malformations of the arteries of the brain, spontaneous rupture sometimes occurs with bleeding into the subarachnoid space and, at times, into the brain. Severe external head injury is sometimes associated with cerebral hemorrhage.

Symptoms. Symptoms develop suddenly, sometimes with loss of consciousness and paralysis. The course is usually fatal, especially if coma persists. If the patient does survive the acute hemorrhagic episode, severe neurologic deficit is frequently present.

Treatment. Occasionally a blood clot within a cerebral hemorrhage is drained surgically, with partial improvement. In some patients a ruptured aneurysm which has produced cerebral hemorrhage is treated surgically to prevent rebleeding.

CEREBRAL THROMBOSIS Cerebral thrombosis is a clot of blood formed within an artery which supplies blood to the brain. Thrombosis of very small arteries may produce only transient symptoms or possibly no noticeable symptoms at all. Thrombosis of a medium-size or large artery will result in a neurologic deficit which is determined partly by the site of the vessel. Damage to the portion of the brain supplied by the particular thrombosed artery is due to the resulting inadequate blood supply (ischemia). If the ischemia is transient, attacks of weakness, loss of sensation, and speech difficulty occur for a few minutes to a few hours, then clear up completely. With prolonged ischemia, death of cells in the area results. A large area of cellular destruction results in a cerebral infarction. The extent of infarction depends upon the adequacy of the blood supply available from neighboring vessels—the collateral blood supply.

The major vessels supplying blood to the brain are the two internal carotid and the two vertebral arteries. From these vessels, blood passes through a circular vascular channel to vessels within the brain. Thrombosis can occur in any of these, but approximately one-fourth of the thromboses occur in the internal carotid and vertebral arteries.

Symptoms. Cerebral thrombosis is the most common cause of apoplectic stroke or cerebrovascular accidents and may result in severe paralysis and sensory change in one arm and leg. One or all four extremities may be involved. Speech disorders, partial blindness, double vision, facial paralysis, or difficulty in swallowing are sometimes associated with it. Drowsiness, confusion, and unconsciousness may occur. With severe brain damage, death may result. In most cases, there is recovery with residual deficit although complete recovery also does occur. Cerebral thrombosis may recur in other vessels.

Treatment. Partial blockage of a vessel in the neck may be corrected surgically. If transient ischemic attacks recur, anticoagulant drugs will decrease their frequency. Physical and occupational therapy are of symptomatic value, and speech retraining is sometimes indicated.

CEREBROSPINAL FLUID   The cerebrospinal fluid fills the spaces between the brain and its covering membrane, the spaces between the spinal cord and its covering, and also the large spaces (or ventricles) within the brain substance. This fluid enters these spaces from the arterial blood system, circulates within them throughout the central nervous system, and returns to the venous blood system. Normally the fluid is clear and colorless.

If the circulation of this fluid is blocked, the ventricles above the block dilate and this interferes with the normal function of the brain.

As a diagnostic procedure, needle puncture of the space containing cerebrospinal fluid in the lower portion of the back is sometimes done. At the time of such examination, the pressure of the fluid contained within the subarachnoid space is measured. Samples of the fluid are also obtained for microscopic and chemical examinations. In certain disorders, the fluid may be bloody or may contain pus. (Occasionally air or oils, which can be seen on X-ray films, are injected into the subarachnoid space for special procedures in the diagnosis of neurological disorders involving the brain or spinal cord.)

CEREBROVASCULAR ACCIDENTS   A cerebrovascular accident is a sudden neurologic disorder which results from thrombosis, embolism, or hemorrhage involving cerebral arteries. The term accident refers to a sudden spontaneous change in the condition of the cerebral artery. This is an internal accident and is not related to any external head injury. The most common type of cerebrovascular accident is cerebral thrombosis, or occlusion of a cerebral artery.

CEREBRUM   The cerebrum is the portion of the brain which occupies the upper half of the inside of the skull. It is divided into two cerebral hemispheres connected by large nerve-fiber bundles. Each cerebral hemisphere is divided into four lobes—frontal, parietal, temporal, and occipital.

The cerebrum is the final destination of all types of sensory information transmitted through the central nervous system from the sensory nerves. Sensory pathways for bodily sensation arrive at the parietal lobes; visual stimuli are transmitted to the occipital lobes; and auditory stimuli are relayed to the temporal lobes.

The frontal lobes are probably the site of initiation of motor impulses under voluntary control, which are transmitted through peripheral nerves to skeletal muscles.

In right-handed individuals, and probably in most left-handed ones, the left cerebral hemisphere is the site for the understanding and expression of language. Complex intellectual functions, memory, and purposeful behavior are functions in which the cerebrum plays a vital role.

Disorders of one cerebral hemisphere result in weakness, decreased sensation, and/or visual loss on the opposite side of the body. With damage to the dominant cerebral hemisphere there is frequently impairment of the ability to understand or use language, thus making a severe communication problem.

COMA   Coma is a clinical state of complete loss of consciousness of more than momentary duration. The onset may be sudden or gradual, and the coma itself may last for hours, days, or weeks. It is associated with various types of serious medical disorders and may occur in the course of fatal or non-fatal illnesses. Among the many possible causes of coma are severe alteration in the content of body fluids; extremely low or high blood sugar contents; kidney failure; meningitis; head injury, cerebrovascular accidents; drug overdoses and brain tumors.

Symptoms. Several levels of decreasing awareness are recognized, ranging from "alert," through "drowsy," "semi-stuporous," "stuporous," and "comatose." A patient may progress in either direction through these different levels. On examination, a comatose patient does not respond to spoken commands nor look about the room (the eyes are usually closed). If an arm or leg is elevated and then released by the examiner, it will drop quickly to the bed. Strong painful stimuli, however, will increase the rate of respiration and may produce some movement of the trunk or extremities. Certain reflex responses, such as the eyelid and gag reflexes, are maintained unless the patient is in very deep coma.

Treatment. Hospitalization of the patient in coma is essential. Various laboratory tests are immediately performed. Treatment includes maintenance of adequate intake of fluids by intravenous injections, maintenance of an adequate airway for respiration, and proper care of bladder and bowel functions. Specific medical or surgical treatment depends upon the cause of the comatose state.

CONCUSSION, BRAIN

Concussion of the brain is produced by head injury and results in transient loss of consciousness. It usually occurs as a consequence of rapid acceleration or deceleration in the motion of the head.

Symptoms. During the brief period of unconsciousness, the patient does not respond to stimulation. Reflexes are temporarily absent. After this initial period of complete unresponsiveness, the individual will respond to painful stimuli; subsequently, purposeful movements and still later volitional movements occur as consciousness is regained. After a brief period of confusion, the individual again becomes oriented and alert. Loss of memory for a brief period preceding and following the injury is usually noted. (The events mentioned above as following a head injury may occur over a period of a few seconds or during several hours.) In the days or weeks following a concussion, the patient may complain of headaches, faintness, nausea, vomiting, or dizziness.

Treatment. Patients with head injuries associated with concussion should be seen by a physician. Hospital care and observation are usually indicated. Further observation in the hospital or at home will enable the physician to exclude the possible development of an associated subdural or extradural hematoma.

CONTUSION, BRAIN

A contusion of the brain is a bruise following head injury. Contusions may occur anywhere in the brain, although they are frequently located in the frontal and temporal lobes. Large contusions may interrupt the function of a large part of one, or both, cerebral hemispheres. In the brainstem, contusions produce severe neurologic damage. All contusions are associated with swelling of the brain, which may result in an increase in intracranial pressure with additional neurologic deficit.

Symptoms. With severe contusion the patient may be comatose. Weakness, paralysis, or alteration of sensation on one side of the body may be present. Difficulties in speech and swallowing may occur. There may be local or generalized convulsions.

Treatment. The patient is placed in the hospital on a course of complete bed rest. Pulse, blood pressure, respiration, temperature, and neurologic status are checked at frequent intervals. (Special X-ray studies may be needed to exclude an associated blood clot.) If the patient is stuporous, intravenous medications are needed. Anti-convulsant drugs are employed to control seizures. Antibiotic drugs are used to treat specific infections if they arise. If unconsciousness is prolonged, nutrition is provided through a gastric tube.

Most of the deaths after a head injury and contusion are due to injury to the brainstem. Recovery may be complete or may be associated with residual weakness, speech disorder, or sensory disturbance.

CONVULSIONS

This is a general term descriptive of the sudden onset of unconsciousness and generalized muscular contractions or spasms, which may or may not be epileptic in origin. In children it can be triggered by a sudden onset of fever.

Symptoms. The afflicted child may cry out, soil himself, stiffen, turn blue, fall down, and then develop twitching and jerking. When due to epilepsy, such major attacks—which are recurrent—are known as grand mal seizures. In the typical epileptic petit mal convulsion or seizure, the patient loses consciousness for only a second or so, but does not stiffen, jerk, nor fall to the floor; rather, he seems merely to stare blankly into space. Other types of seizures can vary all the way from spells of violent anger to mild, uncontrollable spasms of shaking in one arm or leg.

There are many causes for convulsions, and by no means all of them (or even most) are epileptic in nature. Tumors of the brain, blood clots on (or in) the brain substance, scars from old brain injuries, low blood sugar (or other changes in blood chemistry), high blood pressure, and certain drugs and poisons are all capable of inducing convulsive states. The vast majority, in fact, have no known cause, although in some cases a family history of convulsions can be found. It is noteworthy that children who suffer from febrile (fever-induced) convulsions do not continue to have seizures as adults—hence the idea that people sometimes "outgrow" epilepsy.

Treatment. If at all possible, diagnosis of the underlying cause must be made. This is accomplished in most cases by an electroencephalogram (brain wave test) which will help establish the type of seizure and, if a localized lesion does exist, tell where it may be found. In the congenital cases of grand mal without discernible cause, successful treatment is difficult to attain.

When a seizure lasts more than a few seconds, the convulsing person must be removed immediately from any dangerous situation. The airway to the lungs must be opened by placing a gag between the victim's teeth and keeping the tongue out of the throat. If the victim is a child, and if there is a fever, sponging the naked skin is therefore a most important thing to do.

CRANIAL NERVES   Twelve pairs of cranial nerves connect portions of the brain and the brainstem with sensory and motor structures about the head and neck. Many of these nerves have specialized functions. However, they are comparable to the peripheral nerves, which supply the remainder of the body. The numbers and names of these paired nerves are as follows:

I	Olfactory Nerves
II	Optic Nerves
III	Oculomotor Nerves
IV	Trochlear Nerves
V	Trigeminal Nerves
VI	Abducens Nerves
VII	Facial Nerves
VIII	Acoustic Nerves
IX	Glossopharyngeal Nerves
X	Vagus Nerves
XI	Spinal Accessory Nerves
XII	Hypoglossal Nerves

The sensory portions of cranial nerves supply sensory impulses including special visual, auditory, olfactory (smell), and gustatory (taste) information. Motor activities transmitted through the cranial nerves determine movements of the eyes, face, palate, and tongue.

Cranial nerves may be damaged by physical injury or by illnesses such as meningitis or neuritis.

ELECTROENCEPHALOGRAM (EEG)

An electroencephalogram is a graphic record of the electrical activity recorded for the surface of the brain by electrodes placed on the scalp. The electroencephalogram is a valuable diagnostic aid in a number of neurologic disorders. Perhaps the most important application of electroencephalography is in the diagnosis and improved understanding of convulsive seizures (epilepsy), since abnormal electrical wave patterns occur during convulsive attacks. Also, in more than half the patients with epilepsy, abnormal activity is recorded on the electroencephalogram between attacks. Localized brain disorders may be associated with abnormal electrical patterns on the electroencephalogram; hence, these are sometimes a valuable laboratory aid in diagnosis. Absence of electrical activity on an EEG in a persistently comatose patient is a medico-legal criterion for being "braindead."

EPILEPSY   Epilepsy is not a single disease, but a general term for symptoms of convulsive disorders. Epilepsy must therefore be understood as a symptom which may occur in any of a number of brain diseases. Scientific experiments show that the brain produces rhythmic electrical potentials, necessary for normal function. In normal persons, during the waking state these brain waves occur at the rate of nine to fourteen per second and are known as alpha rhythms. In sleep or under conditions of coma, the rhythms slow down to three to six per second and are known as delta waves. Apparently underlying all convulsive disorders is an abnormality of the electric potentials or waves produced in the normal brain. In such disorders therefore occur out-of-step waves (cerebral dysrhythmias) now recognized medically as indicative of epilepsy. Diagnosis of epilepsy, and location of the brain-areas producing abnormal rhythms, can now be positively made with brain-wave (electroencephalographic) equipment available at most modern hospitals.

Symptoms. It was formerly thought that

different forms of epilepsy could be diagnosed by the types of seizure involved. Three main patterns of epilepsy have been identified classically. In grand mal seizures, the person suddenly loses consciousness and falls to the ground in a convulsive seizure involving contraction and relaxation of all muscle groups. Frequently the epileptic bites his tongue or injures himself in other ways, for example, by falling against hot or hard objects. The seizure usually terminates spontaneously within a few minutes, following which there is gradual recovery of consciousness and reorientation. (Some grand mal epileptics report a warning aura—such as unusual visceral sensation—which gives warning of an impending seizure.)

Petit mal seizures usually involve a limited convulsive movement or temporary alteration of consciousness, but the patient does not lose consciousness completely or show generalized convulsion. The convulsive movement or alteration of consciousness may be so slight in petit mal epilepsy that only the patient himself or someone well acquainted with him knows that it has occurred. As in grand mal epilepsy, a petit mal diagnosis can be confirmed by brain-wave analysis (electroencephalography).

Psychomotor epilepsy involves involuntary alterations of conscious mental life, usually without any overt convulsive disorder. The pattern consists of a period of uncontrolled and unpremeditated behavior; the person may perform senseless or atypical actions without knowing why.

In medical circles the term epilepsy has largely been replaced by the designations convulsive disorder or cerebral dysrhythmia.

Treatment. Great advances have been made in chemotherapy of epilepsy, and it is entirely probable that future research will show the abnormal physical and chemical disorders underlying all convulsive conditions. The first step in treatment is to positively identify the cerebral dysrhythmia by means of brain-wave study. After abnormal cerebral rhythms have been found, a large number of very effective drugs are available to control all types of convulsive symptoms.

It is absolutely essential for the epileptic to admit that he has a convulsive disorder. He must accept certain limitations on his life pattern; not engaging, for example, in any activity—driving, swimming, climbing in high places—where the onset of convulsions might be dangerous to himself or others. (*See also* CONVULSIONS in this section.)

EXTRADURAL HEMATOMA An extradural hematoma is a collection of blood between the outer coverings of the brain and the skull due to a tear in an artery which runs just beneath the temporal bone of the skull. Extradural hematomas are due to direct blows to the skull.

Symptoms. Usually the individual will develop a headache, vomiting, and drowsiness within a few hours after head injury. A bruise in one temporal area may be noted and weakness of the arm and leg on the opposite side of the body from the blow subsequently develops. The patient may rapidly become comatose and develop irregular breathing and convulsions.

Treatment. The patient should be hospitalized immediately and surgical removal of the hematoma carried out as soon as possible. Recovery is usually rapid and complete if treatment is prompt. Late treatment may result in partial recovery with residual weakness or speech disorder. If there has been a delay, and if severe damage to the brainstem has occurred, death may result in spite of surgical therapy.

FACIAL NERVES The paired facial (or seventh cranial) nerves supply motor function to the muscles of the face and also carry sensory impulses of taste from the front two-thirds of the tongue to the brainstem. These nerves may be damaged by injury, infection, or neuritis.

FACIAL PARALYSIS (BELL'S PALSY) Bell's palsy, or facial paralysis, is a sudden palsy of the muscles of one side of the face, probably due to a neuritis of the facial nerve.

Symptoms. The muscles of one side of the face become weak or paralyzed without previous warning or illness. The eyelids may not close completely, and it may be difficult to use the lower portion of the face to smile and to chew food. Taste sensation may be lost on the side of the tongue on which the facial paralysis occurs.

Treatment. Most patients with Bell's palsy recover function of facial muscles. Recovery may be complete within a few weeks, or it may occur slowly and partially over a period of six to twelve months. No specific drug is uniformly effective in producing early recovery, although cortisone has been recommended. If function does not return after two years, plastic surgical repair may be required to obtain cosmetic improvement.

GLOSSOPHARYNGEAL NERVES The two glossopharyngeal (or eleventh cranial) nerves carry sensory impulses such as pain and temperature from the throat and also taste sensation from the back one-third of the tongue. These nerves may be damaged by injury or infection.

HEADACHE Headache is a very common symptom that occurs at some time in all individuals and has many different causes. Constant generalized headaches occurring periodically are frequently related to emotional stress, while headaches that throb on one side are characteristic of migraine. Headaches occur in association with a wide variety of systemic diseases. Acute fever (due to many causes) is frequently accompanied by headache, and infections of the ears and mastoids are also associated with local head-pain. Sinusitis, too, is a common cause of headache.

Less commonly, neurologic disorders such as meningitis, encephalitis, brain tumor, disease of cerebral blood vessels, or head injury may also produce headaches of varying severity.

Headache is usually characterized by the dilation (enlargement) of the blood vessels in the head. This dilation exerts pressure upon the nerves that surround the blood vessels, thereby producing the pain of headache.

The most common type of headache is the tension headache. This may be caused by the tightening of the muscles of the back of the neck and the scalp. Prolonged neck strain, for example, during long distance driving may induce tension headache. Emotional stress that causes the neck and scalp muscles to tighten involuntarily is responsible for most tension headaches.

Headache associated with fever is usually generalized and present on both sides of the head, whereas ear and mastoid infections and migraine frequently produce intense one-sided headache. Localized frontal head-pain occurs with frontal sinusitis; with maxillary sinusitis, pain over the cheek is common. Headache caused by neurologic disorders may be either one-sided or generalized.

Treatment. Because headache is a symptom of various health disorders, identifying the underlying cause is important in determining treatment. If headache is associated with acute infection, drug therapy focused at the infection should eliminate headache. Dealing successfully with the causes of emotional stress can remove tension headaches. Minor headache pain often responds to treatment with aspirin, or other non-aspirin analgesics. With severe or chronic headaches, it is important that careful examination is done to determine the cause of the headache. Persistent headache that does not respond to aspirin or a non-aspirin analgesic (such as acetominophen) should be reported to a physician.

HEADACHES, MIGRAINE Migraine headache is an intensely painful type of headache that may last several days and temporarily incapacitate its victim. A migraine attack may bring with it dizziness, chills, and sensitivity to light.

What exactly causes migraine headache is not completely known. A variety of factors that predispose individuals to migraine are known, however. Researchers have discovered a genetic disposition for migraine, as well as a connection to hormonal imbalance. Also twice as many women as men have migraine. Quite a number of migraine victims have personalities that may be characterized as compulsive, tending to be perfectionists with high standards set for themselves and not prone to communicating their anxieties to others.

A migraine attack is an excruciating experience. It may begin with flashes of light or other impairment of vision. The pain is almost always on one side of the head and can be accompanied by nausea, vomiting, and soreness of the scalp. Migraine, like many types of headache, involves painful dilation of cerebral blood vessels but is not caused by organic problems. For many sufferers migraine attacks can be induced by abrupt temperature and air pressure changes and by an allergic reaction to certain foods or drugs.

Treatment. Migraine may be relieved by vasoconstricting drugs, such as dihydroergotamine. Some of the nonsteroidal anti-inflammatory drugs used for arthritis and as pain killers have proved useful. So also have been some cardiovascular drugs such as the calcium channel blockers and the beta blockers. Methysergide maleate is sometimes prescribed in the attempt to decrease the frequency of migraine episodes in very severe cases. Throbbing, suddenly recurrent headache may also be associated with elevated blood pressure, for which the treatment is reduction of blood pressure by use of drugs and by training of the individual to be emotionally calm. Some migraine victims benefit from warm baths and bed rest.

A large percentage of migraine attacks, as well as lesser types of headaches, have psychogenic causes, such as emotional conflicts, psychological instability, and intense anxiety. Two forms of headache characteristically occur in association with emotional instability. These are "belt-like" headaches in the region of the temples, with the sufferer complaining of a constricting sensation around the skull, and occipital headaches involving a dull ache in the muscles at the back of the head and neck. Psychogenic headaches should be treated with psychotherapy directed at discovery and removal of the causes of emotional conflict.

HEMORRHAGE, SUBARACHNOID
Subarachnoid hemorrhage is a bleeding into the spaces between the inner coverings of the brain. Brain injury from external violence is the most common cause. Spontaneous subarachnoid hemorrhage occurs as a result of the rupture of a weakening (aneurysm) in a cerebral artery, or of a vascular malformation. In one-third of cases the cause of bleeding is not found.

Symptoms. Severe headache is usually followed by drowsiness and stiff neck. Vomiting, double vision, weakness of one arm and leg, and other signs of neurologic deficit may develop, particularly if there is associated intracerebral bleeding. The patient may become comatose and show irregular respiration. When a spinal tap is made, the cerebrospinal fluid is bloody.

Treatment. Subarachnoid hemorrhage associated with head injury may result in severe complications. Spontaneous subarachnoid hemorrhage is of the greatest importance due to the threat posed by the leaking arterial aneurism. (The blood in the subarachnoid space itself is absorbed within two to three weeks.) Approximately one-third of patients die after the first episode of spontaneous subarachnoid hemorrhage. Among survivers of the initial attack, the aneurysm may bleed again within a few weeks or months, with an increasing mortality rate. Surgical treatment is recommended for selected cases of aneurysm with rupture. This, however, is a major operative procedure and is associated with a high mortality rate. The aneurysm is located by X-ray studies made immediately after injecting oil, which is opaque to X-rays, into the cerebral circulation. An opening into the skull is then made to expose the aneurysm, to place clips on it, and to prevent it from rebleeding. Hospital care is required for every patient with subarachnoid hemorrhage. Intravenous fluids are frequently needed. If there is difficulty in swallowing, suction is necessary to maintain adequate aeration of the lungs.

HUNTINGTON'S CHOREA
Huntington's chorea is a familial disorder occurring during adult life and is associated with involuntary movements and mental deterioration.

Symptoms. Involuntary movements of the face, arms, and legs are noted, usually when the patient is between twenty and forty years of age; these gradually increase in severity. The patient has difficulty in writing and in performing other precise movements of the hands. The gait has a dancing quality. Together with these involuntary movements, or subsequent to them, the patient undergoes intellectual changes: his ability to remember recent and remote events, his ability to calculate, and similar intellectual capacities decline. Subsequently psychotic behavior may require institutional care.

Treatment. The course of Huntington's chorea is progressively downhill over a period of years and ends fatally. No therapy is yet available to prevent intellectual deterioration.

HYPOGLOSSAL NERVES
The two hypoglossal (or twelfth cranial) nerves innervate

the tongue. If one of these nerves is damaged, the tongue becomes wrinkled and wasted on that side. When the tongue is protruded from the mouth, it deviates to the weak side. If both hypoglossal nerves are affected, the tongue becomes wasted on both sides and its function is lost.

MEDIAN NERVE The median nerve supplies important muscles relating to flexion of the fingers. It also carries sensory impulses from the skin over the thumb, index, and middle fingers.

MENINGES The meninges are three membranes which cover the brain and spinal cord: an outer fibrous membrane, a filmy middle membrane, and a delicate inner membrane. (The space between the middle and the inner membrane is called the subarachnoid space and contains cerebrospinal fluid.) Infections of these membranes result in meningitis. (*See also* MENINGITIS in the section INFECTIOUS DISEASES.)

MULTIPLE SCLEROSIS Multiple sclerosis is one of the common chronic disabling disorders of the central nervous system. It is characterized by recurring symptoms with progression of disability. The white matter of the brain and spinal cord is damaged through spotty destruction of myelin, which coats the nerve fiber. The cause of this malady is unknown.

Symptoms. The initial symptoms depend upon the portion of the central nervous system involved. A frequent early symptom is the rapid onset of blurred vision and decreased visual acuity due to disordered function of the optic nerves. Involvement in the brainstem may produce double vision, facial numbness or weakness, vertigo, or slurred speech. Sudden weakness, numbness, or bladder disorder may be due to spinal-cord damage. Symptoms and findings characteristically progress for a period of days or weeks and then recede, with partial or nearly complete recovery in subsequent months. With recurrence, more residual disability persists. The diagnosis is based primarily on the clinical findings. Many other neurologic conditions present a similar medical picture, however.

Treatment. Although there is no specific treatment for multiple sclerosis, supportive care is most important. It is explained to the patient that a single episode of disability may be followed by complete, or nearly complete, return of function. Then too, the interval between recurrence may vary from less than a year to many years. Thus, the patient may frequently enjoy many productive years before severe disability occurs. With an acute attack, bed rest (followed by limited activity) is important. A nutritious diet and supplementary vitamin therapy are indicated. Steroid drugs are of value in selected cases. Physical therapy enables the patient to improve gait and strength, and occupational therapy is of value in improving hand coordination.

MYASTHENIA GRAVIS Myasthenia gravis is a disorder associated with weakness and easy fatigability of muscles. It is related to a defect in the transmission of impulses from the nerve fiber to the muscle fiber and occurs both in children and in adults. The cause of myasthenia is not known.

Symptoms. The initial symptoms of myasthenia gravis frequently relate to a disturbance in function of muscles supplied by the cranial nerves. Drooping of the eyelids may occur. With weakness of the muscles which move the eyeball, double vision may be a prominent symptom. The facial muscles may be weak. Swallowing may become difficult due to weakness of the throat muscles. The voice may be hoarse. Weakness may also be noted in the muscles of the neck, shoulders, arms, and legs. Characteristically, the muscles become weaker with prolonged use; for example, the patient may initially have little difficulty in chewing, then note progressive weakness as he eats a meal. Such muscular weakness diminishes with rest, and there is no wasting of muscles.

In some patients weakness is confined to only a few muscle-groups, whereas in others generalized weakness is present. During the course of myasthenia, severe attacks of generalized weakness or paralysis may occur, producing weakness of the muscles of respiration. The reflexes remain normal and sensation remains intact.

Treatment. Several drugs are available to improve conduction from the nerve endings to the muscles, such as Neostigmine®, Mestinon®, and Mytelase®. These drugs are taken several times a day, in order to prevent muscle weakness and easy fatigability. Given the proper dosage of medication, the majority of patients with mild or moderate myasthenia are able to carry out their normal activities. Patients with severe myasthenia will show significant improvement but may continue to have partial disability in spite of large amounts of one or more of these medications. Removal of the thymus gland has been the recommended treatment in selected cases.

Patients with myasthenia have spontaneous flare-ups and remissions of their disorders; in severe flare-ups, present methods of therapy may be unsuccessful. The mortality rate in myasthenia gravis is still high.

NARCOLEPSY   This term describes a sudden overwhelming desire to sleep, regardless of where the person is or what he is doing. It is not caused by physical fatigue or sleep deprivation. Unlike syncope (fainting), the sleeping state is natural, lasting from seconds to a few minutes. If the slumberer is wakened, he promptly falls asleep again; upon awakening spontaneously, he feels refreshed. This bizarre affliction usually affects obese young men, who often also complain of sexual impotence. The drug amphetamine controls the condition quite effectively.

NERVE CELL (NEURON)   A neuron, or nerve cell, includes a cell body and long receiving (afferent) and transmitting (efferent) extensions from that body. It is the cellular unit of the nervous system. Nerve cells are designed for the reception and transmission of sensory and motor impulses throughout the entire body. Within the central nervous system, neurons are arranged in networks which transmit impulses from one transmitting extension (axon) across a gap (synapse) to a receiving extension (dendrite), and so on through an entire series of cells.

The primary motor neurons in the spinal cord have their cell bodies located in the anterior grey matter. These cell bodies contain nuclei and cytoplasm. Their dendrites form a network of receptors, which extend locally within the cord. Their axons, or motor fibers, leave the cell-body and pass through the anterior root, the spinal nerve, and the peripheral nerve to the muscle fibers, which they innervate. These axons are covered with a fatty material called myelin.

The primary sensory neurons together with their sensory fibers are the receptors in the skin, the muscles, the viscera, and elsewhere. Secondary and other sensory neurons relay these impulses to the cord and brain.

NERVE FIBERS   Nerve fibers are the long processes which extend from the cell-bodies of neurons. Nerve fibers transmit sensory and motor impulses throughout the nervous system. These fibers are of microscopic diameter, but may be as much as several feet in length.

Columns (tracts) of fibers form the white matter in the brain and spinal cord. The cranial and peripheral nerves consist primarily of bundles of nerve fibers. Each motor fiber in a peripheral nerve connects by way of a microscopic endplate with a muscle fiber, whereas sensory nerve fibers extend from sensory nerve endings through peripheral nerves.

Damage to bundles of peripheral sensory and motor nerve-fibers results in decreasing sensation and weakness of muscles in the area supplied by the nerve.

NERVOUS SYSTEM   The nervous system is a highly integrated mechanism for the central control of the activity of all of the responsive (excitable) tissue of the body. Microscopically, it is composed of millions of nerve cells with their long processes. These cells constitute a conducting system for receiving and sending impulses throughout the body.

Although it functions as a unified system and is an integral part of the body as a whole, the nervous system may be arbitrarily divided into anatomic parts. The two major anatomic portions are the central nervous system and the peripheral nervous system; the central nervous system consists of the brain and the spinal cord, and the peripheral of outlying nerve fibers.

Certain portions of the nervous system are more susceptible to specific diseases than others. For example, certain substances, such as diphtheria toxin and arsenic, primarily damage peripheral nerves. In contrast, poliomyelitis virus involves the central nervous system.

NEURALGIA   Neuralgia is pain which lies along the path of a cranial or peripheral nerve, or posterior root. It is not associated with any change in the function of the nerve.

Symptoms. Trigeminal neuralgia is a recurring, sharp, knife-like pain along the paths of the trigeminal (fifth cranial) nerve. Frequent severe bouts of pain may be temporarily disabling. Periods of recurring pain may last for several weeks or months and may then be followed by periods of remission. (*See* TRIGEMINAL NEURALGIA in this section.) A similar neuralgia, involving the ninth cranial nerve, occasionally occurs and produces severe sharp pain in the throat and spreads to the ear on the same side. Intercostal neuralgia produces pain extending from the back (at the level of the affected segment) to the chest or abdomen.

Treatment. Medicines which relieve pain are needed for relief of recurrent neuralgia. It is important, however, to avoid the repeated use of narcotic drugs. Sedatives to induce sleep are required in patients with prolonged severe attacks of neuralgia. In selected patients, injections of alcohol into the involved nerve are followed by prolonged relief of symptoms. (However, alcohol-injection results in loss of sensation in the distribution of the injected nerve.) In other severe cases, direct surgical treatment is indicated. Dilantin® Sodium, which slows the rate of peripheral nerve conduction, has been recommended in the treatment of trigeminal neuralgia; carbamazepine, an antiepileptic, has also been shown to be of value and is increasingly used.

NEURITIS Neuritis is an inflammation of one or more cranial or peripheral nerves and is associated with disturbance of sensation and strength in the muscles supplied by the involved nerve or nerves. Damage to a single nerve (mononeuritis) is frequently the result of local nerve injury. Involvement of multiple nerves (polyneuritis) occurs with severe nutritional deficiencies often associated with chronic alcoholism or with poisoning by such substances as lead, arsenic, and chemical compounds.

Symptoms. The symptoms of mononeuritis are related to the sensory and muscular (motor) control activities of the particular nerve involved. This neuritis involving the radial nerve in the arm results in weakness of extension of the wrists and fingers; while neuritis of the peroneal nerve at the side of the knee results in foot drop and numbness over the lateral aspect of the lower leg and foot.

Polyneuritis produces decreased sensation and weakness in the distribution of multiple nerves. Usually numbness and weakness occur in both legs or in the arms and legs. With severe weakness, the patient is unable to walk or stand. With severe involvement in the hands and arms, he may be unable to write or to feed himself.

NEURITIS

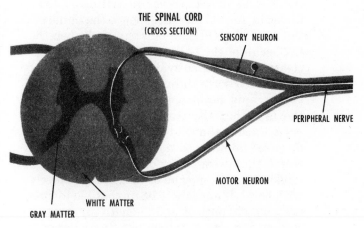

THE SPINAL CORD
(CROSS SECTION)

SENSORY NEURON

PERIPHERAL NERVE

MOTOR NEURON

WHITE MATTER

GRAY MATTER

Treatment. If an external poison is responsible for polyneuritis, this is removed. In arsenic-caused polyneuritis, the drug BAL (British anti-Lewisite) is used to increase urinary excretion of arsenic; to treat lead poisoning, Versene® is used. The administration of pyridoxine will prevent the appearance of polyneuritis in patients who are being treated with large dosages of isoniazid. Nutritional polyneuritis is treated by use of a high-protein, high-caloric, high-vitamin diet, with supplemental oral or peripheral vitamins. Diabetes mellitus associated with neuritis is controlled by diet and insulin. Symptomatic therapy includes physical therapy, occupational therapy, the application of supports and braces, and rehabilitation.

NEUROLOGIST The neurologist is a specialist who deals with organic diseases of the nervous system and is specially trained in the appropriate anatomy, physiology, and pathology. (A neurological surgeon or neurosurgeon is a specialist who combines training both in neurology and in brain and spinal cord surgery.) Competence in the field is recognized by certification by the American Board of Neurology and Psychiatry.

NORMAL PRESSURE HYDROCEPHALUS (NPH)

This is a recently described disorder which accounts for a small number of cases of dementia in the elderly. It results from a derangement in the cerebrospinal fluid production in the brain; this leads to a slowly progressive dilation of the ventricles with signs of neurological damage. Findings include a spastic unsteady gait, urinary incontinence, and impairment of cognitive functioning. A spinal tap reveals the fluid not to be under increased pressure, hence the name for the disorder. NPH can be suspected when the CAT scan of the head reveals dilated ventricles with little or no evidence of brain atrophy apart from some thinning, also by the sometimes rapid development of symptoms, and the fact that the trouble walking appears early rather than late as with Alzheimer's disease. Sometimes a ventriculo-peritoneal shunt, the operation performed for hydrocephalus in infants, may be of value to the elderly with NPH. It appears to be impossible to forecast which patient will benefit by such a shunt. (*See also* WATER ON THE BRAIN [HYDROCEPHALY] in this section.)

NYSTAGMUS

This is an involuntary rapid to-and-fro movement of the eye. It is seen in normal individuals as they gaze at telephone poles from a rapidly moving automobile. Rapid rotation of the body causes nystagmus, as does stimulation of the inner ear with warm or cool fluid. Eyes which have had extremely poor vision since birth also jerk irregularly back and forth, and diseases of the brain may also cause nystagmus. Symptoms may or may not occur. Attention should be directed to the cause.

ORGANIC BRAIN SYNDROME

The human brain is subject to many types of physical injury and disease which can destroy its substance. Organic brain syndrome is a general classification of such conditions, which result in irreversible chronic impairment of mental functions; in extreme degree, such a syndrome produces complete loss of mental functions, a state formerly known as dementia.

It is now known that a large number of diseases and injuries can cause permanent organic damage to brain cells, which unfortunately are unable to reproduce themselves. Organic brain damage to the fetus may occur in pregnancy, if the mother contracts infectious diseases such as measles, German measles, scarlet fever, or whooping-cough. Birth injuries to the central nervous system are estimated to occur in 10 percent of all deliveries, and childhood accidents and diseases may also involve brain damage.

In later life, the most common causes of organic brain damage are cerebrovascular accidents such as "stroke" (embolism or hemorrhage).

Treatment. The main hope in treatment programs consists in teaching the patient to compensate for lost functions by overdeveloping his remaining resources.

PARESIS, GENERAL

General paresis is due to infection of the central nervous system, particularly the cerebral cortex, by syphilis. It is a chronic, infectious process which results in organic mental deterioration. General paresis was much more common in the nineteenth century, before its cause became known; today it is only rarely observed in untreated or inadequately treated syphilitic patients.

Symptoms. The onset is usually gradual and insidious, involving slow changes in personality and character which include deterioration of personal habits and cleanliness. A common symptom is delusions of grandeur, in which the patient, suddenly boastful and grandoise, believes that he has suddenly become very wealthy or powerful. The mood is usually one of euphoria and satisfaction with life. Subtle impairment of memory and judgment may result in irrational behavior and loss of normal self-control and inhibition of impulses.

Relatively late in the disorder, neurological signs begin to appear, including abnormalities in eye-response and generalized skeletal muscle weakness or rigidity. If the syphilitic process also involves the spinal cord, tendon reflexes are disturbed and knee-jerks absent.

Treatment. Successful treatment always depends on definite early diagnosis, easily made by tests performed on the blood and/or spinal fluid for the presence of syphilis. (This is the reason why premarital and prenatal blood tests should be legally compulsory in order to detect the presence of syphilis before marriage and before birth.)

Once a positive Wasserman reaction has been obtained, the patient should be put on intensive anti-syphilitic treatment; this must be continued until repeated spinal-fluid tests are negative. Fortunately, modern treatment is very effective and most cases can be completely controlled if early diagnosis has been made.

PARKINSON'S DISEASE

Parkinson's disease (shaking palsy) is a common chronic disorder associated with rhythmical tremors of the hands and rigidity of muscles. Post-encephalitic Parkinsonism occurs in young adults after encephalitis. Parkinsonism in individuals from forty to eighty years of age is usually due to arteriosclerosis. Damage to large masses of cells in the central portion of the brain also produces this disorder.

Symptoms. With the arm at rest, a rhythmical pill-rolling type of tremor of the fingers is present. When the patient walks, he has difficulty in initiating movements, he takes small steps, and his trunk is flexed. The face shows little expression and the eyelids blink infrequently. If the arm is moved at the wrist or elbow, cog-wheel rigidity is present with increased resistance to passive movement. Although speech and writing are slowed, normal intelligence is preserved.

Treatment. An important advance, with fundamental implications for Parkinsonism, was the introduction of the drug l-dopa. L-dopa passes from the brain circulation into the cells involved in the disease. When given in slowly increasing amounts (thus lessening the troublesome side-effects of nausea and blood-pressure drops), l-dopa is capable in many instances of reversing Parkinsonian symptoms in a manner unrivaled by any other available agent. It is generally administered in combination with another drug Sinemet® which diminishes the side effects. A more recent useful agent is Parlodel® either alone or in combination with Sinemet®.

PERIPHERAL NERVES

Nerve cells in the spinal cord are in contact with muscles and sensory receptors throughout the body by way of the peripheral nerves. Each spinal nerve is formed from an anterior motor and a posterior sensory root. The spinal nerves are divided from above to below into eight cervical, twelve thoracic, five lumbar, and five sacral nerves, plus one coccygeal nerve. In the cervical and lumbar regions, groups of spinal nerves form the brachial and the lumbar plexuses, from which peripheral nerves arise. In these areas, the disturbance of function of muscles and of sensation will vary somewhat, depending upon whether the damage is to the root, plexus, or peripheral nerve. In other areas the spinal nerves continue as the peripheral nerves, and the damage to an individual nerve will result in a uniform segmental loss of function.

Unlike the nerve fibers in the spinal cord, the peripheral nerves are capable of regeneration after interruption. Peripheral nerves may be injured by pressure or may be partially or completely severed. These injuries may be related to fractures of bones in the area. The function of peripheral nerves is also sometimes affected by diabetes mellitus, nutritional deficiency, diphtheria, and other disorders.

With complete damage to a peripheral nerve, the muscles supplied by the nerve are useless, and sensation is lost in the distribution of that nerve. With partial damage, weakness and decreased sensation are observed.

Transection of a nerve may require surgical treatment. Disorders of nerves related to systemic diseases, however, may respond to treatment of the primary disorder, and recovery may be partial or complete.

RADIAL NERVE

The radial nerve supplies muscles in the arm and hand. Extension of the elbow, wrist, and fingers is carried out by muscles supplied by this nerve.

REFLEX ARC

A reflex arc consists of the transmission of impulses across two or more neurons. The simplest type of reflex arc occurs in the spinal cord and involves only one synapse. A sensory impulse is transmitted along a sensory fiber to the cord; this impulse

SPINAL CORD

then crosses a synapse to a motor neuron, whose axon stimulates a muscle fiber. By such simple reflex arcs, the spinal cord carries out certain functions, such as some aspects of the maintenance of posture.

Most reflex arcs involve three or more neurons. Some involve many chains of neurons within the cord and brain.

A reflex arc can be demonstrated by the response to a sharp scratch of the skin on one side of the abdomen. Impulses are thereby sent to the cord, where they pass through several intermediate neurons to the motor cells controlling the muscles of the same side of the abdomen. The axons of these cells stimulate the abdominal muscle, and a visible brief contraction occurs. This skin reflex is called the abdominal reflex.

If the tendon below the kneecap is tapped with a rubber hammer, the reflex response is that of transient extension at the knee. This tendon reflex is called the knee-jerk.

SCIATIC NERVE   The sciatic nerve supplies many of the muscles in the upper and lower leg. It also carries sensory impulses from a large portion of the skin of the lower leg to the spinal cord. Painful disorders of the nerve result in *sciatica*, perhaps the most common of the painful neuropathies. (*See also* SLIPPED DISK in this section.)

SENSORY NERVE CELL (NEURON) Primary sensory neurons are located in the skin, muscles, eyes, ears, nose, viscera, and elsewhere throughout the body. They receive stimuli and transmit impulses along sensory pathways to the central nervous system. Thus, the rods and cones in the retina of the eye are special cells for the reception of visual stimuli from the external environment. Taste buds in the tongue receive and transmit chemical stimuli, which the central nervous system integrates and interprets as sweet or sour. Sensory neurons in the skin receive stimuli such as a pin prick or a light touch. Sensory neurons contained within muscle bundles transmit stimuli relating to movement. Special neurons in the intestines, in the bladder and elsewhere, provide other types of sensory information.

Secondary and other sensory neurons transmit impulses to the cord and brain through relays.

SHAKING PALSY   *See* PARKINSON'S DISEASE in this section.

SLIPPED DISK   This is one of the most common causes of "low-back pain." The vertebrae most often involved are the fourth and fifth lumbar, which have undergone strain and degeneration with resultant displacement of their intervertebral disk. Onset may be acute and sudden (for example, while bending over to lift a weight); it may be gradual, particularly in degenerative vertebral changes when the disk protrudes more and more. Disk protrusion is known as herniated disk.

Symptoms. Pain is the dominant sign, and is one-sided, indicating the direction in which the disk protrudes. In its common location, a disk impinges on the rootlets of the body's largest nerve, the sciatic—a condition generally called sciatica. There is compensatory muscle spasm in all cases, and the sufferer "favors" the painful side. There is tenderness along the sciatic nerve frequently down to the lower leg. If the patient is asked to stand on tiptoe, the pain is immediately aggravated. There are several tests that clinch the diagnosis.

Treatment. During the acute phase, bed rest on a firm surface is indicated. Careful use of heat (electric pads, hot water bottles used intermittently), analgesics (aspirin, codeine, etc.), and gentle massage are prescribed. Many patients are referred to a physical therapist very soon after the onset of pain. The acute attack usually subsides in a couple of weeks at which time attention is paid to correction of postural defects, and a supporting brace or corset may be needed. Sometimes traction is used in recalcitrant or repetitive cases. Surgery is resorted to when the acute attack does not yield to the usual treatment or when attacks tend to be repetitive. The presence of the offending disk may be verified on a CAT scan or nuclear magnetic resonance imaging (MRI). Occasionally more than one such disk may be visualized. The operation consists of the removal of the protruding disk, and the vertebrae may be fused.

CERVICAL

THORACIC

THE SPINE

The spine is the main supporting structure of the trunk of the body. The head rests on the upper end and the bones of the pelvis are attached to the lower end of this strong, flexible column.

LUMBAR

SACRAL

The five sacral vertebrae are fused into one bone (sacrum). The last five coccygeal bones form a rudimentary tail.

COCCYGEAL

SPASTICITY   Literally a drawing in, spasticity is increased tension or tonus of a muscle or group of muscles. It is marked by increase in deep reflex response, often with clonus (movements characterized by alternating contraction and relaxation, commonly referred to as clonic spasm), and a partial or incomplete loss of voluntary control. The examining physician determines the presence of clonus by suddenly putting a muscle on the stretch, for example pushing the foot upwards which puts the Achilles tendon on the stretch; if there is spasticity, this results in contractions. Spasticity is often seen after spinal cord injuries or after a stroke ("spastic paralysis").

SPINAL ACCESSORY NERVES   The two spinal accessory (or eleventh cranial) nerves control the trapezius and the sternomastoid (neck and high-back) muscles. Injury to these nerves results in weakness or paralysis of these muscles. The sternomastoid muscles rotate the head and the trapezius muscles elevate the shoulders.

SPINAL CORD   The spinal cord is enclosed within the bony spine and is protected by meningeal coverings and the cerebrospinal fluid. It is arbitrarily divided from top to bottom into cervical, thoracic, lumbar, and sacral portions. At each segmental level, the posterior roots bring sensory impulses from the sensory nerve endings into the cord, and the anterior roots carry motor stimuli to skeletal muscles.

At the "core" of the spinal cord is the grey matter consisting of nerve cells. This is surrounded by white matter which contains columns of nerve fibers. Some of the closely packed fibers carry impulses from the brain to the spinal cord, while others carry impulses from the spinal cord to the brain.

If the spinal cord is severely injured, the isolated portion of the cord below the level of the injury is capable of a variety of limited reflex activities. However, voluntary motor control from the brain is completely lost, and transmission of sensory impulses to the brain is blocked. If injury to the spine occurs at the level of the chest or abdomen, the patient is paralyzed in the legs, and bladder and bowel control is lost. If the injury occurs in the neck, the arms as well as the legs are paralyzed.

Compression of the cord by tumor results in similar loss of function below that level. Some disorders involve only selected portions of the cord. For example, multiple sclerosis involves only white matter, whereas the virus of poliomyelitis damages the cells in the anterior grey matter.

STROKE This condition is also called cerebral vascular accident. There is an impeded blood supply to some part of the brain, generally caused by
- A blood clot forming in a cerebral artery (cerebral thrombosis)
- A rupture of a blood vessel wall (cerebral hemorrhage)
- A blood clot or other material from another part of the vascular system which flows to the brain and obstructs a cerebral vessel (cerebral embolism)
- Pressure on a blood vessel, as by a tumor.

(*See also* CEREBROVASCULAR ACCIDENTS in this section.)

SUBDURAL HEMATOMA A subdural hematoma is a collection of blood in the subdural space of the meninges located between the skull and the surface of the cerebral hemisphere. One-third of subdural hematomas are bilateral. Bleeding is usually related to an external head injury, although the patient and his family may not be able to recall the injury. Rarely, subdural hematomas occur as a complication of an abnormal bleeding tendency. Usually, however, the bleeding occurs as a result of laceration of veins which bridge the meningeal coverings.

Symptoms. Subdural hematomas may occur acutely within forty-eight hours after head injury; subacutely from forty-eight hours to two weeks after injury; or chronically from two weeks to many months after injury. The variability is explained by rates of bleeding, and rates of healing including diffusion of fluids into the area. The pressure of the subdural hematoma on the brain results in mental confusion, memory defects, weakness, speech disorder, stupor, or other findings of brain dysfunction.

Treatment. The patient is admitted to the hospital for X-ray studies to locate the suspected blood clot. The treatment is surgical, the clot being removed through an opening made in the skull. This procedure frequently results in dramatic improvement in the clinical condition of the patient; but, with some patients in whom the brain is also "bruised" (contused), there may be little clinical improvement noted after removal of the blood clot.

SYNAPSE A synapse is the microscopic space at which the end of an axon of a nerve cell comes in contact with the dendrite or the cell body of another neuron. The axon carries an impulse away from its cell body. This impulse is transmitted across the space, or synapse, to the receiving portion, the dendrite, of a second nerve cell. Transmission (which is probably accomplished by chemical mediators) occurs at the synapse in only one direction. The system of nerve fibers and synapses provides a conduction and insulation system which regulates and controls the spread of impulses throughout the nervous system.

TRIGEMINAL NERVES The two trigeminal (or fifth cranial) nerves carry sensory impulses such as pain and temperature from the skin of the face to the brainstem. These nerves also transmit motor responses to the muscles used in chewing.

Neuralgia of the trigeminal nerve results in severe periodic facial pain. This nerve may also be damaged by tumors or infections.

TRIGEMINAL NEURALGIA Trigeminal neuralgia (tic douloureux) consists of sharp shooting pains in the distribution of one or more branches of the trigeminal (fifth cranial) nerve. It is not associated with any change in sensation in the face. The cause is not known.

Symptoms. The severe bouts of knife-like pain in the face may be temporarily disabling. Pain may occur in any one or all three divisions of the nerve on one side of the face. The lower portion of the face is more commonly involved than the forehead. A "trigger point" is often present in the area of the pain. Light pressure along the lower lip may set off severe pain extending along the lower jaw on the same side. Similarly, touching the gums, chewing movements, or stimulation of the skin over the cheek or forehead may set off pain. Bouts of pain may occur frequently over a period of weeks or months and then subside, with periods of complete freedom for months. Recurrence is the rule.

Treatment. Although pain-relieving medicines are required in severe cases, it is important to avoid the repeated use of narcotic drugs. The anti-epileptic drug carbamazepine is fairly specific and useful for flare-ups. Dilantin® Sodium and vitamin B$_{12}$ have been associated with remissions of trigeminal neuralgia. In selected cases, injection of alcohol into the maxillary or mandibular (jaw) divisions of the trigeminal nerve may provide relief of pain. Alcohol injection will, however, result in loss of sensation in the distribution of the injected nerve. In other severe cases direct surgical treatment is indicated.

ULNAR NERVE The ulnar nerve supplies many of the muscles which regulate hand function. It also carries sensory impulses from the little finger and the adjacent portion of the ring finger.

UNCONSCIOUSNESS Abnormal unconsciousness, occurring when a person would ordinarily be in a waking state and from which one can not be aroused by normal stimuli, may be symptomatic of various disorders of the central nervous system which can be diagnosed only by comprehensive medical examination. Loss of consciousness may occur on several levels of severity, ranging from simple transient fainting (syncope), to stupor from which one can be aroused only with difficulty, to complete unconsciousness or coma from which the patient can not be aroused at all.

Symptoms. Every case of unconsciousness should routinely consider the most common causes: circulatory collapse, including fainting, stroke, head injuries, acute alcoholism, poisoning, diabetic shock, and epilepsy. It is very important to secure a case history clarifying the conditions under which loss of consciousness occurred; often the diagnosis can be made from the history alone. Any evidence relating to reasons for loss of consciousness, such as containers suspected of having held alcohol, drugs, or poisons, should be retained for further examination. In cases where collapse has occurred without apparent cause, diabetes should be ruled out first, by means of laboratory tests of urine and blood sugars.

It is particularly important to rule out an expanding lesion such as hemorrhage or tumor within the skull. In many cases of cerebral hemorrhage following head injury, the person loses consciousness for a few minutes immediately after the injury because of cerebral concussion, following which he appears normal for several hours only to lose consciousness again suddenly. This secondary loss of consciousness suggests an expanding hemorrhage and immediate neurologic examination is indicated.

An important diagnostic problem consists in distinguishing organically caused coma from hysterical reactions. In all emotionally unstable young persons and particularly in women, it is common to observe fainting or apparent collapse which is actually a hysterical reaction to acute emotional conflict. (In such cases, application of painful stimuli such as light slaps results in immediate return to consciousness.)

Treatment. Successful treatment of unconsciousness always depends on rapid and successful diagnosis of its causes. Rapid transfer to an emergency department or physician is primary. Emergency measures should include placing the person flat on his back, loosening tight clothing, checking to see that the nose and throat are clear, keeping the person warm, and oxygen inhalation if available. There should never be any attempt to force fluids such as alcohol on semi-conscious or unconscious individuals.

VAGUS NERVES The paired vagus (or tenth cranial nerves) control the muscles used in speaking and swallowing and have extensive branchings which go on to the heart and visera. These carry impulses regulating the function of the heart and of respiration. If the vagus nerve is damaged, the patient will have difficulty in swallowing and his speech will have a nasal quality. Cutting the vagus nerve, vagotomy, was once a frequently performed operation to help peptic ulcer. Stimulation of the vagus slows the heart rate and is thought to be the cause of some syncopal episodes (faints) of emotional origin.

VOLUNTARY NERVOUS SYSTEM Also known as the motor system and the efferent nervous system, this complex consists of the nerve cells and fibers which convey impulses from the central nervous system to the periphery, chiefly the muscles.

WATER ON THE BRAIN (HYDROCEPHALY)

Although called water on the brain, this condition is more accurately cerebrospinal fluid in the brain. This fluid is found over the surface and within the ventricles of the brain and is manufactured by certain blood vessels inside these ventricles. Normally, the cerebrospinal fluid travels through small apertures at the base of the brain, circulates over the spinal cord and upper surface of the brain, and is reabsorbed by other blood vessels. If formation of the fluid is more rapid than its removal, or if there is obstruction to the flow of fluid, it will accumulate inside the brain in the unborn infant. This accumulation can stretch the ventricles, expand and thin out the brain, and "balloon" the thin skull. The condition may be secondary to a congenital infection such as rubella, toxoplasmosis, syphilis, and various viruses. It may be due to a maldevelopment which produces a large malfunctioning brain. No cause may be found, and the abnormality may be mild.

Symptoms. In some hydrocephalic infants (often before birth) the whole skull and skin will sometimes be stretched to paper thinness; the face, however, stays relatively normal. Most such infants die in the early weeks or months of life. There may be seizures or other evidence of brain damage. Milder degrees of hydrocephaly may show no impairment, and the condition may stabilize with or without an operative procedure.

Treatment. Once the advanced "skull-stretching" stage has been reached, the brain is irreparably damaged. An occasional patient will, however, be aided by very delicate neuro-surgical techniques which employ a catheter to lead the fluid to another area where it will be absorbed, generally the abdominal cavity. Nevertheless, the outlook, especially in the advanced cases, is not good.

(*See also* NORMAL PRESSURE HYDROCEPHALUS in this section.)

RESPIRATORY CONDITIONS

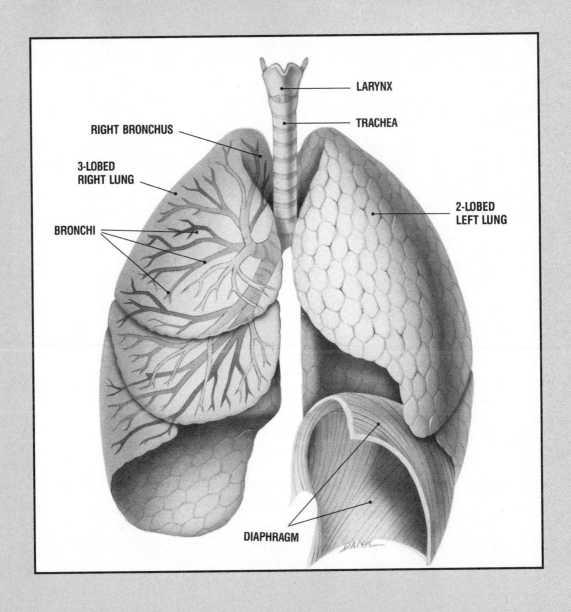

LARYNX

TRACHEA

RIGHT BRONCHUS

3-LOBED
RIGHT LUNG

2-LOBED
LEFT LUNG

BRONCHI

DIAPHRAGM

$\mathbf{T}$he process whereby the body assimilates oxygen for necessary body functions and eliminates carbon dioxide as a byproduct of the process is called respiration. The respiratory system consists of the nose, throat, larynx, trachea, bronchial tubes, and the lungs. As part of the respiration process, the physical ability to speak is possible.

This section examines the process of respiration and the various disorders and conditions which can affect the body's ability to breathe and assimilate oxygen. Conditions affecting respiration which involve the nose and throat are discussed in the section EAR, NOSE, AND THROAT. *See also* the questions on shortness of breath (Q-46, Q-47), cigarette smoking (Q-48, Q-49) in the section QUESTIONS AND ANSWERS ABOUT COMMON SYMPTOMS.

The following is a list of terms identified in this section:

AIR POLLUTION
ALVEOLI
ASBESTOSIS
ASTHMA
ATELECTASIS
BREATH, SHORTNESS OF
BREATHING DIFFICULTY
BRONCHIAL ASTHMA
BRONCHIAL CONGESTION
BRONCHIECTASIS
BRONCHITIS
BRONCHOGRAPHY
BRONCHOPNEUMONIA
BRONCHOSCOPY
COUGH
CROUP
CYANOSIS
DIAPHRAGM
EMPHYSEMA
HEMOTHORAX
HICCUP (HICCOUGH)
HYPERPLASTIC RHINITIS
HYPERVENTILATION
L.T.B. (LARYNGOTRACHEOBRONCHITIS)
LARYNGITIS
LARYNGOSPASM
LARYNX
LARYNX, ABNORMALITIES OF THE

LARYNX, INJURIES OF AND
    FOREIGN BODIES IN THE
LARYNX, TUMORS OF THE
LOBECTOMY
LUNG ABSCESS
LUNG CYSTS
LUNG EMBOLISM
LUNG FIBROSIS
LUNG INFARCT
OBSTRUCTIVE LUNG DISEASE
PHARYNX
PHRENIC NERVES
PLEURISY
PNEUMOCOCCUS
PNEUMOCONIOSES
PNEUMONIA
PNEUMONIA, ATYPICAL
PNEUMOTHORAX
PULMONARY EMBOLISM
PULMONARY INFARCTION
RESPIRATION (BREATHING)
RESPIRATORY TRACT INFECTION
SIDEROSIS
SUFFOCATION
THORACOTOMY
TRACHEITIS
TRACHEOTOMY (TRACHEOSTOMY)

AIR POLLUTION This common phrase refers to excessive accumulation of waste products in the environmental air which may be hazardous to health and safety, interfere with comfort, destroy property, or damage food supply. The quality and quantity of pollutants change with geographical location, the industrial growth of cities, and technological development. Principal air pollutants in the U.S. are smoke, soot, fog, motor exhausts, and radioactive materials acting individually or—more commonly—by interaction.

Medical knowledge has not yet pinpointed the specific pollutants which produce or aggravate disease. (*see* SMOKING in the section MISCELLANEOUS HEALTH CONDITIONS.) Nevertheless, certain facts seem well established. Certain diseases, such as chronic bronchitis, bronchial asthma, emphysema of the lungs, arteriosclerosis, and heart disease (particularly in older and sicker patients) are definitely worsened with an increase in air pollution. At certain times air pollution has produced epidemics of serious pulmonary diseases, as in Donora, Pennsylvania (1948) and in London (1952). Many died and thousands became ill from the excessive fog, and after-effects were still evident years later, reflected in increased mortality rates. Still more intriguing is the relationship of air pollution and tobacco smoking to lung cancer. (*See* the section CANCER.) The statistical evidence points to a definite increase in relation to both offenders.

The problem is but one aspect of man-made pollution of all the natural environment. The dumping of industrial and municipal wastes into lakes and streams has destroyed fish and other aquatic life. Noise pollution, particularly in our urban centers, is also a known hazard to health. The only effective measure against pollution is control of man-made wastes—a civic responsibility.

ALVEOLI Alveoli are the microscopic air sacs in the lungs where the exchange of carbon dioxide and oxygen takes place. The minute air chambers are quite numerous; both lungs contain several hundred million alveoli grouped in clusters. Pulmonary disorders such as emphysema force the alveoli to enlarge and decrease in numbers, thus causing a loss in respiratory efficiency.

The term "alveoli" is also applied to a very different part of the body. Alveoli are the bony sockets of the jaws which serve to encase the roots of teeth.

ASBESTOSIS Asbestosis is a disease of the lungs caused by inhaling minute particles of asbestos. The disease is often contracted by persons whose work causes them to be in direct contact with asbestos.

Because asbestos particles, like many foreign substances, produce bodily reactions such as fibrosis, asbestos worsens other respiratory conditions. Asbestos is a carcinogen and increases the incidence of lung cancer in smokers. Asbestos was once widely used in insulation around heat pipes. In time as the insulating wrapping deteriorates, asbestos particles are loosed into the room air. This has been particularly alarming in schools and public buildings. Extensive programs for removing asbestos wrappings of pipes are currently underway.

ASTHMA This word comes from the Greek word that means panting. This disease is known all over the world, and may affect any person, regardless of age, sex, or race. In the United States it is estimated that there are about five million asthmatic patients. Together with chronic bronchitis and emphysema (*see* OBSTRUCTIVE LUNG DISEASE in this section), asthma is responsible for the loss of about thirty-five million work days annually. A great deal of confusion attends the definition of this disease, and the word asthma often becomes a catchall for many ill-defined respiratory diseases.

Broadly speaking, asthma may be due to either extrinsic or intrinsic factors. Extrinsic asthma (also called allergic asthma) is due to external offenders which sensitize ("set up") the organism to subsequent exposures to the same agents. Let us use pollen as an example. During certain seasons, pollen is carried by the wind and inhaled into the respiratory system, without causing awareness or discomfort in most individuals. In some persons, however, due to the presence of genetically inherited characteristics, a reaction will be established between the "stranger" (pollen), thereafter called an antigen or allergen, and the host body-tissue cells. The latter will not "recognize" the antigen and react by producing defensive substances, called antibodies, which will close around the antigen and create an inflammatory reaction. From then on, every time this particular antigen reaches the body, an encounter takes place in the form of an asthmatic attack. In this instance, the target-cells for the encounter are in the mucous membrane (mucosa) of the respiratory tract. The same allergic phenomenon may express itself in any other part of the body, such as the skin (eczema), and the bowels (diarrhea). Most asthmatics have a past history of allergic episodes of one kind or another.

Basically, the allergic reaction stems from a mechanism of defense set up by the body against intruders, but which in the allergic individual is carried too far and becomes deleterious. The mechanism is a sort of protective "memory" recollection. For instance, after having passed through measles in childhood, the body develops antibodies against the causative virus; if it is again exposed to measles, antibodies are summoned and quietly deter the invader. The antigens capable of producing asthma are large in number and widely distributed. Many physical agents, such as foodstuffs, animals, clothing, cosmetics, and emotional stimuli have been found to be potential allergens. The search for the particular offender in a given person is always difficult and often fruitless.

Intrinsic asthma, on the other hand, is a term coined for the type of asthma which usually starts later in life, for which no obvious allergen can be detected, and which often develops in the wake of a severe respiratory tract infection. Thus, intrinsic asthma is sometimes called infectious asthma. Regardless of the specific cause, the mechanism of the asthmatic attack is always characterized by marked obstruction of the small bronchial tubes. This obstruction is the result of a combination of factors: thickening of the inner bronchial walls (edema) due to increased outpouring of fluid; active constriction of the muscular circular coat present in the walls of the tubes (bronchoconstriction); and production of a very thick phlegm which tends to block the bronchial airways. Under these conditions it is hard to breathe in but even harder to breathe out, and excessive air accumulates in the lungs so that they have become over-inflated.

Symptoms. Regardless of the cause, the classical asthmatic attack has the same typical characteristics. It is manifested by an acute, severe paroxysm of shortness of breath (usually of a choking nature), accompanied by audible chest wheezes, bothersome ineffectual cough, profound exhaustion, anxiety, and fear. The lips become bluish (cyanosis) and the patient perspires profusely. Most attacks develop quickly, often at night, and force the patient to sit up to insure maximal use of his respiratory muscles, including the accessory respiratory muscles in the neck. The patient feels that not enough air is coming in (though the chest is held at maximal inflation) and also that it is hard to push it out. The attack may last from minutes to several days. Spontaneously, or by medical treatment, the paroxysm is reduced and improvement is commonly heralded by expectoration of small plugs of sputum.

The mechanism of the attack is interpreted as due to generalized obstruction of the small bronchial tubes by a combination of factors: contraction of the bronchial wall musculature, thickening of the inner lining, and production of thick tenacious sputum. All factors combined reduce the passageway of the bronchial tubes significantly and obstruct the flow of air. If the attack lasts for more than a couple of days, the condition is called status asthmaticus. The attacks may recur at varying time intervals. At the onset, they may be purely seasonal (e.g., pollen asthma), related to some change in the weather, due to house-cleaning (dust asthma), or the sequel to an emotionally upsetting situation. At this stage the patient may feel perfectly well during intervals between attacks. As time goes on, however, the periodicity of attacks tends to disappear, there are less defined periods of well-being, the attacks are more frequent, and chronic bronchial asthma becomes perennial. This change is attended by new characteristics: shortness of breath does not disappear between attacks and becomes progressively more incapacitating; chronic bronchitis supervenes, with the production of daily expectoration and recurrent episodes of upper-respiratory infection; complications set in—particularly emphysema and eventually heart failure.

In other cases the attacks may repeat themselves for several years and then taper off completely, or they may reappear after several years of "cure." The course of the disease is highly unpredictable. In most cases it will last for many years with up-and-down swings in intensity. In a minority it may cripple the patient relentlessly in a matter of a few months. The popular belief that asthmatic children will "outgrow" the disease when they reach their teens is only partially true and may lure one into unwarranted confidence.

Treatment. Complete cure is possible when the specific offender is detected and can be either avoided completely, made harmless, or treated. For example, avoiding certain foods is feasible, but living in an environment of pure, pollen-free air is not. If the allergen cannot be avoided completely (dust or pollen), injections of such allergens can be given, starting with very small amounts to build up immunity slowly (desensitization). If, on the other hand, one can prove a definite established emotional disturbance, psychiatric treatment should be given.

A word of caution should be spoken about cures: Many of these are only temporary because the potentiality for becoming sensitized to newer allergens, either singly or in combination, is typical of an allergic individual. Moving to a new location may bring only temporary relief since new allergies may be contracted. Specific antiallergic treatment of progressive desensitization has the best rate of success in children and young adults. Symptomatic treatment of the disease can also be highly effective, though not curative. Particularly useful are the medications given by inhalation (bronchodilators), which bring quick relief and are given through small, pocket-sized "vaporizers" (nebulizers). Bronchodilators can be also given by mouth or by rectum.

During severe paroxysms, injections are required, the two most effective drugs being adrenalin and aminophylline. For the most difficult cases, steroid drugs are used. (These drugs are very potent and derived from sub-

stances present in the adrenal gland. It is best to use them only for short periods when simpler, conventional treatment has failed.) Expectorants and drugs to liquefy the sputum are useful adjuvants in treatment, as is reeducation in breathing habits by means of physiotherapy. Antihistamine preparations are of less value than is commonly believed. The patient should have adequate rest and sedation when overtired; control of respiratory infections is most important, particularly in chronic and elderly asthmatics.

Asthma appears to be on an increase especially in urban areas where it is perhaps related to increasing air pollution. And, despite the proliferation of new antiasthmatic measures, mortality from asthma has recently started to increase. Severe asthma should be treated in a hospital and may even call for a respirator. Asthmatics should keep in touch with physicians especially if the condition worsens.

ATELECTASIS This word means incomplete expansion. Commonly the term implies an airless or nearly airless lung which becomes functionless. The degree of atelectasis in any given situation varies considerably and may involve anything from a small segment to an entire lung.

Atelectasis may be caused fundamentally by any of the following three mechanisms: obstruction of the bronchi or blockage of the air passages; inflammation of lung tissue which takes up the space normally used for air; and insufficient chest-wall expansion or lung-collapse due to filling of the pleural space by fluid or air. In any of these conditions, although the affected lung area ceases to be ventilated, the blood continues to flow through it and progressively removes the remaining air in the space. In slow, progressive atelectasis there is always suspicion of bronchial tumors.

Symptoms. The symptoms of this condition depend on the amount of atelectasis present, varying from none, to severe degrees of breathlessness, bluish color of the lips and nail beds (cyanosis), fever, and cough. Furthermore, the symptoms of the original disease (pneumonia, tumor, muscular paralysis) which lead to atelectasis in the first place will also be present. Infection of the airless lung is a serious complication because of the lack of natural drainage from such an area.

Treatment. Treatment is directed toward correcting the original cause, together with restoration of open airways by removal of the obstruction or inflammatory secretions. Artificial respiration may be needed, particularly in cases where the nervous system and muscular mechanisms are insufficient to expand the lung. Antibiotics to combat infection and bronchodilators to expand the diameter of the bronchial tubes are commonly employed. Any tumors blocking the airways (either from the inside or acting by outside compression) are treated by surgical removal or by deep X-ray therapy.

BREATH, SHORTNESS OF Everyone experiences breathlessness now and then. Usually it is a burst of exercise such as running that causes the consumption of more oxygen in the muscle fibers than the circulation is able to supply during the time of exertion. The heart rate quickens, blood going through the heart increases in volume per minute, and the rate (as well as depth) of breathing increases becoming much faster than the usual fourteen to eighteen respirations per minute.

Causes other than extraordinary physical activity can bring about shortness of breath. For example, even with little exertion, disorders of the heart or the circulatory system frequently cause breathlessness; it all depends upon how efficiently blood can run its circuit from the tissues and through the lungs. If for any reason the tissues build up an oxygen deficiency that cannot be corrected quickly, shortness of breath will usually persist until corrective treatment is supplied.

The fault will sometimes be in the lungs rather than the circulation of blood. If, for example, a stab wound of the chest collapses one lung, breathlessness will be experienced because there is not enough exposure of blood to inhaled air, the useful surface of membrane for oxygen-transfer having been halved by the airlessness of the collapsed lung. (Blood still passes through the collapsed lung and reenters the arteries, but it is not refreshed by new oxygen.)

Hemorrhage, severe bleeding, and anemia can also cause breathlessness; since, although the circulation of the blood may be within nor-

mal limits, the number of red cells in the fluid blood may be too small to satisfy the tissues' demand for oxygen. This can be very distressing if the anemic patient has need of additional oxygen in his tissues, no matter whether the increase in demand is due to a little exertion, fever, or tissue-needs after an accident or operation (which may have caused the anemia in the first place).

Occasionally the accumulation of waste products (especially carbon dioxide) in the tissues can produce additional efforts in breathing to bring about efficient elimination of these products. This sort of breathlessness can occur in metabolic acidosis of diabetic kidney, or other origin. It is important that a person stay calm during an acute episode of shortness of breath since heightened anxiety only serves to worsen the problem.

BREATHING DIFFICULTY The most common causes of difficulty in breathing are infections, tumors, paralysis of the vocal cords, foreign bodies, spasms of the muscles of the larynx, and abnormalities of the larynx. (*See also* the Index for ACUTE EPIGLOTITIS; L.T.B. [LARYNGOTRACHEOBRONCHITIS]; DIPHTHERIA; TUBERCULOSIS; SYPHILIS; LARYNX, TUMORS OF THE; VOCAL CORDS, PARALYSIS OF; LARYNX, INJURIES OF AND FOREIGN BODIES IN THE; LARYNGOSPASM; LARYNX, ABNORMALITIES OF; and the section FIRST AID AND EMERGENCIES.)

BRONCHIAL ASTHMA *See* ASTHMA in this section.

BRONCHIAL CONGESTION *See* BRONCHITIS in this section.

BRONCHIECTASIS Bronchiectasis is a disease characterized by extensive anatomical damage to the bronchial tubes, leading to their dilatation and to formation of ballooning pockets which become the seat of chronic infection and suppuration.

The causes of bronchiectasis are multiple and, in some instances, remain unknown. In children, the condition may develop after whooping cough or measles, or may be due to the accidental swallowing of a foreign object which "goes the wrong way" and lodges in the airways instead of in the stomach. Occasionally, in debilitated or alcoholic patients, a large amount of vomited material may be partly sucked back into the lung and cause the disease. In many other instances bronchiectasis is the end result of a respiratory infection (tuberculosis, pneumonia, influenza) which did not resolve completely.

The common denominator of bronchiectasis seems to be the presence of foreign material which becomes "trapped" in the lung. Patients with such conditions are easy prey for infection which cannot find its way out through the normal airway channels. The infection roots itself in the bronchial walls, which become progressively more damaged and tend to dilate and lose their normal characteristics. Damage to the bronchus alters the protective function of the cilia, hairs which normally clean out the foreign material that lodges in the airways. (*See* RESPIRATORY TRACT INFECTION in this section.)

Symptoms. The most characteristic symptom is the coughing up of quantities of purulent material. This is the result of chronic bronchial irritation and continuous formation of such material. Cough characteristics will depend on the degree of infection and virulence, the season of the year (outbreaks are more common in winter), the position of the body, etc. Often the cough comes in paroxyms, or following laughter. The sputum is usually yellow or greyish in color and frequently foul-smelling; red streaks or frank bloody expectorations are common. As a consequence of the chronic infection, the patient may lose his appetite and may weaken and waste. The disease characteristically runs in "ups and downs" over a prolonged course marked by frequent lingering "colds," pneumonia, and bronchopneumonia.

Treatment. It is difficult to clear the pockets of infection completely. Medical treatment is aimed at the following objectives:

- Identification of the type of bacteria present and institution of repeated and prolonged courses of antibiotics
- Liquefaction of the expectoration (if thick and tenacious), to facilitate its discharge through abundant fluid-intake, steam-inhalation, or expectorants
- Best utilization of the normal pathways of bronchial discharge by postural drainage. According to the area of involvement, the patient is advised to assume certain body positions to facilitate bronchial drainage. For the lower lung areas, for example, the patient should lie down with his chest and head hanging down over the side of the bed and also turned over according to the side involved. The physician or respiratory therapist should give detailed instructions on how to perform postural drainage.

Moving to certain geographical areas, particularly to a dry and warm climate, can be useful.

When the disease is circumscribed to a definite lung area, surgical excision may be the treatment of choice.

BRONCHITIS Bronchitis may be described as inflammation or irritation of the inner lining (mucosa) of the bronchial tubes. The disease may run an acute or chronic course, the implications of each being quite different. Acute bronchitis is usually a benign, self-limiting disease which often develops in the course of a severe cold or a generalized inflammation of the nose, throat, larynx, and trachea. (*See* RESPIRATORY TRACT INFECTION in this section.) Chronic bronchitis, on the other hand, is a protracted, insidious, progressive disease, prone to exacerbations and remissions and fraught with many complications.

In recent years a complete reassessment of the serious implications of this disease has taken place. Chronic bronchitis has been recognized as an extremely common disease in the United States, but its exact prevalence is not yet adequately known. It is fair to assume that it is essentially similar to the better studied "English bronchitis" which is known to be responsible for about one-fourth of all male illness, producing the loss of twenty million work-days annually and causing about thirty thousand deaths per year. There is no single cause of chronic bronchitis, and many irritants of the bronchial mucosa have been described. The most common irritants are cigarette smoking and air pollution. Certain diseases, such as repeated upper-respiratory infections, allergy, sinusitis, or influenza are usually discovered in the background history of such patients. Eventually, with progression of the disease, bacterial infection also takes place, becoming chronically imbedded in the respiratory tract and giving rise from time to time to acute exacerbations of the disease as well as to severe complications.

Symptoms. Cough and expectoration are the outstanding symptoms, and when present daily for a period of more than six months, establish the diagnosis. Unfortunately, these symptoms are readily dismissed by most people as "smokers' cough" or "morning cough." The patient may not seek medical attention for many years, and then usually only after some complication has arisen. Expectoration can be variable in amount, character, and color. At the beginning it is clear, scanty, easy to raise, and noticeable only upon arising in the morning. As time goes on, sputum volume increases; the color changes to yellow, greyish, or blood-tinged; and the sputum itself is raised through paroxysms of cough that last progressively longer. The presence of phlegm and inflammation of the bronchial tubes commonly leads to audible respiratory wheeze produced by the passage of air through the narrowed bronchi. This wheezing is sometimes improperly ascribed to asthma, and as a result the confusing expression asthmatic bronchitis has been coined. (*See* ASTHMA in this section.) Concomitantly, shortness of breath insinuates itself progressively until it severely limits the patient's activities. Another common feature is development of protracted, lingering episodes of "colds" of progressively longer duration. Unfortunately, this symptom develops slowly over a period of several years, and most patients adjust subconsciously to the changing symptoms and signs which come to be accepted as part of their normal routine. At some time a severe cold which cannot be "shaken off" will appear, and severe, persistent incapacitation will develop. If such a state has been reached, complications are to be expected—particularly the development of chronic pulmonary heart disease or heart failure secondary to lung disease which marks the appearance of the last stage of the condition.

Treatment. Due to the chronicity of this illness, there is great variation among patients in terms of degree of reversibility of the disease, which bears a relationship to the time when they seek medical attention. With increasing awareness on the part of the public of the meaning of chronic, "innocent" cough, earlier treatment can be instituted and serious incapacitation and complications avoided. Treatment can be divided into hygienic, symptomatic, and specific. Important in hygienic treatment are avoidance of respiratory irritants (particularly cigarette smoking); of dust in all forms; of fumes, fog, smoke; of excessive cold and dampness; and of air pollutants. During the early stages of disease, and before severe incapacitation or complications have set in, these hygienic rules alone can effect a remarkable improvement and sometimes even a complete cure. Symptomatic treatment is directed toward facilitating sputum-expulsion by bronchodilator drugs (opening up of the constricted bronchi) and by liquefaction of the sticky, heavy phlegm; reducing the excessive cough; and, vigorously treating the complications—particularly the respiratory infections. Moderate physical activity is helpful and should be allowed, according to the breathing comfort of the patient; obesity should be avoided. Specific treatment can be effective in cases where the primary offender is known (allergy, tuberculosis, fungal diseases, etc.), or by surgical approach in the few cases where the disease is well-localized. Great emphasis has recently been placed on the use of antibiotics, either for short-term treatment at the time of acute respiratory infections; or as long-term treatment, particularly throughout the winter months.

BRONCHOGRAPHY This term is applied to X-ray visualization of the bronchial tubes after they have been filled with contrast material (iodine dyes). By this procedure any section of the bronchi and their branches can be observed in detail. Bronchography and bronchoscopy may complement each other for diagnostic purposes: the former affords more detailed examination and reaches down to far smaller bronchi in caliber; the latter cannot go as deep, but allows a direct examination and/or obtaining of tissue for analysis.

BRONCHOPNEUMONIA This is a type of lung inflammation similar to pneumonia, but involving such smaller lung areas (usually only millimeters to a few centimeters in size). It also differs from classical pneumonia in that it principally affects individuals whose defenses have already been weakened by other diseases or by toxic conditions. Also, it is more common at the extremes of the age-range: elderly people and children. (*See also* PNEUMONIA in this section.)

Bronchopneumonia can be caused by many bacteria, fungi, viruses, parasites, and by physical agents either as inhalants (toxic fumes) or droplets (oil). It is important to remember that many of these agents are normal inhabitants of the upper respiratory passages and attack the lung only after some disease or condition has weakened the organism, for example, during measles or whooping cough in children, or in the course of chronic bronchitis, after surgical operations, or with malnutrition in the elderly.

Symptoms. The onset is less sudden than in pneumonia, but the main symptoms are the same: marked increase in cough and expectoration (which turns yellow or greenish), moderate rise in temperature (this may be deceptively low or even normal), and general malaise. The patient does not exhibit the markedly "hard-hit" (toxic) appearance characteristic of pneumonia. If bronchopneumonia develops in a patient already affected by chronic bronchitis, the diagnosis may at times be difficult because of the similarity of symptoms. In such cases, one should become suspicious of a relative increase in frequency and severity of the "normal" cough and expectoration.

Treatment. Treatment is essentially similar to that described for pneumonia, modifications being due to the fact that bronchopneumonia often affects previously weakened individuals, so that complications are more frequent and the rate of relapses much higher. By the same token, prevention of bronchopneumonia in such persons is extremely important and depends on continuous proper care of the basic disease or condition that first attacked the patient.

BRONCHOSCOPY This is a procedure which allows direct visual inspection of the respiratory tract down to the level of the larger bronchi. It is performed with a long metallic tube—the bronchoscope—which is passed through the throat, larynx, trachea, and right or left bronchus. Thus the physician can methodically observe these areas, obtain secretions or tissue samples for analysis, and introduce medicines directly to any particular diseased area. Bronchoscopy is usually performed under local anesthesia and in skilled hands is a safe procedure for both patient and physician. The indications for bronchoscopy are many, particularly for diagnosis of suspected malignant disease.

COUGH Cough is a sudden, violent expulsion of air following a deep intake of air, exerted against some degree of glottis (larynx) closure. It is a very common symptom observed in most persons at one time or another. Essentially, it denotes an irritation of some part of the respiratory system and is basically a protective mechanism to expel an intruding object or excessive amounts of body-produced substance.

Of no particular significance is the acute cough, which follows a common cold or upper respiratory infection and progressively decreases in intensity, disappearing over a period of two to four weeks. In contrast, a cough which appears for no particular reason or which is accompanied by expectoration unusual in character or color; or which lingers for more than a month (with or without expectoration) is considered a chronic cough and should not be dismissed lightly. This is often a symptom in smokers, and unfortunately the term "cigarette cough" is widely employed to denote what is believed to be an innocent occurrence of no significance. In fact, any degree of cough which is present daily for more than a month should be considered potentially serious and brought to the attention of a physician.

Cough can be produced by numerous mechanisms acting either directly as irritants of the respiratory mucosa or by reflex action. Thus, the stimulation to cough may be initiated by an inflammation of the nose, throat, larynx (the upper respiratory tract), or below—in the trachea, bronchi, or lungs themselves. These areas may be stimulated by local inflammation, allergy, or the presence of foreign bodies. So it is that nasal discharge may travel downward as a postnasal drip and irritate the lower respiratory tract. Excessive bronchial secretions, heart-failure, airless lung (atelectasis), chronic bronchitis, pneumonia, and pleural disease have cough as an early and prominent feature. In addition, cough (particularly dry cough) may occasionally be of psychological origin either involuntary or as a means of attracting attention.

Specific diseases of the respiratory system in which chronic cough is a prominent symptom are tuberculosis, chronic bronchitis, lung cancer, and bronchiectasis.

Treatment. There is no specific treatment of this symptom itself, but rather of the underlying disease of which cough is a feature; nevertheless, when the cough is excessive, one must artifically reduce or suppress it to insure periods of rest. The best medications for this purpose are codeine, mild sedatives (such as phenobarbitol), and certain newly developed non-narcotic cough-suppressors. It should be understood that in general it is not advisable to suppress a cough entirely, since it accomplishes the function of ridding the respiratory system of offending agents.

CROUP This is an acute infection of the larynx (voice box) which produces spasm and swelling of the vocal cords. The condition usually strikes suddenly at night during cold, dry weather and is seen largely in children.

Symptoms. The child awakens from a sound sleep as if someone were choking him. He produces a deep, barking, brassy cough followed by a prolonged, wheezy rasp (stridor) on inhaling. (This should not be confused with asthma, in which there is a prolonged exhalation.) The condition is always worse at night, and there are apt to be three consecutive bad nights, followed by several days of a cough with loose phlegm.

Treatment. As croup is often due to a virus, there is no specific medication. However, steam inhalations will allow the victim to sleep at least an hour or so between spasms. Lemon juice and honey in equal amounts is a effective cough remedy, as are the codeine and related agents.

If steam and cough remedies do not induce sleep or relieve the spasm and difficult breathing, the condition is obviously more serious than simple croup and may require oxygen and vapor administered in the hospital; an occasional patient requires a tracheotomy (the cutting of a hole and insertion of a metal tube in the windpipe) because the obstruction is so great. In this latter situation the infec-

tion is most probably due to a bacterium, and antibiotics are often necessary. There are occasional patients who suffer from croup because of some allergy to food or inhalants; skin testing is usually required to determine the cause here. (*See also* the section FIRST AID AND EMERGENCIES.)

CYANOSIS A bluish discoloration of the skin, lips, and nail beds, cyanosis is caused by insufficiently oxygenated blood passing through the tiny capillaries and vessels under the skin or mucous membrane. If the oxygen saturation in arterial blood falls below about 75 percent (the normal is 97 percent), a blueness of the skin and mucous membranes appears. This can be a sign of great importance. The blue color is determined by the concentration of unoxygenated hemoglobin in the capillaries of the skin. Cyanosis requires four or five grams of unoxygenated hemoglobin per one hundred milliliters of blood before it can be seen with the unassisted eye. Thus when a severe anemia is present, cyanosis may never appear, even though serious oxygen-deficiency exists in arterial blood, because there is simply not enough hemoglobin to produce the cyanosis. On the other hand, if hemoglobin is much higher than normal, cyanosis may be seen in a patient who is not suffering at all from abnormally low oxygen saturation. In some of the congenital heart diseases, the hemoglobin can rise to twenty grams or above. In these patients, cyanosis indicates the need for careful study of the blood count as well as the heart or lung defect that has caused this high level to appear.

The oxygen concentration of the blood determines hemoglobin saturation, for all oxygen is transported by adding itself into the hemoglobin molecule during passage through the capillaries of the lung.

There are three chief causes for cyanosis originating in the heart-lung system:

Decreased ventilation of the lungs. If for any reason adequate oxygen is not able to reach the lung capillaries, the oxygen-uptake of blood passing through the lungs will be very poor. This can happen in pulmonary diseases, such as emphysema of the lungs, or during an attack of choking on a foreign body lodged in the throat or windpipe that interferes with the in-and-out flow of air to the lungs.

Short-circuiting of blood in heart or lungs. If there is a defect in the chambers of the heart, part of the blood in the right-hand side of the heart can pass into the left-hand side and be forced into the arterial system without having taken the trip through the lungs. This is aggravated if there is, in addition, an obstruction in the pulmonary artery leading to the lungs. Occasionally, there is an inborn "short circuit" in the arteries of the lung itself, so that blood passes abnormally from artery to vein before the respiratory membrane is ever reached; this is called an arteriovenous fistula of the lungs.

Failure of oxygen diffusion across the respiratory membrane (alveoli). An oxygen-diffusion block can be caused by some lung diseases that thicken the respiratory membrane. Thickening or any other abnormal state, including cysts, of the membrane, can prevent oxygen-transfer across the pulmonary membrane into the blood in spite of adequate circulation in the lungs and an adequate supply of oxygen in the alveoli of the lung. (A common example is the hyaline-membrane disease frequently seen in premature babies.)

THE DIAPHRAGM

The diaphragm is the musculo-membranous partition that separates the abdomen from the thorax.

DIAPHRAGM   This is the chief muscle of respiration and separates the abdomen from the thorax.

Diaphragm is also the name of a birth control device. (*See also* CONTRACEPTION in the section FEMALE HEALTH CARE.)

EMPHYSEMA   This word means to inflate. It designates a variety of states in which overinflation occurs in any part of the body. In common usage, emphysema refers to a condition in which the smallest lung sacs (alveoli) become overdistended and lose their normal structure, and in which progressive "trapping" of air in the lung takes place. An additional important characteristic of the disease is the development of severe obstruction to airflow; at the present time it is not clear whether this obstruction precedes or follows the anatomical destruction. Emphysema is a disease much more prevalent in men than in women (ten to one ratio).

Overdistention of the lung may be purely a functional change without significant disease implications, as many otherwise healthy elderly individuals exhibit this feature. Pure emphysema (also called chronic pulmonary emphysema, or obstructive or hypertrophic pulmonary emphysema) is a disease in which overinflation is accompanied by anatomical destruction of lung-tissue, leading to the formation of small or large cavities called bulla; these become functionless, and in turn encroach upon and impair the function of still-normal lung areas. (*See* OBSTRUCTIVE LUNG DISEASE in this section).

The cause, or causes, of emphysema are unknown. Commonly-held theories link the condition to chronic bronchitis, which almost invariably precedes it. It is believed that emphysema is the final result of the sustained irritation to the bronchial tubes which follows in the wake of excessive smoking, air pollution, or repeated episodes of respiratory infection or allergic asthma. The common factor in all these conditions is the development of obstruction to airflow; this may be intermittent and reversible at the beginning (bronchoconstriction) but is eventually superseded by excessive mucous secretions which progressively narrow the bronchial passageway. With progression of the disease, air is allowed to flow in but is partially trapped on its way out, leading to formation of larger and larger air sacs. More respiratory pressure must then be exerted to promote airflow. This, in turn, further contributes to closing down the already narrowed and unsupported bronchial tubes.

Symptoms. Chronic pulmonary emphysema is a disease of insidious and progressive nature. A typical case might be seen in a male in his late fifties who has been a heavy smoker for more than thirty years. He will have had a chronic sputum-productive cough for many years—one which was always dismissed as a "cigarette cough." For the past ten to fifteen years he has given up certain physical efforts which produce uncomfortable breathing (dyspnea), such as fast walking, running to catch a bus, or climbing more than two flights of stairs.

Because of the gradual development of this incapacitation, the typical patient often disregards it and does not volunteer such information until specifically questioned. At some point a respiratory infection develops and the patient becomes acutely ill and overcome by severe shortness of breath which clearly prevents him from performing his common daily activities. Cough and expectoration increase. The chest acquires a barrel shape, the shoulders are thrown forward and the patient gasps for breath. Usually the lips become bluish and the fingernails "clubbed" (similar in shape to drumsticks). Breathing ceases to be an effortless, unconscious mechanism and becomes a struggle.

The respiratory muscles have to perform a tremendous amount of work to get enough oxygen into the lungs and to transfer it to the blood in order to provide for the metabolic needs of the body; here, more oxygen is also required. This creates the following paradox: reduced lung function provides less than the necessary amount of oxygen, which is avidly "fought for" by both the body and the very respiratory muscles whose own need of oxygen is abnormally increased because of excess labor in moving an overdistended and inefficient chest.

Since breathing must continue, the respiratory muscles have "priority" on the available oxygen. Next in line for use of oxygen are the important organs of circulation and digestion, the brain, and others. Thus, very little is left in the end for use by the skeletal muscles, and such activities as walking, for example, have to be severely curtailed. Effective expectoration of sputum is impaired, and mucus "plugs" create more bronchial obstruction. The stage is set for the development of repeated episodes of bronchial infection which acutely reduce the already chronically impaired breathing capacity. Curtailment of breathing capacity (particularly in acute emphysema) throws a burden onto the heart, which is forced to strain itself to maintain circulation through the lungs. Thus, heart-failure or pulmonary heart disease is a common complication in the advanced stages of chronic pulmonary emphysema.

Treatment. At present, treatment is mostly symptomatic and directed toward obtaining "bronchial cleansing." In essence, it is the treatment of chronic bronchitis. During its early stages, effective regimes may considerably delay the otherwise expected downward course of emphysema. Breathing exercises are useful in reeducating the breathing pattern and can ease the work of the respiratory muscles. Slight degrees of physical activity (below the point of marked discomfort) are to be encouraged under a progressive program of rehabilitation. At the beginning of such a program, oxygen may be added to lengthen the training periods. Chronic use of oxygen at the patient's home has to be monitored carefully, because in certain patients it may induce severe respiratory depression—the so-called "carbon dioxide narcosis syndrome." Symptoms of heart-failure are treated with digitalis and other drugs (diuretics) designed to promote urinary output and prevent fluid accumulation in the body.

HEMOTHORAX   Collection of blood in the chest (pleural) space is referred to as hemothorax. This may vary in degree from very small amounts to a massive collection. The condition represents one form of internal bleeding. Hemopneumothorax is a combination of air and blood in the same location.

There are four principal causes of hemothorax: pleural inflammation, either localized primarily in the pleura or most commonly following a lung inflammation such as pneumonia or pulmonary infarct; rupture of a blood vessel following or as a sequel to chest-wall injury of a rib or other penetrating chest wound; tumors which in their progressive course invade and erode blood vessels; as a complication of a partial pneumothorax (air in the pleura) due to rupture of an adhesion-band.

Symptoms. If the collection of blood is small, the condition may go undetected in the course of the primary disease or may be manifested only by mild pain. With increased amounts, the fluid compresses the lung and breathlessness and bluish discoloration (cyanosis) become prominent. Massive collections, beside producing the above, give rise to rapid heartbeat, pallor, drop in blood pressure, and shock (internal hemorrhage).

Treatment. Cases of small hemothorax do not ordinarily require specific treatment other than that for the primary cause. When large, the blood should be evacuated by the same procedures described in the treatment of pleurisy.

HICCUP (HICCOUGH) This is an involuntary spasm of the diaphragm during its inspiratory (inhale-phase) contraction which is checked suddenly by the closure of the voice box (larynx). It is often caused by fast eating. It usually repeats itself for several minutes and disappears spontaneously, or by simple measures such as holding the breath, drinking cold water, or pulling the tongue out firmly. Sometimes, eating granulated sugar will stop it.

Persistent hiccup is of medical significance because of its underlying cause, which may be an irritation of the gastrointestinal tract, the pleura, lung, heart, central nervous system, or of the diaphragm itself. In such cases it is postulated that an abnormal nerve-reflex mechanism is at fault, persistently stimulating the diaphragmatic motor-nerve pathways. Contact a physician if the condition is prolonged.

Treatment. Treatment for this condition should be aimed at controlling the basic underlying cause. In addition, the following measures are occasionally effective: rebreathing into a paper bag; gastric lavage; breathing a mixture of 10 percent carbon dioxide in oxygen, or injecting antinausea

drugs such as chlorpromazine. If all fails, and this is reserved for rare cases where hiccups have been present for a long time, one may have to resort to surgical interruption or temporary paralyzation of the phrenic nerve in the neck.

HYPERPLASTIC RHINITIS After repeated nasal infections or recurrent sinusitis, sometimes at puberty, and temporarily during pregnancy or the menses, the nasal mucosa becomes thickened. It is swollen, secretes mucus excessively, and after a time shows thickening of the bone and bony lining (periosteum). These changes in the structure of the nose cause symptoms of nasal blockage and thick, sticky discharge. Difficult to treat, hyperplastic rhinitis requires finding and successfully treating underlying causative factors for its control.

HYPERVENTILATION Hyperventilation is the rapid exhaling of excessive carbon dioxide and the inhaling of large volumes of oxygen exhibited by individuals suffering from an anxiety reaction or from chronic obstructive pulmonary disease.

Symptoms. Fast breathing (greater than forty times a minute) with accompanying dizziness, lightheadedness, chest discomfort, and tingling in the extremities are common symptoms.

Treatment. Patients are encouraged to take long slow deep breaths or to breathe in and out of a paper bag, as a way to increase the carbon dioxide intake. Treating the anxiety reaction that caused the hyperventilation is generally more difficult and lengthy, though beneficial in the end. Treatment of chronic obstructive pulmonary disease is with specific medications prescribed by a physician. (*See also* OBSTRUCTIVE LUNG DISEASE in this section.)

L.T.B. (LARYNGOTRACHEOBRONCHITIS) This condition usually occurs in a child less than three years of age who has had a cold and cough with hoarseness. As the infection progresses, there is more and more difficulty in breathing, and the larynx, trachea, and bronchi produce heavy, thick mucous secretions.

Treatment. This inflammation of the larynx, trachea, and bronchi responds to high humidity, antibiotics, and maintenance of fluid intake. But tracheotomy may still be necessary.

LARYNGITIS This common term may be defined as inflammation of the larynx (voice box), occurring most commonly as part of, and in the course of, upper-respiratory infections. It may be caused by bacteria, viruses, or an allergy. The main symptom is change of voice, ranging from hoarseness to severe degrees of incapacity to produce sounds. Breathing becomes more difficult and the obstruction may lead to sudden suffocation (asphyxia). The rest of the symptoms will depend on the other organs involved (nose, throat, glands). The laryngeal symptoms are more dramatic and develop faster than those in the other areas because of the relative smallness and unusual irritability of the larynx, especially in infants. The manifestations of diphtheric laryngitis are essentially similar to those caused by other bacteria or even viruses, and may be differentiated only by direct laryngeal examination and study of the secretions.

Another form of acute laryngitis is croup. This condition is due to an acute spasm of the laryngeal muscles. Its symptoms are the sudden onset of harsh, metallic cough (without warning or preceding symptoms, frequently at night) and alarming "rattling" sounds (stridor) during inhalation, accompanied by severe shortness of breath. The disease-picture is very dramatic, but can be quickly controlled by steam inhalations or induced vomiting, the patient being completely relieved the following morning. This should be clearly differentiated from the mild shortness of breath which is part of the symptomatology of common laryngitis, but which may progress (obstructive laryngeal dyspnea) to irreversible asphyxia and require an emergency operation.

Other forms of laryngitis are those chronic forms due to continued irritation (smoking, air pollutants) or caused by specific diseases such as tumors, tuberculosis, syphilis, or nerve diseases.

Treatment. In most cases common acute laryngitis requires only the hygienic measures described for other upper-respiratory infections. If the cause is bacterial, the proper antibiotic should be given. The important exception is diphtheria, which requires quick administration of diphtheria antitoxin if the patient has not been previously vaccinated. If a picture of breathing-difficulty (obstructive laryngeal dyspnea) begins to develop, regardless of cause (aside from the classical croup), an immediate tracheotomy should be performed by medical personnel. (*See also* TRACHEOTOMY in this section.)

LARYNGOSPASM Laryngospasm, or spasms of the muscles of the larynx, occurs chiefly with the use of some kinds of anesthesia in the operating room (where it is readily taken care of) and in children between one and six years of age. In these latter cases the child typically awakens from a sound sleep with respiratory difficulty, although there is no immediate previous history of a cold or fever. Reassurance and deep regular breathing may relieve the problem. Breathing oxygen (if available) mixed with room air may stop the attack. The inducing of vomiting has been used successfully for this problem, but this is probably dangerous since there is a chance of aspirating and sucking in vomited material.

LARYNX The voice box, or larynx, is composed of cartilages held together by ligaments, muscles, and strong sheets of fibrous tissue. It can be felt in the front part of the neck. The most prominent bulge in the neck—approximately where the knot of a man's tie is—is the "Adam's apple": the prominence of the thyroid cartilage of the larynx. Just below this is the only complete ring of the larynx, the cricoid cartilage. (Within the thyroid cartilage, near the Adam's apple, is the attachment to the vocal cords.)

The real functions of the larynx are threefold: as a sphincter—an organ of closure—to prevent fluids and food from entering the lungs; as a rigid structure to permit and assure an open pathway for breathing; and as a voice-producer. The intricate workings of the larynx are indeed wonderful; when not functioning well, however, the larynx gives rise to two recognizable and common symptoms: hoarseness and difficulty in breathing.

LARYNX, ABNORMALITIES OF THE
The most common problem under this cate-

gory occurs in children under two years of age. The cartilages of the larynx—particularly the epiglottis—are frequently very soft and flabby (laryngomalacia). These soft cartilages may be drawn inward on inhaling, thus producing difficulty in breathing. The child usually outgrows this problem by the age of two. Webs, cysts, and vascular rings are less common, but when found can often be relieved by surgery.

Congenital webs are membranous growths which may be partially obstructive within the larynx. Vascular rings are abnormalities in the development of the local blood vessels. All of these, as well as occasional congenital cysts, may require surgery.

LARYNX, INJURIES OF AND FOREIGN BODIES IN THE   Trauma is a general term referring to injury. In its broad sense this can, for example, be injury from a cold or from tobacco.

In the usual sense, trauma refers to an actual physical blow causing injury. This type of direct trauma to the larynx, and the resultant scar it can form, may be a cause of hoarseness. Direct blows to the larynx are dangerous and can break the cartilage. If the cricoid cartilage is broken, or if sufficient swelling and hemorrhage occur, respiration can be severely compromised, resulting in death.

Foreign matter sucked into the larynx can also obstruct the airway or produce swelling and hemorrhage. After an initial period of irritation and coughing, the foreign body may cause no further outward symptoms, but days or weeks later cause serious illness. Furthermore, suction of a foreign body into the lungs can cause pneumonia or blockage of the main bronchus.

Treatment. Location of the foreign body by examination and X-rays, and removal by special instruments, is now performed by both ear-nose-and-throat specialists and by chest specialists. If a child is suspected of having inhaled foreign materials—anything from buttons to beans—he should be examined by a physician. The fact that the child has stopped coughing is no excuse for neglecting the possibility of retained foreign material.

LARYNX, TUMORS OF THE   There are both benign and malignant (cancerous) tumors of the larynx, with the vast majority manifesting themselves through the symptom of hoarseness. Therapy for benign tumors consists of removal of these tumors and of voice-rest. Some benign tumors called papillomas are frequently multiple and tend to recur after removal, although not so readily once adolescence is past. One very common cause of hoarseness results from vocal nodules caused by vocal abuse. These nodules are not true tumors but are called tumors for the sake of convenience. With proper use of the voice and removal of the tumor, the problem can be solved.

Malignant tumors (cancer) have only one early symptom: hoarseness. Pain is not an early manifestation. The diagnosis can be made by your family physician or by an ear-nose-and-throat specialist. Mirror inspection of the larynx, viewed indirectly from the mouth, clearly reveals lesions of the vocal cords, but a small piece of tissue is necessary for absolute diagnosis. This is called a biopsy, and is most often taken with a special forceps through a long, hollow, lighted tube. Brief hospitalization is usually necessary for this procedure.

Treatment. Early cancer of the larynx is curable in a high percentage of people. In very early cancer of the vocal cords, radiation or surgery can provide a cure in 85 percent of cases. In view of the possibly dangerous nature of the symptom, it is inexcusable for the patient to neglect hoarseness.

The position and/or size of tumors causing hoarseness may be such that airway obstruction also occurs. There may be strong objections to surgery on the part of some patients with cancer of the larynx who refuse surgery because they fear voice-loss. In most cases the size of the tumor and the swelling associated with it will eventually necessitate tracheotomy, and tumor-plus-tracheotomy will cause a loss of voice in any event. The patient will have lost valuable time and perhaps sacrificed his life for no good reason.

LOBECTOMY   Lobectomy is the surgical excision of a lung lobe. This procedure is indicated for destructive diseases such as advanced bronchiectasis, tumors or chronically infected areas of the lung. In terms of salvaging as much lung tissue as possible, lobectomy when applicable is preferable to pneumonectomy in which the entire lung of the affected side is removed.

LUNG ABSCESS This term refers to a localized area of inflammatory destruction and suppuration within the lung which enlarges by progressive tissue-death (necrosis) and formation of infected cavities. When the process has been present for more than six weeks, it is considered a chronic abscess. Most abscesses are localized in the right lung, more specifically in its posterior areas. In the past twenty years the incidence of lung abscess has decreased considerably, probably as a result of antibiotic drugs.

Abscess is caused by infectious agents, notably bacteria. Many types of bacteria, fungi, or parasitic infestations are capable of producing an abscess; but most commonly responsible are the bacteria which live in or invade the respiratory system. Interestingly enough, there is frequent association with the bacteria which normally live in the mouth and become virulent due to poor hygienic conditions of the teeth, gums, or throat. In the genesis of a lung abscess, there must exist certain pathological conditions which favor bacterial attack upon the lung: among the most common are the sucking of stomach contents into the lung during prolonged periods of sleep (such as may follow an alcoholic bout); or the accidental inhalation of a foreign body into the lung, thus creating a state of acute bronchial obstruction. In either case, some areas of the lung are insufficiently ventilated and the stagnation of materials favors the growth of any bacteria which may be present. (In other cases, lung abscess may be the result of uncontrolled pneumonia, lung tumor, or injury.)

Symptoms. Temperature peaks, cough, and expectoration are the most outstanding symptoms, and their intensity is related to the severity and toxicity of the infection, the patient's natural resistance, and the freedom of the airways as a coughing-outlet for sloughed material. One can picture lung-abscess evolution by analogy with a deep abscess under the skin, before and after it has opened its way to the surface and draining has started.

Many complications can attend the presence of a lung abscess, notably its extension to the pleura (empyema), its dissemination by way of the bronchi into other lung areas, and development of hemorrhages because of erosion of blood vessels. Even after the abscess is cured, the formation of thick—and sometimes extensive—fibrous tissue may severely restrict future lung activity.

Treatment. Some years ago the prognosis in cases of lung abscess was very poor and hopes were mostly pinned on surgery. Today, however, the treatment is mostly medical, and this should always be attempted first. It consists of intensive administration of antibiotics and maintenance of open airways for discharge of the necrotic, sloughed debris. The latter is accomplished by inhalations of bronchodilator drugs, repeated suctioning of bronchial secretions, and—most importantly—use of postural drainage as described in the treatment of bronchiectasis. It is generally agreed that if the abscess has not been cured or definitely controlled after six weeks of such intensive medical treatment, surgery may be indicated. If feasible, the best surgical procedure is minimal removal of the destroyed area.

LUNG CYSTS These are air-containing spaces or cavities which develop abnormally within the lung and do not follow the ordinary arrangement of normal lung structure. The abnormality may be present from the time of birth (congenital) due to arrested development of certain areas of the lungs. Most lung cysts, however, are acquired during life as the result of destructive lung diseases such as emphysema, bronchiectasis, or traumatic wounds. Thus the nomenclature of air cysts includes such names as bleb, bullae, pneumatocele, emphysematous cysts, and cystic fibrosis.

Symptoms. The nature of symptoms depends on the cause leading to the formation of the cyst, its size, and the condition of the rest of the lung. Congenital cysts, for instance, are usually "silent" and may be discovered only during a routine chest X-ray. Acquired cysts exhibit symptoms characteristic of the causative disease and will tend, when large enough, to decrease breathing capacity and express themselves by breathlessness. This is the result of the fact that the cyst does not itself participate in ventilation and also because its size tends to compress the surrounding normal lung areas and render them airless (compression atelectasis). Three important complications may attend the presence of a cyst: rupture into the pleural space, with formation of a pneumothorax—air in the lung-covering; hemorrhage within the cyst; and infection. If the cysts result from obstruction of the airways, they may enlarge progressively, reach enormous size, and even occupy most of the lung space (giant tension cysts).

Treatment. Surgical removal is indicated only for the very large cysts, tension cysts in which acute complications have arisen, or in chronically infected cysts. Otherwise, the cyst is treated as part of the background disease.

LUNG EMBOLISM A lodgement of a blood clot or other foreign material in a branch of the pulmonary artery, lung embolism (pulmonary embolus) produces interruption of the arterial blood supply to a certain area of the lung and leads to a lung "solidification," usually hemorrhagic in nature, called lung infarction.

Since venous blood from all parts of the body must return through the lung, any abnormal material discharged into the circulation may finally lodge in the pulmonary arterial circulation. The most common cause is the formation of blood clots due to inflammation of a vein in the leg or following an abdominal operation (thrombophlebitis). A failing heart which cannot adequately maintain the circulation may also be the source of blood clots. Other materials, such as large parasites, globules of fat, and even air which accidentally find their way into the venous circulation, may also produce embolization of the lung arteries. Emboli may range in size from microscopic to a huge, long strip. They may be single or multiple, and may occur simultaneously, in regular series, or at irregular intervals.

Symptoms. Diagnosis is difficult or even impossible in the case of small-size embolisms, which may be single or repeated over a period of several years. In such cases, ill-defined symptoms of breathlessness, chest-pain, or heart-failure will focus attention on such a possibility only after multiple embolisms have occurred and curtailed circulation irreparably through more than half of the lung arteries.

On the other hand, a large single embolus produces a dramatic picture of acute chest-pain, cough and blood-tinged sputum, rise in temperature and pulse, and rapid breathing. Bluishness (cyanosis) is also usually present, in addition to the appearance of sudden apprehension. This combination of symptoms and signs leads the physician to search for an inflamed or painful leg-vein or for any of the other possibilities mentioned among the causes. Most episodes of lung embolism are not immediately fatal and will resolve in a period of days or weeks. The most common complications are formation of a lung infarct which may become secondarily infected; pleurisy with or without fluid-formation; and acute heart-failure. Most dangerous, however, is the repetition of small series of emboli which are not clinically recognized until later, when they ultimately lead to an established and progressive chronic heart-failure called cor pulmonale. (*See* the section CARDIOVASCULAR CONDITIONS.)

Treatment. Aside from the rare cases of a very large embolus which is recognized immediately and removed surgically, treatment is mainly directed to the original cause. If this is an inflamed vein, appropriate rest position for the leg and antibiotics are employed. Often, anticoagulants should be used; these are drugs (such as heparin and dicoumarol) which decrease the capacity of the blood to clot. If embolization continues despite these measures, the physician may be forced to tie off a large common vein such as the inferior vena cava. More important is consideration of prevention of embolization. Older, bedridden individuals, patients with any serious prolonged disease, or patients who are being operated upon for any reason should be encouraged to move their legs or should have them moved at frequent intervals. These measures are designed to prevent stagnation of the circulation, the common forerunner of the vein inflammation or thrombosis from which emboli are subsequently released to lodge in the lung.

LUNG FIBROSIS This is a term applied to a number of diseases which lay down appreciable amounts of scar tissue in the lung. Such conditions include tumors, degenerative and allergic conditions of the lung, chronic inflammatory diseases, and pneumoconiosis. To a large degree, lung fibrosis is a token of defense mechanisms, past or present, employed by the lung against multiple offenders. Eventually, however, the residual marks of such fight (scar tissue) are large enough to supplant the delicate elastic network of the lung and become a burden to the breathing or circulation, leading to respiratory or heart-failure.

Symptoms. The amount, distribution and localization of fibrosis in the lung varies considerably, to the same degree as do the symptoms and complications. The fibrosis may be focal (circumscribed) or diffuse. It may encroach preferentially upon the airways, producing symptoms of obstructive lung disease; along the blood vessels, giving rise to pulmonary heart disease; or produce a scarred, rigid pleura that restricts lung expansion. The most common symptom in any given cause of lung fibrosis is breathlessness (dyspnea).

Treatment. Already established fibrosis is irreversible. Treatment may be effective only when the original disease is promptly recognized and further spreading can be controlled, preventing formation of new scar tissue. In a few cases, when a relatively localized amount of fibrosis has distorted the structure of neighboring normal tissue, surgical removal of the worthless area of fibrosis may restore the lost function of the normal adjacent lung.

LUNG INFARCT *See* LUNG EMBOLISM in this section.

OBSTRUCTIVE LUNG DISEASE This is a general term applied to a group of respiratory diseases whose most common prevalent characteristic is the presence of chronic impairment of airflow into and out of the lungs. Most conspicuous in the obstructive lung disease group are bronchial asthma, emphysema, and bronchitis.

Obstruction to airflow may be due to many factors. Some of these are of a physical, anatomic nature, such as tumors, foreign bodies, fibrosis, or postinflammatory scars, which decrease or close down the bronchial passageway. By present-day agreement, however, the term obstructive lung disease is mainly reserved for airflow-obstructing conditions caused by one or more of the following factors: broncho-constriction (active narrowing of the bronchi due to excessive contraction of the

THE LUNGS

RIGHT (3 LOBES)

LEFT (2 LOBES)

muscular coat present in their walls); edema (excessive thickening of the inner layer [mucosa] of the bronchial tubes due to inflammatory or allergic fluid-accumulation); and secretions (produced excessively by the mucosal glands and which mechanically impair the flow of air).

It is characteristic of this group of diseases that they are insidious and chronic in nature. Although the obstruction is usually reversible in the early stages, it becomes fixed as time goes on. The diseases of this group are usually prone to complication by bacterial infection and in their final stages, lead to progressive lung destruction and a parallel decrease in breathing capacity. Symptoms include wheezing, cough, expectoration, shortness of breath, and choking. In advanced states, the right side of the heart is pumping against increased pressure, and cardiac-decompensation may occur.

PHARYNX The pharnyx has three divisions, which may be observed if one looks into the open mouth with the help of a mirror. Following the tongue to the back of the throat, and looking a little beyond, will lead the eye to the very back of the throat, the oral pharynx.

Up above the palate and in back of the nose is the nasopharynx, while the laryngopharynx lies below the base of the tongue.

PHRENIC NERVES The phrenic nerves arise from the roots of the spinal cord in the mid-portion of the neck and descend through the central portion of the chest to supply the muscles of the diaphragm. In normal breathing, the diaphragm contracts on inspiration and allows the lower portions of the lungs to expand. It relaxes during exhalation. With paralysis of the diaphragm, breathing is limited.

PLEURISY The term pleurisy refers to an inflammation of the chest structure known as the pleura. The pleura is a two-ply membrane, one layer of which neatly encloses each lung-surface, the other layer lining the inner side of the chest wall. Normally there is no free space between these two layers; a thin amount of lubricant fluid contained between them allows for free movement of the lung during breathing. So it is that pleurisy may be merely a dry inflammation of the lining or it may progress to the formation of increased amounts of fluids, separating the layers and creating a true space in between.

Pleurisy is usually a complication or extension of diseases affecting the lung or chest wall; but once established, it may run a course independent from the original disease. Pleurisy is most commonly secondary to pneumonia, tuberculosis, lung tumor, abscess, chest wounds, or rib fracture. Primary pleurisy, in which the disease begins in the pleura itself, is rare.

Symptoms. The disease may be acute—the symptoms and course being of short duration—or chronic, lasting for months or years with exacerbations and remissions. The chief manifestation is always pain. In a typical case of pleurisy the pain develops progressively over a period of hours or days, is jagged and shooting in quality and intensified during deep breathing, cough, or sneezing. (Patients instinctively curtail the depth of breathing or lie on the affected side.) The pain is due to the continuous rubbing together of the inflamed pleural layers. As the inflammation continues, fluid begins to accumulate in the pleural space, thus separating the inflamed layers, and thereby somewhat reducing the pain. If fluid-formation is large, the breathing expansion of the lung is decreased and breathlessness may ensue. Fever may or may not be present. (Other concurrent symptoms, such as cough, expectoration, and malaise, are usually features of the primary disease in the lung or chest wall.)

Depending on the cause and nature of the inflammation, the disease may subside completely; if the fluid is clear, it may be reabsorbed without further consequences. In other cases, when the fluid is itself infected (empyema) or bloody (hemothorax) spontaneous reabsorption is difficult and slow, and the ultimate result is formation of adhesive bands which will continue to "imprison" the lung, severely limiting breathing capacity.

Treatment. Fundamentally, treatment is aimed at therapy for the primary disease whether in the lung or the chest wall. In cases of pneumonia, tuberculosis, lung abscess, or penetrating chest-wall injury, which cause the pleurisy, proper antibiotic treatment will take care of the pleural inflammation as well.

Sometimes symptomatic treatment of the pleurisy itself is necessary to relieve pain or breathlessness. If fluid-formation is large, or if it is purulent or bloody, thoracentesis is indicated. This consists of removing the fluid by means of a needle puncture or by inserting a rubber tube which will drain the fluid continuously into a sealed bottle. This process is called closed chest drainage. The latter is usually left in place for several days or weeks until the fluid stops reaccumulating and the lung has re-expanded. In cases where the lung will not re-expand after fluid-removal because fibrous adhesions "imprison" the lung, a decortication should be performed: this operation strips the lung from the pleural peel.

PNEUMOCOCCUS This word refers to a bacterial microorganism (conical or lance-shaped and usually appearing in pairs, which takes on a bluish color when stained by the Gram method [Gram-positive]). About seventy-five types or strains of pneumococcus have been isolated by laboratory tests, the type depending on the composition of the bacterial capsule. Also depending on the capsular material is the differing virulence of various pneumococcal strains.

The pneumococci are normal inhabitants of the upper respiratory tract of most individuals. Under stress situations, they may become virulent, multiply rapidly, invade the lower respiratory tract, and produce disease. The exact reasons for this transformation are not clear at present.

The pneumococcus is responsible for more than 95 percent of lobar pneumonias and is also a common cause of bronchopneumonia. Most pneumococci are extremely responsive to penicillin therapy, the drug of choice in lobar pneumonia. (*See also* PNEUMONIA and RESPIRATORY TRACT INFECTION in this section.)

PNEUMOCONIOSES This word was coined in 1866 to describe all lung diseases caused by inhaled dust. Even at that time several specific "industrial diseases" were already known, including anthracosis (in coal miners), silicosis (in mine, quarry, and road workers), and siderosis (in foundry workers). Early medical studies also indicated that inhalation of any dust in excessive concentrations, if continued long enough, might lead to manifest disturbances of lung function. It was also learned that the lungs of most individuals living in largely populated areas would always show the presence of dust during postmortem examination.

As modern industry expanded, new materials and new means of processing old materials considerably complicated and enlarged the pneumoconioses hazard, either in the form of direct inhalation of comparatively large particles or through fine breakdown and subsequent inhalation as fumes. In the United States, silicosis is still the most prevalent pneumoconiosis, and more than 3,000 cases (chiefly in the mining industry) are reported and compensated annually. Other relatively common pneumoconioses and their causes are asbestosis (magnesium silicate fibers), talcosis (talc), diatomaceous earth pneumoconiosis, berylliosis (beryllium oxide fumes), and byssinosis (cotton).

Different offenders may produce different types of pneumoconioses. The most important factors relating to disease are the physical form, chemical state, and particle-size of the dust, as well as duration of exposure to it. For instance, dust particles greater than 20 microns in diameter will not cause disease because they will be trapped in the upper respiratory tract and will never reach and settle in the lung. (An exception to this is the long, thin asbestos fiber.) The chemical state is important: the more soluble the offender, the greater the chance it has to produce chronic inflammation. Obviously, the higher the concentration of the dust per unit of air volume and the longer the time of exposure, the more likelihood there is of producing disease. An important and variable factor is the biological response of the respiratory system to the ability of the offenders to induce toxic tissue-reactions: some individuals are susceptible and respond early; others, under the same conditions, are more resistant.

Symptoms. Pneumoconiosis is usually a disease of slow and insidious nature, diagnosis of which is generally made only after several years of exposure to the harmful dust. The most common symptoms are breathlessness and cough. Certain types of pneumoconioses do not produce symptoms at all, although considerable deposit of dust has taken place in the lung. (These are the benign or inert pneumoconioses, such as the siderosis of welders, steel-burners, and some grinders.) On the other hand, certain types of dusts tend to produce complications. Complicated silicosis, for instance, is frequently associated with infections, bronchitis, emphysema, and tuberculosis. In such case the manifestations of pneumoconiosis and the respiratory disability become dependent on the course of the superimposed diseases.

Fibrosis of the lung (replacement of its normal elastic structure by nodules and strands of solid, coalescent, inextensible material) is a distinctive characteristic of pneumoconiosis. This material curtails the capacity of the lung to expand and contract and contributes to breathlessness. As time goes on, crippling respiratory invalidism becomes more severe and a bluish color of the skin (cyanosis) and heart-failure appear. This latter is called pulmonary heart disease because heart function fails as a consequence of, and secondary to, lung disease.

Treatment. In the symptomatic or complicated pneumoconioses, both cessation of exposure and treatment of associated disease are mandatory. Any favorable results achieved are due to effective treatment of the infection or bronchitis and not of the dust disease itself (which is usually of a non-reversible nature and whose disability effects tend to increase with time).

Considerable controversy may, from the legal standpoint, arise regarding compensation. To validate a claim, there must be sufficient proof of the relationship between the type of employment and length of exposure to the symptoms, signs, and X-ray manifestations observed in the patient. Not every X-ray shadow, although due to dust deposits in the lung, implies that the person is or will be affected by continuance of his present occupation.

Most important are the preventive measures which are the responsibility of industrial hygienists. It is the responsibility of these persons to collect the proper information concerning the processing and production equipment of industrial concerns and to analyze the physical, chemical, and toxicological properties or harmful materials likely to be present in the air. In addition, they also study the characteristics of exhaust-ventilation and sample and determine the concentration of dust which is representative of habitual working conditions during different shifts or times of day. Based on such studies the degree of hazard can be properly estimated and preventive measures (in terms of general exhaust-ventilation and individual filtering devices) can be instituted.

PNEUMONIA This word comes from the Greek word meaning lungs. The disease is an inflammation of the lung during which the normal "beehive," air-containing lung structure is consolidated into a solid mass. This mass may vary in size according to the structural lung unit it occupies: lobule, segment, or lobe. Not every lung consolidation is a pneumonia. Tumors, non-infectious processes, atelectasis (airless lung due to bronchial obstruction and subsequent air reabsorption), and lung fibrosis (replacement of the normal elastic lung structure by scar tissue) can mimic, or be complicated by, pneumonia.

The classical pneumonia is most commonly lobar in size, but may be bilobar (involving two lobes) or larger. The disease is more prevalent in late winter and early spring and attacks more men than women, particularly in the fifteen to forty age-range. Prior chronic respiratory or cardiac disease, poor nutrition, alcoholism, and exposure to sudden changes in temperature particularly predispose persons to the disease. Although it is not considered highly contagious, pneumonia may spread in small epidemics. There is no absolute immunity against the disease, and healthy individuals may be stricken.

More than 95 percent of all classical primary lobar pneumonias are due to pneumococcus bacteria, of which there are numerous strains of different virulence. This characteristic, together with the previous state of health of the patient, will eventually determine the seriousness of the infection, the capacity of the organism to fight it, the severity of the possible complications, and the effectiveness of treatment. A nonbacterial type of pneumonia, caused by a virus, is called primary atypical pneumonia.

Symptoms. The clinical picture of lobar pneumonia is often dramatic and its onset sudden. Usually a mild head cold has been present for several days; the disease may also strike "out of the blue." The patient is attacked by shaking chills shortly followed by very high fever. Symptoms center in the chest in rapid succession: cough becomes troublesome (first dry and then slightly productive of mucus which may be red or rusty in color); breathing becomes labored (dyspnea); and chest pain may be intense—usually of a stabbing or constricting nature and intensified by deep breathing and by changing position in bed. Air-hunger may be intense and frequently the patient needs to sit up in bed to relieve it. The color of the nail beds and the lips becomes dusky or bluish (cyanosis), reflecting an inadequate supply of oxygen to the body tissues. Serious complications may ensue: local spread of the disease to the pleura (pleurisy) and formation of fluid which may become infected (empyema); invasion of the blood vessels producing a blood infection (bacteremia); subsequent localization of the bacteria in other organs such as the brain-covers (meningitis), and heart (endocarditis, pericarditis). As a result, the patient may become unconscious (coma) or go into shock (blood pressure drop). The diagnosis is usually easy to establish on the basis of physical examination, study of the sputum, and especially the chest X-ray findings.

Treatment. The seriousness of the disease and its potential complications in most cases warrant immediate hospitalization. The basis of modern treatment rests on the antibiotics—in this case particularly penicillin, which will be effective against most strains of pneumococcus. Occasionally, other antibiotics need to be employed because of the patient's allergy to the drug or because of complication of the infection by other bacteria. Under antibiotic treatment the results are usually dramatic: the fever disappears in twenty-four to forty-eight hours and the symptoms (chest pain, cough, malaise, dyspnea) are promptly relieved. Nevertheless, treatment should be continued for at least one week after the fever disappears. Notwithstanding the importance of antibiotics, other supportive measures are also employed, particularly to relieve the pain and cough temporarily, to decrease the fever, and insure rest. Adequate fluid intake is important and oxygen is often needed. The complications should be treated selectively as they appear.

PNEUMONIA, ATYPICAL

Similar to the classical lobar pneumonia in its physical characteristics, this condition differs in other aspects. The cause is a virus, or group of viruses, which spreads from person to person via infected discharges from nose and mouth. This disease is most common in middle age, but has no predilection for race, color, or sex. It produces extensive patch areas of lung consolidation, is hemorrhagic in nature, and tends to regress without complications.

Symptoms. These are similar to pneumonia, but the patient appears less seriously affected. Cough and expectoration is always a prominent feature in addition to fever, malaise, and chest pain. The severity of symptoms varies from a mild feverish illness of a few days' duration to a severe disease with high temperature lasting several weeks. In the average case, the temperature lasts approximately ten days and declines slowly. Convalescence is attended by prolonged weakness; there are comparatively few complications.

Treatment. Some patients respond to the tetracycline group of antibiotics. The patient should receive therapy directed to the prevailing symptoms (particularly the cough and fever), adequate fluid intake, and medicines to insure rest. Thus, aspirin, salicylates, and codeine are commonly employed. Early ambulation (moving or walking about) is to be discouraged because it accentuates and prolongs the weakness which characteristically follows the period of acute illness. However many cases are mild, and uneventful recovery occurs.

PNEUMOTHORAX

Pneumothorax indicates the abnormal presence of air within the two layers of the pleura. (*See* PLEURISY in this section.) Normally the pleura is a virtual space containing only a very small amount of lubricating fluid to favor lung movement during inspiration and expiration. If air (or fluid) occupies this space, lung expansion is impaired, leading to its collapse. Hydropneumothorax, pyopneumothorax, and hemopneumothorax indicate the combination of air with water, pus, or blood respectively in the pleural space.

Pneumothorax may occur spontaneously because of rupture of internal blisters (bullae) or cysts into the pleura of the lung. It may be traumatic, the result of a chest wound; or it may be induced by the physician for therapeutic purposes. Spontaneous pneumothorax may occur in otherwise perfectly healthy individuals, but it is most common in patients already afflicted by chronic pulmonary emphysema, lung cysts, or pulmonary fibrosis.

Symptoms. If pneumothorax occurs suddenly and in large amounts, the onset will be abrupt and marked by severe pain, breathlessness, cyanosis, and a shock-like state. These symptoms may progress rapidly and threaten the patient's life because in some cases, the air continues to enter the pleural space but is prevented from leaving it (tension pneumothorax). Chronic pneumothorax renders the collapsed lung useless, and if left untreated for long periods of time the organ may never re-expand. Any pneumothorax, although composed at the beginning of air only, has the potential for complication by the addition of clear or infected fluid.

Treatment. If the amount of air is small, no active treatment is necessary. With increased amounts immediate suction (aspiration) is indicated, either through repeated needle aspirations or preferably by continuous suction. Early aspiration of the air will prevent chronic lung collapse and failure to re-expand. Artificial pneumothorax is a therapeutic procedure which was very popular in the past for the treatment of pulmonary tuberculosis. The lung was collapsed selectively in the diseased area to arrest the activity of the inflammation. Although the method was effective in many instances, complications were frequent, some of them very serious. Today this procedure is seldom employed.

PULMONARY EMBOLISM If a blood clot (thrombus) is present in the veins of the legs or pelvis, it can break away and migrate in the blood to the right atrium, pass through the right ventricle and pulmonary artery, and then come to rest in a major vessel of the lung, where the diminishing diameter of the vessel finally traps it and prevents further travel.

If a medium-sized vessel is blocked, there is usually sudden pain in the chest over the area of lung involvement, some spitting of blood, and variable signs and symptoms that accompany tissue destruction—for inevitably there will be some death of tissue in the lung that is being denied proper circulation by the thrombus. An X-ray of the chest usually shows the involved area as a wedge of airless lung rather clearly demarcated from unaffected pulmonary tissue.

If very small fragments of clot pass into the lungs at repeated intervals, a somewhat different disease of pulmonary vessels can occur. In this case a progressive pulmonary hypertension appears. When a number of arteries become blocked in the lungs, high pulmonary-artery pressure will be needed to move along the same quantity of blood per beat; because fewer blood channels are available, extra force is needed to push blood through the remaining few pathways.

Occasionally, a very large clot breaks away from a pelvic or leg vein, passes into one of the main pulmonary arteries, and blocks it. When at least two-thirds of all pulmonary blood-flow is blocked, death can occur in a few minutes.

PULMONARY INFARCTION *See* PUL-MONARY EMBOLISM in this section.

RESPIRATION (BREATHING) Although the function of breathing is performed by the integrated mechanisms of the whole respiratory system, respiration itself is accomplished only at the level of the lung, by exchanging oxygen and carbon dioxide between the inhaled air and the blood circulating through the lung. To obtain a total picture of the respiratory process, however, it is pertinent to review briefly the characteristics of the participating organs that accomplish the entire function of breathing.

The respiratory system can be pictured in simple terms as a series of tubes of progressively decreasing width (the airways): the nose, mouth, throat, voice box (larynx), windpipe (trachea), and the bronchi. The bronchi themselves subdivide into smaller and smaller tubes running throughout the lung until they reach the basic respiratory units, the alveoli.

Alveoli can be pictured as small, lobed sacs, microscopic in size, of which there are billions in each lung. Amazingly, if one could continuously "stretch out" all the alveoli in the human lungs, they would cover a surface roughly the size of a tennis court. Paralleling this branching structure, there exists a similar network of subdivisions for the blood vessels, which run throughout the lungs in proximity to the air tubes. Ultimately, tiny blood vessels called capillaries reach the air in the alveoli and it is here that gases are exchanged. Thus, joining together, alveoli and blood capillaries become the actual cross-point of respiration. Here the freshly inhaled air gives off oxygen to the blood and receives in exchange carbon dioxide, which is then expelled while breathing out (expiration). (Incidentally, this expired air passes back through the larynx and makes it vibrate, generating sounds or voice.)

Attention should next be turned to the motor forces involved in the process of breathing. Respiratory centers located in the central nervous system (brain) send orders through the nerves to both the respiratory muscles located in the chest wall between the ribs (intercostal muscles) and the muscular "tent" separating the inside of the chest from the abdomen (diaphragm). The contraction of these muscles forces the lung to "open up" in all directions. This in turn creates a suction force within the lung which produces an inrush of outside air (inspiration). Being elastic in nature, the lung when it fills up behaves like a rubber balloon under tension and will deflate by itself (expiration) as soon as the filling has ceased. Inspiration is therefore normally an active process which requires energy, while expiration is passive. The pump for the circulation of blood through the lung is of course the heart. Venous ("used," dark) blood, which returns to the heart from all over the body, is pumped by the heart to the lung through the pulmonary artery. This blood is "revitalized" (oxygenated) in the capillaries of the alveoli by inspired fresh air, and is returned to the heart by the pulmonary veins as "fresh," bright-red blood, and is thence pumped out to the entire body. There the process is reversed: the body tissues extract the oxygen from the blood and load it with carbon dioxide.

Although the true process of respiration (gas exchange) takes place only within the lung in the lower respiratory tract (at the alveoli-level), the upper airways do perform some specific work in addition to letting air pass through. The upper respiratory tract has a rich network of blood vessels which readily give off heat and bring the temperature and humidity of inspired air instantaneously to optimal levels. In addition, the airways possess numerous glands which constantly produce mucus that acts as a lubricant fluid. On the inner surface of the airways there are also numerous hair-like formations called cilia. These beat constantly, thus keeping the mucus in motion and eventually expelling it. (Another function of the cilia is to act as a trap for some of the dust particles contaminating the air.)

One can see that breathing involves many structures which strike a beautifully designed balance to satisfy changing body needs. Still, breathing is largely an involuntary function performed without our awareness, although we may change it at will. Normally an adult will breathe at a rate of about twelve to eighteen times per minute, each inhalation consisting of about 500 cubic milliliters (30 cubic inches) of air. However, like the pulse rate, this often varies.

Excessive breathing (hyperventilation) can be as deleterious as insufficient breathing (hypoventilation). When breathing becomes noticeable and creates discomfort, under otherwise normal conditions of body activity, one speaks of dyspnea or "shortness of breath."

RESPIRATORY TRACT INFECTION

Because of its easy accessibility to external offenders, the respiratory system is the most common site of infection in the body. Thus, all sorts of viruses, bacteria, and parasites present in the environment or carried by other individuals can easily gain access to any level of the respiratory system in the inhaled air. Many of these agents are normal inhabitants of the upper respiratory tract, where they live in harmony with the body until some disturbing condition creates a favorable climate for their multiplication and attack upon the host.

The lung can also be infected from within; infections in any part of the body may gain access to the circulation and thence be carried to, and eventually lodged in, the lung.

The potential harm of any infectious agent varies with the condition of each individual and the characteristics of the body-system under stress. The respiratory tract has certain anatomical characteristics designed to provide natural mechanical defenses against the entrance and deposit of foreign materials: a temperature-control system provided by a rich network of blood vessels which almost instantaneously equalizes the temperature and humidity of the inhaled air with that of the body; hair-like structures, called cilia, which beat constantly to keep the constantly-produced lubricant fluid (mucus) in movement. This system works as a conveyor belt and prevents the deposit of larger particles at the upper levels of the respiratory tract. In addition, the cilia act as a trap for these particles; and a mechanical "wash-out" provided by the rhythmic exhalation of air.

It therefore becomes obvious that most of the infections attacking the respiratory system will be dealt with primarily by the "first lines of defense" in the upper respiratory tract; namely the nose, throat, larynx, and trachea. This also explains why the development of symptoms usually follows a descending anatomical course.

Much less frequent, but of far greater seriousness, are the infections which localize in the lower respiratory tract: the bronchi and lung tissues. To the extent that the respiratory system suffers anatomical or functional damage to its natural defenses, it becomes exceedingly vulnerable to infectious agents—and particularly to the serious consequences of bronchitis and pneumonia.

Any infectious agent can produce respiratory disease; in practice, however, viruses and bacteria are by far the most common offenders. Although either can attack any part of the respiratory system, some broad distinctions can be made. The viruses are responsible for the largest number of upper respiratory tract infections, which are usually self-limiting in nature, free of complications, and for which no specific treatment is either gradually available or mandatory. Studies in the United States Army classified the upper-respiratory viral diseases in two main clinical groups: Acute Undifferentiated Respiratory Disease; and Non-Streptococcal Exudative Pharyngitis. A particular group of viruses (adenovirus) seems to be the prevalent agent in these conditions. In addition, one should also consider the group of viruses responsible for the disease called influenza.

Bacteria which produce respiratory infections originate more distinctive types of disease, and the agent can easily be identified in the nose and throat, or by examination of the sputum. Bacteria are responsible for such potentially serious diseases of the upper and lower respiratory tract as diphtheria, streptococcal sore throat, pneumonia, and bronchopneumonia. The bacterial diseases are more prone to serious complications, and are not self-limited; they can, however, be effectively treated by presently available specific means. The most common bacteria responsible for respiratory infections are the pneumococcus, hemophilus influenza, and streptococcus. A respiratory disease of viral origin may be complicated secondarily by a bacterial invader, but the reverse is rare. Furthermore, any initial bacterial agent may be eventually superseded in the course of the same disease by a different bacterium. Viral respiratory diseases are usually diagnosed on clinical grounds alone, because their precise recognition and identification require highly specialized laboratory techniques. Fortunately, despite the large number of viruses hitherto identified as capable of producing respiratory infection (more than one hundred different types and strains), they all tend to exhibit similar clinical characteristics. They are worldwide in distribution and appear in epidemic outbreaks involving in a short period of time many individuals in the family, at school, or at work, without regard for age or sex.

Symptoms. The most common viral symptoms are itchy and watery secretions from the nose, throat, or eyes, accompanied by pains or discomfort in the neck glands, headaches, and malaise. Fever, if present, may be high but usually lasts no more than forty-eight hours. Often these symptoms are followed by hoarseness and cough—at first dry, and later productive of sputum.

Treatment. In most cases the only treatment required for virus infections is abundant fluid ingestion, mild analgesics (such as aspirin), and simple nasal decongestants. If the symptoms are severe or the patient is debilitated, bed rest is advisable. Widely advertised "miracle drugs" have not been proven to be superior to the regimen mentioned here. Prevention of these diseases is primarily a matter of avoidance of the human source of infection. Vaccines are at present of very limited use because of the large number of viruses involved, each requiring a specific different vaccine.

The bacterial respiratory diseases primarily affect the lower respiratory tract—with the important exceptions of the streptococcal sore throat and diphtheria. In the bronchi and lung the bacteria may produce bronchitis, bronchopneumonia, pneumonia, tuberculosis, lung abscess, and pleurisy (*see* the respective entries). These are serious conditions which may last from several days to weeks and longer, and are prone to complications. Most of them are characterized by fever, prostration, and productive cough. Frequently they produce respiratory difficulty leading to shortness of breath (dyspnea) and dusky lips and nails (cyanosis). The bacteria are usually easily recognized by microscopic examination of the secretions, and specific antibiotic treatment is highly effective.

SIDEROSIS *See* Pneumoconioses in this section.

SUFFOCATION Suffocation, asphyxiation, strangulation, choking, and hanging cause coma due to insufficient oxygenation in the body.

Blockage of the air passages (windpipe, bronchi) may result from water in the lungs from submersion or a foreign body in the throat. Carbon monoxide blocks air passages by keeping air from the lungs and replacing oxygen by itself. Cessation of breathing may result from paralysis of the respiratory center in the brain by tumor, injury, drugs, electric shock; it may result from pressure on the chest and/or abdomen as when a person is caught beneath rubble from a collapsed building.

Choking, particularly due to a foreign body lodged in the throat (such as insufficiently chewed meat), or strangulation due to hanging requires prompt dislodgement of the foreign body in the former and cutting of rope in the latter. In either case, an emergency tracheotomy performed by a physician (cutting directly into the windpipe and installing a rubber tube to allow air to enter) may have to be done. Artificial respiration is then used as in suffocation. (*See also* CHOKING and THE HEIMLICH MANEUVER [Plates F8B-F8C] in the section FIRST AID AND EMERGENCIES.)

THORACOTOMY The surgical opening of the chest wall and exposure of the inside structures, thoracotomy may be done as a diagnostic (exploratory) procedure to view the area directly and/or to obtain a specimen for microscopic examination (biopsy), or it may be followed by an actual removal of rib, pleura, lung, or tissue between the two lungs (mediastinum). These procedures have different names: thoracoplasty and pleurectomy refer to removal of tissue in rib and pleural areas respectively. Segmentectomy, lobectomy, and pneumonectomy refer to the cutting-out (excision) of progressively larger divisions of the lung.

TRACHEITIS *See* RESPIRATORY TRACT INFECTION in this section.

TRACHEOTOMY (TRACHEOSTOMY) These terms are applied to the surgical opening of a small aperture in the forward wall of the windpipe (trachea) through which a tube is inserted to maintain access to air. The procedure is designed to relieve certain types of airway-obstruction, and for many years it was mainly indicated in cases of diphtheric croup. With time, the indications have broadened to incorporate other conditions such as tumors of the upper respiratory tract and, more recently, relief of obstruction in the lower respiratory tract. In the latter case, the operation is obviously not intended to by-pass any point of blockage—the obstruction being on the far side of the tracheal opening—but provides a means to give direct access for cleaning out secretions and for connecting apparatus to produce effective mechanical ventilation (artificial respiration); many different diseases and conditions which threaten or preclude normal breathing may therefore be benefited by temporary or prolonged periods of artificial ventilation through a tracheotomy. Among these are poliomyelitis, chest injuries, extensive burns, tumors, severe respiratory infections, and so forth.

As an emergency procedure, the tracheotomy may be a truly life-saving operation, particularly in children where the complete closure of the larynx may take place in a period of hours. The length of time a tracheotomy is maintained depends on the nature of the underlying disease, and may vary from several days to the occasional case in which it has to be maintained for months, or even indefinitely. Upon removal of the tube and bringing-together of the skin surfaces, the wound will generally close by itself without after-effects.

SKIN CONDITIONS

The skin does more than merely cover the body parts: it functions in respiration, in maintaining body temperature, and in the manufacture of Vitamin D. Diagnoses of many diseases are first made upon examination of the condition of the skin. The skin secretes certain antifungal agents as well, which ward off certain types of infections.

This section examines the physiology of the skin and the symptoms, diagnosis, and possible treatment of common skin disorders. Specialists in the field of dermatology are concerned with treating diseases of the skin. *See also* the questions on acne (Q-55); excessive perspiration (Q-56); itchy skin (Q-58); itchy scalp (Q-60); and sun exposure (Q-57) in the section QUESTIONS AND ANSWERS ABOUT COMMON SYMPTOMS.

The following is a list of terms identified in this section:

ACNE
ALBINISM
ALLERGIC SKIN DISEASES
ALOPECIA AREATA (GENERALISATA, UNIVERSALIS)
ANGIOMAS
BALDNESS AND HAIR REGROWTH
BEDBUG BITES
BEDSORES (DECUBITUS)
BERLOQUE DERMATITIS
BIRTHMARKS
BLACKHEAD
BLISTER
BODY ODOR (BROMHIDROSIS)
BOILS
CALLUS
CARBUNCLE
CHAPPED SKIN
CHEILITIS
CHIGGER BITES
CHILBLAINS
CONDYLOMATA
CORNS
CREEPING ERUPTION
CYST, SEBACEOUS
DANDRUFF
DERMATITIS
DERMATITIS HERPETIFORMIS (DUHRING'S DISEASE)
DERMATOLOGY
DERMATOMYOSITIS
ECZEMA

ERYTHEMA
FLEA BITES
FRECKLES
FROSTBITE
GOOSE FLESH (GOOSE PIMPLES)
GRANULOMA PYOGENICUM
HAIR, EXCESSIVE
HAIR LOSS
HANGNAIL
HIRSUTISM
ICHTHYOSIS
IMPETIGO
INFANTILE ECZEMA
INSECT BITES
INTERTRIGO
ITCHING (PRURITUS)
JUVENILE WARTS
KELOID
KERATOSIS, SEBORRHEIC
KERATOSIS, SENILE
LICE
LICHEN PLANUS
LIVER SPOTS
LUPUS ERYTHEMATOSUS, ACUTE DISSEMINATE
LUPUS ERYTHEMATOSUS, CHRONIC DISCOID
MELANIN
MOLES, PIGMENTED
MOLLUSCUM CONTAGIOSUM
MYCOSIS FUNGOIDES
NEUROTIC EXCORIATIONS

ACNE Beginning in early adolescence, and often the first symptom of glandular change, acne is a disease of varying intensity and unpredictable duration. It can remain an insignificant condition consisting of scattered blackheads and some greasiness of the face for its entire course. Papules, pustules, cysts, and scars can develop at a very early age or appear suddenly in the late teens; recurrences after a seeming cure are not uncommon; absence of any evidence of acne in adolescence is rare. Severe eruptions are not necessarily of lengthy duration, and mild cases are not necessarily short-lived. Because it is impossible to predict with any certainty either the degree of involvement of the skin or the length of time the condition can be expected to last, it is advisable to treat even mild cases of acne in an attempt to control the eruption and minimize residual scarring.

Occurring as it does at a crucial time in the lives of young people already burdened with problems arising from rapid growth, both physical and emotional, the patient's reaction to the various degrees of unpleasantness of appearance ranges widely from feigned or real indifference to arrogant insistence on "immediate cure" to complete social withdrawal. The emotional response to acne depends more on the personality of the patient than on the severity of the condition. So, because it may be possible to avoid permanent damage to the skin and, just as importantly, to improve the immediate disfigurement with its emotional and social consequences, treatment is necessary and is usually effective.

Overactivity of the sebaceous (oil) glands causes the many types of lesions comprising the acne syndrome: blackheads, whiteheads, papules, and cysts. Any of the types of lesions may occur in combination or may appear as the only manifestation of the disease. Because the sebaceous glands are so abundant on the face, chest, and back, these are the usual sites of involvement. Oiliness of the skin is also usually present as a result of the heightened activity of the sebaceous glands. Scarring is commonly the aftermath of large destructive lesions, but scars may follow even uncomplicated blackheads or be the result of self-induced injury (picking).

Acne of the newborn is an infrequent but nevertheless well-known condition which disappears in a few weeks with little or no treatment when the causative maternal hormones are completely excreted. A more common form of acne, and longer lasting, is that found in middle-aged women. In this condition, the lesions are usually cystic and pustular and are likely to be concentrated on the chin. Acne lesions are also found in rosacea, in forms of tuberculosis of the skin, and constitute one of the undesirable side-effects of cortisone therapy.

The fundamental cause of acne is almost certainly an imbalance in hormone secretion, the nature of which is not presently known. Adding to the difficulties of ascertaining the basic mechanisms in acne are "secondary" factors such as foods, stress, and the psyche, which often sustain or enhance or possibly even initiate the condition. The often-observed benefits of season (summer) and climate (seashore) are probably the result of the drying effect of sunlight, the freedom from stressful school situations during the summer recess, the change of dietary and sleep habits, subtle differences in metabolism, etc. The significance of menstrual-related flare-ups in girls is not clear, but this occurrence does afford a clue to the type of hormonal imbalance and a possible therapeutic approach. Similarly, flare-ups during pregnancy, and disappearance of otherwise persistent acne during pregnancy, are also suggestive of the endocrine causation of this disease.

Treatment. Mild cases can be benefited by the use of simple drying measures including frequent washing with ordinary soap and with the application of drying lotions and pastes (containing resorcin, precipitated sulfur, etc.) now available "over-the-counter" in the pharmacy; dietary restrictions (avoiding chocolate, nuts, shellfish); adequate sleep; medical supervision to check on foci of infection, on anemia, on constipation, etc.

More extensive or persistent involvement may necessitate treatment to reduce activity and infection in sebaceous glands; antibiotics and sulfonamides for control of the pustular lesions; vitamin A to relieve the plugging of the blackheads; surgical drainage of destructive cystic lesions; dermabrasion, dry-ice peeling or other repair of residual scars.

ALBINISM This is a rare disease in which there is an inherited inability to produce visible pigment (coloring) in the skin. The condition does not necessarily result in an absence of pigment of the entire skin; but when there is a total absence of pigment, there is a concomitant absence of pigment in the retina of

SEBACEOUS GLAND

HAIR ROOT

1 Acne usually begins as a comedo (blackhead), a blocked accumulation of sebaceous gland secretion.

2 If the comedo becomes inflamed, a prominent hard, red papule develops.

3 If the papule becomes infected, pus-filled pustules develop which finally burst.

the eyes, which gives the pupils a red appearance. The skin is not otherwise affected.

Treatment. No treatment is available except a cosmetic covering if the areas of involvement are small. However, because the skin is unprotected from the damaging effects of the sun's rays (in the absence of pigment) it is necessary to use protective ointments on the uncovered parts of the body and to wear clothing made of materials and colors which are least likely to permit absorption of sunlight.

ALLERGIC SKIN DISEASES The several kinds of skin disease which are caused by, or are evidence of, an allergic mechanism differ considerably. Nevertheless they have in common the important criteria implicit in the term allergic, and are identifiably different from diseases caused by mechanisms of another nature. The concept of allergy as a mechanism of the production of disease is necessary not only for purposes of describing and recording certain clinical findings, but also for purposes of seeking treatment and prevention. The adoption of the word allergy to denote a unique medical happenstance was an act of great significance in medical history and provided a basis for the study of heretofore inexplicable diseases and a working tool for an entirely new biologic field, immunology.

Allergy is an acquired, specific alteration in the capacity to react. To be the result of an allergic process, a condition must be the result of an alteration, a change—one that is not present at birth and hence is noted by the fact that the response is different on a subsequent exposure to a causative substance (an allergen) than was the response to the first exposure. Moreover, the causative substance must not only be proven capable of producing the alteration noted but must not have produced it at the first encounter, since this would indicate that the reacting person would not have had an "altered" or changed capacity to react. The alteration in capacity to react must be specific (directed at a particular chemical structure, a particular wave length of light, a particular drug, food, weed, dander, pollen, etc.).

The allergic skin diseases are comprised of two major categories: the atopic and the nonatopic. The latter group consists of contact dermatitis, urticaria (hives), drug eruptions, and infectious diseases of allergic mechanism. The atopic type of allergic response is evident in the skin as a dermatitis, in the lungs as asthma, and in the eyes and nasal passages as hay fever. Migraine, sinusitis, and some forms of epilepsy are considered to be some of the other manifestations of atopy. In atopic persons, there is usually both a family and a personal history of other atopic diseases; scratch and intradermal tests give positive reactions; there is a high eosinophil count of the blood; circulating antibodies are demonstrable; and the allergens (here called atopens) are usually proteins or protein-bound substances. The nonatopic allergic diseases differ from the atopic in almost every detail, except in the basic mechanism of their common causation; the acquired, specific alteration in the capacity to react. (*See also* the section ALLERGIC CONDITIONS.)

ALOPECIA AREATA (GENERALISATA, UNIVERSALIS)   This type of hair loss, occurring either in single lesions or in varying-sized patches predominantly on the scalp (but capable of remaining confined to another area such as the bearded portion of the face) is of unknown causation. Although considered a disease primarily of young adult life, it occurs in all age groups, including infancy, in both sexes, and is not associated with any "disposition" on the part of the patient, inheritance, or environmental influence.

Symptoms. The appearance of an area in which there is a complete loss of hair is marble- or billiard-ball-like. The single lesion can enlarge and become very extensive; or several lesions, appearing either simultaneously or progressively, can merge with each other to form bizarre patterns. When the hair of a considerable portion of the skin surface is lost, the disease is known as *alopecia generalisata* and when all of the body hair is lost, the condition is termed *alopecia universalis*. There are usually no sensations of itching or burning in the affected areas. When there is a return of hair, either spontaneously or as a result of treatment, the new hair first appears as fine, silky, gray-white shiny threads (lanugo hair). There is a gradual replacement of this forerunner of hair with hair that has the patient's usual hair texture and color.

Treatment. Not until the advent of the cortisone drugs was treatment available for this distressing condition. While not universally effective, the variety of types of these drugs (corticosteroids) makes relief possible for a significant percentage of affected patients. Until treatment makes it unnecessary, the wearing of a wig for patients with extensive loss of scalp hair can be helpful to the patient for cosmetic reasons.

ANGIOMAS   Blood vessel tumors (hemangiomas) of several types, including both superficial and deep lesions, may be seen at birth, but are more often noted several days to weeks after birth. They occur on any part of the skin, can be single or multiple, and each tumor can comprise several types of vessel growth. Almost all types of angiomas are said to be capable of spontaneous disappearance. Almost none of them are of medical significance except for their interference with function and cosmetic deformity depending on their size and the part of the skin involved.

Symptoms. The superficial hemangiomas (strawberry marks) appear as intensely red elevated lesions grouped like berries, grow by extension, and tend to clear irregularly in the center. The color of the lesions becomes intensified on coughing or crying and can become quite dusky and purple. About 25 percent of the superficial angiomas are accompanied by deep (cavernous) lesions of much larger size, the superficial lesion appearing to "cap" the dome-shaped deeper lesion (cavernous hemangioma). Cavernous lesions can be present with no covering superficial lesion, are irregularly dome-shaped, purplish in color, and of varied size. Their rate of growth often determines the advisability of active treatment or of awaiting spontaneous disappearance. The lesions rarely bleed or ulcerate. Another type of hemangioma, the port-wine stain (nevus flammeus) is discussed under a separate heading.

Treatment. Many factors play a part in determining the type of treatment most effective for a particular lesion at a particular site. Most cases of strawberry angioma disappear without treatment, but for the rapidly growing ones, prednisone treatment by mouth may be used. This usually produces regression. Dry-ice applications, laser treatment, injection of sclerosing solutions, simple excision, and plastic repair are the most frequently used means of treatment for cavernous hemangioma. Both the dry ice and sclerosing methods are used to initiate shrinkage rather than to destroy the lesions, and therefore are likely to leave little residual scarring. Simple excision of very small lesions can successfully forestall growth, but is usually done with reluctance because of the size and age of the patient. Although there is a considerable body of evidence demonstrating the disappearance of these tumors, to permit a tumor to grow in the hope of eventual disappearance and then to be faced with an atypical situation—nondisappearance of the lesion—becomes regrettable for the patient, the parents, and the physician.

BALDNESS AND HAIR REGROWTH

Over the years male baldness has resisted all efforts at hair regrowth. However, patients taking minoxidil, an oral preparation for high blood pressure, noted unexpected increase in facial hair growth. This led to research to determine whether minoxidil applied to the bald scalp might reduce baldness, without affecting blood pressure in patients with normal pressure. The research demonstrated that in the majority of the test-patients who used the preparation on a continuous basis, baldness decreased. However, if application of the drug was discontinued hair regrowth stopped. Because minoxidil is new, as a hair-growth drug, the long-term side effects of the preparation are unknown, although no significant ones so far have developed. (*See also* HAIR LOSS in this section.)

BEDBUG BITES   The bedbug *(Cimex lectularis)* resides in the crevices of furniture, including the seams of mattresses, and emerges for purposes of feeding. It punctures the skin, producing a usually visible puncture mark around which develops a small but persistent hive, probably the result of a deposition of insect fluid.

Symptoms. The insect bites are usually grouped in a line or in an arc shape made up of three lesions. Most commonly affected sites are the ankles, buttocks, and parts of the body usually covered by night-clothes. Diagnosis is occasionally made difficult by the absence of skin lesions in one of two people sharing a bed. This may be the result of the person's immunity to the insect toxin, or due to some metabolic substance in the person's skin which either rejects or "detoxifies" the offending material.

Treatment. Eradication of the bedbugs by fumigation (but first check with local authorities about available legal methods) will eliminate further skin response since the bedbug does not live on the body. The existing lesions can be treated with soothing lotion (calamine) and the itching minimized with the orally administered antihistaminic drugs.

BEDSORES (DECUBITUS)   These lesions appear in areas of persistent pressure to the skin of chronically ill or debilitated patients as a result of poor circulation in the mechanically restricted area.

Symptoms. First the lesions may appear blanched and then as an area of redness, the skin becomes macerated, denuded, and ulcerated. Pustular infections, including boils, are common. Similar lesions can occur under restrictive dressings, such as casts, in an otherwise healthy person.

Treatment. Frequent movement of the patient in whom bedsores can be expected to occur, and the use of air, water or egg-crate mattresses to provide more resiliency, will afford some protection. The skin should be kept dry and dusting powder applied to the sheets to reduce friction against the linens. The sores or ulcers are treated with antibiotic ointments and surgical removal of dead tissue (debridement). A variety of occlusive, absorptive and specialized dressing are also available.

BERLOQUE DERMATITIS The result of a unique type of photosensitization, this deep brown hyperpigmentation occurs in sharply defined bizarre configurations in sites of deliberate or accidental application of substances containing essential oils such as oil of lemon (rind), oil of orange (rind), and the most frequent offender and common ingredient of perfume, oil of bergamot. The areas affected are usually those to which perfume and perfume-containing preparations are applied and which are ordinarily exposed to light.

Symptoms. The back of the neck and forehead (from hair preparations running onto the skin), sides of the neck, anterior chest, upper arms and bends of the elbows (from perfume, cologne), demonstrate spherical, elongated, or splattered brown lesions with no apparent preceding redness or swelling or blistering. The eruption fades gradually, although remnant stains have been known to last for years.

Deliberate experimental sensitization of this type has been difficult to produce, and the mechanism of this occurrence is not known.

Treatment. Avoidance of light will prevent further darkening of the affected sites. Avoidance of the application of the offending oil at least to exposed areas of the skin will prevent recurrence. Treatment of the lesions is unnecessary.

BIRTHMARKS *See* Moles, Pigmented and Angiomas in this section.

BLACKHEAD A blackhead is formed from the oily material (sebum) secreted by the sebaceous gland and the horny keratin which lines the opening of the gland. The resulting waxy substance becomes blackened on oxidation and gives the classic appearance of a blackhead. Often this pluglike material causes further overactivity of the sebaceous gland and irritation which results in redness, papule formation, and pus characteristic of the acne lesion.

Blackheads are most frequently found on the face, chest, and back. They are less prevalent but often of much greater size in the ears, where they cause scarring and painful infection. They can exist as the only manifestation of acne or in association with the several other types of lesions. Scarring can result from mechanical distention of the skin by the plug, or as the result of secondary infection.

Treatment. Drying agents (lotions) exert a peeling effect on the orifice permitting extrusion of the plug; vitamin A taken orally is known to alter the putting down of keratin and permit the flow of sebum without opportunity to harden at the surface; proper removal (lifting out) of the horny plug prevents further distorting and possible scarring. Lack of cleanliness is no factor in the production of blackheads, though over time frequent washing with soap and water exerts a drying and gentle peeling of the skin and releases the blackhead.

BLISTER Caused by the seeping of serous fluid within the skin, usually under the epidermal layer, a blister can exist as an integral part of a complex reaction comprising a disease entity (poison ivy dermatitis, pemphigus, cold sores) or result from local trauma (friction, burn).

Depending on the mechanism of production, a blister can remain small and uninfected until it is finally absorbed, leaving a brownish crust which falls off spontaneously if left alone; or it can become enlarged to almost any size or shape, drain, refill, become jellylike, peel off, or become infected.

Treatment. Aside from blisters which are present as part of a skin disease, treatment will vary according to the site affected, the number and size of the lesions, and the discomfort and disability of the patient. Small blisters dry up quite rapidly if treated with applications of cold water, either by immersion or by compresses. Large lesions can be emptied by ripping with an alcohol-sterilized needle. If the blister is not opened adequately, it will refill. The opened lesion should be covered with an antibiotic ointment such as bacitracin or neosporin. It is often useful to apply cold water compresses to opened or spontaneously draining blisters at intervals of three or four hours, following each wet dressing with drying and with the application of an antibiotic ointment.

BODY ODOR (BROMHIDROSIS) The term body odor invariably refers to unpleasant body odor and can be a problem in both health and disease. Among the diseases giving rise to perceptible and unique body odors are diabetes, gout, pemphigus, typhoid fever, and scurvy. Foods and drugs can give a body odor on being excreted in the sweat (garlic, onions, asparagus, arsenic). But more commonly, unpleasant body odor is derived from the apocrine sweat glands of the armpits, long considered the source of the "scent" of our species (as it is in other animal species). Recently it has been demonstrated that armpit odors are probably due solely to the luxuriant growth of bacteria in the presence of much sweat. Hence efforts at preventing body odor should be directed not only at reducing the sweat, but more importantly at removing the bacteria. This is accomplished by shaving off the hair which harbors the bacteria; using antibacterial soaps and the local application of the numerous masking and deodorizing cosmetic items available in drug stores.

BOILS This term refers to intensely red, tender, painful nodules which are initially hard and finally soften, rupture, and drain. Variously called furuncles, carbuncles, or boils, depending on their size and number, the infection may be single or multiple, chronic or recurrent. The causative bacteria are usually staphylococci, but streptococci may be present. The many predisposing factors may not be present in an individual case, but these must be considered when ordinary care does not result in cure. Included among the conditions thought to contribute to the recurrence or persistence of boils are diabetes, anemias,

malnutrition, obesity, poor hygiene, excessive sweating (occupational or athletics), and drugs (iodides and bromides). Boils also occur as a secondary problem to already-existing skin conditions such as insect bites, scabies, louse infestation, and eczemas.

Treatment. Antibiotics such as erythromycin and some of the penicillins are effective for the individual attack of boils and may also be useful in attempting to prevent recurrences. Locally, the application of hot-water compresses and local antibiotics until there is spontaneous drainage, or until surgical incision is indicated, are helpful in hastening the course of the lesion. Treatment of any predisposing causes and restriction of diet (chocolate, nuts, shellfish) and the halogen drugs (iodides and bromides) in addition to improving the hygiene by washing with antibacterial soaps, may avert the occurrence of new lesions. When excessive sweating is a predominant factor, as in athletes, at least temporary interruption of sweat-inducing activity may become necessary.

CALLUS This abnormal thickening of the skin is the result of chronic and repeated friction to the affected part. It occurs most commonly on the feet, but can be produced on almost any other part of the skin. Calluses of the palms (in laborers, tennis players) and of the finger tips (violinists), or of the knuckles, ankles, and knees may differ somewhat in appearance, but are produced in the same way as those of the feet.

Treatment. Removal of the friction causing the thickening will result in spontaneous disappearance of the callus. Application of salicylic acid plasters and lessening the thickening by scraping with a file will afford some relief. For calluses of the soles of the feet, properly fitting shoes and thick socks to minimize friction are essential for continued improvement and cure. Resistant cases should be seen by a podiatrist.

CARBUNCLE A carbuncle is caused by the staphylococcus germ. It is like a furuncle or boil except that it penetrates to deeper tissues. It is larger than a boil (usually it is several boils that have coalesced) and may go on to extensive sloughing of tissue. It heals slowly and a large scar may ensue. Prevention and treatment are the same as for a boil. Occasionally, surgical incision of a deep and/or extensive lesion is required.

ANTHRAX

Anthrax is an infectious disease of cattle and sheep, due to the Bacillus Anthracis. It can occur in man. It is characterized by the formation of hard edema or ulcers at the point of inoculation. The disease can be fatal.

CHAPPED SKIN This condition results from the deliberate or inadvertent removal of oil from the surface of the skin. The usually low humidity of winter weather induces rapid evaporation of water from the skin surface and has a drying effect. Coupled with reduced production of oil, the drying can be intense enough to induce redness and scaling and a leathery feel. Contact of cleaning solutions and fat solvents with the skin can produce the same effect even in the presence of normal oil production and high humidity.

Treatment. The wearing of gloves outdoors in wintertime affords protection both against evaporation of surface water and reduction of oil production because of chilling of the skin. The application of simple greases like vaseline or lanolin is useful in relieving the condition and the burning sensation usually accompanying the reddened and roughened skin.

CHEILITIS This term applies to any inflammation of the lips of whatever causation. The lips are subject to allergic sensitization to many substances including lipstick, mouthwashes, dentrifice, bubble gum, mangoes, fruit dyes, perfumes. Some disease processes can specifically affect the lips (lupus erythematosus, lichen planus), causing dryness, peeling, scaling, or atrophy (loss of tissue). Often, but not always, as the result of an existing disturbance of the lips, the patient is inclined to pick the free peeling edges, or to lick them to relieve the smarting sensation. Both the picking and the licking may produce further irritation. Excessive exposure to wind or to sunlight can induce inflammation with swelling and drying.

Symptoms. Except as the result of allergic reaction, a burn, or cold sores, inflammation of the lips does not often cause blistering. There is usually an intensification of the normal redness, swelling, wrinkling, peeling associated with burning, smarting, and occasional itching.

Treatment. Removal of the causative agent(s) and application of soothing ointment (vaseline, lanolin) will often suffice. Protection from excessive exposure to wind and sun may prove difficult but may be essential in chronic cases.

CHIGGER BITES Caused most commonly by *Eutromobicula alfreddugesi* (the red bug or harvest mite) which lives on grasses, shrubs and vines, chigger bites occur most frequently on the legs, just above the shoes and along the belt line. The lesions are produced by larvae, which become attached to the skin for feeding. In addition to intense itching, chiggers produce large papules which persist for about two weeks.

Treatment. The intense itching can be relieved by application of ice-cold water and soothing lotion (calamine). Antihistaminic drugs taken orally are also effective for the relief of itching. Prevention is possible if insect repellants are used around the ankles and wrists before exposure. Clothing of closely woven material, fitting snugly around the ankles and wrists, is also a deterrent to the bite of the chigger.

CHILBLAINS Caused by exposure to excessive cold, and more especially wet cold, this disease affects the hands, feet, face, and ears. The lesions consist of red or purplish plaques, flat or slightly elevated. On even slight warming of the affected areas, there is considerable discomfort from the smarting, burning, and occasional itching. If the exposure is more prolonged and the cold more intense, the lesions are aggravated and resemble burns with blistering and ulceration.

Treatment. Contrary to popular legend, gradual warming of the area, either with gentle dry massage or with lukewarm wet dressings, *will* restore normal circulation. Rubbing with ice and snow can only induce more damage, and it is difficult to understand how this "remedy" continues to enjoy popularity. For severe cases, treatment for the general symptoms of exposure and local blisters or ulcers is the same as for severe burns. (*See also* FROSTBITE in the section FIRST AID AND EMERGENCIES.)

CONDYLOMATA These are warts, varying in number and size and appearing around the genital organs (occasionally inside the vagina) and the anus. Condylomata are produced by a virus and are more common in women with poor habits of cleanliness and multiple sexual partners.

Symptoms. The symptoms are usually itching, burning, and excessive discharge. The warty tumors may become quite large.

Treatment. The condition responds fairly well to treatment with application of caustic and antibiotic drugs, although surgical removal may be required for excessively large and obstructive growths. Recent trials with the antiviral drug Interferon have been successful.

CORNS Caused by ill-fitting shoes, both soft and hard corns are the result of repeated friction. Soft corns differ in appearance from hard corns only because the moisture in the area between the toes macerates the lesions. Both types of corns are painful and require removal.

Treatment. Other than going barefoot, wearing shoes of proper fit is the only certain way of preventing recurrences. The corns can be lifted out. Slicing them with a razor blade is ineffective. Removal is made easier by the application of a salicylic acid plaster or ointment, which is available over the counter, for several days. Large recurring corns may need medical attention.

CREEPING ERUPTION This disease is caused by several species of roundworms (nematodes) commonly found in the southern portion of the United States and in many other parts of the world. The larva of the worm (present in the soil) can enter the skin through even slight abrasions.

Symptoms. The eruption is found on the feet of children whose barefoot habits and inattention to small scratches or cuts make them especially susceptible to the disease. At the point of entry of the larva, a small papule forms and the larva tunnels its winding way into the skin, forming more papules and blisters in the form of arcs, circles, and hyperbolas. Itching is often intense. Secondary pustular infection is uncommon.

Treatment. Freezing with ethyl chloride spray, and taking care that the advancing "head" of the larva is frozen, are usually completely effective. When local freezing methods fail, systemic medication must be prescribed by the physician.

CYST, SEBACEOUS These dome-shaped tumors range in size from that of a small pea to that of a small lemon. Occurring usually on the face, scalp, and behind the ears, they are commonly also found on the chest and back. They can disappear spontaneously as the result of pressure or other injury, but it is more usual for them to persist, to become infected from time to time, and occasionally but rarely to become calcified. Multiple lesions are common.

Treatment. Surgical excision, though curative, is not often necessary, and should be avoided if possible for cosmetic reasons. Drainage of the sebaceous material through the pluglike opening which is usually present, and removal of the sac through this opening, is likely to leave little or no scarring. In instances in which the cyst has become infected and removal of the sac is difficult, simple drainage of the lesion may cause disappearance. If the cyst is not infected or bothersome, removal is not essential.

DANDRUFF *See* SEBORRHEIC DERMATITIS in this section.

DERMATITIS The word dermatitis merely denotes inflammation of the skin. It is often mistakenly used to denote a specific condition of the skin, but the word dermatitis has little meaning without a modifying word or phrase to describe either the appearance of the dermatitis (exfoliative, exudative), the location of the dermatitis (palmaris, plantaris), the causative agent of the dermatitis (medicamentosa, plant, occupational, diabeticorum), or a factor in the mechanism of production of the dermatitis (varicose, allergic, atrophic). The term is also used as part of a compound name for a specific disease caused by infecting microorganisms, as in infectious eczematoid dermatitis, dermatitis blastomycetica, streptococcic dermatitis; and by physical agents, as in roentgen dermatitis or dermatitis calorica or solare.

DERMATITIS HERPETIFORMIS (DUHRING'S DISEASE)

Of unknown causation, this disease is most common in adults but is occasionally also present in children. It is primarily a disease of the skin and is not associated with any other condition. Many variants of the usual skin lesions and distribution of these lesions sometimes make the diagnosis difficult, and a biopsy (study of a microscopic specimen of the skin) may be necessary.

Symptoms. The lesions consist of papules and vesicles (small blisters) arranged in groups situated over the eminences of the back (shoulders and buttocks) and distributed also over the rest of the trunk and the extremities. The groups of lesions can vary considerably in size, and also in duration (weeks to months), with fresh crops of lesions appearing irregularly and periods of remission unpredictable. The involution of a lesion is often succeeded by an area of increased pigmentation which can remain for years. The condition is accompanied by severe itching.

While the cause of the disease is not known, an attack can be induced or worsened by certain foods, notably those containing free iodine (shellfish) and drugs containing bromides or iodides. A diagnostic skin test with potassium iodide is often used in questionable cases.

Treatment. The two most commonly employed remedies are dapsone and sulfapyridine. Either of these can be very effective; but treatment, because it is usually prolonged and repetitious, must be under the physician's surveillance. Avoidance of iodide- and bromide-containing foods and medicines is essential.

DERMATOLOGY Dermatology is the science of the skin in health and in disease. Historically, dermatology is the oldest discipline in medicine, not only because its overt display of disease could be contemplated before even the crudest instrumental aids were invented, but also because the skin was available for observation over varying periods of time. This has permitted documentation of many diseases of lengthy duration and tortuous course such as syphilis and leprosy; of swift and devastating infections such as smallpox, diphtheria, gangrene; and of slow and unremitting conditions such as lupus, cancer, and scleroderma.

Dermatology is the oldest discipline, and the most challenging. One can see the disease process directly; not indirectly by a shadow cast on an X-ray film, or by looking at a blood smear and interpreting from it what the bone marrow is doing, or by testing with dyes and deducing from this the function of the liver. The dermatologist can observe the details of the disease process—then can alter the process and study it. The skin can be excised and looked at under a microscope; it can be transplanted to another site, to another person, to another species; it can be stained and observed; chilled and observed; heated and observed; peeled and observed; or even treated and observed. The disease can be smelled as in pemphigus and in sweatiness (bromhidrosis); it can be felt (leathery, nutmeg-grater-like, horny, velvety, marble-like, doughy, woody). Readily observable for study are the colors and the shades of color of different diseases, the many shapes and configurations of the lesions, each unique for each disease, or at least for each disease of similar dynamic mechanism.

And for all its availability, there remain unanswered the myriad questions seemingly capable of ready answer. Why is most itching worse at night and, as a matter of fact, why do temperatures rise at night in most febrile diseases? Where in its growth does kinky hair get its kink and how does it retain it for its full growth for its entire life; how do "circles" under the eyes get to look that way; why does a person seemingly not changed in any other way suddenly develop an allergy to something he has been exposed to with no reaction for many years, as for instance poison ivy, shoe leather, or aspirin; how do warts disappear overnight after being present for years; why does no one contract leprosy in a temperate climate; what has happened to make scabies such a rare disease when only a few years ago it was endemic (prevalent)?

As in other fields of medicine, so too in dermatology, the physician today practices with a host of therapeutic modalities undreamed of a few short years ago. With their causes not yet established, treatment is nevertheless now available for a great variety of both serious and inconveniencing diseases such as pemphigus, cancer, lupus erythematosus, scleroderma, vitiligo, alopecia areata among others. And diseases of known cause, such as boils, leprosy, fungous infections, erysipelas, allergies, syphilis, diseases of vitamin deficiency and of hereditary disarrangement, are among those for which cure is now possible where prevention is not possible.

DERMATOMYOSITIS This poorly understood syndrome occurs at almost any age and in both sexes. The skin lesions consist of varying-sized red plaques which are occasionally slightly elevated and hive-like. The lesions become atrophic or hardened (scleroderma-like). Concomitant changes in the muscles result in swelling, pain, and tenderness, followed by atrophy of the muscles and crippling contractures. Other changes include puffiness of the eyelids, enlargement of the liver and spleen, fever, and anemia. A significant number of patients have cancer (adenocarcinoma) of an internal organ at the time of diagnosis of dermatomyositis.

Treatment. Eradication of the cancer in patients in whom this appears to be the cause of the dermatomyositis usually results in remission of the skin and muscle symptoms. For patients in whom there is no malignancy, cortisone drugs afford a high percentage of remissions, some of them permanent.

ECZEMA *See* the section INFANT AND CHILD CARE.

ERYTHEMA Erythema is skin redness due to blushing, emotional stress, exposure to sun, X-ray, and ultraviolet emanations, drugs, certain diseases (particularly of the skin), and local injury.

FLEA BITES The common flea *(Pulex irritans)* and the flea endemic to cats and dogs *(Ctenocephalus canis)* cause hive-like lesions in groups of two or three, arranged in a line or arc, with a tiny central puncture point. Any area of the body can be affected, and the eruption is accompanied by considerable itching. There appears to be variable susceptibility in responsiveness to the bite of a flea, and the diagnosis cannot be ruled out in the absence of similar lesions in other persons residing in the household of the affected member.

Treatment. Eradication of the fleas by fumigation, and de-fleaing the domestic animal are essential to a cure. It must be remembered, however, that if a dog or a cat is the source of the infection, the animal should not be removed lest the fleas attack the human being for nourishment in the absence of the prime host. The animal can be treated by a variety of household measures. For the existing bites, soothing lotion (calamine) and orally administered antihistaminic drugs, both for the relief of itching and allaying of the swelling, are effective. If the insects cannot be readily eradicated, the use of locally applied insect repellants may be necessary for persons highly reactive to the flea-venom.

FRECKLES Almost universally prevalent, and resulting from a simple dominant inherited characteristic, freckles are both elicited and made more prominent by exposure to sunlight. In identical twins, freckling will appear in identical distribution and intensity. Except when this condition is very intense and is part of a very rare disease of photosensitization (xeroderma pigmento sum), there are no indications for altering the process. For cosmetic purposes, however, bleaching applications, notably ointments containing monobenzyl ether of hydroquinone, can be effective but are attended with some risk of producing allergic dermatitis, and should be supervised by a physician. Retin A ointment as a follow-up to hydroquinone treatment may be of further help, as are sunblock agents.

FROSTBITE   *See* the section FIRST AID AND EMERGENCIES.

GOOSE FLESH (GOOSE PIMPLES)
This common symptom of rapid and simultaneous elevation of myriads of tiny papules of the skin on sudden and extreme joy, sorrow, cold, or fright is the result of the contraction of muscle fibers (erectores pilorum) attached to the outer lining of the hair follicle just below the attachment of the sebaceous gland. The muscle extends from this point in a diagonal manner to an area just below the epidermal layer, at which point the "puckering" or goose pimple forms.

GRANULOMA PYOGENICUM   A growth of proliferating blood vessels resulting from an infection in which the pus formation is minimal, the globular tumor mass of granuloma pyogenicum is characterized by bleeding on slight injury. Because the blood vessels have little or no elasticity, the bleeding is difficult to control. The lesion is usually the size of a pea, intensely red and glistening, and occasionally crusted. Any part of the skin can be affected, although the condition occurs most commonly on the face.

Treatment. The lesions can be readily destroyed by electrocautery performed by a physician. Only rarely does the lesion disappear without being deliberately destroyed. The persistent bleeding can be alarming; it can be controlled by applying pressure until treatment is available.

HAIR, EXCESSIVE   *See* HIRSUTISM in this section.

HAIR LOSS   There are several types of loss of hair in addition to the oft-encountered male baldness and the distinctive hair loss of alopecia areata.

Hair can be lost by reason of chemical, physical, or mechanical damage; or as the result of infections having a unique affinity for hair involvement; and, as a result of chemotherapy used to treat cancer. Aside from singeing the hair by the application of very warm or hot instruments, hair can be so "softened" by

chemical or physical agents designed to straighten, curl or color it that it can break off. Hair damaged in this manner is no different from hair that had been cut off. Regrowth will take place at the usual rate—providing no injury was sustained by the scalp.

Hair can also be broken off mechanically as the result of a habit mechanism not unlike that of fingernail-biting. This condition can only be alleviated by the patient's being made aware of the condition and seeking help in breaking the habit. Cure of this condition is especially difficult in those patients in whom the eyelashes are the site of the pulling-out, the twisting, or the breaking-off. It is usually not necessary to probe the original cause of the habit which, as with fingernail-biting, has long ceased to matter. Breaking the habit can be accomplished with devices (greasing the hair to make it impossible to get a grip on it), rewards (in addition to the obvious one of improvement of appearance), and—rarely—threats (infection, deformity of hair regrowth).

Other apparent loss of hair is encountered in ringworm infection of the scalp, in which the hair shaft is invaded by the fungus and the hair breaks off and gives the appearance of bald spots. (*See* RINGWORM OF THE SCALP in this section.) Loss of hair in the secondary stage of syphilitic infection gives the scalp a "moth-eaten" appearance.

Probably even more common than baldness in men is the loss of hair in women, either as a result of pregnancy or in relationship to some change in endocrine activity. The hair loss of pregnancy usually ceases after delivery, or after the menstrual cycle is reestablished. While it is usual for only a portion of the hair to regrow, there is sufficient regrowth to reassure the patient that she will not be bald even if the condition recurs with each pregnancy. The most distressing loss of hair is that which occurs in young women and appears not to be related to hair appliances like curlers, styling lotions, or permanent waves, and seems also not to be related to the metabolic rate, menstrual cycle, or other organic or psychic distress (except as a result of the loss of hair). In spite of the absence of findings of any significance in recent extensive investigations, there is a continuing impression that this type of hair loss is related to some malfunctioning of the endocrine glands. To this end, the patient is well-advised to seek help from the internist. Correcting even minor defects in the general health may possibly result in the cessation of the hair loss, though not ensure its regrowth. (*See also* BALDNESS AND HAIR REGROWTH in this section.)

HANGNAIL Resulting from an injury (tear) of the skin around the nail which affects the nail fold, a hangnail almost always causes infection at the site of the injury. When not induced by the biting of nails, these lesions are caused by an irritation from the irregular shedding of the cuticle or by repeated injury sustained in active use of the fingers or toes.

Treatment. To prevent further irritation from friction of the torn epidermis or cuticle, the torn skin should be cut as close to its attachment to normal skin as possible, and an antibiotic ointment should be applied. To prevent frequent recurrences, the cuticle should be kept soft and pliable with the application of simple lubricants like vaseline or lanolin.

HIRSUTISM Excessive growth of hair on the face (and other areas) of women is frequently first seen in early adult life, but is an almost universal occurrence in women of middle age. Both the time of onset and the distribution of facial hair growth are governed to some degree by an inheritance factor. Other factors, including endocrine activity and metabolic imbalances, may be of significance in some patients. Tests for blood levels of androgens (male hormones) may be elevated. A medication used in treatment of high blood pressure, minoxidil, may produce hirsutism and is now available as a topical agent in the treatment of baldness.

Symptoms. Dark, relatively stiff hairs may be confined to the upper lip, the chin, the anterior chest or the breasts; or they may be present in all or in several of these areas. More rarely, the forearms and the thighs are the sites of excessive hair growth. The appearance of a diffuse growth of fine, light-colored "down," usually on the cheeks, is not necessarily a forerunner of a growth of real hair, the color and texture of this hair almost always remaining unaltered. Hair is rarely found in the ears of women, usual as it is in the ears of men.

Treatment. Permanent removal of hair can be accomplished by electrolysis or by electrocautery. Both processes are tedious and seemingly endless, requiring repeated treatment; but both are finally effective. Temporary removal with depilatories is a practical procedure for excessive hair of the extremities. Removal with wax applications or with tweezers affords longer periods of relief because removing the hair with its root prolongs the time before reappearance of the hair at the surface of the skin. With both these methods it is necessary for the hair to be long enough to permit its being clutched without injuring the skin.

While the elimination of unwanted hair may be difficult, future hair growth can not be prevented. The commonly held view that pulling out, or otherwise removing, hair induces further growth probably stems from the fact that early appearance of hair is the first evidence of the likelihood of more growth; and the removal of this first growth is erroneously cited as the cause of later-appearing hair.

It is impractical to attempt removal of the fuzz type of downy hair except under extraordinary circumstances. Wax depilation is probably the most useful for this purpose.

Bleaching of excessive hair growth is most often used for the forearms, legs, and upper lip. Usually no problems are encountered except in people who have an allergic sensitivity to the bleaches and dyes. (*See also* BALDNESS AND HAIR REGROWTH in this section.)

ICHTHYOSIS Ranging from mild, generalized dryness of the skin to severe fish-scale-patterned peeling, ichthyosis is first noted in infancy and early childhood. Not infrequently, there is some spontaneous improvement during and after adolescence. It is almost always congenital and tends to be more common in some families.

Symptoms. More prominent on the outer sides of the extremities, ichthyosis also involves the face and trunk; on the palms there is a thickening which results in exaggeration of the "lines." The upper arms and thighs often are also the site of plugging of the follicles and give the appearance and the feeling of a nutmeg grater. The condition is much less apparent and less inconveniencing in the summer months, largely because of the increase in sweating of the otherwise reduced number or the usually reduced activity of the sweat glands.

Treatment. Maintaining a comfortable environment may be difficult, but avoiding extremes of cold and of humidity is necessary, at least in the more severe cases. Bathing should be kept to a minimum; and water softeners or bath oils should be used in hard-water areas. Ordinary cold creams, liniments (lime water and olive oil combined), and mild peeling ointments are helpful. Medication with thyroid extract and vitamin A is occasionally indicated.

IMPETIGO   Common in childhood, and sometimes in adult life, this infectious and contagious disease is caused by bacilli (streptococci and staphylococci). It is characterized by pinhead to bean-size crusting and occasionally oozing lesions. The crusts are the color of honey, crumble easily, and can be removed with slight friction. Since the crusts themselves contain the infecting organisms, they carry the infection to surrounding areas directly and to remote areas by contact with clothes or by contact with other skin areas. The disease cannot be contracted except by direct contact with the affected part. No perceptible injury to the skin is necessary to initiate the eruption, and uncleanliness is not the cause except to the degree that washing with soap and water tends to remove, or alter the vitality of, possibly causative organisms.

In infants this disease not only has a different appearance, but also a different course. The lesions appear as blisters which often become very large before breaking; the patient is acutely ill even if no general symptoms are apparent. Early antibiotic therapy, usually by injection, is urgent and usually effective.

When the disease affects a hairy portion of the body (beard, armpits, groin), deeper infection of the hair follicles may occur together with the superficial crusting lesions, and may constitute a source of reinfection.

An impetigo-like eruption may be present as a complication of many other skin diseases, usually as a result of scratching, and appears as a diffuse crusting rather than a discrete, sharply defined lesion.

Another variant of this disease occurs in the skin at the site of other draining infec-

tions; in pustular drainage of a middle-ear infection; on the eyelids and surrounding skin from "pinkeye"; or around a draining surgical wound. This condition is known as infectious eczematoid dermatitis. The yellowish crust forms in the area exposed to the infected draining exudate as a result of an allergic response to the bacteria. Curing the pre-existing infection and usual treatment with antibiotics for the skin involvement are both necessary for cure.

Treatment. Because the crusts of impetigo are the site of growth of the causative bacteria, and also because the crusts are so easily removed, wherever possible they should be removed and the remaining glistening, reddened area covered with an antibiotic ointment (bacitracin, neosporin). The crusts are formed again very quickly; it is therefore necessary to remove them repeatedly. An effective regime is to apply the ointment every two hours during the day, wiping off the crust before each application. Washing with soap and water should not be excessive lest the skin be irritated and further infection induced. In extensive cases it may be necessary to administer antibiotics systemically, but local treatment will have to be carried out in addition. Other than the blistering impetigo of infancy, all other eruptions, whether primary or a secondary complication of other skin diseases require the same basic treatment.

In children it is well to cut the nails short and apply the antibiotic ointment to the fingertips so that they do not contribute to spreading the infection. Patients should be instructed to use their own towels. Contaminated clothes should be boiled or dry-cleaned.

INFANTILE ECZEMA   Eczema in the infant results from a variety of causes. Encountered in earliest infancy is seborrheic eczema with greasy scaling of the scalp (cradle cap) and red scaly plaques of the brows, the cheeks, shoulders, back, and chest, and the skin behind the ears. Soon after birth, too, the infant is subject to eczema from excessive moisture in the groin and in the armpits. This condition, often associated with the previously mentioned seborrheic dermatitis, constitutes a hazard to the infant because of the frequent presence of yeast infestation (monilia), a condition common also to the mouth and tongue of the infant (thrush). A third type of eczema in the infant is that of allergic contact dermatitis, caused most often by the application of "baby oil," powders, medication applied for a preexisting condition; or, in older children, from contact with toilet seats (plastic) or materials in toys or clothes (dyes, finishers). This condition is no different in infants and children from that of adults except that the causative agents are unique for the age group.

Still another group of patients, small in number, suffers from eczema induced by infectious organisms which cause an allergic rather than an infecting response. The most important of the infantile eczemas is that of atopic dermatitis in which the eruption is the beginning evidence of an allergic state and indicates that the patient may require medical management of this and related conditions for some time. Eruption of atopic dermatitis is not unlike that of seborrheic dermatitis in the infant, although there is a greater tendency for the lesions to appear on the arms and legs and, after a relatively short period of time, to be confined to the bends of the elbows and knees.

Treatment. Although treatment is somewhat modified in the infant and very young child, symptomatic relief is sought through the application of soothing lotions (calamine), water-softened baths (starch, oatmeal, salts), oral antihistaminic drugs (see under specific diseases). The infant's nails should be cut short to prevent damage from scratching. Restraints (splints) are usually not necessary and are indeed often irritating to the infant in his attempts at moving about in the crib. Socks sewn (not pinned!) to the shirt and worn over the hands will deflect some of the trauma of scratching.

In connection with eczema in infancy and early childhood it is necessary to emphasize the warning that these patients may not be vaccinated against smallpox. Every small damage of the skin is vulnerable to the pox inoculation, no matter what care is taken to keep the site of intended vaccination covered. Accidental inoculation into many skin areas results in a general infection. Although this disease is much milder than smallpox, it can be very serious and can involve the eyes sufficiently to cause much damage. Not only should children suffering from eczema be protected from the inoculation of smallpox virus, but their siblings or other persons in contact with them should also be removed from the environment lest accidental vaccination occur.

INSECT BITES   The large zoologic division of Diptera includes several types of mosquitoes, night-flying moths, and gnats.

Symptoms. Almost all the members of this group of insects produce hive-like lesions with central puncture and occasional small local hemorrhage, the result of reaction to the contents of the insect's saliva deposited into the skin. The contents of the saliva vary according to the species. It is quite likely that almost all species produce saliva containing both an irritating substance and a material which is capable of producing an allergic response in susceptible persons. Both types of substances can be the cause of the usual insect bite reaction. However, it is probably only the allergenic material which is capable of producing the large hives with disfiguring swelling of ears, eyelids, and other affected areas, along with general symptoms of varying degrees of shock (chills, sweating, faintness).

Treatment. Soothing lotion (calamine), antihistaminic drugs, and application of ice-cold water will control the usual mosquito bites. Symptoms of shock should be treated as in any other condition. For prevention, it is advisable to apply insect repellants to skin and clothes. Patients who are very susceptible to insect bites may find it necessary to take antihistaminic drugs by mouth prior to expected exposure to insects to render the bites innocuous.

INTERTRIGO   This eruption occurs in areas of the body where one skin surface is in contact with an adjoining skin surface and causes a retention of sweat and moisture, affording opportunity for the skin to become macerated (softened) and for resident microorganisms to flourish. The most common areas for adults are the under-surface of the breasts, the groin, and the armpits. In infants, the folds of the neck and the bends of the elbows and knees are often affected. These warm, moist sites are highly suitable for the growth of the causative organism, a yeast *(Monilia)*, which is also the organism causing "thrush" in the infant.

Symptoms. The eruption is usually confined to the areas where skin "meets" skin and has an intensely red, moist, shiny and often dusky appearance, with a sharply demarcated border.

Treatment. Wherever possible, repeated drying of the area and avoidance of restricting and warming clothing are effective both in prevention and in implementing treatment. Drying lotions (calamine) carefully applied so that excessive amounts do not further macerate the skin may suffice in mild cases. In persistent or severe eruptions, specific antibiotic therapy (mycostatin) administered systemically or applied locally may be necessary. Solutions of gentian violet are also specific and effective and can be used when mycostatin is either unavailable or contra-indicated. However the great inconvenience of purple staining on skin and clothes is a deterrent to the use of this otherwise excellent remedy.

ITCHING (PRURITUS) Itching is not a disease but a symptom and is best described as the need to scratch to obtain relief. Itching can be elicited by a large number of substances and situations. The sensation can occur in the absence of any obvious change in the skin, as for instance in liver disease with no visible jaundice. The degree of itching and the extent of area response to itch stimuli vary greatly with the disease giving rise to the symptom and with the individual response of the patient. The pattern of itching is also variable. Thus patients with louse infestation produce long scratch marks of the torso; scabies infestation produces scratch marks of the papules only (and almost exclusively at night); patients with atopic dermatitis or with dermatitis herpetiformis rub the skin with the back of the fingers and produce shiny nails (from the buffing). Itching can occur as a continuing low-grade symptom or as a crisis relieved only by gouging the skin (or by sedation). The severity of itching may far exceed the importance of the disease producing the symptom and may be the predominant factor in prognosis and treatment.

Preeminent among the several types of localized itching is that which occurs in the anus (pruritus ani), in the vulva of women (pruritus vulvae), and the scrotal sac of men. Although these conditions are extremely common, the cause is usually not known except in instances of recognizable diseases such as contact dermatitis, seborrheic dermatitis, moniliasis. Although often discouraging, treatment for relief of the itching should be pursued because continued scratching or rubbing of the site causes thickening (lichenification) which in itself produces itching.

Treatment. In addition to the specific therapy indicated for the causative disease, generalized itching is best controlled by tepid, water-softened (starch, Calgon®, oil) baths, oral antihistaminic drugs, soothing lotion or liniment (calamine), and cortisone remedies, both locally and systemically administered. When small areas are involved (eyelids, hand, foot) application of ice-cold water affords rapid relief. It should be mentioned that extremes of temperature afford relief from itching; and that it is apparent that cold applications are preferable since damage from excessive cold is less likely than damage from excessive heat (burn) in a patient already distressed and given to extremes in seeking relief. In blistering eruptions, opening the blisters by a physician may afford some relief from itching. Persistent itching in the absence of a skin eruption should be investigated by the internist.

JUVENILE WARTS The term juvenile refers to the size rather than the age of a certain type of warts. These warts, usually the size of the head of a pin, occur in groups and are found on the face and on the extremities. Because they often occur in such large numbers and in areas in which scarring would be cosmetically unacceptable, only the application of mild acids, oral medication or other nondestructive measures are suggested. Furthermore, the duration of this disorder, while very variable, is not lifelong, and the patient can be assured of the ultimate spontaneous disappearance of the warts. (*See also* WARTS in this section.)

KELOID This disease is the result of the depositing of an unusual form of connective-tissue fibers in areas of the skin which have been either accidentally or deliberately penetrated.

Symptoms. Firm nodules, pink in color, conforming to the site of disruption of skin and sometimes growing beyond it, appear at varying times after the injury and are accompanied by itching, burning, and sometimes pain. The nodules can become pale and occasionally even decrease in depth if not in extent after some time. Rarely does complete deterioration occur, and even then a marble-like disfigurement of the skin remains. The lesions have a tendency to occur in patients for varying periods of time (years) after even slight trauma (scratch). The condition also has a tendency to be more prevalent in some families, although no specific hereditary pattern has been noted. This condition can result in serious cosmetic disfigurement. Reports of malignant degeneration of the lesions are extremely rare. The disease is, however, one of great concern because of the distortion of the skin. Avoidance of all but essential surgery is a necessity of prevention.

Treatment. Repeated application of dry ice with minimal blistering, local injection of the cortisone drugs, and irradiation (radium, X-ray, Grenz ray) are among the available forms of treatment. In some instances it has been found useful to excise the involved area and administer X-ray immediately after surgery. The results of treatment vary considerably, and consideration should be given to the possibility of not treating lesions that do not constitute serious cosmetic problems.

KERATOSIS, SEBORRHEIC These warty lesions begin to appear in middle age and usually increase in both size and number. There appears to be a familial tendency, though the lesions can be of limited number and occur in a single member of a large family.

Symptoms. The keratoses occur most commonly on the chest, face, and scalp. They first appear as small buff-colored or brown raised lesions covered with a greasy scaling and are sharply defined. They increase in diameter and in depth and often attain the size and shape of a walnut. The greasy scales peel off easily, leaving early lesions barely perceptible for a while. The large lesions often crack and bleed.

Although these lesions are almost always benign no matter what the size or duration, removal of seborrheic keratoses is necessary both for comfort and for aesthetic reasons.

Treatment. Destruction of the lesions by electrocautery performed by a physician is both simple and effective. It is possible to destroy early lesions by repeated applications of several types of acid with little or no scarring. Surgical excision is usually not necessary.

KERATOSIS, SENILE Occurring most commonly in people past middle age, these lesions develop on areas of skin exposed to the sun (the face and back of the hand) and are often accompanied by other evidence of sunlight change. They are precancerous, and if left untreated for a sufficient length of time undergo malignant degeneration. Because they so invariably do become cancerous, they are considered by some to be true cancers even in their earliest stage. Aging of the skin, whether because of occupational exposure to the sun as encountered by farmers and sailors, or because of inherited disease (xeroderma pigmentosum, hydroa aestivale), is an important factor in producing this condition regardless of patients' age in years.

Symptoms. The lesions are grayish black, small, sharply outlined flat papules, often covered with a dry tenacious scale. There is some reddening of the surrounding area which varies and gives the lesion a different appearance from time to time. Some early lesions remain undefined, red, scaly and unpigmented, making diagnosis more difficult. Even in a single area, the size of the lesions may vary greatly.

Treatment. Destruction by electrodesiccation is the treatment of choice. When removal of a lesion for biopsy study is indicated, surgical excision may be more practical. Repeated biopsy study is usually neither practical nor necessary when many such lesions are removed from a single area, but the procedure should be done when possible malignant degeneration is suspected.

LICE   *See* PEDICULOSIS (LICE INFESTATION) in this section.

LICHEN PLANUS Lichen planus is of unknown causation but is thought to be related to stress, emotional crises, or worry. Lichen planus can occur as an acute, widely disseminated disease including lesions of the mucous membranes of the mouth and eyes; or it can appear gradually, persist, and become a thickened, horny and plaque-like condition usually of the shins. Occasionally drugs (most notably Atabrine®) produce this type of eruption.

Symptoms. The lesions consist of shiny, octagonal-shaped papules, purplish in color and with slightly depressed centers. They usually remain discrete, although they are often arranged in circles or parts of circles along a line of trauma (scratch or burn) and are most commonly found on the wrists, the flexor surfaces of the arms and legs, and the mucous membrane surfaces (mouth, eyelids, penis, vulva). Itching is both severe and persistent. Other forms of the disease include blistering, hyperpigmentation and atrophy. Although the incidence of recurrences is high, the disease constitutes no threat to the general health other than the unsightly appearance and the disability caused by the itching.

Treatment. The cortisone drugs are effective in some cases, and the older remedies (bismuth, arsenic) are worthy of trial in the absence of more specific therapy. Sedation, tranquilizers, relief from stress, and other supportive measures should be used. Local treatment consists of soothing lotions, but they are of limited value except in the hypertrophic cases. Injection of steriods into the lesions may be of value.

LIVER SPOTS   These flat, discrete and confluent lesions of excessive pigmentation occur most commonly in women, on the face, along the margin of the brow and on the cheek bones. They are sometimes so joined together as to seem to form a rim around the eyes. The eruption neither resembles the liver nor is it caused by diseases of the liver. The most usual condition alleged to precede this eruption is pregnancy. Many cases are also thought to be due to some functional ovarian disturbance, the exact nature of which is not known.

Treatment. Several types of local bleaching applications designed to interfere with the production of pigment or to alter already existing pigment are commercially available and may be of some benefit. Peeling of the affected sites can be tried by a physician with acid, or with blistering dry ice, or with abrasives like brush-planing. Great care must be taken that the irritation from treatment does not in itself induce further hyperpigmentation and therefore worsen the condition.

LUPUS ERYTHEMATOSUS, ACUTE DISSEMINATE   Previously thought to be a predominantly dermatologic disease, it has in recent years become clear that the cutaneous manifestations of acute disseminate lupus erythematosus may appear many years after the disease has been present in other organs and has given rise to a multiplicity of symptoms. Long-standing fatigue, low-grade fevers, joint pains, epileptiform seizures, abdominal cramps, chest pains, recurrent attacks of pneumonia are among the symptoms that can precede involvement of the skin, and may indeed remain undiagnosed and unattended until the skin lesions afford a clue for investigation.

Occurring in all age groups and in both sexes, this condition is so much more common in young women that many investigators have fruitlessly looked into the possibility of a causal connection with some ovarian disturbance. The cause of the disease remains unknown, except for the observation that exposure to ultraviolet light almost invariably worsens the condition or precipitates an attack. Prior to the advent of cortisone, the condition was fatal after a few months, or at most two years. Treatment with one of the many available cortisone drugs has afforded years of productive life to many patients with this disease. It has also been possible, through the relief of symptoms and the prolonging of life, to better differentiate this disease from the subacute form, a vastly different disease of almost identical appearance but with no systemic involvement.

Symptoms. The lesions are usually symmetrically on the "exposed" surfaces of the body (face, neck, arms, and legs), but in severe cases occur over the entire body, including the palms and soles. The reddened swollen papules appear diffusely in these areas and only seem to have a border of demarcation on the face, giving a butterfly appearance. In addition to feeling moderately or acutely ill, the patient has symptoms reflecting the presence of the disease elsewhere (joints, lungs, kidneys). Diagnosis can be confirmed by several types of studies of the blood (lowering of the white-cell count, disturbance of clotting, changes in gamma globulin) and in the finding of the lupus erythematosus cell in the bone marrow and the blood. The lupus erythematosus cell is formed when an unusual substance in the blood (probably an enzyme) causes a disintegration of lymphocytes (a type of white blood corpuscle). The disintegrated nucleus is quickly surrounded by neutrophiles (another type of white corpuscle) which engulf the material and form an abnormal but characteristic cell, the lupus erythematosus cell. The discovery and elucidation of the lupus erythematosus cell constitute a great advance in the diagnosis and the treatment of this disease.

Treatment. Except under unusual circumstances, treatment consists of administration of the cortisone drugs, the selection and dosage of which can vary considerably not only with the phase of the disease, but also with the response of the particular patient. In addition to strict avoidance of exposure to ultraviolet light, avoidance of fatigue and stress, appear to be essential both to effectiveness of treatment and to maintaining improvement.

LUPUS ERYTHEMATOSUS, CHRONIC DISCOID   A disease of young and middle adult life, and more common in women, chronic discoid lupus erythematosus can nevertheless begin at any age. Of unknown causation, both the initial appearance of the eruption and subsequent flareups may follow excessive exposure to the sun. The relationship of this disease to ultraviolet light has not yet been established; but it is very clear that patients already affected must avoid any deliberate sunning and must seek protection from even casual sun exposure encountered in ordinary daily activity. The condition is often difficult to differentiate from polymorphous light eruption and from acute disseminate lupus erythematosus, both of which have entirely different courses and prognosis. It is therefore essential that insofar as possible a definitive diagnosis be established.

Symptoms. The eruption is most commonly found on the face (cheeks) and anterior chest, and on the exposed surfaces of the arms. The lesions first appear as small plaques of reddened papules and scales with sharp, slightly elevated borders. As the lesions become more extensive, the central portions become depressed from atrophy (loss of tissue). When this process has stopped, the area appears scarred and not infrequently is hyperpigmented at the borders. The course and extent of the disease are very variable, lasting from months to years, and consisting of a single bean-size lesion to extensive involvement of all the susceptible areas.

Treatment. Although this is not a disease of specific photosensitivity, the regularity of exacerbations following exposure to ultraviolet light (sun or artificial) make avoidance of such exposure urgent. The antimalarial drugs (Chloroquine®, Atabrine®, etc.) have largely replaced the previously used bismuth, gold, and arsphenamines. However, the latter group of drugs are of some benefit and can be used when the antimalarial drugs are not tolerated or are ineffective. Local treatment consists of using sun screens in an attempt to avoid the sun exposure of ordinary living. The sun screens, applied as lotion or cream, can also be used to cover the lesions and achieve some cosmetic improvement. It is possible to destroy small lesions with the application of carbon dioxide (dry ice) in the hope of forestalling progression. In rare cases, when destruction of the skin has been extensive and the disease appears to be "burned out," reconstructive surgery may afford the patient cosmetic improvement.

MELANIN   Produced in the basal cell layer of the epidermis of the skin by the pigment-producing cells, the melanocytes, this pigment is largely responsible for the color of human skin. It is a relatively inert protein substance produced by the amnio-acid tyrosine through the intervention of the enzyme tyrosinase, both of which substances are themselves colorless. The intensity of skin color is governed by the amount of melanin distributed in the cells of the basal layer, since the number of pigment-forming cells (melanocytes) is relatively constant in all people.

The activity of the melanocytes is governed by the anterior pituitary gland through the action of its hormone (melanocyte-stimulating hormone).

Disturbances of melanin production can be either that of increase or of decrease, and can be of local or systemic causation. Although the primary function of this pigment is protection against the damaging effects of solar radiation, changes in pigmentation can be symptomatic of specific (systemic) diseases, such as vitiligo, chloasma, and Addison's disease.

MOLES, PIGMENTED   Often referred to as birthmarks, but rarely present at birth, pigmented moles, or nevi, are tumors made up of pigment-producing cells (melanocytes). The lesions begin to appear in childhood and continue to grow in size and number through adult life. They range from flat to warty, dome-shaped, and hanging brown tumors of various shades, some of which also contain hair.

The problem of classifying the large variety of tumors in this group, many of which have overlapping characteristics, is complicated by the fact that nonpigmented moles are of the same basic structure as the pigmented ones, but without evident pigment to help in the differential diagnosis. It is obviously neither practical nor useful to remove the literally countless moles as a prophylactic measure against the rare occurrence of malignant change which occurs almost exclusively in the "junction type." Differentiation between the three main classes (intraepidermal, junction, and compound) can be made with a high degree of accuracy, and changes in the pigmentation with fuzziness at the borders, irregular coloring with speckling, or change to black or very dark brown, are indications for considering surgical removal. Hairy pigmented nevi almost always remain benign. Moles situated in areas of trauma (feet) should be removed unless removal will itself cause disability. So large a percentage of the population has moles of the toes and feet, and so low is the incidence of malignancy at these sites, as to afford a statistical reassurance and warning against unnecessary (and possibly disabling) surgery.

The intraepidermal type of nevi are more likely to be dome-shaped, globular, and hanging, as contrasted with the flat or slightly elevated junction type (with the exception of warty lesions which are usually junction type also). It must be emphasized that classification of nevi is possible only after it has been determined that the lesion concerned belongs to this group of growths. The skin abounds in different kinds of growths of various size, shapes, and degrees of pigmentation having no relationship in structure or significance to moles. Since it is well within the ability of the layman to recognize the common mole, expert advice should be sought either when a long-standing lesion becomes altered in appearance, or when either a new or an old lesion does not readily lend itself to a diagnosis. Warty lesions which are obviously not really warts; bleeding lesions which are not really the result of immediate injury; and inflamed lesions with no apparent explanation for the inflammation present the type of situation requiring professional diagnosis.

Treatment. Moles known to be benign and known not to undergo malignant degeneration can be removed for reasons of convenience and for improved appearance by surgery or electrocautery. Moles of known potential danger or of undetermined classification should be excised surgically and sent to the pathologist for review. Prophylactic removal of warts is neither practical nor desirable except in instances of known potential danger.

MOLLUSCUM   CONTAGIOSUM   This condition occurs most often in children. When its incidence is high in a community, the "epidemic" is usually attributed to contacts in swimming pools, gyms, and dormitories. It also occurs both in children and in adults as an isolated happenstance, without the source of infection being detected.

Symptoms. The lesions are characteristically button-shaped papules with hard rims and relatively large depressed centers. The smaller lesions are more dome-shaped. They are skin-colored and appear on almost every part of the body, including the eyelids. Other than the continued growth of the individual lesions and the spread of the eruption, only occasional secondary pustular infection is a bothersome feature.

Treatment. The molluscum body, that self-contained mass under the upper-most layer of the skin which gives the lesion its form, disintegrates on even slight injury. Pricking the lesion with a sterile needle is usually sufficient to cause its disappearance. Catharidin applied to each lesion or freezing may also be curative. More destructive measures such as electrocautery are rarely needed for cure.

MYCOSIS FUNGOIDES This disease belongs to the lymphoma group whose characteristic disturbance is that of the reticulo-endothelial cells which are present in the skin, lymph nodes, bone marrow, and spleen. Unlike other lymphomas, mycosis fungoides is always seen in the skin first, and remains predominantly though not exclusively in the skin throughout the course of the disease. Much more common in males, this disease rarely begins before the age of forty.

Symptoms. The lesions first appear as oval-shaped, pink, slightly scaly plaques of the face, torso, and extremities. The number of lesions can be very variable. Gradually there is a thickening of the areas, and the color becomes more intense and tends to have a violet hue. Finally, the lesions enlarge and take on the appearance of tumors, reddish-brown in color, and often ulcerated.

Treatment. Localized irradiation of small individual tumors with X-ray and generalized beta ray irradiation for patients with more general involvement constitute the current treatment for this disease.

NEUROTIC EXCORIATIONS These lesions are usually present on the face, shoulders, arms and legs, and consist of small ulcers usually covered with a bloody crust. They are produced by the patient's picking, digging or scraping the skin in an attempt to remove a real or imagined substance from the skin. Whatever the initial cause of the need to excoriate the skin, a habit of doing this becomes established. As in nail-biting, the habit is difficult to break. The psychologic mechanisms capable of inducing neurotic excoriations are numerous but this condition is made even more difficult to resolve because both the patient and the accessibility of the skin are conducive to a habit mechanism. Whereas at first the patient picks a pimple while washing the face in the bathroom, soon the turning on of the bathroom light results in an almost reflex picking of the skin.

Treatment. Seldom can the patient be convinced of the damaging effect of excoriating the skin, nor is the patient often convinced of the need for psychiatric care. Occasionally the patient can be persuaded to try devices for avoiding picking while the skin is being treated. The use of gloves securely fastened with adhesive tape, low-watt bulbs in the bathroom, and handiwork while looking at television can be suggested to the willing patient.

PARONYCHIA This infection of the skin surrounding the nails is much more common on the fingers than the toes, and is usually the result of invasion by two types of organisms: pus-forming staphylococci or streptococci and a yeast *(Monilia albicans)*.

Symptoms. It is likely that there is injury to the nail fold, which is followed by redness, swelling, and the formation of pus. Simultaneous involvement of several fingers is common. Recurrence of the condition is also common in susceptible persons.

Treatment. Soaking in hot water and frequent applications of antibiotic ointment in the intervals between the soakings usually effectively relieve the infection. Occasionally it becomes necessary to release the pus by means of surgical incision. Recurrence of paronychia may require investigation to determine the cause(s) for susceptibility to this infection. But often care of the hands with special attention to avoiding injury to the cuticle will suffice in removing the provocative factor of infection.

PEDICULOSIS (LICE-INFESTATION) There are several different forms of pediculosis, including pediculosis capitis, or louse-infestation of the head. This is more common in children than in adults. Both the adult louse and the nits (eggs) can be found without much difficulty. Itching can be intense, secondary infection common, and enlargement of the lymph glands of the neck or groin, a common complication.

If the hair is long and thick, there is considerable advantage in cutting it prior to the application of remedies. Various shampoos are available which attack both the adult forms and the eggs (nits), such as Nix®, and R&C®. The manufacturers' directions should be followed regarding length of application and second treatments.

Another form, pediculosis corporis, is that in which the body louse lives in the seams of clothing and attacks the skin only to feed. Pinpoint marks are produced, followed occasionally by small hive-like lesions. The intense itching and consequent scratching result in deep excoriations and in irritation of the skin.

Removal of the infested clothing is necessary. The clothing, if it is to be used again, should be boiled or cleaned or ironed with a hot iron. For the occasional remaining nits of the hair of the armpits, soap and water washing or the application of pyrethrins solution are effective. Soothing lotions are useful for the remaining irritation and itching.

Pediculosis pubis, except for the difference in location (genital area, abdomen, and occasionally the eyebrows and lashes), has the same symptoms as those produced by the body louse.

Soap-and-water washing and application of the above-mentioned remedies are effective.

PEMPHIGUS   A disease of unknown causation, occurring almost exclusively in adult life, pemphigus primarily affects the skin and the mucous membranes. Prior to the advent of cortisone therapy no treatment was effective in altering the usually—but not invariably— fatal outcome after a course ranging from several months to two or three years.

Symptoms. Usually gradual in onset (though occasionally rapid and fulminating), blisters appear on any part of the body including the mouth and nose. The blisters enlarge rapidly and become sagging, finally breaking and becoming emptied of fluid, leaving a stretched, folded mass of skin. The blisters arise on normal-appearing skin and can be produced in unaffected areas by gentle stroking of the skin. Other than a feeling of weakness, the patient presents no complaints. Secondary infection, pneumonia, and severe anemia are encountered in the terminal phase of the disease, and death is usually attributed to these although the actual cause of death is not known.

The disease is neither contagious nor inherited, and there is no sex preponderance. Variants of the disease also occur, most common among them being a scaling and crusting eruption.

Treatment. The cortisone drugs (corticosteroids) act in an almost specific manner and are life-saving. Patients have been sustained for many years and have been able to pursue a normal life. Occasional change in the particular drug may be necessary, and the precautions usual in the use of these drugs must be maintained. Length of use of the drugs is determined by the physician.

PERSPIRATION, EXCESSIVE   Excessive perspiration or hyperhidrosis is observed in fevers, when a high fever breaks (especially in influenza), with or following physical exertion or emotional stress, when induced by physiotherapeutic apparati such as inductothermy, steam baths, and heat lamps, in hot weather and climates, or in a humid atmosphere. Severe pain, such as colic, and shock and collapse may also cause sweating. The sweat-producing drugs (diaphoretics), ipecac, camphor and pilocarpin, cause profuse sweating. Excessive perspiration occurs in hyperthyroidism, chronic tuberculosis of the lungs (especially nocturnally, the so-called "night sweats"), psychoneurosis, acute rheumatic fever, bacterial invasion of the bloodstream, malaria, chronic myocarditis, and, less commonly, in bronchiectasis (also at night), epilepsy, gout, morphinism, and other minor conditions.

Hyperhidrosis due to emotional stimulation is often localized (perspiration under the armpits, the palms of the hands, the face, feet, etc.). In this type of sweating the stimulation to sweat glands originates in the sympathetic nervous system which responds to emotional stimuli.

Human sweat is odorless. The unfavorable scent, often referred to as body odor or "b.o.," is due to the bacteria which flourish in perspiration. A good deodorant measure (and the safest) is a bath followed by thorough toweling and dusting susceptible areas of the body with powder that tends to promote dryness of the skin regions commonly affected by perspiration odors (armpits, crotch, etc.).

PLANTAR WARTS   Plantar warts are painful warts on the sole of the feet and can be confused with calluses of the soles and not infrequently the two conditions coexist. The virus which causes plantar warts is apparently "triggered" into producing the lesions by irritation (from shoes, pebbles, splinters).

Other than eliminating the most usual precipitating factor of friction from shoes (either by going barefoot or by wearing shoes molded to the exact shape of the foot, thus simulating the barefoot state), treatment must necessarily be left to the specialist.

POISON IVY (OAK, SUMAC) *See* DERMATITIS in this section.

POLYMORPHOUS LIGHT ERUPTION
This eruption occurs at all ages and in both sexes. It can make its first appearance notwithstanding the patient's previous uneventful exposure to ultraviolet light. Not infrequently, however, the initiation of the photosensitivity may have been preceded by the taking of drugs capable of inducing or eliciting the eruption. Among the known photosensitizing drugs are the sulfonamides, antibiotics, and tranquilizers, and no doubt a host of other substances less well known and less frequently encountered (for example, diagnostic fluorescent dyes).

Symptoms. The lesions appear on the parts of the body usually exposed to the sun (upper chest, face, neck, arms, and legs). The eruption consists of red papules irregularly distributed and giving a measles-like appearance. The course is short, the eruption lasting a few days or weeks after removal from ultraviolet light exposure (and elimination of the drug in cases in which this has been an eliciting factor). There are usually no concomitant systemic findings.

Treatment. On eliminating the provocative agent(s), palliative soothing lotions suffice in treatment. Because of the possible photosensitizing potential of many drugs, some presently unknown, the usual remedies for sedation and control of itching are better avoided. In some patients the physician with the use of proper instrumentation is able to determine the particular wavelengths of ultraviolet to which the patient has become sensitized, and it is then possible to find lotions containing sunscreening substances (to screen out the offending bands of ultraviolet light) for the patient to apply before exposing himself to the sun. Difficulties attend such a procedure, and the patient must continue to be cautious in further exposing himself to ultraviolet light.

PORT-WINE STAIN (NEVUS FLAMMEUS) This type of blood-vessel birthmark is extremely common on the nape of the neck and occurs less commonly over the bridge of the nose, on the forehead, and elsewhere. The bluish-red, flat, irregularly shaped lesion of varying size becomes exaggerated on crying, coughing, or blushing. Not infrequently the smaller and less intensely red lesions will completely disappear. Some lesions extend and grow in size in proportion to the growth of the child.

Treatment. Because this type of birthmark is of importance only as a cosmetic defect, it is essential that no treatment be undertaken which might produce further disfigurement. Hence surgical procedures which necessarily produce scarring are not useful, since scars cannot be covered with makeup as effectively as the smooth surface of the lesion. Even a very young child can accept the application of a cosmetic lotion or cream, and should be instructed in the use of one early in order to avoid disturbing comments from playmates. The possibility of treatment with the recently developed laser method may be considered for some cases.

PRICKLY HEAT (MILIARIA) Prickly heat is a plugging of the openings of the sweat glands which results in the damming back and enlargement of the glands and the consequent formation of pus from resident bacteria. This condition has always been an important occupational disease in industries of high environmental humidity caused by geographic conditions (tropics, sub-sea level) or the nature of the industry (steam process or other heat mechanisms). It also occurs in infants.

Symptoms. The lesions can appear singly or in groups evenly or irregularly distributed over the body, but chiefly on the face, neck, and upper chest. Each lesion consists of a tiny pustule surrounded by a flush of redness. In infants, the redness of adjacent lesions merges, especially in the folds of the neck, and forms a confluent mass of redness and moisture. This also happens in adults where moisture accumulates in folds of skin (under the breasts, in the groin).

Treatment. Care consists of drying each lesion by using simple agents, such as corn starch, talcum powder, or plain calamine lotion. If the pustular portion does not respond to the drying agents, local antibiotics (bacitracin, neosporin) will be required. Removal of the patient from the humid (for him) environment is essential. Also frequent sponging, the use of air-conditioning, dehumidifiers—and where the condition is endemic in an industry, changes in the industrial process—may be necessary for prevention.

PRURITUS   *See* ITCHING (PRURITUS) in this section.

PSORIASIS   The cause of psoriasis is unknown. This noncontagious disease occurs in both sexes and usually first appears in adults but is occasionally present in very young children. Although the hereditary nature of the disease has not been established, there is a tendency for it to be more prevalent in certain families. Psoriasis is not associated with any other medical condition (except for the rare combination of arthritis and psoriasis known as psoriasis arthropathica). The accumulated information on the influences and mechanisms of what psoriasis is not related to is so extensive that it is often referred to as a disease of persons in good health—a view not shared by those with the disease.

Symptoms. The silvery-scaled red lesions range from pinhead to silver-dollar size and larger, and are most often present on the outer sides of the elbows and knees and on the scalp. The areas are sharply outlined and the skin is thickened and raised. When the body and other portions of the arms and legs are involved, it is usual for the lesions to begin small and very slightly raised. They then become enlarged, join with adjacent lesions, and become so thickened and leathery that the skin can "crack" and bleed on little provocation. The disease is accompanied by itching of varying degree. Aside from the tremendous inconvenience that an even limited form of the disease imposes, the patient suffers no concomitant disorders and there are usually no secondary complications unique to this disease.

One of the more distressing features of psoriasis is the presence of the disease in the nails. This can occur at any time in the course of the disease and is occasionally present in patients with no other evidence of this condition on the skin. Diagnosis is often made difficult, not only when the disease is not evident elsewhere on the skin, but also because lesions of the nails of the toes are often complicated by infection with fungi. Psoriatic nails are characterized by pinpoint depressions arranged in fairly symmetrical horizontal and longitudinal pattern throughout the nails, and greyish heaped-up scaling in small plaques under the nail at the side margins. Except for irradiation (X-ray, Grenz ray), local remedies are not effective.

The course of psoriasis is quite varied, as is the response to treatment. Its duration is from months to years to a lifetime, with similar periods of remission. Recurrences are more common in the winter, or in climates in which exposure to the sun is not possible. Recurrences have also been attributed to many generalized conditions including tension, changes in diet, infection, and pregnancy.

Treatment. In spite of the patient's quick discouragement—usually the result of well-intentioned lay opinion—control of the eruption is possible in most cases. Types of management of the disease are numerous, though the response of the patient to a particular type of treatment unpredictable. It is not unheard-of, for instance, for a previously much-treated patient suddenly, for no apparent reason, to respond to an old and simple

PSORIASIS

Psoriasis is a chronic, inflammatory skin disease. The elbows, knees, and scalp are favorite sites. The lesions are reddish, dry, rounded, or sharply defined patches covered with abundant scales.

remedy like mercury ointment. Conversely, even the most sophisticated and well-designed course of treatment may fail. Among the effective remedies are ultraviolet light, tars, combinations of ultraviolet light and tar application, vitamins given singly and in combination (A, B, D), local and systemically administered cortisone drugs, arsenic in the form of Fowler's Solution, irradiation (X-rays, Grenz ray), nonspecific immunization (autohemotherapy, immune globulin), hospitalization or other environmental change, baths for the softening of the scales, antihistaminic drugs for control of the itching, supportive measures (sedatives, stimulants, tranquilizers), and finally the newer drugs which are toxic to cellular proteins (Methotrexate®).

What should be made eminently clear is that an energetic and diligent pursuit of relief from the symptoms can be rewarding. The fact that cure is not obtainable under current circumstances should not be a deterrent to the seeking of relief in this disease, any more than it is in such other diseases of unknown cause and long duration as stomach ulcer, with its need for continued therapeutic vigilance.

RETIN A

A derivative of vitamin A, Retin A has long been used as a treatment for acne and more recently to improve the appearance of aging and wrinkled skin. Skin that has been exposed for long periods to the sun tends to become wrinkled and thin. Application of Retin A on a daily basis has been found to improve the skin's appearance with varying results. Some find the disappearance of small wrinkles and lightening of "old age spots" very pleasing. While others find the side effects of blotching, redness and bursting of small capillaries not worth the treatment. Because of the side effects, physicians are still very selective in recommending Retin A.

RINGWORM OF THE SCALP

This still-common condition is due to a fungus which gets into the hair shaft and causes brittleness; the hair then breaks off, leaving quite an obvious bald spot. (The skin at the base of these short hairs may be slightly scaly.) A special ultraviolet filter (Wood's light) at the doctor's office will show these diseased hairs, and a culture can be made to confirm the diagnosis.

This type of ringworm is called the human type because it comes from other infected children.

Treatment. Treatment of scalp ringworm is more satisfactory than it once was, thanks to the new drugs which destroy the fungus. Many doctors still advocate plucking the hairs out and applying ointment in addition to giving internal medication, continuing this treatment until no more diseased hairs are found under the Wood's light. They argue that unless this is done the diseased hairs may spread the infection to healthy ones. Others argue that the same oral medication which destroys the fungus will also take care of the overall situation, preventing spread. Before the oral fungicides were developed, curing a case of ringworm of the scalp usually required at least a month or two of treatment. Today a child is given medicine for only one day; the cure, however, is not effected for two and a half weeks.

ROSACEA

This chronic reddening of the center portion of the face (forehead, nose, chin) is often accompanied by the papules and pustules of acne. More common in women of middle age, it can nevertheless occur in both sexes and almost any age. The reddening worsens on exposure to extremes of temperature, and gradually the intensity of color becomes persistent with no periods of lightening. Tiny superficial vessels become visible in the skin. When the nose is the area most dominantly affected, as is often the case in men, an overgrowth of all the components of the skin takes place, giving the lower portion of the nose a grotesque appearance.

Rosacea is often associated with lesions of the eyes (conjunctivitis, keratitis) at the same time that the skin becomes involved with blackhead formation, dilated pores and much greasiness.

Probably of multiple causation, the condition flares up on eating hot foods (both from condiment and temperature), iodides (shellfish), bromides (sedatives), chocolate, and nuts, and is thought to be associated with a lowering of the stomach's hydrochloric acid.

Treatment. Avoidance of extremes of temperature, alcohol, and spicy foods, is essential in treatment. Drying lotions, antibiotics for pustules, suitable hydrochloric acid therapy, and, finally, electrolysis or electrocautery of the enlarged vessels and surgical removal of excess tissue (nose), can prove effective. (*See also* ACNE in this section.)

SCABIES An intensely itchy, highly communicable disease occurring in all age groups and both sexes, scabies is caused by a mite, *Sarcoptes scabiei,* and is transmitted by direct contact from person to person. Other varieties of mite, parasitic to fowl and to domestic and wild mammals, occasionally attack human beings, but produce eruptions of less intensity and shorter duration. It is interesting to note that prior to about 1950, scabies was a common disease, both endemic and epidemic in the urban communities of the United States.

Symptoms. The mite produces small papules in which a darkened horizontal shadow (a burrow) is noted. The lesion may give the appearance of a small blister, and in young children the condition may indeed be a blistering one. The lesions occur most commonly in the bend of the wrist, the webs of the fingers and over the entire torso, but not on the neck, face, and head. In children, the palms and soles are frequently affected. Secondary pustular infection is usual. The itching is always intense, but characteristically is much worse at night (perhaps because of the warmth of bed covers).

Treatment. Sulfur ointments, solution of benzyl benzoate, Qwell® or Nix ointment applied before bedtime and left on the next day are among the effective remedies. Reapplication of the remedy for five to seven days, and boiling or cleaning the clothes and bed linens, are necessary for cure.

SCARS Of considerable variety and of many causes, scars are evidence of a disruption of the connective tissue of the dermis subcutaneous layer of the skin, with a loss of the elastic elements, hair follicles sebaceous and sweat glands, a scarcity of blood vessels, much fibrous tissue, and a thin epidermal covering. The fibrous tissue can be so excessive as to give the lesion the appearance of a keloid, and then become flattened spontaneously (hypertrophic scar). The smooth, glossy appearance of scars and the absence of contours of surface "relief" is the result of the absence of certain tissues (gland and hair structures) in the normal skin.

Many scars can be identified as resulting from a specific preceding condition (acne, chickenpox, striae of pregnancy, neurotic excoriations, burns, lupus erythematosus, syphilis, surgery).

Treatment. Except when scarring is extensive and interferes with function, or when a scar is injured and "breaks down," treatment is unnecessary. For aesthetic betterment, scars can be excised, abraded, or treated with acids, depending on the configuration of the scarring and the area involved. Plastic surgery may successfully transform prominent or unaesthetic scars into almost imperceptible ones.

SCLERODERMA, LOCALIZED (MORPHEA) This benign disease affects both children and adults, but it is rare in the elderly.

Symptoms. Confined to the skin, it consists of a disturbance of the connective tissue and is first noted as bluish discoloration occurring on any part of the skin surface, though most commonly on the face and neck. The area becomes enlarged, feels hard to the touch, loses its violet-blue color, becoming yellow or alabaster-like. As the lesions become firmer they also become elevated. Succeeding flareups produce a purplish halo around the existing lesions. The eruption can consist of a single lesion stationary in size, or the lesion can extend—usually in linear fashion—over the entire extremity. Remission can result in a moderate depression in the center of the lesion, but the hard, firm texture almost always persists, even when the lesion is "burned out" and presents a brownish hyperpigmented, and occasionally scaling area. Itching is not common.

Localized scleroderma is not associated with any known condition. While the prognosis is good, disfigurement and incapacitation can be severe and constitute a significant handicap.

Treatment. The many suggested remedies including massage, local administration of mecholyl, cortisone, and PABA (para-aminobenzoic acid) afford only questionable relief.

SEBORRHEIC DERMATITIS This is a disturbance of the hair follicle-connected sebaceous (oil) gland in which the eruption consists of round and oval-shaped plaques located chiefly over the mid-portion of the chest, the middle of the back, the shoulders, the eyebrows and eyelids, the sides of the nose, behind the ears, and the margin of the scalp where it joins the skin of the face and neck. This term also applies to a similar condition of the scalp, which in a mild form, and present in a very high percentage of persons in certain populations, is the well-known dandruff.

Symptoms. Ranging from the earliest "cradle-cap" of the newborn, and the simplest mild scaling of the scalp noted by almost everyone from time to time, to a recurrent and often persistent widespread eruption, the disease is associated with considerable itching. Remissions are common especially in the summer (during vacations, and under conditions of an improved state of health). No specific cause has been assigned to this malfunctioning of the sebaceous glands.

Treatment. For the uncomplicated dandruff confined to the scalp, there is an abundance of effective and harmless remedies available over-the-counter in the pharmacy. These remedies contain (either singly or in combination) such remedies as sulfur, mercury, tars, and salicylic acid. Dandruff which does not respond to the commercially available remedies may be relieved by prescription drugs. Seborrheic dermatitis, found on areas other than the scalp which does not respond to simple drying agents like calamine lotion, requires a physician's care.

SHINGLES (HERPES ZOSTER) This condition, often attributed to "nerves," is actually an affliction of a particular nerve. The site of the pathology is at the point of emergence of the nerve from the spinal column or the skull, as the case may be. The inflammation of the nerve is caused by a virus closely related to the virus of chickenpox; and, indeed, the disease occurs either in people who have never had chickenpox and have therefore not had an opportunity to become immunized to the virus (and to related viruses); or in people who have lost their immunity either partially or completely. Therefore this disease occurs in senior citizens who are exposed to children with chickenpox and no longer have sufficient immunity to withstand the related virus of shingles. Also, in elderly and in the extremely and often terminally ill, activation

of the virus is evidence of a general loss of immunity, hence of a poor prognosis.

Symptoms. The eruption consists of groups of blisters surrounded by some redness. The blisters are deep-seated and therefore not easily broken. The groups are found in the general distribution of a nerve. For instance, groups of blisters will form around the chest in the approximate location of one rib, or in an irregular line down a thigh or leg. There can be a scattering of smaller groups beyond the ordinary position of a particular nerve, because very small nerve-ends extend into areas seemingly beyond that of the involved nerve. And so one occasionally sees shingles appear to be present on "both sides." The legendary fatal outcome for this situation is not based on fact. Pain may precede the eruption by several

SHINGLES

days. The pain is similar to a dull toothache but with occasional sharp, knife-like sensations. The skin condition lasts from two to three weeks, somewhat longer when the face is involved. The pain may last a much longer time. Often patients having known somebody with prolonged post-shingles pain are apprehensive about this aspect of the disease. It should therefore be noted that prolonged pain is the exception, and that patients usually recover in three or four weeks from both the skin eruption and the pain.

Treatment. Vidarabine (Zovirax®) is an antiviral drug shown to be of value for shingles. It shortens the course of the disease and decreases the severity of the post-herpetic neuralgia. It is taken every four hours around the clock for up to ten days. Steroid drugs also diminish pain and shorten the course of the disease. If the disease is mild with little discomfort and eruption, which sometimes happens, no special measures need be called for.

SKIN, FUNCTION AND STRUCTURE

The skin is not only the largest organ in the body, but also probably has the largest number of different functions, in addition to the pre-eminent one of enveloping and containing all the other organs. Its soft and elastic structure permits voluntary and involuntary motion and at the same time withstands physical trauma. Its highly impermeable outer layer seals off the body from noxious agents in the environment, and yet permits the excretion of sweat and oil for the maintenance of even body temperature by the former and lubrication of the surface by the latter. Its pigment, melanin, protects against actinic radiation, and yet permits sufficient absorption of ultraviolet light to ensure the skin's production of vitamin D. The skin protects against excess of heat and of cold, and gives notice of many forms of danger by its sense of pain. The sense of touch affords communication with the environment and fills a variety of needs, organic and emotional. The immunologic role of the skin (manifest in its reactions to substances conveyed to it directly by application or indirectly by the blood vessels after injection, ingestion, or inhalation) is another facet of its protective function. And probably most impressive of all is the skin's "memory" and

"record-keeping," as revealed in the individuality of fingerprints, life-time specific allergic responses, genetic precision of distribution of pigment, hair, and texture, and the reliability of the cells to reproduce seemingly identical cells during the whole span of life.

The skin is made up of three readily identifiable parts: the epidermis which is comprised of the vital stratum germinativum and stratum spinulosum, and the non-vital stratum granulosum, stratum lucidum, and stratum corneum; the cutis which consists of a network of collagenous supporting tissue through which the blood vessels and nerves reach the epidermis; and the subcutaneous layer composed of fat and connective tissue, and interspersed blood vessels and nerves.

The thickness of the epidermis varies considerably in different body sites, depending partially on the thickness of its four component parts. However, the stratum germinativum or basal layer always consists of a single layer of cells, except in disease. The cells of this layer constantly reproduce themselves, and in this layer are found the pigment-forming cells which produce melanin and give the unique and varying color to the skin. The epidermis also contains a varying number of nerve fibrils. This outermost portion of the skin is nourished by fluids derived from the blood vessels of the underlying cutis since there are no blood vessels in the epidermis.

The cutis is also of varying thickness and density. The blood vessel supply is of a dual nature, superficial and deep, and is augmented by a lymphatic system made up largely of "spaces" and few identifiable vessels. The two major types of nerves are seen in the cutis: the autonomic (vegetative) nerves which service the tissue themselves, blood vessels, glands, hairs, and the cerebrospinal nerves (perceptive organ) which convey sensation.

The subcutis, or subcutaneous layer, like the epidermis and the cutis is of varying thickness in different regions of the body. In addition to the blood vessels and nerves which traverse it, the connective tissue network enmeshes clusters of fat which provide padding for absorption of mechanical shock, insulation against heat and cold, and storage for food and water. The apparent difference of distribution of fat in the sexes is probably based on biologic usefulness, a factor of which is undoubtedly its aesthetic satisfaction.

Of the same tissue of origin (the ectoderm) as the epidermis, and indeed an extension of epidermal development, are the skin appendages: hair, nails, sweat glands, oil glands.

Hair arises from an invagination—or dipping down—of the epidermis which extends into the cutis, and occasionally into the subcutis, at an oblique angle and is apparent at its emergence at the surface of the skin as the shaft. At its deepest portion, the epidermal lining of the shaft is enlarged to form the bulb in the convexity of which is the nourishing blood vessel network, the hair papilla. The hair-bulb is made up largely of germinating or reproductive cells which undergo cyclic periods of activity and of rest, depending on the type of hair and the area in which the hair is situated. For example, the long hair of the scalp grows for about three years, is loosened and lost when a new active cycle of hair-growth replaces the loosened hair. The rate of growth, the texture of the hair, the color, and the contour are considerably dependent on inherited characteristics.

The portion of the hair contained in the cutis is comprised of an inner root sheath attached to the hair cuticle and an outer root sheath coated by a vitreous (glossy) layer. The entire structure is encased in a dense mass of connective tissue to which are attached strands of "involuntary" muscle (arrectores pilorum), one of the functions of which is to aid in the secretion of the sebaceous glands.

The three types of hair (long, bristle, and lanugo) begin to replace the fetal hair at birth, and the replacement is complete at puberty. But even within the groups, there are apparent and functional differences. The long hair of the scalp differs from that of the beard, the armpits and the pubis; and they each differ from each other. The same is true of the eyelashes, the eyebrows, the hair of external openings of the nose and of the ears. Only the lanugo or downy hair varies little from area to area. Lanugo-like hair is also seen as the first hair growth preceding the appearance of the normal hair in alopecia areata, a disease of complete loss of hair in circumscribed areas.

The color of the hair is largely derived from the pigment melanin present in the shaft and

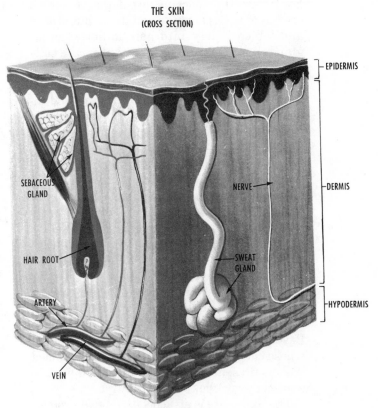

THE SKIN (CROSS SECTION)

EPIDERMIS

DERMIS

HYPODERMIS

SEBACEOUS GLAND

NERVE

HAIR ROOT

SWEAT GLAND

ARTERY

VEIN

synthesized in the upper portion of the hair bulb.

The sebaceous glands are situated in the upper part of the cutis and secrete sebum (oil) into the hair follicles to which they are attached just beneath the epidermis. Only the sebaceous glands of the border of the lips, the foreskin, and the vaginal labia (mucous membrane surface) are "free" of hair follicle association. The glands, which are grape-like in structure, vary in size inversely with the size of the follicles to which they are attached—a small gland being connected with a large follicle and a large gland being connected with a small one. Over-activity of the sebaceous gland, with thickening of the orifice, results in the horny plug (blackhead) of acne; overactivity and occlusion of the orifice results in cyst formation; uncomplicated over-activity of the gland results in excessive oiliness of the skin.

The sweat glands are tubular coiled structures situated chiefly in the lower part of the cutis and occasionally in the subcutis. They extend in a vertical fashion and penetrate the cells of the epidermis to empty at the surface of the skin in very small openings, the pores.

Except for the apocrine sweat glands which are found in the armpits and in the pubic area and which empty into hair follicles, sweat glands are of eccrine nature, that is, the cells secrete sweat without shedding themselves in the secretion. Disturbances of activity of these glands result in local irritation and infection and in systemic reactions resulting from interference with the sweating mechanism.

The nail consists of a nail-plate which is firmly attached to the nail bed except for its outermost portion which has a free, unattached edge. Composed entirely of closely packed keratin and growing continuously, nail is almost colorless except for the shades of color resulting from light reflection on the three different-appearing portions of the nail-plate. The moon-shaped portion closest to the cuticle is the matrix, that portion of the nail which produces the keratin nail substance. Beyond this is the pink-appearing nail bed whose color is attributable to the many blood vessels present in this area. The free edge is white or gray, the color of keratin.

The nail-plate is attached to lateral grooves at the sides and a posterior groove at the base. These are covered by nailfolds, the anterior portion of which is visible and is known as the cuticle.

Changes in the nail often reflect specific alterations in the functioning of the matrix, although distortion or infection can disturb nail growth without matrix involvement.

The blood vessels of the skin, whose primary function is the conveying of necessary materials and removing noxious agents, consist of minute capillaries and only slightly larger venules. Much of the exchange of materials is accomplished by "shunts" or "joinings" of arterioles (slightly larger than capillaries) and venules (A-V shunts).

In addition to the autonomic nerves (motor nerves) which control sweat, the skin is supplied with sensory nerves which afford the skin perception of touch, temperature, and pain. Itching is not a "primary" sensation, but is probably a low order of pain produced by tissue injury of small magnitude.

SKIN HYGIENE In health, the skin is in an exquisite state of balance: with myriads of microorganisms living on its surface; with the gaseous and water content of the enveloping air; with its own lubricating mechanisms giving varying textures to its different areas, depending on the local needs (compare palms and soles with eyelids, armpits, knees, ears); with radiation effects of light (tanning to protect); and environmental temperature, noxious agents, allergens, etc.

The problems arise largely from excesses: excesses of bathing, excesses of sunning, excesses of control of environmental temperature (overheating in winter and overcooling in summer); and excesses of cleansing, lubricating, de-sweating, deodorizing; and others.

We bathe for many reasons unrelated to the requirements of skin health. We bathe to rid ourselves of normal "animal" odor, having trained our sense of smell to respond to man-made, perfume odors, or at worst, to no odor at all. We bathe to maintain a status symbol of affluence (being able to afford the plumbing, the time, and cosmetic accoutrement of the bath). We bathe to remove the stigma of the soil of labor.

But bathing does have merit. A bath supplies privacy and relaxation which are not only pleasant but also often therapeutic. Bathing cleanses the skin of air-borne industrial contaminants, the grime of urban and commercial areas, the dust of the arid areas. Modern soaps are designed for frequent bathing and are not usually irritating to the normal skin. Sometimes soap-substitutes or super-fatted soaps may be necessary even for skin not obviously disturbed. Excessive drying of the skin from bathing can be modified by the use of water-softeners or bath oils, especially in areas of hard-water supply. The use of after-bath oils is unnecessary, except in areas prone to dryness (shins, arms, ankles), and in cases of generalized dryness unrelieved by specific therapy. Excessive oiliness is usually confined to the face and can be controlled with frequent washing and with the use of astringents.

The frequency of hair-washing is a matter of individual taste. In most climates, weekly shampoos serve to cleanse the hair of accumulated oil and dust; but more frequent washing is not harmful. Hair oils, waving solutions, dyes, sprays, and the like do not affect hair growth. They can cause damage to the hair, the scalp, and the surrounding skin under circumstances of excessive use (breaking of hair) or allergic sensitization (eruption of the skin and scalp and occasionally burn-like irritation from prolonged application). Mechanical devices (curlers, clips, rubber bands, brushes) can cause breaking of hair; but the damage is only to the portion of the hair that was injured and does not affect the basic growth of the hair. The wearing of wigs does not seem to alter the growth or texture of the natural hair. (*See also* the section HOME NURSING CARE.)

Sunbathing is undeservedly popular. Notwithstanding the attractiveness of a "tan" and the luxurious circumstances under which it is acquired, no certain benefits accrue from the deliberate exposure of adults to the sun, other than the enforced rest necessary to the achieving of the desired result. Actinic radiation (sun or sunlamp) causes an aging of the skin in excess of that of the chronologic age and hastens deterioration of the skin, with resultant keratoses and skin cancer in susceptible individuals.

Sweating is variously managed by the wearing of porous and absorptive clothing, the use of local antiperspirants, and the oral administration of sweat-inhibitors (Banthine®) in aggravated cases. Associated "strong" body odor is relieved by frequent bathing, avoidance of strong perfumes to which the body odor can cling, restriction of odor-producing foods (and consequent restriction of their excretion in sweat), removal of the hair of the armpits (and a consequent removal of resident odor-producing bacteria), the use of deodorants, and the use of pleasant perfume odors to alter or displace remnant unpleasant body odor.

Hand lotions are widely used and are often necessary for prevention of hand irritations resulting from occupational (both gainful and non-gainful) exposures to abrasives, cleansers, oils, etc. A high percentage of hand eczemas are the result of repeated washing and inadequate drying of the hands. The busy housewife, the pediatric nurse, the dentist, the bartender, are all likely to have constantly moist hands as they go from chore to chore meticulously washing but not taking the time to dry their hands. The skin tolerates wetness (total immersion) or dryness, but reacts to remnant moisture which interferes with the mechanism of sweating and evaporation. Es-

pecially in cold, wet climates, careful drying of hands, the use of mild soaps, hand lotions for excessive dryness, and gloves on exposure to the outdoors will be helpful in preventing eczema of the hands.

The large array of wrinkle creams, youth-giving lotions, mud packs, fresheners, and restorers are of no known merit in retarding aging changes in skin. Possibly the Vitamin A-like substance, tretinoin (Retin A) applied topically may be of value in improving skin damage due to the sun and to aging.

SKIN TAGS (SKIN POLYPS)   These small outpouchings of skin occur chiefly on the neck, upper chest, armpits, and occasionally the face of middle-aged women, and also in men. The bases of these lesions are thread-like and often do not bleed when cut off. While the usual tag is skin-colored, some are variously brown-colored. Other than being irritated or torn from the skin (with some bleeding), no serious consequences result from leaving them untreated. Simple excision or cautery is useful in this unimportant, but occasionally very disagreeable, condition.

SPIDER NEVUS   Occurring at any age, but not infrequently also in early childhood—most commonly on the face—the lesion of spider nevus consists of a pinhead-size enlargement of a blood vessel, surrounded by very small tentacle-like vessels. Sometimes the central raised vessel can be seen to pulsate.

The occurrence of lesions on the chest and neck is often noted during pregnancy and after sunburn in susceptible patients. Although spontaneous disappearance of the lesions is possible, it is more likely that they will persist and that new ones will appear during subsequent pregnancies and on subsequent episodes of sunburn. The condition is also noted in patients with diseases of the liver.

Treatment. The lesions can be obliterated with electrocautery or with electrolysis. It may be necessary to repeat either procedure several times for final removal of the vessel.

SUNBURN   Caused by excessive exposure to ultraviolet light (sun or artificial), sunburn is an increasingly common disability resulting from greater opportunity for exposure to sun (ease of travel to distant places), increased open-air activity (skiing, fishing, mountain climbing), and the current social acceptance.

No portion of the body with the possible exception of the palms and soles is immune to the burning properties of sunlight. The eyelids, armpits, and the like are more readily affected because of the sparseness of the horny protective skin layer. Highly pigmented skin offers protection but no guarantee of freedom from possible sun damage. Seemingly similar exposures to sun may vary widely depending on elevation (sea level), time of day, wind, reflection (sand, water), and available shade.

Even mild redness of the skin may result in extensive blistering and be accompanied by dizziness, nausea, and much discomfort.

Treatment. Aside from the obvious wisdom of prevention, early application of wet dressings, either by immersion in a tepid bath or by placing cold water-soaked cloths on the affected parts for as long and as often as practical, is the single best remedy for sunburn. Aspirin by mouth seems helpful in reducing the inflammation in its early stages. Addition of a water softener (salts, starch) is useful but not essential. During the intervals between wet applications, thin, mild lotions (preferably unmedicated and unperfumed) can be used. Large blisters can be opened under antiseptic conditions; this should be followed by application of an antibiotic ointment (bacitracin, neosporin).

SUNSCREENS Sunscreens, also referred to as sunblock lotions, are chemical products applied to the skin to reduce the amount of damage caused by exposure to the harmful ultraviolet rays of the sun. Repeated sun exposure causing sunburn results in wrinkling, color changes and premalignant and malignant growths. Commercial sunblock lotions are rated by their Sun Protective Factor (SPF) numbers. The number signifies the length of time one can spend outdoors with protection versus no protection. An SPF 15 extends by a multiple of fifteen the amount of time one can safely spend outdoors. Perspiration and water tend to remove sunscreen so reapplication of the lotion is necessary. As the amount of skin

cancer has increased dramatically due to sun exposure it is prudent to apply sunscreen lotion whenever one intends to spend more than a few minutes outdoors.

SWEATING, EXCESSIVE Excessive sweating is a source of great inconvenience to many people. It constitutes an occupational hazard in a variety of types of work, especially those in which the hands or feet are in primary use, for instance, the work of musicians, mechanics, typists, dentists, artists, construction workers, dancers, and models. The condition also can cause great embarrassment when it occurs in other areas, such as the face, the armpits, and the chest. Sweating is worsened by physical exertion, fatigue, and a variety of emotions including fear, anxiety, and states of stress.

Treatment. Mild sedation, rest, and the use of sweat-inhibiting drugs (Banthine®, Prantal®) will afford some relief. However, the patient must also be made to understand the underlying emotional factors for effective management of the problem. Astringents and anti-perspirants are available commercially and have a limited usefulness.

SWIMMER'S ITCH This is caused by a larvae (cercariae) of several species of the worm Schistosoma (known also as Bilharzia) which are hatched from snails found in water which has been polluted by the parasite-laden feces of the mammalian and avian hosts. In the U.S. unlike the situation in the Orient or Africa, the disorder is uncommon and the larvae do not develop into adults. Water contamination is thought to come about from the droppings of migratory birds.

Symptoms. The eruption appears on portions of the body which were submerged in the water. A few minutes after the patient leaves the water, there is a burning sensation, followed by the appearance of small, flat, reddened areas, in turn followed by several crops of similar lesions. These enlarge and are covered by crusts. The burning and smarting is followed by itching. Secondary infection is not uncommon. The lesions last about two weeks, leaving reddish-brown stains.

Treatment. Immediate washing with soap and water followed by thorough drying of the skin serves to remove the larvae, or to prevent their penetrating the skin. Penetration of the larvae is facilitated in the process of evaporation of the water, and quick drying effectively prevents this. Subjective symptoms are controlled with soothing lotion (calamine), oral antihistaminic drugs for the itching, and antibiotic drugs for the secondary infection. Control of further infestation from the polluted water depends on removal of the parasite's vector, the snails.

SWIMMING POOL GRANULOMA   This relatively new disease entity, which apparently results from injury incurred in swimming pools, has been noted with increasing frequency. The causative organism, *Mycobacterium balnei,* either survives or thrives in swimming pool water, and closely resembles the organism causing tuberculosis of the skin.

Symptoms. The lesion appears three or four weeks after even minor injury. The most common sites for the appearance of the lesions are the bridge of the nose, elbows, knees, and feet. One or more small brownish-red nodules appear, grow slowly, extend somewhat, and usually disappear in several months. It is possible, though not usual, for other sites to become infected from the original lesion.

Treatment. Small lesions can be destroyed with electrocautery if spontaneous disappearance seems unlikely. Prevention can be achieved by lining roughened pool surfaces with smooth tile and by adequate chlorination of the water.

TATTOO   A tattoo is commonly thought to be solely the result of deliberate decoration of the skin (with a variety of substances deposited deep into the skin). However, a tattoo may often be the result of accidental deposition of such substances as lead (from pencils), dye (from pens), gravel (from brushburns), and from medicinals like mercury and gentian violet applied to abraded skin.

Treatment. Extirpation by some form of surgery, electrocautery, application of acids, or blistering with the application of dry ice yield varying degrees of success. Because the tattoo is in the deep portion of skin, scarring is an inevitable result of removing the lesion. Depending on the area involved, reconstruction of the tattooed area by means of plastic

surgery may be necessary to achieve cosmetic betterment.

TRENCH FOOT   Rarely encountered in civilian life, trench foot results from long exposure to cold and moisture of the extremities encased in restricting footgear. Obvious damage to the skin is rarely noted except as a secondary and ominous effect.

Symptoms. Hemorrhage of the small vessels of the skin, ulcers, blisters, and gangrene constitute an extension of the primary condition, in which the damage appears to be the deep blood vessels and nerves, giving the skin a blanched appearance at first, and then a reddening and swelling. The condition is accompanied by a sensation of "pins and needles" and marked sweating. The sweating may indeed worsen the condition by producing more of the wet-cold local skin environment.

Treatment. Prevention is afforded by the far-sighted wearing of roomy and sturdy footgear in circumstances where this condition can be anticipated. Repeated drying of the feet and gentle massage (under a shirt or outer garment) may seem to be a luxury in military situations conducive to producing trench foot, but they are essential precautions. Treatment consists of bed rest, elevation of the feet, systemic antibiotic remedies, and supportive measures.

VITILIGO   This disease is characterized by a progressive loss of pigment occurring most often on the face, neck, arms, and the back of the hands, but no portion of the body is exempt from involvement. The lesions appear first as small round or oval alabaster-white spots which grow larger and join with adjacent lesions. When the skin is tanned on exposure to the sun, there appears to be an increase of the pigment at the border of the white lesions. Whether the increase is "real" or whether it is "relative" and due to a larger differential in color (from the border's ability to become tan from the sun) is still an unresolved question. There is no known cause for the disease and there are no significant concomitant symptoms.

Treatment. Before treatment can be started it is necessary to differentiate this disease from several quite similar conditions, namely albinism (congenital loss of the ability to produce pigment, which is not susceptible to treatment), chloasma (partial and irregular hyperpigmentation, in which the paler areas may resemble vitiligo), and pseudoachromia parasitica (or tinea versicolor, a fungous infection causing lesions of both lessened and increased pigmentation). Because spontaneous remission is uncommon, treatment, limited though it is, may afford relief. Among the many and varied kinds of treatment, the recent revival of an ancient remedy, the plant-derived ammoidin which is now synthesized as the psoralenes, has stimulated extensive clinical research of great promise. The psoralenes are worthy of trial, especially in patients with extensive involvement of the skin.

VITILIGO
Vitiligo is an acquired pigmentary disease characterized by irregular, sharply defined, milk-white patches. Except for the loss of pigment, the skin is normal. The condition lasts throughout life.

WARTS This well-known condition, especially common in children, is caused by an identifiable filtrable virus. What is so curious and so baffling about a wart is that even though the condition is that of a tumor mass, it can resist all forms of destructive treatment including irradiation, surgery, and acids, and can regrow in the identical site after seeming

total removal and complete healing. Conversely, the most persistent, obdurate, extensive warty masses can disappear overnight for no apparent cause and with no attempt at treatment. There is considerable evidence indicating the importance of psychic influences in therapy. But the nature of effective psychogenic modality (anger, indifference, acceptance, resentment) is not known.

Treatment. Since the largest number of warts disappear without treatment, it is desirable to treat only those that are easily removable or that are so large as to interfere with function of the affected part. Treatment which may result in permanent damage (scarring, distortion) is almost never indicated because the wart itself is never a threat to life, and because it not only can, but most often does, disappear without treatment. Treatment (aside from patience) varies from the highly skilled administration of irradiation (X-ray, Grenz ray) and "alteratives," whose function it is to change the immunity to the virus, to the application of local remedies like silver nitrate, and bi- and trichloracetic acid. A plant extract, podophyllin, and inteferon also may be utilized.

WRINKLES Degeneration of the connective tissue of the dermis (subcutis) of the skin results in both a loss of elasticity of this tissue and a lessening of the number of connective tissue fibers. Almost always the result of senile changes, the process is irreversible. Relief from the undesired changes in the skin-surface patterns, laxness, and folds, can be achieved by reconstructive plastic surgery.

XANTHELASMA Occurring in both sexes between forty and fifty years of age, although occasionally in younger people, too, this disease is often a manifestation of disturbance of fat (lipid) metabolism or of diabetes. Although sometimes accompanied by fatty tumors elsewhere, xanthelasma usually affects the upper and lower eyelids near, and sometimes extending onto, the nose.

Symptoms. The lesions consist of yellowish or buff-colored, velvety, firm plaques, ranging in size from one-eighth inch to one inch and often joining to form irregularly shaped masses. Occasionally they become large enough to interfere with vision. There are no accompanying subjective symptoms.

Treatment. Because of the high incidence of fat-metabolism disturbance and of diabetes in patients with xanthelasma, examination for the possible existence of these conditions is essential. The lesions can be removed surgically, destroyed by desiccation, or peeled with acids. Recurrence is not uncommon. Marked reduction of fat (plant and animal) intake may cause the lesions to disappear. However, the necessary drastic reduction and attendant monotony and impalatability of diet may be impractical.

XANTHOMATOSIS Disturbance of fat metabolism resulting in fatty deposits in the skin may occur as a primary, inherited disease (incomplete dominant trait), or may result from the increase of fat in the blood serum from diabetes, nephrosis, pancreatitis, etc. Determining the type of xanthomatosis present in a patient often necessitates extensive observation and investigation.

Symptoms. The lesions consist of yellowish brown tumors or plaques of varying size, usually occurring in groups over the joints, on the buttocks, in the creases of the palms and on the heels, but sometimes scattered elsewhere on the body. They can enlarge and interfere with movement of the hands and feet; and occasionally they can become ulcerated.

Treatment. Drastic reduction of fat in the diet will cause a diminution, and even disappearance, of the lesions. The necessary reduction of fat (both vegetable and animal) intake is difficult to maintain because of the resulting monotony of diet. In cases in which the disease is a secondary result of another condition, treatment of the causative condition in addition to restriction of fat intake is essential. Surgical removal of lesions interfering with function is feasible, especially if recurrence can be avoided by treatment of the causative systemic condition.

XERODERMA PIGMENTOSUM An inherited disease of the skin in which there is an accelerated and persistent reaction to even small exposures to light, with a resultant excessive freckling and aging of the skin.

Symptom. This condition is usually noted soon after the first or second summer of infancy and may first appear as a vague dermatitis accompanied by freckling and by tearing of the eyes. Dryness and wrinkling of the skin of the exposed areas of the face, chest, and upper extremities are followed by the production of warty growths; finally, skin cancers of several types develop in the affected areas. The intolerance of the eyes to light may be severe. Deafness and mental deficiency are sometimes associated with this disorder.

Treatment. Rigid avoidance of sunlight is essential in the care of the patient. Protective creams (with ultraviolet-light filters) should be used when even minimal exposure to light is necessary. Removal of warty and malignant growths should be done early to avoid excessive surgery.

URINARY CONDITIONS

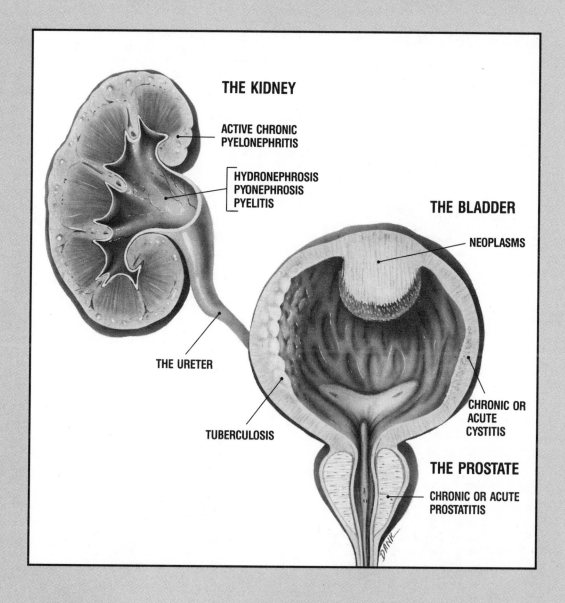

THE KIDNEY

ACTIVE CHRONIC
PYELONEPHRITIS

HYDRONEPHROSIS
PYONEPHROSIS
PYELITIS

THE BLADDER

NEOPLASMS

THE URETER

TUBERCULOSIS

CHRONIC OR
ACUTE
CYSTITIS

THE PROSTATE

CHRONIC OR ACUTE
PROSTATITIS

The urinary tract (kidneys, ureters, bladder, urethra) determines the chemical composition of the blood, the body and its water excretion. All the blood in the body passes through the kidneys, is filtered, and superfluous and/or toxic matter passed out, returning unneeded material for the urine. The kidneys also manufacture hormones and blood pressure regulators as well as improve the efficiency of vitamin D. A system of ingenious tubes, a receptacle (the bladder), and sphincters enable us to pass water at appropriate and controlled intervals. As with other organs, inflammation, tumors, and blockages can occur that require medical attention.

This section examines the physiology of the urinary tract and common disorders of the system. *See also* the questions on binary colic or renal colic and stones (Q-10); pelitis (Q-23); frequent urination and other problems with urination (Q-24, Q-25, Q-26); and jaundice (Q-27) in the section QUESTIONS AND ANSWERS ABOUT COMMON SYMPTOMS.

The following is a list of terms identified in this section:

ACUTE KIDNEY FAILURE
ALBUMINURIA (PROTEINURIA)
ARTIFICIAL KIDNEY
BLADDER, URINARY
BRIGHT'S DISEASE
CATHETER
CHRONIC KIDNEY FAILURE
CYSTITIS
CYSTOCELE
CYSTOSCOPY
DYSURIA
ENURESIS
HEMODIALYSIS
INCONTINENCE
INCONTINENCE, STRESS/URGE
KIDNEY
KIDNEY TRANSPLANT
KIMMELSTIEL-WILSON SYNDROME
NEPHRITIS

NEPHROLITHIASIS
NEPHRON
NEPHROSIS AND NEPHROTIC
   SYNDROME
PERITONEAL DIALYSIS
PYELITIS
UREMIA
URETER
URETHRA
URETHRITIS
URINALYSIS
URINARY OBSTRUCTION
URINARY-STONE FORMATION
URINARY TRACT
URINATION (MICTURITION)
URINE
URINE, RETENTION OF
UROLOGICAL STONE

ACUTE KIDNEY FAILURE   In this condition of rapid onset the kidney can no longer maintain the balance of water and other substances in the body. Usually reversible, acute kidney failure may require the temporary use of hemodialysis or peritoneal dialysis. (*See also* HEMODIALYSIS and PERITONEAL DIALYSIS in this section.)

ALBUMINURIA (PROTEINURIA)   Filtration of blood plasma through the walls of the tiny blood vessels in the glomerulus of the kidney produces a clear watery liquid which passes down the kidney tubule to form urine. If blood proteins leak through, chiefly albumin, they may appear in the urine; this condition is called albuminuria. Albumin is routinely tested for in all urinalysis and is an important indication of kidney disease.

ARTIFICIAL KIDNEY   *See* HEMODIALYSIS and PERITONEAL DIALYSIS in this section.

BLADDER, URINARY This structure lies just behind the pubic bone and connects directly to the exterior of the body through the urethra. It is the collecting and storage sac for urine, which comes to it through the ureters from the kidneys. The urinary bladder is able to hold as much as two or three quarts of urine; ordinarily, however, a sensation to urinate occurs when four to eight ounces of urine is present. The precise amount that will send out the signal of need is variable in different persons.

BRIGHT'S DISEASE *See* NEPHRITIS in this section.

CATHETER The catheter is a rubber or plastic tube which is inserted in the bladder to provide urinary drainage when there is obstruction of the urethra or inability to control urination. One type of catheter (the Foley catheter) has an inflatable balloon at the inserted end which may be filled with liquid once the catheter is in place. The inflated balloon prevents the catheter from slipping out. A urethral catheter may be used to allow for healing following certain types of surgery in the pelvic area. It may also be used to obtain specimen (sterile) for diagnostic purposes.

A catheter is routinely inserted in men undergoing prostatic surgery, often in women having pelvic surgery, and often in many other surgeries. It may simplify nursing in very ill patients or in others incontinent because of stroke or other conditions of brain damage.

Although, when not otherwise specified, the term refers to a urinary catheter, there are specialized catheters for other purposes—such as the balloon catheter used to open up coronary arteries.

CHRONIC KIDNEY FAILURE Chronic kidney failure occurs when the kidney can no longer maintain a balance of water and other substances in the body. This condition is slow in onset and may progress over many years. Treatment is necessary to replace kidney function, or death will occur. Kidney function is replaced by hemodialysis, peritoneal dialysis, or kidney transplant.

CYSTITIS Cystitis is an infection of the urinary bladder and almost always occurs in females. It is assumed the immature female is more susceptible because of the shortness of the tube joining the bladder to the outside of the body (urethra) and the consequently short distance from the anal opening to the inside of the bladder. Furthermore, the secretions of the girl are more alkaline than those of the adult woman, thus making this site more suitable for bacterial growth than the more acid environment of the adult female bladder.

Symptoms. There is usually a burning sensation and unusual frequency of urination, occasionally associated with fever or blood in the urine. A soreness of the abdomen below the naval is frequent. Since it is easy to see the pus cells in the urine under the microscope, rapid diagnosis can be made by bringing a specimen to the doctor. (Clouded urine is seldom due to pus—more often to harmless crystals.)

Treatment. Neglect of cystitis may result in the migration of the infection upward through the ureters (pyelitis) to the kidneys (pyelonephritis). Drug-treatment may be easy if the causative bacteria are not resistant to the medication prescribed. Some doctors will take a culture and identify the germ more accurately, actually testing to find what medication kills it quickest.

The treatment, often a sulfa, is usually continued for ten days to two weeks at full dosage, then halved for another week or two. If the child has more than three episodes of this disease, it may be assumed that there is something wrong with her urinary tract. In such cases a more thorough investigation should be made by a urologist who will look inside and/or X-ray the urinary system and make cultures of the bacteria obtained.

CYSTOCELE This is a form of hernia in which the bladder drops into the female birth canal (vagina). It is the result of a weakening of the structures that support the bladder and is usually secondary to childbearing. It is much more common in the white race, especially in women who have given birth to several children and have lost most of the normal anatomical support for the birth-canal.

Symptoms. Even large cystoceles may remain totally without symptoms. A large number of them, however, will result in stress incontinence—the involuntary loss of urine under minimal stress, such as laughing, coughing, standing up.

Treatment. Treatment is surgical and consists of repair of the cystocele via the vaginal route, with or without hysterectomy. Removal of the uterus will ensure fewer recurrences and may be recommended to women who have completed their families.

CYSTOSCOPY This is an instrumental procedure in which a tube with a system of lights and mirrors is inserted into the bladder through the urethra. The doctor can observe the interior of the bladder, including the openings of the ureters through which urine is discharged from the kidneys, and can evaluate the condition of the bladder wall. In men, cystoscopy makes it possible to sight enlargements of the prostate gland and to detect bladder tumors. Cystoscopy is often done in the doctor's office. Cystoscopy is often accompanied by the passage of tubes into the ureters so that opaque (contrast) material may be sent into the body (pelvis) of the kidneys for the purposes of X-ray observation.

DYSURIA The term refers to the painful or difficult act of urination. Often the first clue to disease in the urinary tract, dysuria is commonly associated with urethritis and cystitis.

Treatment. Antibiotics are usually effective in treating the condition.

ENURESIS *See* BEDWETTING in the section MENTAL HEALTH: PSYCHIATRIC AND PSYCHOLOGICAL CONDITIONS.

HEMODIALYSIS This is a treatment for the replacement of kidney function which utilizes an artificial kidney. The process of hemodialysis involves pumping blood through an artificial kidney and back into the body. A special bath surrounds the artificial kidney which allows excess water and poisons to be removed from the blood before it is returned to the body. Hemodialysis can be performed in a dialysis unit or, in some special cases, at home.

INCONTINENCE When the sphincter muscle which closes the urethra is weak, torn, or damaged by disease, there is an intermittent or constant flow of urine from the bladder. This is much more common in women than in men and is prone to occur in aged people who are confined to their beds and have lost some of their faculties. In women it is commonly due to the damage that may occur in childbirth, and in men may occur after surgery on the prostate gland. Treatment of incontinence is dependent on the cause.

Control of urination involves not only the integrity of pelvic structures but also of higher centers. Thus damage to the brain or spine from stroke, Alzheimer's disease, multiple sclerosis, or injury may lead to incontinence. Incontinence may be reversible; for example, older debilitated but otherwise intact persons who are encouraged or helped to get out of bed and to urinate may establish a schedule of urination and thus regain continence.

INCONTINENCE, STRESS/URGE Involuntary loss of urine is a condition which can be classified as stress incontinence, in which the patient leaks urine with minimal stress, such as coughing, laughing, or sneezing; and urge incontinence, in which the patient suddenly feels that she must void immediately or she will lose urine. One cause of stress incontinence is an anatomical defect of the bladder and urethra, often brought about by repeated vaginal deliveries. It is corrected by surgery with generally good results. Stress incontinence may be improved or cured by a number of measures: emptying the bladder on a schedule which prevents overfilling; use of drugs which diminish bladder contractibility; use of antibiotics in the presence of infection; programs which use female hormones either locally or by mouth; use of Kegal exercises, a regimen of repeated contraction of the outlet muscles of the pelvic region.

KIDNEY The kidneys are among the most important organs in the body; without them life is impossible for more than a few days. They are set under the last ribs, lying against the large muscles of the back on each side of the spine. They are shaped roughly like beans (hence the term kidney beans) and are normally about the size of a clenched fist.

The kidneys are essentially filters which remove poisonous substances from the blood and carefully regulate the amount of minerals, acids, and certain food substances in the bloodstream. For example, they keep the blood just slightly alkaline through their ability to transfer acid into the urine. They very efficiently prevent the collection of too much urea and other nitrogenous products in the body and carefully regulate the level of calcium, potassium, and sodium. They also permit the excretion of certain substances such as sugar only when its level is too high in the blood.

The actual filtering apparatus of the kidneys is known as the glomerulus. Blood is brought to this structure by an artery which divides from the abdominal aorta and breaks into many tiny branches. The first step in urine formation is the collection of a filtrate from the blood. This is then passed along a system of tubules which twist and turn through the inner portion of the kidney. During the passage of the blood-filtrate through the tubules, a good deal of water is extracted and substances which the body desires to dispose of are concentrated and eventually gathered in larger collecting ducts. The urine is next directed into a funnel-shaped structure (the kidney pelvis), from which it is passed down the ureters into the bladder, and from there through the urethra to the outside.

KIDNEY TRANSPLANT By surgically removing a kidney from one person and placing it into another person, a kidney transplant allows a person with chronic kidney failure to lead a longer life. The person who receives the kidney must take medication for the rest of his life in order to keep the kidney functioning. The success rate of kidney transplants is about 85 percent.

KIMMELSTIEL-WILSON SYNDROME This syndrome is a type of kidney disease associated with diabetes mellitus. There is a characteristic abnormality seen in the filtering portion (glomerulus) of the kidney tubule when examined microscopically. The condition, when present, is usually found in individuals who have had diabetes for many years. Leakage of protein from the serum into the urine (proteinuria) is characteristic of this disease. There may be high blood pressure and distinctive blood-vessel disease in the ret-

ina as seen on ophthalmologic examination. Advanced cases may show an accumulation of nitrogen compounds in the blood (uremia). The disorder is also known as diabetic glomerulosclerosis, and K-W disease.

Treatment. Good glycemic control is important in prevention or progression of the disease. Low protein, low potassium, low phosphate diets are applicable to the abnormalities that become manifest with K-W disease. As the disorder advances renal or peritoneal dialysis may become necessary. Many renal transplants have been performed in diabetics with K-W disease. The transplanted kidney may itself develop diabetic glomerulosclerosis.

NEPHRITIS Inflammation or destruction of the interior of the kidney by disease is known as nephritis. If the disorder is chiefly in the glomerulus, the term employed is glomerulonephritis; if in the collecting portion of the kidney and caused by infection, the term employed is pyelonephritis.

Nephritis produces a complex of symptoms composed of high blood pressure, weakness, easy fatigability, swelling of the tissues of the body (edema), and hemorrhages—especially in the interior of the eye. Glomerulonephritis is often caused by an allergic-type reaction to the streptococcus; it is treated by steroid drugs, careful regulation of diet, and general health measures. Pyelonephritis is treated by identification of the infectious agent and its elimination by means of antibiotics. In pyelonephritis there may be an obstruction somewhere in the urinary tract which must be treated by surgery before there can be permanent healing.

NEPHROLITHIASIS This is the medical term for the presence of kidney stones. (See Urinary-Stone Formation in this section.)

NEPHRON The microscopic functional unit of the kidney is the glomerulus, a filtering device and tubules. This consists of a small bundle of blood vessels and a cup-like structure which accepts blood plasma and passes into a tubular structure. This tubule has straight and looped portions and ends in the collecting duct which empties into the pelvis of the kidney.

The function of the nephron is to clear the blood of poisonous substances and products of normal metabolism which the body excretes as waste. It also functions as a regulator of the level of blood alkalinity. It also controls the balance of water in the body.

NEPHROSIS AND NEPHROTIC SYNDROME   Damage to the kidneys from disease or toxins results in an inability of the kidney to prevent loss of protein from the blood; examination of the urine will reveal large quantities of albumin. This condition is known as nephrosis. The nephrotic syndrome includes systemic effects of this disorder. Because of loss of protein from the bloodstream, fluid collects in the tissues of the body, giving rise to a condition called edema (dropsy). This is particularly apt to occur in the face and about the eyes, helping to distinguish it from heart conditions, in which edema of the lower extremities is more common.

PERITONEAL DIALYSIS   This is a process in which a tube is surgically placed in the abdomen. Fluid is run through the tube into the abdomen where it acts to filter excess water and other poisonous substances out of the blood before the fluid is drained out of the abdomen. This procedure can be done at home.

PYELITIS   The term pyelitis applies to the presence of an infection (pus) in the kidneys. The disease is almost exclusively seen in females. (*See also* CYSTITIS in this section.)

Symptoms. Pyelitis often begins suddenly with a chill followed in an hour or so by a high fever. It may or may not be accompanied by backache (just below the floating rib), or frequent and/or burning urination. Usually the patient is prostrated and has a headache. A urinalysis will reveal pus.

Treatment. Because these patients are nauseated and often vomit, they often need antibiotic injections for the first day or so of treatment (which treatment is much the same as that given for cystitis). Patients with pyelitis should have a urological examination when the condition has subsided.

UREMIA   When the kidney is unable to excrete poisons from the body in a normal fashion, these substances—mostly organic acids or nitrogenous substances—collect in the bloodstream and produce characteristic symptoms of uremia. This condition is due to decreased function of the kidneys and may be due to disease in the kidney itself, interference with the blood supply of the kidney, or disease infection or blockage in the lower part of the urinary tract.

Symptoms. Symptoms of uremia are usually those of change in mental status with nausea, vomiting, or general malaise.

Treatment. Uremia due to kidney failure may be potentially reversible by medical or surgical measures. Chronic uremic states may be managed by dialysis on the artificial kidney or, even better, by a donor kidney. The transplantation of a single kidney can completely reverse all of the disturbances found in uremia.

URETER   The ureter is a muscular tube approximately a foot long which passes from each kidney to the base of the bladder and carries urine to the bladder for storage until its ultimate excretion from the body. Its walls are muscular and are capable of contraction. When the ureter is obstructed, spasm may ensue with resulting severe pain. This occurs with passage of a stone.

URETHRA   This is the tube which carries urine from the bladder to the exterior (via the penis in the male, and to the opening just above the vagina in the female). Lubrication of the tube is accomplished by glands which secrete slippery mucus along its course.

URETHRITIS   Inflammation of the passage from the urinary bladder to the exterior (urethra) is spoken of as urethritis. Since the urethra is short in the female, infection is readily spread from the vagina or the rectum when proper toilet hygiene is not used. The walls of the urethra become inflamed, and passage of urine becomes difficult and painful. Because in the male the urethra traverses the interior of the penis, it may be the site of infection from gonorrhea or other bacterial organisms acquired during sexual intercourse. Over recent years, chlamydia has received increasing recognition as a frequent cause of urethritis in both sexes. In some sexually active women it becomes clear that urethritis (and cystitis) frequently follow intercourse.

Symptoms. Common symptoms are the same as for cystitis—frequency of urination and dysuria.

Treatment. Suitable antibiotics as prescribed by the physician are often curative; although some types of sexually transmitted diseases are not curable.

URINALYSIS   A urinalysis is a laboratory investigation of urine. Routine examination reports on the color, turbidity, the acid reaction, specific gravity, the presence or absence of albumin, sugar, ketone elements, pus, or crystals, and a microscopic investigation for casts, blood cells, and epithelial cells. Abnormal findings are followed by special quantitative and qualitative tests.

URINARY OBSTRUCTION   Obstruction to the flow of urine may occur in the ureter because of a stone, a blood vessel which passes across the ureter, or a kink in the ureter due to misplacement of the kidney. Usually, however, the term urinary obstruction refers to inability to pass urine through the urethra. In men this is most commonly caused by an enlarged prostate or a stricture of the urethra due to infection. In the days before modern antibiotics, strictures of the urethra were very commonly the result of attacks of gonorrhea.

URINARY-STONE FORMATION   Various kinds of stones are found in the urinary tract. Calcium phosphate stones are the most common and are formed when there is an excess of calcium in the urine, alkaline or neutral urine favoring deposits of additional calcium phosphate on an already extant tiny stone. Calcium phosphate stones are usually small and round, of a white or yellow-white color, and show evidence of layering.

The presence of infection in the urinary tract favors the growth of uric-acid stones which form around cellular fragments or uric-acid deposits. These stones are often very soft and crumble easily, accounting for the fact that they are frequently passed from the body in the form of small bits of gravel.

A hereditary condition results in stones made of cystine, a sulphur-containing amino acid.

Urinary stones containing calcium are visible on X-ray films, while uric-acid and cystine stones are not directly visible and may require the use of X-ray opaque (contrast) material given either intravenously or injected directly into the ureters.

Urinary stones are generally passed down the urinary tract and out of the body. This passage is painful and is called renal colic. A stone may obstruct a ureter and this can lead to a swelling of the kidney on that side. The condition is termed hydronephrosis and may require surgical relief.

Lithotripsy is a new methodology by which surgery for stones may become unnecessary. Instead of surgery, the stone is broken into tiny fragments by shock waves and passed out as a sort of gravel.

All persons with a history of a stone should be under specialized care.

URINARY TRACT   The entire system through which urine is made and passes is referred to as the urinary tract. This includes the kidneys, the ureters, the bladder, and the urethra.

URINATION (MICTURITION)   This is the process of expelling urine from the bladder. Voluntary relaxation of the sphincter muscle in the urethra is accompanied by contraction of the detrusor muscle of the bladder, which forces the urine in a stream through the urethra. This process is not ordinarily painful but may become so with the presence of obstructions, constrictions of the urethra, or in the presence of infectious processes.

URINE   The urine is a solution of waste products and water excreted by the kidneys. Passing from each kidney down the ureter into the bladder, it is expelled by the process of urination (micturition). Urine is usually yellow in color but will be darker or lighter depending on the concentration of dissolved pigments. It usually shows an acid reaction except for a short period after meals or during the presence of urinary infection, at which time it may be alkaline. Normally, urine does not contain either protein or sugar. There is often a small amount of mucus present. The color of the urine may be affected by the ingestion of various kinds of dyes found in some foods or medicines and its odor by dietary substances.

URINE, RETENTION OF Urinary retention is an accumulation of urine, with inability to pass it and distention of the bladder. The patient complains of pain, an overwhelming desire to urinate, and frequently attempts to do so without satisfaction. Retention of urine is common in enlargement of the prostate gland, stricture of the urethra (the urinary excretory channel leading from the bladder), prostatic cancer, tabes dorsalis, stone or foreign body in the urethra, dislocation and/or fracture of the spine, inflammatory disease of the spinal cord, tumor of the bladder, in certain emotional states and psychoneurotic conditions. In infants, elongation of the foreskin to the extent that it cannot be pulled back may cause urinary retention. Treatment in this instance is, of course, circumcision.

   Treatment. Immediate relief of obstructed urinary flow is catheterization. This consists of the passing of a sterile flexible, very thin tube into the bladder via the urethra. In extreme bladder distention, all urine is not immediately permitted to escape; otherwise the radical change in intraabdominal pressure, particularly in the aged or those with impaired or weak hearts, may cause unpleasant reactions; often a small amount is permitted to pass every twenty to thirty minutes until the bladder is emptied. If catheterization cannot be done (as in complete urethral block), surgery is the only answer. Treatment of the various basic causes, as listed above, is presented under the respective headings.

UROLOGICAL STONE A stone anywhere in the urogenital tract is referred to as a urological stone. Such stones may be present in the kidney, ureter, bladder, or urethra. The recent development of special shock wave machines which break up stones (lithotripsy) was a revolutionary advance in this field.

THE URINARY SYSTEM

RIGHT KIDNEY

LEFT KIDNEY
(CROSS SECTION)

URETER

BLADDER
(CROSS SECTION)

PROSTATE
(CROSS SECTION)

URETHRA
(SECTION)

The organs concerned with containing or secreting urine are the kidneys, ureters, bladder, and urethra. The fluid secreted by the kidneys is stored in the bladder and discharged by the urethra.

AGING: GERIATRICS AND GERONTOLOGY

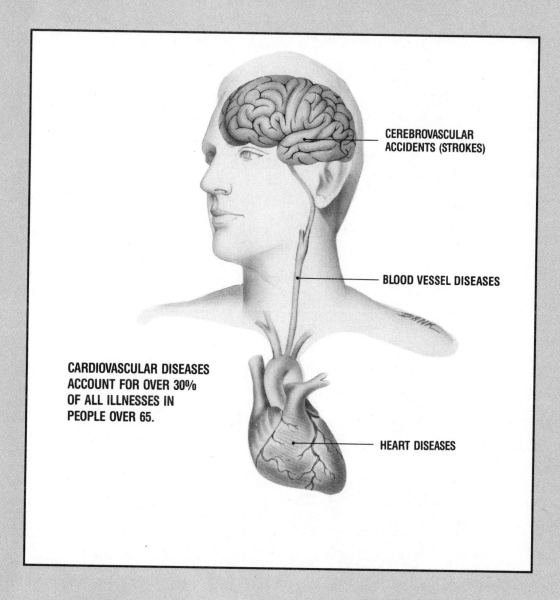

CEREBROVASCULAR ACCIDENTS (STROKES)

BLOOD VESSEL DISEASES

CARDIOVASCULAR DISEASES ACCOUNT FOR OVER 30% OF ALL ILLNESSES IN PEOPLE OVER 65.

HEART DISEASES

The numbers of the elderly, defined as those age 65 and above, are growing both in relation to other age groups and to their medical, social, and political importance. This section is devoted to those changes which help to distinguish this important age group. Physical, psychological, and social changes are discussed along with their implications for the aging. And, an overview of Alzheimer's disease is included due to the growing importance of this disease.

The following is a list of topics identified in this section:

ALZHEIMER'S DISEASE
GERIATRICS

GERONTOLOGY
SENESCENCE AND SENILITY

See also the following topics in these sections:

Ear, Nose and Throat Conditions
Hearing Aids
Presbycusis
Vertigo

Eye Conditions
Cataract
Eye, Dry
Eyelids, Twitching of the
Presbyopia
Retina Macular Disease
Tears, Excessive

Gastrointestinal Conditions
Achlorhydria
Swallowing Difficulties

Musculoskeletal Conditions
Arthritis, Degenerative, or Osteoarthritis
Leg Cramps

Nervous System Conditions
Cerebrovascular Accidents
Normal Pressure Hydrocephalus (NPH)
Stroke

Respiratory Conditions
Emphysema

Skin Conditions
Bedsore (Decubitus)
Keratosis, Senile
Shingles (Herpes Zoster)

Urinary Conditions
Incontinence

ALZHEIMER'S DISEASE A German physician, Alois Alzheimer, in 1907 described the case of a 52-year-old woman who developed a dementing disease which progressed over a few years and resulted in death. Examination of the brain revealed unusual cell loss and replacement by plaques and tangles of filaments. For years this condition was referred to as presenile dementia and distinguished from the more common, generally slowly progressing brain impairments seen in persons age 65 and older. It is now known that these two forms of dementia are essentially similar in both age groups and are placed together in the category of Alzheimer's disease. Though memory loss is one of the chief complaints in early Alzheimer's disease, testing reveals other deficits that are more widespread than would be found in normal aging. Recognition may be severely impaired—Alzheimer's patients do not recognize persons they could reasonably be expected to and often get lost on what should be familiar streets. In Alzheimer's disease progression leads to confusion, increasing difficulty in activities of daily living (ADL), such as shopping, handling money, dressing, bathing, eating and finally even walking. Wandering and reversal of the day-night cycle compound the difficulties for both patient and caretaker. Incontinence of urine and of stool may appear and the nursing problems that result often exhaust caretakers and lead to institutionalizing of the patient. About half of the 1.4 million persons in U.S. nursing homes are there primarily because of Alzheimer's disease. The cause of Alzheimer's disease is basically unknown. In the small number of families which have many members with Alzheimer's disease, there may be an inherited tendency to develop the disease.

Drug research is concentrated on those drugs which improve memory. There is some hope that memory can be improved for some patients in the early stage of the disease with a few experimental drugs. Current drug therapies, however, are not effective for every patient, do not halt the progression of the disease, and have serious side effects. The search continues to find the cause or causes, treatment, and ultimately a cure for this devastating disease.

GERIATRICS The branch of medicine devoted to the special considerations of aging changes and illness in the elderly is called geriatrics. Physicians who specialize in this area are called geriatricians, and there is now a qualifying examination for such doctors. Additionally, since the population as a whole is getting older, physicians in all branches of medicine are seeing an increasing number of older persons. As an example, the most rapidly growing segment of the U.S. population consists of women over the age of 85. And for the first time in human history, many societies have more than 10 percent of their population in the over-65 age group.

There are no sharp divisions between the middle and later years though certain illnesses grow more common in the older years. Human beings are peculiarly subject to atherosclerosis, the abnormal collection of fatty plaques on the inner wall of the arteries. This leads over the middle years and more so in the later years to such disorders as stroke, heart attack, and peripheral vascular disease (PVD). But atherosclerosis is a disease process, and the fact that it is widespread should not be construed as meaning that it is a normal aging event or that it is inevitable. Indeed recent developments in this area indicate that atherosclerosis is a disease produced by multiple interacting factors, almost all of which can be successfully controlled. Increasingly we can anticipate that people will grow old and escape the ravages of this disorder.

The same may be said for cancer, the second most common cause of death in older people.

There is a strong age relationship to cancer; its incidence peaks in the elderly, but it is entirely clear that this disease can be found in childhood and rises through the middle years as well. It is well established that the cause of the most common kinds of cancer are caused by chemical agents to which the body has to be exposed over many decades.

The clearest case would be the relationship of cigarette smoking to lung cancer. We know that it takes at least 20 years of persistent smoking before the first cancers of the lung begin to appear. But in any population of smokers there are some, who because of native resistance or the slow nature of the cancer-inciting process itself, will reach their 60's and 70's before the lung cancer becomes manifest. The time needed for the development of the cancer and for aging of the individual overlap although at first glance it would appear the aging process itself is causally linked to the emergence of cancer, yet these are separate processes that happened to occur at the same time.

The variability in the onset of these important diseases, but especially their absence in many older persons, has led to the belief that aging and disease can logically be separable. It follows that none of these common major causes of death (cardiovascular disease, cancer, lung disease, etc.) are inevitable with aging, and that healthy aging can be regarded as the norm.

In separating aging from illness, one need not deny that a considerable number of declines do occur in the aging human body. When these declines occur in 100 percent of all individuals, one can perhaps talk about a universal aging change. An example might be the loss of height with aging that sooner or later is seen in both males and females. Individuals followed over the life span universally show some loss in height, on the order of one to two inches in males and somewhat more in females. Much of this is attributable to increased thinning of the disks, the cartilage that separates the vertebra of the spinal column. Over a lifetime the disks lose some of their moisture, are compressed by the impact of weight bearing, and ultimately become thinner. Since there are more than two dozen of these, even an average 1/16 of an inch shrinkage could lead to a one and a half inch loss of height over the lifetime. In actuality the situation is more complex and indeed a given disk may virtually disappear while others shrink little.

Another example of a universal aging change is the increasing thickness of the lens of the eye. In the embryo the lens of the eye is derived by an outpouching from the same tube of tissue that gives rise to the skin. Like skin cells, the cells that compose the lens of the eye tend to multiply with the passage of the years, but they are not shed as are the cells of the skin. As a result, as individuals age the lens of the eye becomes thicker and heavier. For many of us, this produces an increasing inability to focus on nearby objects and leads to a need for glasses by around age forty. The thickening of the lens seems to be a universal and, therefore, a true aging change. Not so with the reduced transparency in the lens known as a cataract. This becomes more common as people age into their 60's and 70's, but there are some who escape cataract formation and come to the end of their lifespan without having a cataract. It is therefore not clear whether cataract is a necessarily inevitable and "true" aging change. Indeed there are some who believe that if the eyes were protected against strong light, (especially the ultraviolet B component of light) and that if blood sugars could be kept lower that it might be possible for many more to escape cataracts.

Thus one must be cautious in unqualified assertions as to what true aging changes are. With this provision in mind one may go on to consider the following as probable aging changes in some bodily systems:

Skin. Some thinning of the skin with diminution in blood vessels, loss of hair follicles and sweat glands are to a variable degree universal. There is a loss of elastic fibers so that the skin tends to be lax, and wrinkling sooner or later occurs. There is variable loss and shifting about in the fat just below the surface of the skin. It is often lost from the hands and forearms, the face and the legs. Loss of pigmentation and graying of the hair are classic markers for aging.

Muscle. Shrinkage in muscle mass is a constant phenomenon in aging. It occurs earlier and to a greater extent in males than in females. Loss of muscle mass is accelerated past age sixty and doubtless contributes to the increased complaints of weakness and fatigue heard from older people. Studies in both man and animals indicate that individual muscle cells die and are partly replaced by fibrous tissue. Muscle strength can, however, be increased with exercise even in the very elderly.

Heart. The heart is a unique muscle which, unlike the skeletal muscle, does not shrink with aging. Indeed the reverse is true: with normal aging, the heart muscle perceptibly increases in thickness and the heart becomes heavier. The heart rate tends to be slower in older people, and the maximal heart rate on exercise is lessened. However, the volume of blood pumped from the normal heart per minute at rest or with moderate degrees of exercise does not decrease with aging, except perhaps towards the very end of the life span.

Lungs. There is a loss of elasticity in the lung tissue with aging. In addition increased stiffness of the tissues and muscles of the chest wall leads to a decline in the breathing function over the life span. From youth to old age this may amount to a 25 percent decline in the vital capacity (the total amount of air moved in and out on maximum inspiration and expiration).

Upper Gastrointestinal Tract. Perhaps because of built-in margins of safety, digestive capability should remain more or less unimpaired over the life span. This is not to deny the existence of some significant age-related change: in many aging persons secretion of acid from the stomach declines considerably and may even reach the level known as achlorhydria, in which no free stomach acid is found. (*See* ACHLORHYDRIA in the section GASTROINTESTINAL CONDITIONS.) A significant amount of shrinkage may take place in the mass of the liver and with it some functional declines such as an apparently lower level of synthesis of albumin, an important protein of the blood. The basic function of such organs as the gall bladder continues into old age. Age-related changes in the pancreas are seen in a decreased glucose tolerance with advancing age.

Colon. Frequently the colon undergoes structural and functional changes. One of the most common structural changes is the development of the little outpouchings known as diverticula. These however are not characteristic of aging, and it has been pointed out that in societies where there are larger amounts of roughage and fiber in the food, people escape diverticula formation. The common complaint of constipation that many older people have may reflect some intrinsic tendency of the colon to slow down.

Kidney. A significant amount of shrinkage in the number of nephrons (the working units of the kidney), size and weight does occur over the life span. As a result, certain of the "normal kidney chemistries" found in other age groups have to be revised upwards in dealing with an older population. Because of a reduction in the reserve capacity of the kidneys, the aging person is more vulnerable when the increased demands of a trauma or disease are added to the changes due to aging. This is especially evident in the aging kidney's reduced ability to eliminate drugs from the body.

Bone Mass. Even in normal healthy males there is some decline in the total bone mass over the life span. In the case of the female, particularly after menopause, major declines in the bone mass generally occur. This can be corrected by the administration of female sex hormones; exercise also maintains the bone mass and may even add to it through the menopausal years. Some experts have described a "senile atrophy" of bone that occurs in both sexes in old age, much like the atrophy of muscle or skin. It is generally agreed that the severe bone loss that afflicts many women is attributable to many factors including sedentary existence and genetic background and is made considerably worse by inadequate calcium in the diet, smoking, and alcohol. Thus, decline in bone mass with aging results from a complex of interacting factors many of which respond to intervention. Subjects at greatest risk for osteoporosis are white women of northern European background with light builds.

Brain. There is an age-related loss of brain cells (neurons) over the life span. From its maximum in youth to its minimum in advanced old age, the loss may amount to as much as 100 grams of tissue even in the absence of such evident disease as Alzheimer's, or the damage produced by stroke. Changes in brain due to aging do not necessarily affect thinking, knowing, and awareness. Loss of neurons, coupled with slowed conduction of nerve impulses, do affect reaction times and the ability to recover from stress.

Blood Cell Function. The bone marrow which manufactures blood cells functions throughout the life span. There is no specific anemia of old age, and most of those that are found are generally due to poor nutrition, iron deficiency, or to the impact of various kinds of chronic illnesses. On the other hand, some white blood cells involved in the immune processes do decline. There are multiple evidences of declining immune function with aging. There is also a loss of the ability to fight off pneumonia and influenza, both of which can be compensated for by appropriate vaccinations.

Drug Responses in The Elderly. Drugs are potent and have the ability to do harm as well as cure disease or ease the symptoms of a disease. Elderly persons are at risk for adverse drug reactions due to the number of drugs they take and the diminished efficiency of the aging body in eliminating drugs. Older people are more likely to receive a prescription from the physician than other ages. Women receive an average of 19.6 prescriptions per year (new and refills) compared to 15.3 per year for men. This is in addition to over-the-counter drug purchases. Taking a greater number of drugs increases the chance of having an adverse drug reaction. Most drugs are excreted by the kidneys which have a lessened capacity to excrete drugs. This results in an accumulation in the body and an overdosage.

The aging brain is particularly susceptible to some drugs, especially alcohol, analgesics, antihypertensive agents, tranquilizers, narcotics, and digitalis preparations. A major adverse effect of these drugs (and others) is confusion; stopping the drugs or reducing the dosage will allow the confusion to clear.

Society values technology and the quick fix. Prescribing drugs rather than simpler solutions to problems has become so commonplace that many elderly feel slighted if the physician does not prescribe a new drug. Tactful questioning of the physician is the order of the day: What is this drug? What will it do for me? What are the side effects? Do I really need it—is there another option? These are questions that can help to reduce the number of drugs taken and the risk of adverse side effects.

GERONTOLOGY Gerontology is the science which deals with all the other aspects of the aging process. Among the broad disciplines that belong in this area are the biological, psychological, and the sociological. Because of the growing numbers of elderly as a percent of the total population, gerontology also considers economics, politics, and cultural attitudes towards the elderly. Here we can only briefly touch on some of the highlights:

Biological. Important genetic components determine longevity. There are long-lived families in which octogenarians (80's) and nonogenarians (90's) occur to an unusual extent. It also appears that there are some families that are shorter-lived than most; studies of such families indicate predisposition to disease processes which are life-shortening, such as combinations of hypertension and stroke, heart attack, and cancer predisposition.

The lifespan of the different species seems to obviously have a fixed genetic component. Consider the contrast in life expectancy exhibited by the mouse, 1.6 years; the dog, 9.9 years; the horse, 17.3 years; and the U.S. white female, 75.9 years. The basic reason for these differences is unknown, but a number of variables have been studied. The cells of a long-lived species such as man have better repair mechanisms. An injury to the nucleus (DNA) which might destroy the cell of the shorter-lived species can be repaired in the longer-lived one. It has been shown that a number of enzymes involved in repair processes are present in greater amounts in the longer-lived species. It has been well established (contrary to the former belief), that all normal cells in tissue culture are limited in the number of their reproductions. The sole exception occurs in cancer cells which are immortal in tissue culture. Of interest also in the normal connective tissue cells of different species, the number of doublings in tissue culture is characteristic of the species and is related to the total lifespan. This is referred to as the Hayflick phenomenon, after the well known American gerontologist who first described it.

One factor that has direct impact on the lifespan is caloric restriction. The American nutritionist McCay reported in 1935 that the lifespan of the laboratory rat could be almost doubled by underfeeding. The underfed animals had a marked postponement of the onset of puberty, but were alive and reproducing long after their well fed controls had died. The McCay effect has been demonstrated for other species and there is good reason to believe that subnutrition may be life prolonging. There is evidence that considerable prolongation occurs even if there is no restriction of calories during the phase of growth and development. Not only is the rate of aging slowed, but also the onset of deterioration and disease processes characteristic of a species is postponed.

Sociological. Gerontology is concerned with shifting trends in the number of the elderly together with considerations of their competence and fates. This is an area that is also of great concern in the financing and planning for health care, medicare, institutional care, and Social Security. Thus the proportion of the total population over 65 in the U.S. has risen from around 4 percent in 1900 to over 11 percent in 1980. Some projections indicate that persons over 65 will number about 32 million and constitute about 12 percent of the population by the year 2000. Actually the recent declines in mortality among the elderly have been so marked that if the trend continues the number of persons over age 65 can reach 38 million by the year 2000 and constitute 13.6 percent of the population. Within the various age groups constituting the elderly the most rapid percentage increase over recent years has been in the population 85 and over, predominantly women.

Obviously the graying of America will put more strains on the health care system and its financing. Even as the threat of certain disease entities is diminished, the facts of aging mean that the survivors will inevitably show a variety of significant impairments. One method of measurement is evaluation of aging persons in terms of their capability in activities of daily living (ADL). These are the basic activities that represent ability for independent living. In the elderly there are many degrees of dependence, ranging from complete independence, to needing supportive services such as Meals-on-Wheels or transportation, to complete dependence requiring 24-hour care. With aging, especially past 75, there is increased loss of capability in ADL. Some of the chronic impairments limiting activity are obvious: there will be an increasing need for long term care programs including institutionalization at the nursing home level. It is also apparent that severe strains will be imposed on aging individuals and the society with respect to financing the care of an increasingly debilitated population.

Psychological. There is no doubt about the universality of the aging processes, including those in the brain. Psychological testing designed to study the effects of aging often involves comparing the elderly with college students whose sole purpose in life is to prove their intellectual capacity. Young adults are used to being tested and have usually developed "test wisdom," a skill either never learned or long forgotten by today's elderly. Intellectual performance which relies on verbal functions declines very little with age, if at all. On the other hand speeded tests for reaction time have a great decline.

Psychologists have defined two types of intelligence: fluid and crystallized. Fluid intelligence is related to the ability of the neurons (the working units of the brain) to react to a stimulus. Fluid intelligence is thought to be related to creative and innovative behavior. It is at its peak in youth and declines with age. Crystallized intelligence is related to education and culture. It uses past experience as a standard for problem solving. Crystallized intelligence grows consistently through life until just before death, when a slight decline can be seen.

The psychological aspect of aging is also concerned with the aging person's ability to adapt to his particular environment. The capacity for change is governed by many factors in addition to intelligence, including motivation, attitude, and personality.

Finally attention should be called to the stability of personality and personality characteristics over the lifespan. Indeed personality is perhaps the most enduring and least changing of bodily characteristics over the lifespan. Warm, extroverted persons of twenty are still likely to be warm, extroverted persons of seventy in the absence of organic diseases affecting the brain. There are also other important faculties that can be relied on to stand up quite well with aging. Verbal facility is maintained well, as are many of the thought processes that one might refer to collectively as judgment or wisdom. Recognition of the maintenance of important capacities underlies the historical respect for the wisdom of the aged and accounts for the fact that in many different periods of human history, faith has been placed in the thinking and leadership of a society's elders.

SENESCENCE AND SENILITY   Studies of biologic development indicate that a peak of physical health, strength, endurance, resistance to disease, and virility is reached in the late teens and early twenties, following which a slow process of aging begins to exert progressive limitations on both physical and mental functioning. Evidence from studies of the growth of intelligence in childhood indicates that maximum development of innate abilities is complete by age fourteen or fifteen, after which any improvements in performance are achieved by training rather than by further increases in native ability. However, any person can compensate for the gradual decline of physical and mental powers through increasing experience and perfection of learned controls over behavior.

Although the brain loses cells, mass, and weight with aging, senility is not necessarily a normal result nor is it inevitable. There is little relationship between the brain's shrinkage and the process of thinking, understanding, and reasoning. Older adults do not do well on timed tests, but given sufficient time they do as well as their younger counterparts. Lack of use does more harm to the function of the brain than the actual fact of aging, especially with respect to memory.

The process of aging cannot be stopped; however, a great deal can be done in preserving and rehabilitating functions. There is considerable evidence that mental as well as muscular function can be retained by means of constant daily exercise and use. The older person who makes every effort to retain the habitual activities of his working life remains useful, continues to learn, and is in full contact with reality. Many older people make no plans for retirement and then feel lost when forced to give up their habitual routine, only to be left without anything interesting to do.

The modern geriatric movement has made great progress in organizing activity programs and stimulating conditions of living for older people.

MEDICAL ASSISTANCE

Medicare

This health insurance program is designed to serve everyone over 65 years of age and disabled persons under 65 years of age who:

(1) have been entitled to receive Social Security disability benefits for a total of 24 months; or

(2) who need dialysis treatments or a kidney transplant because of permanent kidney failure.

The program is not based on income, but is available regardless of financial need.

The Medicare program has two parts:

Part A: Hospital insurance at no cost that helps pay for care while in the hospital and for related health care services after leaving the hospital.

Part B: Voluntary medical insurance at a monthly premium that helps pay doctor bills and other approved medical services.

More information about Medicare is available from your local Social Security Office, or by writing to:

Health Care Financing Administration
Inquiries Branch
Rm. 1–N–4, East Lowrise Bldg.
Baltimore, MD 21235

Medicaid

Medicaid (Medical Assistance Programs) is a joint Federal/state program to provide physical and related health care services to persons with low incomes. Disabled persons may be eligible for Medicaid on the basis of their income.

Because eligibility is determined by your state program of public assistance (welfare) on the basis of broad Federal guidelines, there are geographic differences between eligibility requirements and types of services covered. Generally, persons may be eligible for Medicaid if they are receiving welfare or other public assistance benefits or Supplemental Security Income or are blind or disabled. Medicaid services are available in all states except Arizona.

Individuals with higher incomes may be eligible for Medicaid Supplemental Medical Care Assistance, or their children may be eligible if medical expenses exceed a given percentage of their annual income.

Each state establishes its own eligibility requirements for Medicaid.

Further information on Medicaid and assistance in applying is available from your local or state welfare or public assistance office.

If you cannot get information locally, write to:
Health Care Financing Administration
Inquiries Branch
Rm. 1–N–4, East Lowrise Bldg.
Baltimore, MD 21235

WHERE THE MEDICAID DOLLAR FOR THE ELDERLY GOES: 1984

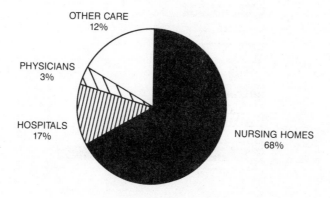

OTHER CARE 12%

PHYSICIANS 3%

HOSPITALS 17%

NURSING HOMES 68%

Source: Health Care Financing Administration, Office of Financial and Actuarial Analysis.

PERSONAL HEALTH CARE EXPENDITURE FOR THE ELDERLY BY SOURCE OF PAYMENT: 1984

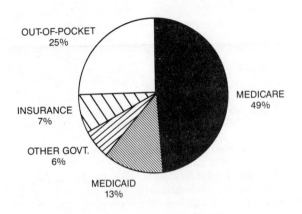

OUT-OF-POCKET
25%

INSURANCE
7%

OTHER GOVT.
6%

MEDICAID
13%

MEDICARE
49%

Source: Health Care Financing Administration, Office of Financial and Actuarial Analysis.

WHERE THE OUT OF POCKET DOLLAR FOR THE ELDERLY GOES: 1984

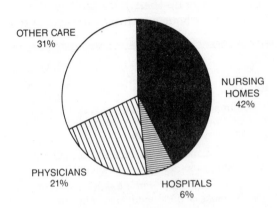

OTHER CARE
31%

NURSING HOMES
42%

PHYSICIANS
21%

HOSPITALS
6%

Source: Health Care Financing Administration, Office of Financial and Actuarial Analysis.

PROPORTION OF MEDICAL EVENTS BY CONDITIONS PERSONS AGE 65 AND OLDER 1982

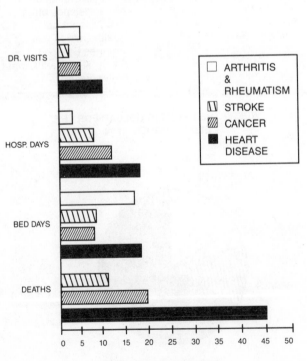

ARTHRITIS & RHEUMATISM

STROKE

CANCER

HEART DISEASE

PERCENT OF EVENTS

Source: Health: The United States, 1982. National Center for Health Statistics.

Some organizations and agencies that deal with the health-related concerns of the elderly:

U.S. Administration on Aging
3303 C St. SW
HHS South
Washington, D.C. 20024

National Council on the Aging
Suite 504
1828 L St. NW
Washington, D.C. 20036

Center for the Study of Aging
  and Human Development
Duke University
Durham, NC 27710

Alzheimer's Association
70 E. Lake St.
Suite 600
Chicago, IL 60601-5997

Family Service Association of America
44 W. 23rd St.
New York, NY 10010

American Cancer Society
219 E. 42nd St.
New York, NY 10023

Andrus Gerontology Center
University of Southern California
Los Angeles, CA 90007

American Association of Retired Persons
1909 K Street, N.W.
Washington, D.C. 20049

RESOURCES*

Action for Independent Maturity, 1909 K St., NW, Washington, D.C. 20049

American Association of Homes for the Aging, 1050 17th St., NW, Washington, D.C. 20036

American Association of Retired Persons, 1909 K St., NW, Washington, D.C. 20049

American Geriatrics Society, 10 Columbus Circle, New York, NY 10011

American Health Care Association, 2500 15th St., NW, Washington, D.C. 20015

American Physical Therapy Association, 1740 Broadway, New York, NY 10019

American Red Cross, 17th and D Sts., NW, Washington, D.C. 20006

Association of Rehabilitation Facilities, 5530 Wisconsin Ave., NW, Washington, D.C. 20015

Center for the Study of Aging and Human Development, Duke University, Durham, NC 27710

Elderhostel, 100 Boylston St., Suite 200, Boston, MA 02116

Family Service Association of America, 44 W. 23rd St., New York, NY 10010

Gerontological Society, 1 Dupont Circle, Washington, D.C. 20036

National Council on the Aging, Suite 504, 1828 L St., NW, Washington, D.C. 20036

National Council for Homemaker-Home Health Aide Services, 67 Irving Place, New York, NY 10003

National Council of Senior Citizens, 1511 K St., NW, Room 202, Washington, D.C. 20005

National Interfaith Coalition on Aging, Inc., P.O. Box 1986, Indianapolis, IN 46206

U.S. Administration on Aging, 3303 C St., SW, HHS South, Washington, D.C. 20024 (Administers ten regional offices. Each state has its own Department, Office or Commission on Aging, usually located in the state capital.)

*Excerpt from John Gillies, *A Guide to Caring For and Coping With Aging Parents* (Nashville: Thomas Nelson, Inc. Publishers, 1981), pp. 207–208.

MALE HEALTH CARE

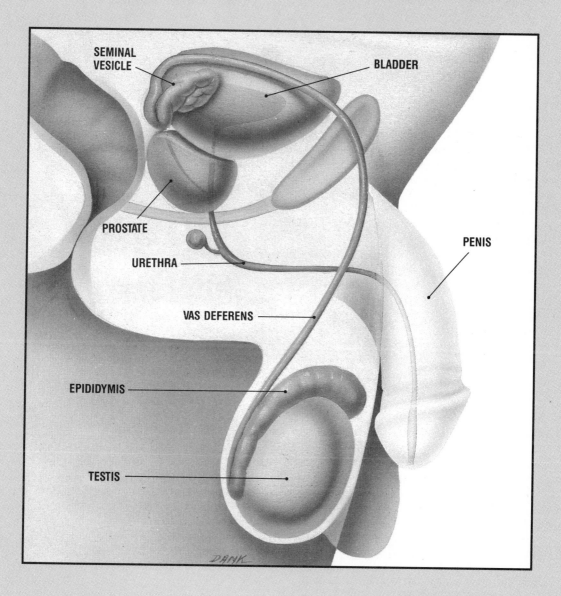

SEMINAL VESICLE

BLADDER

PROSTATE

PENIS

URETHRA

VAS DEFERENS

EPIDIDYMIS

TESTIS

DANK

The male organs are involved in both reproduction and in removal of urine from the body; thus, conditions of one can have an effect on proper functioning of the other. Most commonly, physicians who specialize in the field of urology are concerned with the diagnosis and treatment of male health care issues.

This section examines the anatomy and physiology of the male, as well as specific medical disorders encountered. The terminology, specific discomforts and diseases, and possible treatments are discussed. *See also* the question on bloody discharge in seminal fluid (Q-21) in the section QUESTIONS AND ANSWERS ABOUT COMMON SYMPTOMS.

The following is a list of terms identified in this section:

CLIMACTERIC, MALE
EJACULATION
EPIDIDYMIS
EUNUCHOIDISM
FORESKIN
GONADS
HYDROCELE
IMPOTENCE
KLINEFELTER'S SYNDROME
NOCTURNAL EMISSIONS
ORCHITIS
PENILE HYGIENE
PENIS
PRIAPISM
PROPHYLACTIC
PROSTATE
PROSTATIC CANCER

PROSTATIC HYPERTROPHY
PROSTATITIS
SCROTUM
SEXUAL ABSTINENCE
SMEGMA
SPERM(ATOZOA)
TESTICLES (TESTES)
TESTOSTERONE
TORSION OF TESTIS
UNDESCENDED TESTICLE
  (CRYPTORCHIDISM)
VARICOCELE
VAS DEFERENS (SPERMATIC CORD)
VASECTOMY
VESICLE, SEMINAL
WITHDRAWAL (COITUS INTERRUPTUS)

CLIMACTERIC, MALE The male climacteric is a rare event, as there is not usually a sudden decrease in hormone production during the middle or later years. When it occurs, however, it is associated with hot flashes, irritability, and decrease in sex drive. Response to male hormone therapy is good. Many men feel their sexual powers waning after the age of forty or fifty and become quite concerned that they will become impotent. If medical examination fails to reveal impaired hormone secretion, diabetes or other medical disorders, assurance may be given that the fears of complete impotence are probably groundless. Because successful completion of the sex act is so dependent on a healthy emotional outlook, concern about aging and the male climacteric (change of life) may produce anxiety and psychological impotence.

EJACULATION The forceful discharge of semen (sperm) from the urethral opening at the tip of the penis is known as ejaculation. This process is rhythmic and begins at the base of the penis, where the ejaculatory duct enters on each side mixing the sperm with the secretion of the prostate gland. Intravaginal ejaculation is the necessary first step in reproduction. It is possible to have ejaculation without erection as the spinal cord centers involved in each process are quite distinct. Following a prostatectomy much of the ejaculate may go into the bladder; this is termed retrograde ejaculation.

EPIDIDYMIS This structure lies adjacent to the testes and is a collecting duct for the sperm. It is frequently the site of infection which may be acute or chronic. An acute infection (epididymitis) with symptoms of painful swelling, and fever, is usually quite responsive to antibiotics. The most common chronic infection of this structure is tuberculosis.

EUNUCHOIDISM A male who has been castrated is referred to as a eunuch. When castration is accomplished before growth has been completed, the individual may become excessively tall because the androgens, which normally cause bone-growth to stop, are absent; or he may develop effeminate characteristics and become excessively fat. Many years ago it was a practice of rulers in the Far Eastern countries to castrate slaves who were placed in charge of harems. Today eunuchs are seen only when there is congenital absence of the testes or failure of testicular development due to an endocrine disturbance, and rarely after severe injuries to the testicles. Injections of male hormone, testosterone, restores male sexual characteristics and sexual drive.

FORESKIN *See* PENIS in this section.

GONADS *See* TESTICLES (TESTES) in this section.

HYDROCELE A collection of fluid in the small sac which partially surrounds the testicle is known as a hydrocele. It may be either congenital or acquired. (When acquired, it is often the result of infection or injury.) Hydrocele causes swelling of the scrotum and is easily treated by puncture of the sac with a needle and withdrawal of the fluid into a syringe. It often recurs, however, and may require surgical removal of the sac.

IMPOTENCE Inability of the man to complete the sexual act satisfactorily is called impotence; the analogous situation in the female is spoken of as frigidity. Impotence may be caused by diseases and injuries which produce damage to the testicles. On the other hand, damage to the nerves which supply the male sex organs results in inability to achieve penile erections.

Impotence due to lack of sufficient male hormone in otherwise normal males is extremely rare. In younger men the most common cause of impotence is psychological. It is likewise the most difficult type to treat. Another common cause of impotence is diabetes. Injuries to the brain and spinal cord are less common causes.

The incidence of impotence rises with aging and is certainly a frequent complaint in men past 60 years of age. Recent studies indicate that narrowing of penile arteries and changes in the draining veins are causative. Injections of the drug papaverine into the base of the penis may produce a firm erection in such men. A vacuum assistive device or penile implants are of value and are increasingly employed.

KLINEFELTER'S SYNDROME This is a condition characterized by small testes and various degrees of eunuchoidism. In almost all cases spermatozoa are absent in the ejaculate, and there is some enlargement of the male breast. The condition becomes obvious at puberty with the failure of normal pubertal changes. In recent years it has been discovered that many men with this condition have a cell chromosome pattern similar to that seen in the female, (double X chromosomes). In other respects most of them appear to be normally masculine.

Treatment. Injections of testosterone (male hormone) will bring out the usual pubertal changes such as hair, penile enlargement, and libido. The injections have to be given indefinitely and do not correct the absence of sperm or infertility.

NOCTURNAL EMISSIONS When sexual activities or masturbation have not been engaged in for a period of time, an automatic discharge of semen may occur during sleep. This is often accompanied by dreams of an erotic nature and is sometimes referred to as a wet dream.

ORCHITIS Inflammation of the testicles is known as orchitis and is most commonly seen in mumps. When inflamed, the testes becomes exceedingly painful and tender. Orchitis is usually treated by rest, application of cold packs, and occasionally by the administration of hormones. It may be of infectious origin, in which case it is often combined with epididymitis, and is responsive to appropriate antibiotics.

PENILE HYGIENE   The uncircumsized penis should by cleansed periodically by completely pulling back the foreskin (prepuce) and washing the secretion known as smegma from the glans penis and the indented area behind it. Infrequently the foreskin may be too tight to do this, a condition referred to as phimosis. A simple slit or a circumcision (performed by a physician) will cure the condition.

PENIS   The male sexual organ is known as the penis. It contains large spaces (sinuses) that are capable of filling with blood and producing a state of erection. The expanded tip of the penile shaft is known as the glans penis. Erotic sensations in the organ are due to specific nerve endings called genital corpuscles. Surprisingly, sensitivity to heat and cold is less developed in the penis than in the skin elsewhere. The fold of skin that covers the glans is known as the prepuce (foreskin) and is removed by circumcision in some males. The adult penis varies considerably in size; an average penis is about four to six inches in length, increasing somewhat in length and diameter when erect. Sexual ability and function bear no intrinsic relation to penile size.

PRIAPISM   Persistent erection of the penis, unrelieved by sexual intercourse or masturbation, is abnormal and is spoken of as priapism. It is a rare complication in patients with leukemia and blood disorders in which the blood collects in the large channels of the penis and is unable to return to the normal channels. Priapism may also occur in spinal-cord injuries, and is a rare complication of certain medications. Priapism may be painful and is now seen more often since the advent of papaverine injections into the penis in treatment of impotence. It generally responds to withdrawal of penile blood with a hypodermic syringe, a procedure administered by a physician.

PROPHYLACTIC   The term "prophylactic" generally refers to any device or method that is used to prevent disease. Thus, vaccines can be considered prophylactic measures. The term may also be used in a specific sense referring to a device or technique that prevents pregnancy. The condom, a sheath usually of rubber, which is worn over the penis during sexual intercourse, is an example of a prophylactic device in that it protects against the spread of venereal disease as well as being a device used to prevent pregnancy.

PROSTATE   The prostate is an accessory gland of the male reproductive system. About the size and shape of a chestnut, it is located at the base of the urinary bladder. Innumerable fine tubules make up the mass of the prostate and produce its characteristic secretion. This opaque white secretion is contributed to the semen at the time of orgasm, but the exact role of the secretion is unknown. The size, shape and consistency of the prostate are easily determined by a digital rectal examination. Because of the high frequency of prostatic disease, such an examination is an

THE BLADDER AND THE PROSTATE GLAND

URETER FROM KIDNEY

BLADDER

SEMINAL VESICLE

PROSTATE GLAND

URETHRA

DUCTUS DEFERENS
FROM TESTIS

important part of the male physical examination.

PROSTATIC CANCER   Cancer of the prostate rises progressively with aging and therefore is sometimes referred to as the old man's cancer. It is a disease distinctly different from benign hypertrophy, though the two can coexist. On rectal examination the cancer is felt as a localized area of unusual hardness. Such an area may require a needle biopsy, also done via the rectum for confirmation of the diagnosis. When the cancer is localized to the gland, a complete prostatectomy will assure a cure. Unfortunately the cancer may be more widespread at time of discovery, spreading initially to the local lymph nodes and to the bones of the pelvis. In such cases, since the tumor is usually hormone-dependent, removal of the testes and its secretion of the male hormone, testosterone, may produce a gratifying improvement. Although remission may last for months to years, there may then be a resurgence of tumor growth. Irradiation, use of feminizing hormones such as stilbestrol, and other forms of chemotherapy may then be employed. (*See also* the section CANCER.)

PROSTATIC HYPERTROPHY   One of the most frequent disorders of the prostate is a benign progressive enlargement termed benign prostatic hypertrophy (BPH). It is found in more than 60 percent of U.S. men past the age of sixty. Because of its close anatomical relationship to the bladder and the urinary canal, prostatic enlargement may produce an encroachment on these structures with consequent problems in emptying the bladder.
    Symptoms. With certain degrees of BPH, the bladder cannot empty itself completely so that there is always a constant residue of urine in it. This may lead to frequency of urination both by day and by night. The stream may be weak, with much hesitancy and dribbling. Complications of BPH include progressive distension, not alone of the bladder, but of the kidneys, a condition termed hydronephrosis.
    Treatment. Recent research has brought forth several medicines which may shrink the enlarged prostate, but at the cost of hot flashes and loss of sexual capacity. Hence the

most frequent approach remains surgical. Much of the prostate may be removed through the urethra, thus leaving no scar. Larger glands require removal through an incision generally quite low in the abdomen. Urinary obstruction is thereby relieved, and the operation is one of the most common in aging men.

PROSTATITIS   A variety of inflammations involving the prostate gland are termed prostatitis. Acute prostatitis is marked by sudden onset of pain in the perineal region—the area between the scrotum and rectum—with a number of associated urinary difficulties, especially pain and frequency. There may be chills, high fever and toxicity depending on the virulence of the bacteria responsible for the infection. More often prostatitis is less severe and more chronic.
    Symptoms. Common symptoms include frequency of urination, nocturia—frequent urination at night—and various degrees of discomfort on passing urine.
    Treatment. Antibiotics may have to be taken for many weeks even with a low grade of chronic prostatitis. This is attributed to the difficulty in getting a sufficient amount of the antibiotics into the prostatic tubules. Temporary relief from symptoms may be obtained by sitting in a tub in about six inches of warm to hot water (the sitz bath) and avoidance of alcohol, spices and long auto rides. In some cases changes in sexual habits may be suggested by the physician.

SCROTUM   The sac suspended below the penis in the male is known as the scrotum. It contains the testicles, epididymis, and seminal vessels, as well as nerves and blood vessels. In the adult it has a somewhat corrugated surface which is capable of contraction and expansion. In a cold environment the scrotum will be markedly contracted, and in a warm environment it will expand permitting the testes to hang further away from the warm body surface. Both of these reactions are designed to provide a stable temperature for the heat-sensitive testes and the sperm.

SEXUAL ABSTINENCE   The term refers to the voluntary abstaining from sexual relations. Abstinence has been affirmed as an approach to birth control by the Catholic Church, with sexual abstinence applied to the most fertile period of the female cycle.

In part because of the rise in sexually transmitted diseases, abstinence has been recommended as a control measure in some quarters. It has also been invoked in connection with teenage pregnancies and as an approach to premarital sexuality in general. Medically speaking, abstinence has no effect on the life span but may produce some symptomatology, especially in the older male. An example is the so-called "widower's prostatitis" complaints of urinary frequency and prostatic congestion in the sexually active male whose spouse has died.

SMEGMA   This term generally refers to the cheesy substance which collects between the foreskin (prepuce) and the glans penis in the male. Actually small amounts may occur also between the labia minora and the clitoris in the female. It is composed of the secretions of the glands in the area, together with shed cells.

SPERM(ATOZOA)   The normal spermatozoon is a microscopic structure consisting of an oval-shaped head and long tail, somewhat resembling a tadpole. The spermatozoa are able to propel themselves about in a liquid medium, and after ejaculation are able to travel into the body of the uterus. It is important for fertility that there be a normal number of spermatozoa present in the ejaculate; adult males should have at least fifty million sperm per cubic centimeter. (The normal average count is one hundred twenty million per cubic centimeter.) A few of the sperm may be abnormal in shape or size or may lack the head or part of the tail. Infertility problems may exist when these abnormal sperms comprise a larger than normal percentage of the sperm count.

TESTICLES (TESTES)   These rounded, elongated organs reside in the male scrotum in adulthood. They are firm and covered by a tough capsule. Internally, they are composed of thousands of tiny pockets in which sperm are manufactured. At body temperature, the process of sperm-manufacture is incomplete, but at the somewhat lower temperature of the

scrotum (outside the body) conditions are favorable to it.

A testicle may become twisted on the spermatic cord producing enlargement, congestion, and tension. Not uncommonly, mumps affects the testes—especially in males past the age of puberty. It is therefore important that rest and a close medical regime be carefully followed to prevent permanent damage after recovery from mumps.

Tumors of the testicles are relatively uncommon but are almost always malignant; they are usually painless, and the only clue to their presence may be a hard lump in the testicle. At an early stage, testicular tumors may be removed with a high likelihood of cure. The most malignant of these tumors, however, spread rapidly, but may be responsive to chemotherapy.

TESTOSTERONE   This is a hormone secreted by the testicles directly into the bloodstream. It is responsible for production of a masculine body configuration and other male characteristics. Output of testosterone greatly increases at the time of puberty, and it is this substance which induces growth of the penis and scrotum, as well as distribution of hair in the pubic, underarm, and facial areas. Testosterone is also a potent stimulator of muscle growth and power, as well as growth and length of the long bones since it influences closure of the cartilage plates (epiphyses) which are responsible for growth of the long bones.

TORSION OF TESTIS   When the testis becomes acutely twisted on the spermatic cord, it may become greatly swollen because the blood supply is cut off. This condition is an acute emergency, calling for surgery, but is completely relieved by opening the scrotum and returning the testis to its proper position.

UNDESCENDED TESTICLE (CRYPTORCHIDISM)   Before birth the testicles are developed in the lower abdomen. Prior to birth they normally descend to the scrotum. One or both testes however, may remain within the body. In such cases descent usually occurs in the first few years of childhood or may be delayed until puberty. If the testicle has not migrated to the scrotum by the age of nine or ten, it is usually considered advisable to institute treatment.

Treatment. Surgery is considered by the majority to be the recommended treatment, although some physicians consider the use of gonadotropic hormone injections. Frequently, surgery is necessary before the testis can be placed in its proper location in the scrotum. It is important to treat undescended testes to assure fertility, because development of the sperm is incomplete at the higher temperature within the body. There is also an increased incidence of tumors in undescended testes.

VARICOCELE   The veins along the cord inside the scrotum often become twisted and enlarged. This both looks and feels like a "sack of worms" within the scrotum. The condition in and of itself is painless and not serious; when developing suddenly in adult life, however, it may be an indication of a tumor in the genitourinary tract.

VAS DEFERENS (SPERMATIC CORD)
The vas deferens is a cord-like structure which runs within the scrotum from the testes up to the inguinal region and enters the prostatic urethra at the base of the bladder. It carries sperm, which mature in transit, from the testes to be ejaculated into the urethra through the ejaculatory duct. It is sometimes the site of tuberculosis, which produces a beading of the tubular structure.

VASECTOMY   Cutting of the vas deferens with surgical tying-off of the severed ends is known as vasectomy. It is a common procedure in operations to remove the prostate gland. This procedure reduces the risk of infection reaching the epididymis and testis; it is also an effective means of producing permanent sterility in the male.

VESICLE, SEMINAL   The seminal vesicles lie adjacent to the base of the bladder. They secrete a thick, glairy material, a normal component of the semen; sperm are not stored in them.

WITHDRAWAL (COITUS INTERRUPTUS)   When conception is not desired, the male partner may withdraw the penis during sexual intercourse just before ejaculation. This is a problematic practice because it often results in failure to reach orgasm, with consequent build-up of tension in either partner or in both. It is likewise risky as a birth-control measure because it may not always be accomplished in time to prevent deposit of sperm in the vagina.

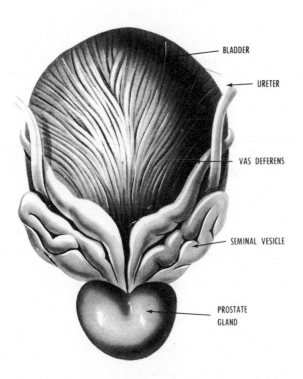

BLADDER

URETER

VAS DEFERENS

SEMINAL VESICLE

PROSTATE GLAND

FEMALE HEALTH CARE

FALLOPIAN TUBE

OVARY

UTERUS

BLADDER

CERVIX

LABIA

RECTUM

VAGINA

$\mathbf{W}$omen's health care issues require an understanding of the basic anatomy of a woman. The reproductive cycle functions for a major portion of a woman's life. Although these reproductive organs are small in size, they have the ability to adapt to accommodate the growing size of the fetus. Gynecology is concerned with a woman's sexual and reproductive function, diseases of the reproductive organs and the breasts, birth control, and fertility, while the field of obstetrics deals specifically with pregnancy, labor, and delivery. Obstetrician-gynecologists (OB-GYNs) practice both medical specialties.

This section examines the anatomy and physiology of women, common conditions and possible courses of treatments, as well as pregnancy. *See also* the questions on side effects of birth control pills (Q-15) and menstrual problems (Q-16, Q-17, Q-18, Q-19, Q-20) in the section QUESTIONS AND ANSWERS ABOUT COMMON SYMPTOMS.

The following is a list of terms identified in this section:

ABORTION, INDUCED
ABORTION METHODS
ABORTION, SPONTANEOUS
ABRUPTIO PLACENTA
AFTER-BIRTH PAINS
AMENORRHEA
AMNIOCENTESIS
AMNIOTIC FLUID
ANALGESIA AND ANESTHESIA
  IN LABOR
BARTHOLIN'S GLANDS
BIRTH CERTIFICATE
BLEEDING IN PREGNANCY
BLOOD PRESSURE IN PREGNANCY
BREAST CANCER
BREAST ENGORGEMENT
BREAST SELF-EXAMINATION (BSE)
BREECH
CAESAREAN SECTION
CEPHALOPELVIC DISPROPORTION
CERVICITIS
CERVIX
CHILDBED FEVER (POSTABORTAL AND
  PUERPERAL SEPSIS)
CHILDBIRTH, PREPARED
CHLOASMA (MASK OF PREGNANCY)
CHORIONIC VILLI SAMPLING
CLIMACTERIC
CLITORIS
COLOSTRUM

CONCEPTION
CONIZATION, CERVICAL
CONTRACEPTION
CONTRACTION, UTERINE
CROWNING
D & C (DILATION AND CURETTAGE)
DELIVERY
DIABETES IN PREGNANCY
DIET IN PREGNANCY
DOUCHING
DYSMENORRHEA
DYSPAREUNIA
DYSTOCIA
ECLAMPSIA
ENDOMETRIOSIS
ENDOMETRITIS
ENDOMETRIUM
ENGAGEMENT, OBSTETRICAL
EPISIOTOMY
FALLOPIAN TUBES
FETAL PRESENTATIONS
FIBROADENOMAS
FIBROCYSTIC BREAST DISEASE
FIBROIDS (FIBROMYOMATA
  OF THE UTERUS)
FORCEPS
GESTATIONAL AGE
GONADS
GYNECOLOGY
HEREDITY

HERPES, GENITAL, IN THE FEMALE	PELVIS (FEMALE)
HYDATIDIFORM MOLE	PLACENTA (AFTERBIRTH)
HYDRAMNIOS	PLACENTA PREVIA
HYMEN	POSTPARTUM
HYSTERECTOMY	PREGNANCY
HYSTEROGRAM	PREMENSTRUAL SYNDROME (PMS)
(HYSTEROSALPINGOGRAM)	PRENATAL CARE
INFERTILITY	PROGESTERONE
IN VITRO FERTILIZATION	PSYCHOSES IN PREGNANCY
IRON-DEFICIENCY ANEMIA	PUERPERIUM (POSTPARTUM)
IN PREGNANCY	"QUICKENING"
LABIA	RH FACTOR AND RH SENSITIZATION
LABOR	SALPINGITIS
LACTATION	SEXUAL ACT
LEUKORRHEA	STERILITY AND INFERTILITY
LOCHIA	STERILIZATION, SURGICAL
MAMMOGRAPHY	STILLBORN
MASTITIS	"STRETCHMARKS" (STRIAE
MEMBRANES	OF PREGNANCY)
MENARCHE	TEMPERATURE CHARTS
MENOPAUSE	TOXEMIAS OF PREGNANCY
MENORRHAGIA	TOXIC SHOCK SYNDROME (TSS)
MENSTRUAL CYCLE	TUBAL (ECTOPIC) PREGNANCY
MENSTRUATION	TUBAL LIGATION
MISCARRIAGE (SPONTANEOUS	TWINS
ABORTION)	ULTRASOUND
MORNING SICKNESS	UMBILICAL CORD
OBSTETRICS	UTERINE BLEEDING, ABNORMAL
OVARIAN CYSTS	UTERUS, SUBINVOLUTION OF THE
OVARIES	UTERUS (WOMB)
OVULATION	VAGINA (BIRTH CANAL)
OXYTOCICS	VAGINAL DISCHARGE
PAP SMEAR	VAGINITIS
PELVIMETRY	VULVA

ABORTION, INDUCED The intentional termination of a pregnancy—either because of complications that threaten the well-being of the mother or because the woman chooses not to complete her pregnancy—is called an induced or therapeutic abortion. In its 1973 ruling in Roe vs. Wade, the U.S. Supreme Court established the legality of abortion "on request." The ruling permitted a woman to have an abortion from a licensed physician without restriction in the first three months of pregnancy and allowed states to regulate where and by whom second-trimester abortions can be performed in order to protect the woman's health. States were permitted to regulate and even prohibit abortions in the third trimester except when the mother's life or health was endangered. The Supreme Court decision has led to a protracted battle between groups who want the ruling overturned and those who seek to preserve it. The Supreme Court did not rule on the matter of when life begins, and much of today's debate focuses on that issue. Recent Supreme Court rulings have required that physicians test a fetus at twenty weeks to determine if it can survive outside the uterus and have given states more latitude in legislating abortions.

ABORTION METHODS The methods used to induce an abortion vary according to the length of gestation. Each has certain risks and possible complications, which increase the later in the pregnancy that the abortion is performed.

Suction (vacuum) curettage. This method is most commonly used in the first seven weeks of gestation. A small spoon-shaped instrument called a suction curet is inserted into the cervix; the fertilized egg and uterine lining (endometrium) are withdrawn using either a hand-held syringe or a hand or electric pump. Dilation of the cervix may not be required if the procedure is carried out before the seventh week of gestation. If this method is used in the first few weeks of pregnancy, it is sometimes called menstrual extraction. After seven weeks, the procedure usually requires dilation either mechanically or using special sterile material derived from seaweed called laminaria. Suction curettage is not always effective and may require a second procedure. Possible complications include infection, excessive bleeding, and injury to the cervix and uterus.

Dilation and Curettage. The cervix is dilated either mechanically or using laminaria; the curet is inserted through the cervix; and the uterus is scraped to remove the fetus and placental tissue. A general anesthesia is often required. Greater dilation is required than for suction curettage and the danger of cervical tears and blood loss is increased. As with suction curettage, other complications include infection and injury to the uterus and the cervix.

Dilation and Evacuation. After twelve weeks, dilation and evacuation is the most common abortion method. The cervix is dilated using the same methods as in the D&C. Forceps are used to break up and remove the fetus. The uterus is scraped, and amniotic fluid, the placenta, and remaining fetal tissue are suctioned out using an electric pump. Infection, hemorrhage, and injury to the cervix, intestines, and uterus are possible complications. Extensive uterine injury may require a hysterectomy.

Medical induction. Abortion in the second trimester can be brought about by injecting certain fluids through the abdominal wall into the uterus and the amniotic sac. Saline solution and prostaglandin, an agent that stimulates contractions, are the most widely used substances. The patient goes into labor and the fetus is delivered. Complications include hemorrhage, infection, and retained placenta. Accidental injection of the saline solution into a vein may cause kidney, heart, and blot-clotting difficulties, and cerebral convulsions. Side effects of prostaglandin include nausea, vomiting, and diarrhea. It may also cause bronchial spasms.

Hysterotomy. This major surgery is rarely performed and carries great risk. Similar to a caesarian section, it is performed under general or spinal anesthesia. The lower segment of the uterus is cut into, and the fetus and the placenta removed. A live fetus may be born.

Hysterectomy. Even more rarely, the fetus and uterus are removed through hysterectomy, usually because of some abnormality of the uterus. As with any major surgery, complications include infection and hemorrhage. Because the uterus is removed, the procedure results in sterility.

Most recently a nonsurgical approach has been developed in France to bring about an abortion. First, an antiprogesterone medication is given followed a few days later by a drug belonging to the group of prostaglandins; this produces uterine cramping and expulsion of the fetus. The ease and effectiveness of this approach produced controversy: the prostaglandin drug was withdrawn in France by the manufacturer but restored after a public outcry. It is not available in the United States.

ABORTION, SPONTANEOUS *See* Mis-CARRIAGE in this section.

ABRUPTIO PLACENTA This is the partial or total separation of the placenta from the uterus before or during labor.

Symptoms. This condition results in the loss of large amounts of blood, usually becoming evident in the form of severe vaginal bleeding. The patient experiences sudden severe abdominal pain, the uterus becomes tense and irritable, and the patient is continuously uncomfortable. Vaginal bleeding usually follows. The baby may die or be seriously compromised because of lack of oxygen.

Treatment. Caesarean section is often performed for the sake of the baby, the mother, or both. If more than 30 percent of the placenta becomes separated, the baby usually succumbs.

AFTER-BIRTH PAINS These are usually mild to severe lower abdominal pains due to the continuing contractions of the uterus after delivery. They last for a few days (commonly two to three) after birth and are not as common following delivery of a first baby as in subsequent deliveries. They are usually stronger while the mother is breast-feeding the baby, but respond well to relatively mild analgesics.

AMENORRHEA This term refers to the lack of menstrual periods. The condition may be primary, when no period has ever occurred in a woman after puberty; or secondary, when a woman who has regular periods suddenly stops menstruating.

The most common cause of secondary amenorrhea is pregnancy, and this diagnosis should be ruled out before any other cause is suspected. The other most common causes of amenorrhea are congenital abnormalities of one or more such glands as the ovaries, the adrenal glands, the thyroid, or the pituitary. Anatomical anomalies of the uterus and the vagina, as well as mixed sex (hermaphroditism), may also account for some of the primary amenorrheas. Psychosomatic factors are very often the cause of secondary amenorrhea, as are eating disorders and exercise.

Treatment. Treatment will depend on the cause and may be surgical, medical (hormones), or psychiatric. A woman with primary amenorrhea should be evaluated for congenital or anatomical abnormalities; a woman with secondary amenorrhea should be evaluated for the other conditions.

AMNIOCENTESIS Amniocentesis is the procedure by which amniotic fluid is extracted from the uterus. Using local anesthesia a small hypodermic needle is placed through the abdominal wall directly into the uterine cavity and amniotic fluid is extracted. The amniotic fluid, containing fetal cells, is then analyzed, possibly revealing abnormalities such as rubella virus infection and congenital diseases, such as Down syndrome and spina bifida.

When a finding is made that the fetus is abnormal, doctors may offer the woman the option of terminating the pregnancy. Amniocentesis is recommended in cases where abnormal fetal development is suspected; it is not a routine procedure. Although infrequent, complications caused by amniocentesis may include continued leakage of amniotic fluid from the puncture site, bleeding, injury to the fetus or placenta, and miscarriage.

Because the incidence of Down syndrome increases with age of the mother, amniocentesis is most often performed in women 35 years of age or older. It is not mandatory of course, and the pregnant mother may decline the procedure.

AMNIOTIC FLUID While the fetus is carried in the mother's uterus, it is surrounded by the amniotic fluid contained in the fetal membranes (bag of waters). The fluid varies in amount, usually equalling one or two pints when the mother is close to delivery (term). Its purpose is to supply a sort of water bath for free movement of the fetus inside the uterus and to protect the baby from violent external injuries. When the bag of waters breaks, the amniotic fluid leaks through the vagina; this usually happens during labor.

Premature rupture of the bag of waters, occurring before onset of labor, should be reported to the doctor because of the risk of infection.

ANALGESIA AND ANESTHESIA IN LABOR Analgesia refers to the temporary reduction or absence of pain without the loss of other sensations. Anesthesia is the absence of sensation, including pain. These effects can be produced during labor through a variety of drugs. However, there also are methods of reducing pain without medication. The most popular of these are hypnosis and prepared or natural childbirth, which combines relaxation and breathing techniques to lessen discomfort. Any drugs that produce analgesia and anesthesia involve some risk to the unborn child, since they are carried through the placenta to the unborn child. However, a number of analgesics and anesthetics have been developed that offer reasonable relief from the pains of labor while protecting the fetus from undue exposure to heavy sedation. Each patient reacts differently to pain and therefore requires an individual plan for pain relief.

Analgesics. Tranquilizers such as Valium® may be administered to lessen pain by reducing anxiety and allowing the patient to relax. Sedatives such as Seconal® and Nembutal® produce the same effect and may also allow the patient to doze between contractions without actually going to sleep. These may be used in combination with narcotics. They may be administered by mouth or by injection.

Narcotics such as Demerol® or Nisentil® may be used in small doses to allow the patient to remain awake and participate in delivery while easing discomfort. Some women complain that Demerol®, which is administered early in labor, interferes with their ability to concentrate or relax. Nisentil® is more commonly administered late in labor when only short-term relief is needed and generally does not result in a loss of control. Narcotics are usually administered by injection or intravenously.

Inhalation analgesia once was commonly self-administered during early labor, but now it is more often administered by specially trained professionals during the later first stage and second stage of labor. It does not offer complete analgesia and is usually supplemented with a local anesthetic if an episiotomy or forceps delivery is required.

Regional Anesthesia. Saddle block anesthesia is achieved through a low-dosage injection into the spinal cord and numbs the buttocks, perineum, and inner thighs. It is used primarily just prior to delivery. It can cause a loss of the urge to bear down, but it does not prohibit the patient from bearing down voluntarily when prompted. It may produce spinal headaches.

Epidural anesthesia is administered through a catheter into the space surrounding the spinal cord. It eliminates pain from near the waist to the toes without prohibiting movement. If dosage is properly regulated, a woman may still feel the urge to bear down and can assist in her delivery. Great care must be taken to ensure that the membrane surrounding the spinal cord is not punctured, resulting in spinal headache and a more extensive area of anesthesia.

Pudendal block is achieved by injecting the anesthetic into the pudendal nerve in the vagina or buttocks. It numbs the vagina and perineum, but provides no relief of uterine pain. It often is used to perform a forceps delivery.

Paracervical block is produced by injection into the cervix after active labor is well under way. It results in complete and instantaneous pain relief in the cervix and uterus. This technique is thought to have serious effects on the child, and, therefore, is used only when other methods are not available.

General anesthesia. General anesthesia is achieved through inhalation and results in unconsciousness. Because the mother is unable to participate in the delivery and because of the risks to the mother and baby, this method is seldom used in normal births. However, general anesthesia may be needed under certain circumstances, such as breech deliveries, patients with severe bleeding, or high blood pressure.

BARTHOLIN'S GLANDS These structures are located, one on each side, at the entrance of the vagina. They may become infected, whereupon they become swollen and tender. Treatment is incision and drainage, or complete removal of the inflamed glands.

BIRTH CERTIFICATE All states require that a birth certificate be prepared by the physician after each delivery and promptly submitted to the local municipal or county authorities. The information is also sent to the Bureau of Vital Statistics in Washington, D.C., where valuable data are coded and permanently maintained. Statistical analysis of these data offers valuable records for medical, socio-economic, military, and other purposes.

BLEEDING IN PREGNANCY Vaginal bleeding at any stage of pregnancy should immediately be brought to the attention of the physician and thoroughly investigated. Often the cause is not serious, but at other times it can be the sign of a condition that may endanger the life of the mother or fetus. Some women continue to have bleeding at the normal time of their menstrual period during the first few months of pregnancy, although the discharge is rarely as heavy as a normal menstrual period.

Some light bleeding or spotting early in pregnancy is quite common. In many cases the bleeding stops by itself and its cause is unknown. However, bleeding can be an indication of a threatened miscarriage or of an ectopic pregnancy. Spotting, especially after intercourse, may be the result of inflammation of the cervix. Later in pregnancy, bleeding may be an indication that the placenta is implanted over the mouth of the uterus (placenta previa) or that it has separated from the uterus (abruptio placenta). Both are serious conditions that require immediate attention.

Blood-tinged discharge late in pregnancy is usually a sign that labor will begin soon.

BLOOD PRESSURE IN PREGNANCY
See TOXEMIAS OF PREGNANCY in this section.

BREAST CANCER This is the leading cause of death among women, with one of every eleven women developing the disease in her lifetime. It occurs most often after the age of 35, with the risk steadily increasing with age. Because of the high incidence of breast cancer, women are advised to examine their breasts monthly for changes. Monthly breast self-examination, regular examination by a physician, and mammography according to the American Cancer Society's recommended schedule are the chief means of combatting the disease. The earlier the cancer can be detected, the greater the odds of less radical treatment.

In its early stage, a cancerous breast mass is usually small, firm, dense, painless, and irregular in shape. Later, it may be accompanied by nipple discharge, nipple retraction, and dimpling of the skin. Mammography and biopsy are used to diagnose the disease. If the diagnosis is confirmed, it must be determined if the cancer is confined to the breast or has spread to other tissue. This will influence the treatment choice. Surgical treatment options include simple excision of the tumor (lumpectomy); removal of the tumor and a large segment of surrounding tissue (partial mastectomy); removal of the affected breast and surrounding lymph nodes (modified radical mastectomy); or total removal of the breast, surrounding lymph nodes, and surrounding muscle (radical mastectomy). Radiation therapy and chemotherapy are often used as adjuncts to surgery. (*See also* the section CANCER.)

BREAST ENGORGEMENT One or two days after delivery, mothers usually notice considerable swelling of their breasts, which at the same time become warm and sore. Contrary to popular belief, this is not due to abundant milk-production and storage, but to obstructed blood- and/or lymph-flow from the breast. This condition should not be confused with mastitis, which is an actual infection of the breast, with much higher fever, and which may occur a week or more after delivery.

Treatment. Treatment of engorgement consists of initiation of breast feeding or proper support of the breasts and application of ice bags.

BREAST SELF-EXAMINATION (BSE) Breast cancers are most often felt by the woman or her spouse. A monthly schedule of breast self-examination can increase the chances of detecting breast cancer at an early stage. A woman should examine her breasts at the same time each month and become familiar with what is normal for her. She should feel for any lump or thickening.

The proper technique consists of feeling the breasts with flat fingers while standing and while reclining and inspection of the breasts in a mirror.

The shower is an ideal place for examining the breasts while standing. The fingers are gently moved over the wet breasts, beginning with the outer region and continuing in a circular motion until the nipple is reached. The arm next to the breast that is being examined is placed behind the head.

In front of a mirror and with arms at the sides, the breasts should be inspected for any changes in shape, including swelling, puckering, or changes in the nipple. The same inspection is followed with hands overhead. Next, with hands on hips, the breasts should be examined to compare them. They will not look the same, but regular examination will enable the woman to determine when there is a change in either.

To examine the breasts while lying down, a pillow or folded towel should be placed under the shoulder on the side of the breast that is to be examined. Each breast should be examined using the same circular movement employed while standing up. Finally, the nipple should be squeezed. If there is any discharge, it should be reported to the physician.

A woman's physician or nurse practitioner can show her how to perform her monthly breast self-examination.

BREECH   Approximately 3 percent of all babies are delivered with the feet or the buttocks coming first. This is known as breech presentation. There are two main varieties of breech: the footling breech, in which one or both feet come first through the vagina during labor; and the frank breech, in which the buttocks appear first. Before the onset of labor, a breech baby can turn headfirst and vice versa; however, this is highly unlikely. Breech deliveries are, as a rule, more difficult for the physician and require more skill and experience than normal deliveries do. This is the reason a few obstetricians prefer to deliver all full-term breeches by caesarean section, especially if the breech is the patient's first baby. This is not generally recommended, however —at least not in places where such good hospital facilities and staff are available as prompt anesthesia, sufficient and well-trained personnel, a blood bank, etc.

A warning of particular importance to the patient who knows that she is carrying a breech baby is to watch for rupture of the bag of waters, whether she is in labor or not. If this occurs, she should immediately be taken to the hospital, because of the increased danger of prolapse of the cord. (*See also* UMBILICAL CORD in this section.) In such cases an immediate operation will usually be required for the delivery of the baby. (*See also* FETAL PRESENTATIONS in this section.)

CAESAREAN SECTION   About 15 percent of all pregnancies are today terminated by caesarean section for the benefit of the baby, the mother, or both. Caesarean section actually means the delivery of the baby through surgical incision of the wall of the abdomen and the uterus. The term "caesarean" is derived from the Latin verb *caedere* (to cut) and not—contrary to popular belief—because Julius Caesar was delivered in this manner. The operation, as performed in our modern hospitals by well-trained obstetricians, with all proper surgical facilities at their disposal, is a relatively simple technical procedure, and the overall prognosis for the mother is excellent. Babies delivered by caesarean section have generally higher mortality rates; this, however, is not due to the operation per se, but to the many and often serious pre-existing complications which make the section necessary. In fact, many of these babies would not survive unless delivered promptly with the help of surgery. Everything else being equal, babies delivered by caesarean section have the same chances for survival and normal development as the ones delivered vaginally.

Indications for caesarean section are numerous, some of them permanent and some temporary. The most common ones are contracted maternal pelvis—always in correlation with the size of the baby (*see also* CEPHALOPELVIC DISPROPORTION in this section); previous caesarean sections; distress of the baby in the uterus (in either the presence or absence of labor); excessive bleeding from the afterbirth before the delivery; prolapse of the umbilical cord; an abnormal position of the baby inside the mother's uterus; and tumors of the uterus and ovaries.

The choice of anesthesia will depend on the general condition of the individual patient and the indication for caesarean section. In most cases, epidural anesthesia is indicated and is perfectly adequate for the operation, but occasionally the patient has to be put to sleep through other anesthesia. On the average, the patient is ready to leave the hospital in five to seven days after the operation.

Should a patient who has been delivered once by caesarean section always be delivered in the same manner? Whenever there is a permanent indication for the original caesarean section—and the only permanent indication is small maternal pelvis—subsequent pregnancies should also be terminated by caesarean section. Whenever the original indication is temporary (such as vaginal bleeding, abnormal position of the baby, prolapsed cord, etc.)

the majority of obstetricians will allow the patient to go into labor and have subsequent babies vaginally, always under close medical observation, however. There are numerous studies and reliable statistical records to back up this approach and, no matter how safe a caesarean section in general can be today, we should not forget that it is still a major surgical procedure and should not be utilized lightly in place of a more natural and safer alternative, that is, vaginal delivery.

Unless there are special indications for the termination of pregnancy before term (such as diabetes or Rh disease), the patient with a previous caesarean section should be allowed to advance as close to term as possible. Prenatal testing will aid in establishing a time for a caesarean. Occasionally, because of lack of proper hospital facilities in close vicinity to the patient, or because the obstetrician estimates that the baby is large enough to be delivered, a repeat caesarean section may be planned and performed before labor begins.

How many caesarean sections can a patient have? Actually, a patient may have as many babies by caesarean section as she wants. It should, however, be realized that with each subsequent pregnancy and operative delivery, the patient is assuming the same and probably increased risks and possible complications.

CEPHALOPELVIC DISPROPORTION

This is a term used in obstetrics and implies that the mother's pelvis is too small in comparison with the size and position of her baby, and that difficulty in labor and delivery might therefore be anticipated. Such a disproportion can be due either to normal-size pelvis and an abnormally large baby, a normal-size baby and a mother with an abnormally small pelvis, or any intermediate combination of these two factors. Most caesarean sections done today are primarily performed for cephalopelvic disproportion alone, or in combination with supervening complications of labor.

CERVICITIS This is an inflammation of the mouth of the uterus. It is a very common infection in the sexually active adult female.

Symptoms. This condition is characterized mainly by abnormal vaginal discharge, itching or burning, and occasional "spotting" after intercourse or between menstrual periods.

Treatment. Diagnosis of this condition is not difficult, and treatment usually consists of special vaginal suppositories, creams, or sprays and douches. Occasionally the doctor will have to resort to electrocautery (burning), which can be easily performed in the office.

CERVIX The cervix is the neck of the uterus; it is located at the top of the vagina, and connects this organ with the cavity of the uterus. The cervix is a vital part of the uterus and plays a very important role both in the transfer of sperm for conception and in the maintenance of pregnancy (by remaining closed for nine months and then gradually opening when labor starts, allowing the baby to pass through and be delivered). The most common diseases of the cervix include cervicitis, cervical cancer, and cervical polyps.

Lasers can be essential instruments in the treatment of certain cancerous and precancerous conditions of the cervix. They allow the surgeon to destroy the abnormal tissue with minimal effect on the surrounding normal tissue. The procedure normally can be performed during an outpatient or office visit.

THE FEMALE ORGANS
(CROSS SECTION)

CHILDBED FEVER (POSTABORTAL AND PUERPERAL SEPSIS) The genital canal of a healthy female adult is sterile above the inner opening of the cervix of the uterus. A woman is protected from infection by the acid vaginal secretion (due to lactic acid normally secreted); "policing" by the white blood cells of the circulating blood; the mucous plug in the cervix; during and after labor by additional safeguards such as the descent of the amniotic fluid, the infant's body, and other discharges; and the diminished virulence of any pathogenic bacteria resident in the vagina. Infection is introduced from the vaginal and genital skin area by vaginal examination, by unclean hands or instruments. Ordinary douches cannot be depended on as a prophylactic measure since they do not destroy pathogenic germs and do destroy the natural safeguard of acid secretion. The most common germs that cause sepsis are the streptococcus, staphylococcus, colon bacillus, gonococcus, and the Welch organism (which causes gangrene).

Symptoms. The first sign is usually a chill followed by fever which rises over the next few days. The pulse becomes rapid, there is extreme weakness, the breath is foul, and the tongue is coated. There may be a skin rash and diarrhea may ensue. The patient has a foul vaginal discharge; the vaginal lips are swollen and red. Later, infectious involvement of the uterus and its ligaments is inevitable.

Treatment. The prompt initiation of antibiotic therapy will most usually check the sepsis and prevent other complications. Antibiotics generally make local treatment (during the acute illness) unnecessary; the less examination and manipulation of the genital tract the better. Sedative and tranquilizing drugs may be given. Women who have had incomplete or unsanitary abortions performed and fail to reveal their post-operative illness until the infection is overwhelming may require abdominal surgery, for example, removal of the uterus.

CHILDBIRTH, PREPARED In this approach to labor and delivery, the parents have undergone preparation so that they can be involved in the birth of their child. The mother is awake and the father assumes an active role. Various methods have been developed that seek to eliminate or reduce the amount of medication the mother needs during labor and delivery. They are based on the belief that pain is intensified if the patient is tense and fearful. In special classes, couples learn what to expect during labor and delivery, exercises to improve muscle tone, and techniques to enhance relaxation. During labor and delivery, the father is at the mother's side, offering encouragement, coaching her in her breathing, and offering comfort.

CHLOASMA (MASK OF PREGNANCY) In this condition irregular brownish patches appear over the skin of the face and neck. They generally disappear soon after delivery. Chloasma may also be a reaction to birth-control pills. The pigment deposits are apparently a reaction to an altered hormonal environment and may be worsened by exposure to sun. It is not known why the phenomenon is so much more marked in some women than others.

CHORIONIC VILLI SAMPLING This new method of diagnosing fetal abnormalities is performed during the first trimester of pregnancy. A thin flexible tube is guided through the cervix and a small sampling of the placenta is removed, cultured, and analyzed. The test can reveal the same abnormalities as amniocentesis, except for neural tube defects, such as spina bifida. Chorionic villi sampling is currently performed in relatively few medical centers and carries a greater risk of miscarriage than amniocentesis.

CLIMACTERIC The cessation of ovarian function in women is called the climacteric. In women there is a gradual decrease in ovarian efficiency after the age of thirty-five. When ovulation ceases, menstrual bleeding may become irregular and cause concern. Bleeding usually decreases gradually in amount, due to lowered secretion of estrogen and progesterone. Normally cessation of menstruation (menopause) occurs around fifty years of age.

Symptoms. A number of troublesome symptoms may occur at this time of life. The most common complaint is periodic "hot flashes," or feelings of warmth flooding the face and neck, often accompanied by excess perspiration. Nervous irritability is common, as are feelings of depression and fears that sexual attractiveness is being lost. Of serious import is the development of bone softening (osteoporosis) which may result in loss of stature due to collapse of vertebrae, accompanied by severe bone pain.

Treatment. When careful medical examination assures the physician that serious mental disturbance is absent, he may simply reassure the woman that her symptoms will be temporary. There is no basis for the fear that sexual interest and responsiveness will be impaired during or after the menopause, if sex life was previously well-adjusted.

Small doses of estrogen by mouth or transdermally are often prescribed and effectively relieve menopause symptoms. Some physicians elect to continue this therapy for extended periods of time to help prevent aging of skin, muscles, mucous membranes, and bone. To treat or prevent osteoporosis in women female hormones are often used, with large doses of calcium.

Of some concern is the effect on mother and child of babies born in the menopausal years. It is a fact that the incidence of Down syndrome and other congenital abnormalities is higher in babies born during late reproductive life, probably due to aging of ova. (*See also* MENOPAUSE in this section.)

CLITORIS   The clitoris is located in front of the entrance to the vagina, just above the urethra (opening of the bladder) and consists of erectile tissue. Its size varies and it is an important organ for the development of sexual orgasm in the female. Except for abnormal enlargement, which is usually accompanied by other endocrinological abnormalities, diseases of the clitoris are rare.

COLOSTRUM   A yellowish fluid, colostrum is discharged from the breasts of some pregnant women from the early months of pregnancy but in most women not until several days after delivery. Its nutritive value is questionable; however, it acts as a mild cathartic and may provide increased amounts of antibodies for the baby.

CONCEPTION   The fertilization of the ovum (egg) by the spermatozoon, is conception and in the human usually occurs in one of the fallopian tubes, which the sperm reaches, through active motion, from the place of their deposition. Only one spermatozoon fertilizes a given egg.

CONIZATION, CERVICAL   Conization is the removal of a very small cone-shaped segment of the neck of the uterus (cervix) for diagnostic and—occasionally—therapeutic purposes. This is a very valuable procedure for the diagnosis of cancer of the cervix and can be done either in the presence or absence of pregnancy. Lasers have recently been used for cervical conization.

CONTRACEPTION   A variety of methods exist to prevent pregnancy. Among the most popular are the following:

Birth control pills. Two types of oral contraceptives are available. One is a combination of the female hormones estrogen and progestogen and the other contains only progestogen. Taken once a day as directed, they prevent the ovaries from manufacturing eggs (ova) every month, so that conception cannot occur. If used properly, these pills are considered to be nearly 100 percent effective.

A recent study indicates that there may be an increased risk of breast cancer in pill users, especially if a woman has taken the pill as an adolescent.

Diaphragms. The diaphragm is a round rubber dome with a flexible rim that is inserted through the vagina and covers the cervix. When used with a spermicidal jelly or cream, it is about 98 percent effective. The jelly or cream is applied to the center of the diaphragm on the side that touches the cervix and, as an extra precaution, around its rim. Diaphragms come in a variety of sizes and must be properly fitted by a physician or nurse practitioner, who also will instruct the user on how to insert the diaphragm. Patients may want to insert the diaphragm in the doctor's office and have the physician or nurse practitioner check to be sure that it has been properly inserted. A woman should not feel the diaphragm once it is in place. If she can, it is either the wrong size or improperly inserted. The diaphragm can be inserted up to two hours before intercourse and must remain in place at least six hours after intercourse to protect against sperm, which remain active in the vagina for some time after intercourse and which may travel into the uterus if the diaphragm is removed too soon. If a woman has more than one episode of intercourse within the six hours, additional jelly must be applied to the vagina using a specially designed applicator. To reduce the possibility of developing toxic shock syndrome, the diaphragm should be left in place no longer than 24 hours.

Vaginal jellies, creams, and foams. These spermicides which are inserted into the vagina are about 90 percent effective in preventing conception. These are available without a prescription.

Intrauterine devices (IUDs). These include several small plastic devices of varied shape which are inserted into the uterus by a physician and can be left in place for several years. Some devices contain the female hormone progesterone and must be replaced annually. It is unclear how IUDs work, but it is generally believed that they prevent implantation of the fertilized egg. They offer a maximum effectiveness of 97 percent. In some women they may cause irregular or excessive bleeding, so that removal may become necessary. Occasionally one may be expelled without the patient's knowledge. IUDs also may cause infection of the pelvic organs.

Vaginal sponges. These disposable rubber devices provide a barrier between the sperm and the cervix by trapping the sperm and releasing a sperm-killing agent. The sponge, which can be bought without a prescription, is inserted at the time of intercourse and offers protection for up to 24 hours. No additional spermicide is required for repeated intercourse. To protect against toxic shock syndrome, the sponge should be removed within 30 hours and should not be used during menstruation. Sponges are slightly less effective than diaphragms.

Condoms (prophylactics). These are fine rubber (or latex) sheaths which the male puts over the penis before intercourse. They are highly effective provided they are of good quality.

Rhythm method. This is based on the fact that most women ovulate around the fourteenth day of a normal twenty-eight-day cycle, so that if intercourse is avoided between days ten and seventeen, the chances are that

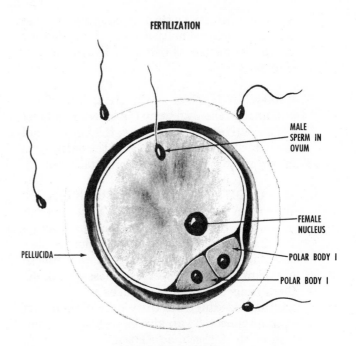

FERTILIZATION

MALE SPERM IN OVUM

FEMALE NUCLEUS

POLAR BODY I

POLAR BODY I

PELLUCIDA

THE EVENTS OF FERTILIZATION

The female ovum (egg), surrounded by a thick, transparent Zona Pellucida, divides unequally, producing Polar Body I. At this point, a single sperm penetrates the Zona. The ovum again divides, producing Polar Body II. The female nucleus migrates toward the male sperm. The union of the two completes fertilization.

pregnancy will not occur. The overall effectiveness of this method is, at best, estimated to be in the vicinity of 50 percent. This low figure is due to the fact that, even in women with normal menstrual patterns, the time of ovulation is quite unpredictable.

Interrupted intercourse (coitus interruptus). With this method, it is up to the male to control the situation—he must make sure to "withdraw" and ejaculate his sperm away from his partner. This is a highly archaic, emotionally unsatisfying approach to birth control, which has little to recommend it in view of the fact that it is not even reliable. There is always the danger of a little sperm penetrating the vagina in spite of the precautions taken.

Surgical sterilization of the male or female. (*See* STERILIZATION, SURGICAL in this section.)

CONTRACTION, UTERINE Involuntary periodic tightening of the muscle of the pregnant uterus, uterine contractions are experienced by pregnant women as labor pains. (*See also* LABOR in this section.) Actually there are uterine contractions throughout pregnancy at a level which are neither painful nor do they reach consciousness (Braxton Hicks contractions).

CROWNING This is the stretching of the entrance to the vagina by the baby's head just before delivery. At this stage, the baby's head is visible from the outside, and the delivery is only a matter of a few more minutes.

D & C (DILATATION AND CURETTAGE) This is an operation consisting of opening or enlarging the cervix (dilatation) and scraping the uterus (curettage). It is done either to clean out the womb after an incomplete abortion; or for diagnostic purposes, as in determining the possible causes of irregular vaginal bleeding, infertility, or in diagnosis of uterine cancer. It can also be used as an abortion method. (*See also* ABORTION, INDUCED in this section.)

DELIVERY Delivery, or childbirth, is the expulsion of the baby from inside the uterus to the outside world.

Vaginal delivery takes place during the second stage of labor. We will describe it briefly here, together with some simple instructions on how to assist in an emergency delivery.

When the cervix becomes wide open as the result of uterine contractions and the baby's head (occasionally the feet or buttocks) is ready to appear, the mother will experience a 'bearing down sensation,' as though she were going to have a bowel movement. This is a sign that delivery of the baby is imminent. The person or persons helping should bear one important point in mind: Let the baby be born by itself. Do *not pull* and do *not* push on anything. Just scrub your hands thoroughly with plenty of soap and warm water, and have several clean towels ready to take care of the baby after it is born. While waiting, sterilize by boiling scissors or a knife as well as some string or heavy-duty thread.

Once the mother gets the 'bearing down feeling,' she should be allowed to push until the baby's head appears and stretches the opening of the vagina. At this point she should be instructed to take deep breaths, panting quickly, and thus allow the baby to be delivered *slowly*—otherwise considerable

harm may result to herself and the baby. She should keep her thighs and legs wide open, and there should be adequate space in front of her for the safe deposition of the baby after birth. Most babies are delivered face down, or turned to one side. After the head has appeared, do not be tempted to pull the rest of the baby out. The only thing you have to do now is check whether or not the cord is around the baby's neck; if it is, you should try gently to slip the cord over the baby's head and leave it there. If the cord is too tight to slip over the head, leave it alone; ask the mother to push the rest of the baby's body out: you may then unwrap the cord from the baby's neck.

Your attention now should be turned to the baby. Having wrapped a towel around its ankles, get a firm grip on its feet and raise them, letting the head and the rest of the body hang down while you gently wrap the baby's back. There is no need for the traditional slap on the bottom—most babies will cry at this time. You may then put the baby down beside the mother, making sure that the cord is slack. Using a clean (preferably boiled) piece of string, tie the cord five or six inches away from the baby's navel; then tie it again an inch or so further away and cut between the two ties with a pair of clean (preferably sterilized) scissors. Then make sure that the part of the cord connected with the baby is not bleeding; if it is, put another tie close to the first one. Wrap the baby in a warm towel and leave it alone. A normal healthy baby will need nothing else at this time.

The afterbirth is still inside the uterus, which now looks like a hard, pear-shaped mass with the top just above the mother's navel. Do *not* pull on the cord. You may, however, apply some gentle massage with one hand to the top of the uterus, above the mother's navel. Do *not* push. The uterus will get harder again and ten to fifteen minutes after delivery of the baby you may notice a small gush of blood coming through the vagina. This means that the afterbirth has become detached from the uterus and is ready to be delivered. Indeed, soon afterward you will see it coming through the vagina and finally being expelled. Continue applying gentle massage of the uterus for thirty to forty-five minutes following delivery of the afterbirth. This will help the uterus remain tight, and prevent excessive bleeding.

Remove the wet and bloody bedcovers and keep the mother clean and warm. If she asks for something to drink, she may be given water or juice. The mother will need rest now; see that she gets it, and keep an eye on the amount of vaginal bleeding. If no tears have occurred in the vagina and the mother's womb becomes nice and tight, no active bleeding should be present.

In case of a breech delivery, the course will be about the same as described above. The only difference is that one or both feet may be seen protruding through the vagina for a considerable time before the baby is really ready to be born. The temptation to pull them is great—be sure to resist it. When the right time comes, the baby will be born of its own accord.

In general, it should be remembered that a normal delivery requires little or no help from an outsider. If something does go wrong, only experienced and qualified persons can help. The amateur is liable to cause more harm than good to both mother and baby.

UTERUS
BAG OF WATERS
CORD
PLACENTA
CERVIX

Figures 1–3. Anatomy of pregnancy, delivery, and umbilical cord.

Figure 4. Umbilical cord wrapped around baby's neck.

TIE
TIE
UMBILICAL CORD

Figure 5. Tying and cutting the umbilical cord.

DIABETES IN PREGNANCY Although most women with diabetes have a very good chance of bearing normal children, there is a definite hazard to the mother and child. Diabetes is almost invariably more difficult to control during pregnancy. Insulin requirements are more variable and diet is more difficult to regulate. Of greater importance from the long-range standpoint is the fact that the effects of diabetes on the kidneys may be aggravated by the increased burden of pregnancy.

The effect of diabetes on the unborn child is also potentially harmful. Prematurity is common in diabetic pregnancies, and stillborn infants are more often encountered than in mothers who do not have diabetes. Furthermore, many newborn babies of diabetic mothers have a very high birthweight.

In general, it is wise for diabetic women who know they also have either high blood pressure, kidney disease, or eye complications to avoid pregnancy.

DIET IN PREGNANCY One of the most disturbing and occasionally dangerous complications of pregnancy is excessive weight gain. The appetite in general is improved during pregnancy and, unless the pregnant woman watches the quantity and quality of her caloric intake, she may gain tremendous weight and endanger both her life and that of the baby.

The total weight gain during the entire pregnancy should probably be about twenty to thirty pounds. This can be accomplished without much difficulty provided the patient's intake does not exceed 2,000 to 3,000 calories daily. The quality of the food should be checked in order to make sure it provides more proteins, vitamins, and minerals than the average diet. Sufficient quantities of meat, fish and poultry, fruits and vegetables as well as an average of one quart of milk daily should be the basis of a proper diet for the pregnant woman. In addition, the expectant mother will require extra amounts of iron and calcium and several vitamins. All these requirements are easily met today, with special multi-vitamin and mineral preparations usually taken in one-a-day oral form.

Sudden weight gain during the last few weeks or months of pregnancy should be con-sidered a danger sign, especially if accompanied by swelling ankles, puffiness of the face, and headaches, and should be immediately reported to the physician.

DOUCHING Medical opinion is not unanimous on whether douching should be part of a woman's hygiene during her reproductive years. Some doctors believe that frequent douching may disturb the natural (benign) flora of the vaginal region and should therefore be avoided except in some infections.

Douching should always be done in a reclining position, preferably in a bathtub. Plain vinegar (two tablespoons to a quart of warm water) is as good a douching solution as any of the commercially prepared ones, and costs practically nothing. If there is persistent vaginal discharge which continues in spite of douching, this is usually due to infection and should be treated by a physician.

DYSMENORRHEA Dysmenorrhea is the severe, sometimes incapacitating, pain accompanying the monthly menstrual flow. Whether the cause is anatomical, hormonal, or psychosomatic, the fact remains that dysmenorrhea is a very painful experience for the patient. Its monthly recurrence may tremendously affect the personality of its sufferers.

Symptoms. Symptoms vary from an acute, colicky type of lower-abdominal (pelvic) pain lasting for the first one or two days of the menstrual flow, to milder but steadier pelvic soreness, not infrequently affecting the patient's thighs, knees, and legs. The patient may also complain of sensations of heaviness and fullness in the lower abdomen, with mild or moderate nausea and (occasionally) vomiting. Headaches, nervousness, and a general feeling of being "unwell" may be a part of the total picture. Part or all of these symptoms usually disappear one or two days after the beginning of menstrual flow.

Treatment. Such a complex and poorly understood entity as dysmenorrhea requires a carefully planned and individually suited program for its relief. Sympathetic understanding and cooperation between physician and patient are a prerequisite for the treatment. Relatively mild analgesics (aspirin or equivalents) will suffice for the milder cases. Stronger analgesics (narcotics) may be required for a day or two in more severe cases. Mild sedatives (in addition to the analgesics) will make it easier for the patient to withstand moderate discomfort. Quite successful also are diuretic drugs given for two to three days before the onset of menstruation; they help relieve the sensation of heaviness and fullness of the lower abdomen, while nausea and vomiting is usually much improved or disappears. In some persistent cases, dilatation of the cervix and scraping of the uterus (D&C) may help temporarily or permanently.

In very resistant cases, temporary interruption of the menstrual periods by the use of hormones will definitely rid the patient of her symptoms, and quite often she will not require further treatment after her periods are allowed to occur normally.

DYSPAREUNIA   Pain experienced by the female during intercourse, dyspareunia may be caused by a variety of conditions. Often the male is responsible, either because of an excessively large penis, or because of ignorance of the act of proper sexual relations. In the female, the most common causes are infection of the vagina or the adjoining structures; an extremely narrow or tight hymen, or too small a vagina (atrophic vagina being a relatively common cause of dyspareunia in postmenopausal women); congenital anomalies of the vagina; abnormal placement of the uterus, so that it is turned backwards and sits on top of the vagina; abnormal placement of the ovaries or infection of the tubes; endometriosis; or psychosomatic factors—alone, or in coexistence with one or more of the above.

Treatment.   Treatment depends on the cause. Infections should be treated; congenital anomalies, acquired malpositions, or tumors should be corrected surgically; a tight hymen must be cut or stretched; and atrophic vaginas of older women can be treated with hormones. Younger, inexperienced couples should be intelligently instructed about the physiological methods of intercourse and the usefulness of lubricants. Psychosomatic factors should be eliminated through careful analysis and some form of counseling. The overall prognosis is very good, and the majority of patients can be helped through specialized professional care.

DYSTOCIA   This term applies to difficulties in labor and delivery. The most common causes are large babies or small pelvic-size of the mother, inability of the pregnant uterus to contract normally, pelvic tumors. Treatment will depend on the cause of dystocia. Quite often caesarean section is required.

ECLAMPSIA   *See* TOXEMIAS OF PREGNANCY in this section.

ENDOMETRIOSIS   This disease is due to the presence of endometrial tissue in areas other than the cavity of the uterus. During menstruation this "out-of-place" (ectopic) tissue undergoes the same changes as the normal endometrium, growing, then bleeding, and causing severe pain. The mechanism through which this endometrial tissue becomes ectopic is still an unsettled question. It becomes commonly implanted on the ovaries, tubes, ligaments of the uterus, top of the vagina, and occasionally in such unusual places as the rectum, lungs, etc.

Symptoms.   Depending on the organ involved and the extent of the lesions, endometriosis is marked by severe pain at, or just before, the onset of the menstrual flow. Acute intermittent cramps in the lower abdomen, or a constant "achy" feeling in the pelvis with dyspareunia, nervousness, and irritability are common.

The ovaries are sometimes involved in extensive endometriosis, resulting in sterility and therefore the loss of the only natural way of treatment of endometriosis: pregnancy. If the bladder is involved, the patient may experience burning on urination during menstrual periods, while involvement of the rectum will result in difficulties of defecation and occasional rectal bleeding. Involvement of the lungs (very rare) may result in "spitting of blood" during the menstrual period.

Treatment.   Conventional surgical treatment of endometriosis has largely been replaced by the use of lasers, which can remove areas of endometriosis and open adhesions caused by scarring with less risk to surrounding tissue. Hormone therapy also is effective. The purpose is to prevent the ovary from ovulating and the uterus from menstruating; in this way, the ectopic endometrial tissue remains dormant, not undergoing the monthly cyclic changes. When hormone therapy is continued for at least six months, most of the patients obtain permanent, or at least prolonged relief. Pregnancy accomplishes the same end by a natural process. Some patients (about 20 percent) may need to take more than one course of treatment, while others are better candidates for surgery. The hormones used for treatment of endometriosis are progesterone-like drugs, taken daily by mouth. The prognosis is generally good, and some of the patients may become pregnant.

ENDOMETRITIS Endometritis is an acute or chronic infection of the endometrium. The most common type of acute endometritis occurs three to four days after childbirth and is characterized by lower-abdominal pain, fever, and bloody foul-smelling vaginal discharge. The infection responds to treatment with antibiotics, and the prognosis is good.

ENDOMETRIUM The tissue lining the inside of the uterus, the endometrium is under the constant influence of the ovarian hormones during the reproductive life of a woman. It undergoes hypertrophy (growth) and is eventually shed, together with blood, in the form of menstrual flow. If pregnancy occurs, the endometrium serves for the implantation of the afterbirth (placenta) and the nourishment of the fetus.

ENGAGEMENT, OBSTETRICAL In obstetrics, engagement of the baby's head means the descent of the head into the true bony pelvis of the mother. It occurs much more commonly in mothers carrying their first baby, and may take place several weeks before term. The mother feels the change, observing that her "uterus has dropped," about the beginning of the ninth month.

EPISIOTOMY The cutting of the tissues between the vagina and the rectum during delivery, episiotomy facilitates the passage of the baby. Some obstetricians advocate episiotomy as a routine, especially for first deliveries arguing that in addition to allowing the baby to be born without too much squeezing through the birth canal, it protects against irregular tearing, and overstretching of the vagina.

FALLOPIAN TUBES Approximately four inches in length, the fallopian tubes extend on each side of the uterus and serve to connect the cavity of the uterus with the two ovaries. The tubes are necessary for transporting the egg from the ovaries to the uterus, and fertilization of the egg by a spermatozoon usually takes place in one of them. If both tubes are obstructed, fertilization is impossible. Tying of the tubes (tubal ligation) is a simple and popular method for surgical sterilization; it is successful in preventing pregnancy in approximately 99 percent of the cases.

Development of the fertilized egg in any location other than the uterus is called an ectopic pregnancy. The most common such abnormal location is the tube, a "tubal pregnancy." Such a pregnancy cannot go on for more than a short time before abnormal bleeding from the implantation site and possible rupture of the tube occurs. This necessitates surgical intervention.

FETAL PRESENTATIONS The part of the fetus that lies against the mouth of the cervix determines its presentation. *Head* or *cephalic presentations* are the most common, occurring in about 96 percent of all deliveries. In breech presentations, the baby emerges feet or buttocks first. *Breech presentations* may be *complete* or *full* (the thighs are against the abdomen and the feet are alongside the buttocks), *frank* (the buttocks are down, the legs are straight up and the feet are at the shoulders) or *footling* (one or both feet are the first to exit the uterus). Rarely, the fetus will lie across the uterus with the shoulder as the presenting part (shoulder presentation or transverse lie). Unless the fetus can be turned in the uterus, a caesarean section must be performed. (*See also* BREECH in this section.)

FIBROADENOMAS Most often occurring in women in their teens and early twenties, fibroadenomas are noncancerous solid, slippery, round lumps in the breasts. They do not seem to be associated with the menstrual cycle and usually are not painful. If any suspicious characteristics exist, they should be biopsied or a mammogram performed. They may be surgically removed.

FIBROCYSTIC BREAST DISEASE

This noncancerous condition is characterized by clusters of liquid-filled cysts, usually firm, mobile, well-defined, and painful, that may grow in size just before the menstrual period. Because the lumps usually do not appear after menopause, it is believed that ovarian hormones are involved. The condition may require no treatment; however, if any of the lumps are of questionable size, shape, or nature, they should be biopsied. In addition, a baseline mammogram may be recommended to distinguish the lumps from early breast cancer.

FIBROIDS (FIBROMYOMATA OF THE UTERUS)

These benign tumors are more prevalent in women between the ages of thirty-five and fifty. They are usually multiple tumors, quite firm, and their growth is slow—especially after the menopause, when they practically cease growing. Fibroids vary from marble-size to huge tumors weighing up to fifty pounds. The cause of these nonmalignant growths is unknown, although there has been definite association between their development and high levels of estrogenic hormones.

Symptoms. The symptoms of fibroids depend on their location and size. If they are located inside or very close to the cavity of the uterus, they cause abnormal vaginal bleeding as well as infertility. When located at the outside surface, they may not be noticed until they grow very large; a feeling of fullness and heaviness in the lower abdomen and constant backache may then occur because of their size. Very often fibroids press the top of the bladder and cause difficulties in urination, kidney infections, etc.

It is rare for fibroids to change into malignant tumors. Fibroids may also be responsible for infertility, or for abortion if pregnancy occurs. Often such tumors, growing from a small cord (pedicle), become twisted and inflamed, and severe abdominal pain follows. If fibroids are present during a full-term pregnancy, they may cause difficulties in labor and delivery.

Treatment. Treatment of fibroids will depend on the symptoms. Fibroid tumors located very close to the cavity of the uterus and producing bleeding will have to be removed, usually by removing the whole uterus; if they are outside the uterus and the patient is young, able, and willing to have children, then the tumors only are removed sometimes through laser surgery, and the uterus is left intact. Truly large tumors are usually removed together with the uterus.

Fibroid tumors in patients who have passed the menopause are removed only if they are too large and cause pressure difficulties; or if they cause bleeding, regardless of their size. The choice will have to be left to the gynecologist who, during the operation, will use his best judgment in deciding whether the uterus can be saved for a useful purpose, or whether everything should be removed. The patient should always be prepared to face the fact that childbearing may become impossible for her.

FORCEPS   These are several types of long, spoon-like obstetrical instruments, made of stainless steel or aluminum and used for the extraction of the baby's head from the patient's birth canal. When used under the proper circumstances and by experienced obstetricians, forceps deliveries may simplify and shorten an otherwise difficult delivery. The patient is usually given some type of satisfactory anesthetic, and the baby's head is delivered with forceps, under the physician's control; in this way the baby as well as the mother are less liable to be injured by very rapid delivery. The slight marks left on the baby's face and scalp disappear very promptly.

GESTATIONAL AGE   Each newborn is classified as premature, full-term, or postmature. These refer to the length of gestation and not to weight.

An infant born before thirty-seven full weeks of gestation is considered premature, usually weighs less than five and a half pounds, and is at risk for many complications. However, a full-term infant—delivered between 38 and 42 weeks of gestation—may weigh less than five and a half pounds and be considered small for gestational age. Although having a low birth weight, the infant usually will have fewer problems than the premature infant, because generally its organs are more developed than the premature infant.

An infant is considered post-mature if it is born after 42 weeks of gestation. Labor may be induced to avoid fetal distress.

GONADS   The gonads are the sex glands; in the female they are the ovaries, and in the male the testes.

The ovaries are located in the pelvic region of the abdominal cavity, one on each side of the uterus. They produce the eggs (ova) which travel along the fallopian tubes to the uterus. If fertilized by a male sperm-cell (spermatozoon), an egg is implanted in the uterine wall and grows to form the fetus. The ovaries are also the site of production of estrogen (female hormone) and progesterone (pregnancy hormone). (*See also* TESTICLES (TESTES) in the section MALE HEALTH CARE.)

GYNECOLOGY   This is the medical specialty concerned with the diagnosis and treatment, both medical and surgical, of diseases of the female genital organs. In recent years great progress in gynecology has been made through intensive research, mainly in the field of hormones, and the early detection and treatment of genital cancer. Lasers, devices that transform light energy into heat, have proven effective in diagnosing and treating a number of gynecologic conditions.

Specialists practicing gynecology are called gynecologists; most of them are given combined training in both gynecology and obstetrics.

HEREDITY   Heredity is the endowment of offspring by parents (beginning with the fertilized egg) with physical and psychological characteristics. Reproduction never results in an exact replica of either progenitor although there may be a remarkable resemblance. Variation in offspring actually opposes heredity. The germ cells arising from sexual reproduction bear certain substances which account for inheritance. Of paramount importance are the carriers of hereditary factors, the chromosomes. Research indicates that there are 46 in each human cell, except in the mature sperm and ovum in which there are 23 in each. Thus, a child inherits 23 chromosomes from each parent. The chromosomes carry genes which are hereditary factors.

Neither natural science, nor anthropology, nor medicine, nor any other division of science has ever fully explained how a single fertilized egg can develop into an organism with billions of differentiated cells, with the capacity to reproduce itself, and with an almost endless number of functions, complex organs, and feelings. Molecular biologists seem to have the answer in the extremely complex cellular substances DNA (desoxyribonucleic acid) and RNA (ribonucleic acid).

DNA and RNA are found in every living cell, animal and vegetable. In brief, DNA transmits orders from cell to cell (through its "executive officer" and "roving ambassador," RNA), and from one generation to another. DNA builds proteins in the cells, and without amino acids (derivatives of proteins) life is not possible. The endless permutations that DNA undergoes in its fissuring explains inheritance; the unusual and even recessive combinations in DNA particles that can suddenly pop up in one generation (never seen before or existing in generations before) strips the mystery from the "sport" which geneticists have never been able to explain in their otherwise set theory of mutation.

In psychiatry, there is no proof that all mental illness or retardation can be inherited or that they are familial in nature. Nevertheless certain types of mental retardation are known to be inheritable, for example, amaurotic family idiocy (Tay-Sachs disease). It is also true that an inherited constitutional predisposition does appear to play a role in some mental afflictions, but the emergence of a psychosis or a psychoneurosis in a given individual is determined by many factors. It has also been shown that a predisposition to epilepsy is inheritable, since normal children of epileptic parents may produce epileptic brain rhythms in electroencephalographic tracings.

HERPES, GENITAL, IN THE FEMALE
If a woman has ever had genital herpes or if her current (or past) sexual partner has genital herpes, she needs to tell her doctor when she becomes pregnant. Babies can get herpes during delivery if the virus is present in the birth canal. Tragically, more than half of the babies who become infected during delivery will die or suffer severe damage.

Babies can also get herpes if they are kissed by someone with a cold sore. A young baby can not fight off infections as easily as an adult can, so serious problems may result. It's important that you do not kiss a baby when you have a cold sore.

Some studies suggest that women with genital herpes may be at greater risk of developing cervical cancer than other women. Since early cell changes can be detected by Pap smears, all women with genital herpes should have regular Pap tests—at least once a year. Early detection and treatment of cervical cancer can usually prevent the spread of disease.

HYDATIDIFORM MOLE This is a disease of early pregnancy in which the fetus undergoes degeneration and takes the form and appearance of a bunch of vesicles (grape-like structures) which are eventually aborted. The disease is much more common in people of Asian origin. It becomes dangerous only when it changes to its malignant form, chorionepithelioma; this occurs in approximately 7 to 8 percent of the cases.

Symptoms. The uterus is usually much larger than in a normal pregnancy. The patient's blood pressure rises quite rapidly, and there are severe headaches, nausea and vomiting. The patient looks puffy, and eventually bleeding starts through the vagina. Labor pains usually follow, the bleeding becomes worse, and the patient may notice pieces of grape-like tissue filled with fluid coming out of the vagina.

Treatment. Treatment of hydatidiform mole consists of complete evacuation of the uterus, followed by thorough scraping. The patient should be checked for at least a year, with special tests to make sure that the mole does not change to a malignant chorionepithelioma. (More than one scraping of the uterus may be required, and blood transfusions may be necessary.) When tests are negative on three successive occasions, the patient may be considered cured, and another pregnancy can be permitted without fear that the same thing may happen again (at least with no more chance than in any other pregnancy). In certain cases, removal of the uterus (hysterectomy) will be indicated; this will depend on the patient's age and the number of children she already has, as well as on pathological examination of the mole.

HYDRAMNIOS This term refers to the production of excessive amounts of amniotic fluid ("baby's water") during pregnancy. The patient's abdomen will look huge, distended, and shiny; her weight will increase rapidly; and there may be swelling of the ankles and high blood pressure. What is more significant, and a real cause for concern, is the fact that hydramnios is usually associated with severe congenital malformations of the baby.

HYMEN This anatomical structure of the female consists of a membranous formation located at the entrance of the vagina. Its location and (usually) delicate consistency have made this organ so notorious a proof of virginity that many otherwise-harmonious marriages have been doomed to failure, especially in more conservative and less informed societies, if the bride's hymen is found missing. The ironic fact is that intact state of the hymen is far from being a reliable evidence of virginity. Its size and structure may vary from a very thin and fragile membrane which easily tears upon first intercourse, to a very thick and ring-like structure which occasionally remains intact even after delivery. (The majority of hymens, however, do rupture after normal sexual relations.) It is even possible for the hymen to rupture as a result of accidents (falls, traumas in that area, etc.). Occasionally the hymen is completely closed (imperforate hymen), so that, when the menstrual flow of the female first begins, it has no way to escape, accumulates in the vagina, and causes discomfort. The cure is simple: incision of the hymen. One reason for a routine gynecological exam prior to marriage is for the physician to assess the hymen. A simple procedure, hymenectomy, can prevent unnecessary discomfort during the woman's first intercourse.

HYSTERECTOMY The removal of the uterus, hysterectomy may be done either through the abdomen (abdominal hysterectomy) or through the vagina (vaginal hysterectomy). Whenever the womb is enlarged or there is indication for removal of the ovaries, or when exploration of the abdomen is indicated, the abdominal route is preferred. On the other hand, when the uterus is small—and especially when repair of the vagina and the bladder is indicated—the vaginal approach is much more practical. In addition to avoiding a scar on the abdomen, a vaginal hysterectomy usually makes postoperative recovery of the patient faster and more comfortable.

HYSTEROGRAM (HYSTEROSALPINGOGRAM) This is an X-ray picture of the uterus and tubes, after injection into the uterus of a liquid impenetrable to X-rays. The purpose is to demonstrate whether the tubes are open or obstructed, and whether the cavity of the uterus is normal or deformed because of congenital malformations or acquired abnormalities (usually fibroid tumors).

INFERTILITY *See* STERILITY AND INFERTILITY in this section.

HYSTERECTOMY

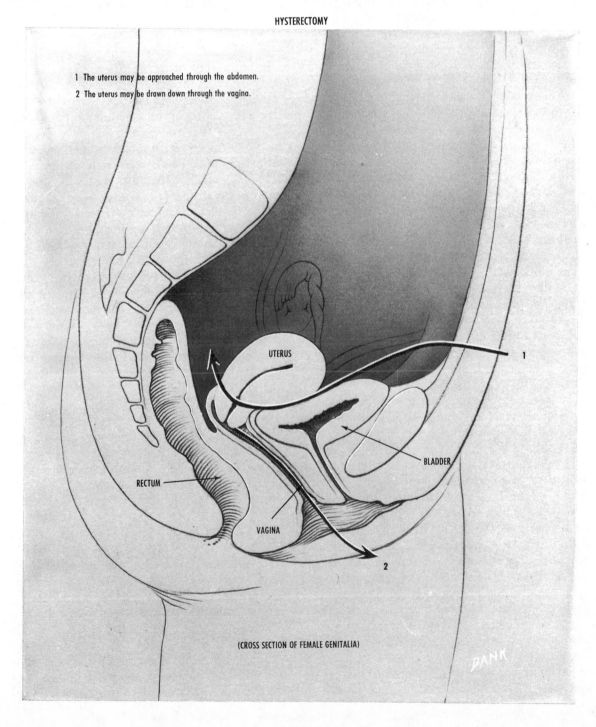

1 The uterus may be approached through the abdomen.

2 The uterus may be drawn down through the vagina.

UTERUS

RECTUM

VAGINA

BLADDER

1

2

(CROSS SECTION OF FEMALE GENITALIA)

DANK

IN VITRO FERTILIZATION Through this procedure, an egg is removed from the mother's ovary, transferred to a laboratory dish, where it is fertilized by the father's sperm and cultured, and then transferred to the mother's uterus. In vitro fertilization is used principally in women whose fallopian tubes are damaged or missing. The first successful in vitro fertilization was in 1978, and since that time hundreds of children have been born using this method. Although the procedure offers hope to couples who might not have been otherwise able to conceive, questions have arisen about its appropriateness, specifically its use by unmarried couples and women (surrogate mothers) hired to carry another couple's child.

IRON-DEFICIENCY ANEMIA IN PREGNANCY This type of anemia is quite common in pregnancy because the baby takes up a large amount of iron from the mother's reserves in order to build up its own blood. Also some women may have had some degree of pre-existent anemia. It may then be advisable that pregnant women, in addition to vitamin preparations, take iron pills regularly after the first three months of pregnancy. Today there are many preparations which combine iron and vitamins in one-a-day form and, if these do not suffice, supplementary iron pills must also be given. For the occasional patient who cannot tolerate iron given by mouth, there are special iron solutions available by injection.

LABIA These are two pairs of folds of skin, one inside the other, at the entrance of the vagina. The inside pair (labia minora) is smaller than the outside pair (labia majora) and, unlike the latter, has no hair.

LABOR Active labor consists of regular contractions of the pregnant uterus, which cause the cervix to open wide and allow delivery of the baby. These contractions are felt by the mother as labor pains and should not be confused with the irregular, short, and slightly uncomfortable pains which the mother experiences for several weeks before term. These latter are known as Braxton-Hicks contractions and may be the cause of false labor; they are useful in preparing the cervix for active labor, but do not accomplish any dilatation of the cervix. When contractions are at regular intervals of fifteen minutes or less, and the mother starts to feel them as labor pains, then she enters the phase of true labor; the doctor or nurse or midwife should be notified and/or the patient taken to the hospital if this is where she plans to deliver.

The duration of labor varies considerably, depending on the number of previous pregnancies and on the constitution of the individual patient. On the average, it lasts fifteen to eighteen hours in patients laboring on their first baby, and approximately six hours less in patients who have already had one or more children. For practical purposes, the entire length of labor is divided into three stages.

The first stage of labor starts with the onset of regular uterine contractions and ends with the complete dilatation of the cervix. This covers about 90 percent of the total length of labor. During the first stage, the labor pains become gradually stronger, longer, and closer together, and the patient may require drugs for relief. The patient may notice pink vaginal discharge, which is mucus from the cervix mixed with some blood. This is known as bloody show. The bag of waters (membranes) may or may not rupture during this stage.

The second stage covers the period between complete cervical dilatation and delivery of the baby. In patients having their first child, this stage lasts one to two hours; while in subsequent pregnancies it only lasts twenty to thirty minutes. During this stage the patient experiences a bearing-down sensation and she pushes voluntarily, using her abdominal muscles. Using breathing techniques learned buring childbirth preparation classes or through the use of anesthesia, the patient is able to control the urge to bear down until she is instructed to push, and the baby is delivered.

The third stage of labor starts after the delivery of the baby and ends with the delivery of the afterbirth (placenta). This phase is approximately fifteen minutes in duration.

Under certain circumstances labor is induced artificially (induction of labor) for the benefit of the baby, the mother, or both. Induction of labor may be accomplished by stripping the membranes from the cervix. The only reliable means for induction of labor, however, are the so-called "oxytocin drugs"—hormones produced by the pituitary. When administered to the pregnant patient, these cause regular uterine contractions. These drugs are administered by continuous intravenous drip, diluted in large amounts of fluids. Intramuscular administration of oxytocic drugs should be avoided before the delivery of the baby.

In some instances labor starts normally, lasts for several hours, and—for a variety of reasons—may then slow down. (This is called uterine inertia.) In some cases the doctor will either resort to stimulation of labor with the same oxytocic drugs, or to caesarean section, depending on the individual case.

LACTATION Lactation, the secretion of normal milk from the mother's breasts, starts two to three days after the delivery of the baby. At this time the mother notices her breasts becoming enlarged and painful; milk may leak from the nipples.

Large amounts of nutritive substances and antibodies are secreted in the mother's milk. The diet of the lactating mother should therefore be improved in quality and quantity (about 1,000 more calories than before pregnancy will be required in her daily diet). Drugs, alcohol, and other toxic substances are promptly secreted in the milk, and the mother should avoid them and consult a physician before taking any type of medication.

Menstrual periods are usually absent for several months during lactation; however, lactation is not a reliable form of birth control. Ovulation can occur, and pregnancy may follow without a preceding menstrual flow; this creates difficulties in the recognition of early pregnancy, and not infrequently the mother becomes aware of a new pregnancy only when the baby starts moving. When this happens, nursing should be discontinued.

LEUKORRHEA Often referred to as vaginitis this condition represents excessive vaginal discharge, whitish or yellowish in color, often due to infection of the vagina by trichomonas or monilia organisms. Treatment consists of vaginal or oral medications and vaginal douches. (*See also* VAGINITIS in this section.)

LOCHIA This is a term applied to the vaginal discharge that follows delivery of the baby and placenta. For the first two to four days after delivery, the lochia are bloody, becoming pink for the next few days, and finally turning whitish.

MAMMOGRAPHY This low-dose X-ray examination is used to diagnose certain breast abnormalities, especially cancer. It can often detect a cancerous tumor at a very small size, long before it can be felt. A negative mammography result may not necessarily rule out the possibility of cancer; if a suspicious lump exists, it should be biopsied. Mammography is also not intended as a substitute for monthly breast self-examination. The American Cancer Society recommends that women have a baseline reference mammogram between the ages of thirty-five and thirty-nine, a mammogram every one to two years between the ages of forty and forty-nine, and a yearly mammogram after that.

MASTITIS Inflammation of the breast is known as mastitis. It usually occurs in mothers who are breast-feeding and is generally caused by bacteria that enter the mammary gland through a break in the nipple. Symptoms include swelling, redness, tenderness in a particular area, fever, and general weakness. It can be treated with antibiotics. If the infection is not treated early, it may cause an abscess that will have to be surgically drained and treated with antibiotics.

MEMBRANES While the baby is carried in the mother's uterus it is surrounded by the amniotic fluid, which is contained within a thin sac (the membranes, or bag of waters). The membranes may rupture before or during labor; it is very important that the patient notifies her doctor as soon as the bag of waters breaks and fluid runs out through the vagina. Once the membranes have ruptured, sexual relations, douches, or other vaginal manipulations are contraindicated.

MENARCHE This is the onset of menstrual periods. (*See also* MENSTRUATION in this section.)

MENOPAUSE   Termination of the reproductive period in the life of a woman—the "change of life"—is called the menopause or female climacteric. The average age for the menopause is fifty, although it may occur a few years earlier or later. The menopause is caused by cessation of the normal function of the ovaries, resulting in gradual or sudden disappearance of menstrual periods. Surgical removal or sterilizing irradiation of the ovaries will result in an artificial menopause.

Symptoms. The symptoms of menopause vary. In some cases cessation of menstrual periods may be the only change. On the other hand, the change of life may be accompanied by excessive physical, functional, and emotional disturbances that require prompt recognition and therapy. The commonest symptoms are sudden or (more often) gradual cessation of menstrual periods; hot flushes—or flashes as they are sometimes called—with the patient feeling a wave of heat passing over her body, sometimes accompanied by actual flushing of the face and neck followed by sweating; weight-gain; atrophic changes of the genital organs, the change sometimes being experienced in the form of itching in the genital area and dyspareunia (pain during intercourse); and psychological symptoms, headaches, dizziness, depression, and insomnia. The symptoms become worse because of inherent fears that the patient is getting old, is losing her sex appeal, and is no longer able to bear children. Most of these fears are unfounded. A menopausal woman with a healthy attitude towards this physiological stage of her life may be as happy and active in all her activities as before. *Warning:* Any amount of vaginal bleeding or spotting occurring after the definite cessation of the menstrual periods should be considered abnormal and potentially dangerous; the woman should seek medical advice immediately, to check for the possible presence of cancer of the female organs (usually uterus or ovaries).

Treatment. The fact that menopause is a normal biological phenomenon should not be taken for granted, and all means available for the well-being of the patient should be utilized. All the symptoms of menopause can be relieved with a daily intake of one of the ovarian hormones available commercially at very low cost. Used properly, they offer a sense of well-being to the postmenopausal woman for many more years. Many patients, of course, can do quite well without hormone therapy or without sedative and antidepressant drugs. Some controversy persists about estrogen therapy so it is important to use the lowest effective dose and continue only under a physician's supervision.

MENORRHAGIA   *See* Uterine Bleeding, Abnormal in this section.

MENSTRUAL CYCLE   This recurring cycle of change in the lining of the uterus varies in duration, but it lasts an average of 28 days. The cycle begins on the first day of menstrual bleeding and ends on the day before the next menstrual period. From the gynecologist's point of view, the menstrual cycle is divided into three phases: the menstrual phase, three to five days in duration, represents the days of active menstrual bleeding; the early or proliferative phase, which on a normal twenty-eight-day cycle covers the next nine to ten days; finally the late or secretory phase which covers the last thirteen to fourteen days, just before the next menstrual period.

Ovulation (release of the egg) occurs between the early and late phase, on about the fourteenth day of the cycle. This is the optimal time for conception. (*See also* Menstruation in this section.)

MENSTRUATION   Menstruation begins with puberty, usually between the ages of nine and sixteen, continues throughout the woman's childbearing years and terminates with the onset of menopause (usually between the ages of forty-five and fifty but normally, as late as 60). Several factors affect the onset of menstruation: race, nutrition, genetic inheritance, etc. Beginning of menstrual function under the age of eight or its delay beyond the age of eighteen should be considered abnormal and should be investigated.

The menstrual flow usually occurs every twenty-eight days and lasts for three to five days; the amount of flow is relatively heavy for the first two days and then gradually decreases. It is not abnormal for a woman to have menstrual periods closer together or further apart (ranging from twenty to thirty-five days or more), so long as they come at regular intervals. During the first year or two after the onset of menstruation there may be considerable irregularity in the interval, duration, and amounts of menstrual periods; this is due to the lack of ovulation, and corrects itself over time.

The monthly menstrual periods (menses) are the result of a very complex interaction of hormones from several glands, mainly the ovaries and pituitary. With the approach of puberty, the pituitary produces special hormones which make the ovaries and the uterus mature and become ready for subsequent cyclic changes that will enable the female to start her reproductive career. The rhythmic changes of the pituitary, ovaries, and uterus that result in the monthly menstrual flow may be outlined as follows: The pituitary secretes follicle-stimulating hormone (FSH) and stimulates the ovary to produce estrogens, which in turn stimulate the lining of the uterus (endometrium) to proliferate (grow thicker). The high levels of estrogens then act as a block for the further production of FSH by the pituitary, which now produces another hormone, the luteinizing hormone (LH), which promotes maturation of one out of thousands of eggs (ova) in the ovary. Ovulation then occurs, usually on the fourteenth day after the last menstrual period. If conception takes place, the menstrual periods stop for the next nine months.

In the absence of pregnancy, the pituitary secretes still another hormone, the luteotrophic hormone (LTH), which results in the formation of the corpus luteum in the ovary; this new glandular structure starts producing another hormone, progesterone, which again stimulates the endometrium to further growth. At this point estrogen levels have dropped to their lowest levels, and the pituitary once more secretes more FSH and less LTH; progesterone levels drop; and the endometrium (which is now at the peak of its growth), losing its hormonal support, breaks down and is expelled from the womb together with blood in the form of menstrual bleeding. By this time the pituitary again produces large amounts of FSH, the estrogen levels rise once more, and the endometrium starts a new

cycle. (*See also* PREMENSTRUAL SYNDROME [PMS] in this section.)

MISCARRIAGE   (SPONTANEOUS ABORTION)   A pregnancy that ends naturally before twenty weeks is considered a miscarriage, or a spontaneous abortion. An estimated 10 to 12 percent of all pregnancies end in miscarriage, with the majority occurring in the first trimester. Defects in the fetus are the principal cause for a miscarriage that occurs at this early stage. Second trimester miscarriages are generally caused by maternal factors, such as diabetes mellitus, acute infection, or inability of the cervix to hold the fetus (incompetent cervix).

Vaginal bleeding or spotting, perhaps accompanied by cramplike pain, is the first sign that a miscarriage is threatened. The physician should be notified immediately. Rest may be sufficient to prevent the miscarriage. If the bleeding is heavy, the cervix has begun to dilate, or the bag of waters has ruptured, the miscarriage is considered inevitable. The miscarriage may progress without any intervention. However, in some instances, not all of the products of conception will be expelled, requiring the physician to intervene, usually with curettage or suction.

MORNING SICKNESS   This is a very common symptom of early pregnancy. It usually disappears after the first three months, although in some cases it may last throughout the entire duration of pregnancy. Morning sickness may vary from mild nausea to very severe and persistent vomiting in which the patient cannot retain any food, and a dangerous degree of dehydration may develop because of the loss of body fluids and minerals. This last condition is called hyperemesis gravidarum and may require hospitalization and administration of intravenous fluids.

The cause of morning sickness in pregnancy is not definitely known. In some cases psychosomatic factors are the cause. Whether the physiological changes of pregnancy, and the adjustment of the body to a new balance of hormones and electrolytes, are manifested in the form of nausea and vomiting is not known.

Treatment. Most cases are mild and the symptoms improve after the first trimester.

Eating small amounts in more frequent meals or eating a small amount before arising may help. Old suggestions include eating a cracker or olive first or having a few sips of a cold carbonated fluid or a few chips of ice. No drugs for morning sickness are approved by the FDA.

OBSTETRICS Obstetrics is the medical specialty concerned with the management of pregnancy, labor, and delivery—both normal and complicated. Physicians specializing in obstetrics are known as obstetricians. Today obstetrics and gynecology are combined in one specialty, known in abbreviation as OB-GYN.

OVARIAN CYSTS Usually benign, these liquid-filled sacs within the ovaries may disappear without any treatment. If, however, they are of sufficient size and persist for more than a month, surgical removal may be necessary to ensure that they are not cancerous. In some cases, they may collect more fluid and grow, another indication for surgery. Dermoid cysts, frequently containing hair, teeth, fatty material, and other tissue, are common in young women and are thought to be embryonic remnants. They require surgical removal. Lasers can be used to remove some cysts by uncapping the sac and vaporizing its interior. Ovarian cysts may cause discomfort, heaviness, or aching. However, they often have no symptoms and are discovered through pelvic examination.

OVARIES Two in number, one on each side close to the uterus, the ovaries are the main female glands, responsible for the production of eggs (ova) and the two major female hormones: estrogen and progesterone. Through these hormones, the ovaries are responsible for the development of the girl into a woman; for the maturation of her uterus; and for the further response of the uterus to changing hormone levels in the form of menstrual flow. The ovaries produce the ova and (after conception has occurred) will help maintain the pregnancy for the first few months.

As all other organs, the ovaries may be involved in a variety of acute and chronic diseases. Infections, cysts, and other tumors—

both benign and malignant—are liable to involve them. Most ovarian tumors are benign, but can become enormously large in size.

Cancer of the ovary is usually discovered in advanced stages, too late for it to be treated. This is one reason why every woman should have regular gynecological examinations. This is true both *before* and *after* the menopause. Many ovarian tumors arise postmenopausally. Thus, unlike the common fibroid tumors of the uterus, which often produce changes in the menstrual cycle, ovarian tumors can grow silently and first become manifest by pressure on the adjacent bladder or bowel.

OVULATION This term means the production of eggs (ova) by the ovary. During the reproductive span of the woman's life (from onset to cessation of menstrual periods), one egg is usually released by one of the two ovaries on alternating months. In the majority of women, ovulation occurs approximately fourteen days before the onset of a menstrual period. This is the most fertile period for a woman—in fact it is believed to be the only fertile period—and if pregnancy is desired, sexual relations should occur regularly or frequently during the period of six to seven days in the middle of the menstrual cycle. It is currently believed that the ovum is capable of normal fertilization for no more than twenty-four hours after ovulation.

Many women can actually pinpoint the day of ovulation by a sudden acute pain felt in the lower abdomen, sometimes on the left and sometimes on the right side. There are several methods of discovering whether ovulation has occurred or not; the most convenient and popular of these methods is the basal body-temperature record, which will show a sustained elevation of temperature of about one degree from the time of ovulation until the beginning of next menstrual period. Other methods consist of special tests carried out by the physician, such as vaginal smears, analysis of mucus from the cervix, and examination of uterine (endometrial) tissues by biopsies.

OXYTOCICS These are drugs used to produce contractions of the pregnant uterus. Since they can be very dangerous to both the

THE FEMALE PELVIS
(CROSS SECTION)

1 UTERUS
2 CERVIX
3 VAGINA
4 FALLOPIAN TUBE
5 OVARY
6 BLADDER
7 URETHRA
8 RECTUM
9 ANUS
10 PERINEUM
11 COCCYX
12 PUBIS
13 LABIA MINORA
14 LABIA MAJORA
15 ABDOMINAL WALL

mother and the baby if improperly used, their use is limited to the medical profession.

PAP SMEAR   The pap smear or pap test is a method for detecting cancer or precancerous conditions principally in the cervix. During a pelvic examination, cells are gently scraped from the cervix and placed on a glass slide, for laboratory examination.

PELVIMETRY   Pelvimetry is the measurement of the dimensions of the female pelvis. External pelvimetry consists of measurements of bony landmarks of the pelvis and gives rough measures of whether the pelvis is of adequate size. Pelvic capacity can also be evaluated while doing an internal bimanual examination during which, as an example, the size of the pelvic cavity, fore and aft, from pubic symphysis to sacrum, can be measured.

Because there is always some reluctance to use X-rays during a pregnancy, X-ray pelvimetry is now used much less frequently. It can, of course, be used prior to a pregnancy in assessing whether inadequate size or distortions in the way the pelvis developed may make a normal delivery problematic or impossible, in which case caesarean section may be necessary.

PELVIS (FEMALE)   This represents the lowest part of the abdominal cavity and is formed by a rigid bony girdle which is firmly

attached to the spine at the back, being hinged on the sides to the bones of the thighs (femoral bones). The floor of the female pelvis is formed by several layers of muscular and connective tissues and is penetrated, from the front backwards, by the opening of the bladder (urethra), the vagina, and the rectum. The floor of the pelvis is known as the perineum.

In addition to the bladder and loops of intestines, the female pelvis contains the uterus and ovaries. When pregnancy occurs, the pelvis plays a particularly important role in the accommodation and protection of the pregnant uterus.

The size of the bony pelvis is an all-important factor for the normal progress of labor and delivery. Disproportion between the size of the pelvis and that of the baby's head will cause difficulties in labor and delivery, and caesarean section will often be required for the baby's delivery.

PLACENTA (AFTERBIRTH)   The placenta is an irregularly round, flat, spongy organ attached to the inside of the pregnant uterus and connected with the fetus by the umbilical cord. The placenta is essential for exchange of nourishing substances and oxygen between mother and unborn child and for removal of waste products. Abnormalities of the placenta, such as premature separation from the uterus or atrophy and fibrosis, will affect the welfare of the baby and if the function of this organ is severely impaired, fetal death will occur. The placenta is the last of the products of conception to be expelled from the uterus; if parts of it are retained in the uterus after delivery, prolonged bleeding, pains, and infection may follow. Retained placenta may necessitate a dilatation and curettage (D&C).

PLACENTA PREVIA This is the implantation of the placenta over the mouth of the uterus. The placenta may cover the opening of the cervix entirely (total placenta previa) or partially (partial placenta previa). This abnormality results in vaginal bleeding, ranging from slight to very profuse and usually appearing in the absence of labor (when labor starts the bleeding becomes worse). The dangers for the fetus and the mother are not as severe as with abruptio; nevertheless this is a very serious complication of pregnancy and caesarean section is almost always required for the delivery of the baby.

POSTPARTUM *See* PUERPERIUM in this section.

PREGNANCY Pregnancy is the result of conception and subsequent implantation of the fertilized egg (ovum) inside the uterine cavity. The tubes, ovaries, or even the abdominal cavity are occasionally sites of implantation and development of the fertilized ovum (*see* TUBAL PREGNANCY in this section). The average duration of the human pregnancy is 280 days (ten lunar months or nine calendar months).

Signs and symptoms of early pregnancy are cessation of the monthly menstrual periods; morning sickness; enlargement and soreness of the breasts, with or without milk discharge; enlargement of the uterus; perception of fetal movements. None of these subjective symptoms is a definite sign of pregnancy, and the presence of one or more of them is merely suggestive, but not diagnostic, of pregnancy. Probable diagnosis of early pregnancy can be made by uterine palpation and verified by laboratory tests available for this purpose. The most widely used are chemical tests performed on a small amount of urine placed on a slide. Unlike the older biological tests using mice or rabbits, the new tests can give diagnostic results in a few minutes.

PREMENSTRUAL SYNDROME (PMS) The condition of mental tension, irritability, headache, depression and a feeling of "bloatedness," with some evidence of edema, usually begins in the week prior to menstruation and usually resolves completely the day after a menstrual period's flow has begun.

PMS is a common condition which causes a good deal of distress to those affected by it—which includes women of all ethnic and age groups. It may occur before the menarche, after the menopause and even after a hysterectomy. Hormonal origins are the obvious cause, with water and salt retention as the consequence of a hormonal imbalance; but psychogenic causes play their part in initiating a behavioral response to physical changes in the body.

Treatment. In severe cases, treatment is often effective with hormonal supplements of the progesterone type, with the initiation of anovulatory cycles by use of the oral contraceptive pill and with diurectics ("water pills") taken for the immediate premenstrual period.

PRENATAL CARE Most of the serious complications of pregnancy which may endanger the health and even the life of the baby and the mother, can today be prevented or controlled with regular prenatal care. Facilities ranging from private obstetricians to municipal or county prenatal clinics, are available for every socioeconomic group, and there is hardly any excuse for the expectant mother who neglects to register for prenatal care. The benefits for both the mother and the baby are numerous, while the potential risks of neglect can be truly dramatic. On the average, a total of ten to twelve visits during the entire nine months of pregnancy are adequate as excellent preparation of the expectant mother for a smooth pregnancy and delivery. Initially, monthly visits suffice; during the seventh and eighth months, they should be scheduled every two or three weeks, and during the last month every week. Important conditions that may call for treatment are the development of high blood pressure and of diabetes.

In the course of the visits, several important blood and urine tests are done by the obstetrician and repeated if necessary; the baby's growth is carefully followed; the mother is given instructions on diet, exercise, and rest;

vitamins and mineral preparations are prescribed, and any deviation from normal is thoroughly investigated and properly treated. The return on this very intelligent investment of time is an expectant mother who is physically and emotionally well prepared to go through the wonderful experience of childbirth with the least possible risks for herself and her baby.

To meet the nutritional requirements of pregnancy, to ensure that the newborn will have had available the best dietary constituents, and to correct any existing dietary deficiencies, it is recommended that a prenatal diet be of wide variety and well-balanced. (*See also* DIET IN PREGNANCY in this section.)

PROGESTERONE This hormone is secreted by the corpus luteum (yellow body) of the ovary and is commonly known as the hormone of pregnancy because it is produced after ovulation—during the second half of the menstrual cycle. If conception occurs, this hormone is essential for the maintenance of pregnancy. Eventually the placenta also participates in the production of progesterone and of the other hormones necessary for the normal development of pregnancy. Progesterone deficiencies may be a cause of occasional or habitual abortions. This abnormality can be detected through special laboratory tests and the patient treated with progesterone, orally or through injections, to achieve full-term delivery. Progesterone is available in tablet form and, combined with a small amount of estrogen is being used, under various trade names, as a birth-control pill.

PSYCHOSES IN PREGNANCY Pregnancy involves many alterations in metabolic status, hormonal balance, physical status, and specific stress factors: childbirth, and psychological conflicts associated with motherhood. The appearance of a psychosis during pregnancy is generally unusual; disturbed behavior is more likely to appear during the weeks and months following childbirth. It is generally agreed, however, that these reactions, including psychotic reactions, do not differ in kind from other mental disorders— although they may be triggered by the hormonal changes following delivery.

It is also true that for many young women with underlying personality disorders and unfavorable views of themselves as women, pregnancy may come as something unwanted, with resultant emotional conflict and ambivalence. For the woman who is psychologically unprepared for pregnancy because of psychological immaturity, marital stress, or the demands of caring for an additional child, lack of existing social support heightens vulnerability for illness.

Symptoms. Psychoses following pregnancy may take the form of reactive psychoses with withdrawal from an intolerable situation, agitation, delusions, guilt, and inability to take care of the child. Major depressive reactions also occur with similar symptoms. In the psychoses following childbirth both aggressive impulses toward the baby and suicidal impulses are common; the young mother may be afraid to be alone with her child for fear that she may harm the baby. Also common are feelings of anger and resentment toward the husband, who is often perplexed by the intensity of the woman's disability. These conditions should be distinguished from a mild and transient postpartum condition known as "baby blues," characterized by crying, irritability, and labile mood.

Treatment. Treatment for the psychoses following pregnancy is the same as for similar disorders not associated with childbirth. While the postpartum "baby blues" is a self-limited disorder, disappearing spontaneously within a few days or weeks, medication is generally required for the more severe disorders. It is very important that the young mother be protected from her own self-destructive impulses, but if at all possible, the mother should be encouraged to care for the baby— while treatment is initiated. Psychotherapy may be helpful when directed toward resolution of the woman's underlying emotional conflicts, or resolving marital stress. Once a woman has had an episode of psychosis following childbirth, her risk for a subsequent episode is markedly heightened.

PUERPERIUM (POSTPARTUM) This is the interval between delivery and the reversal of all the changes caused by pregnancy to normal levels. The process takes approximately six weeks, and the interval has been traditionally set for the medical reevaluation of the mother and the detection of any persisting changes or abnormalities connected with her recent pregnancy and delivery. Resumption of normal menstrual periods usually takes place seven to eight weeks after birth, unless the mother is breast-feeding the baby, in which case several months may elapse before menstruation begins again.

"QUICKENING" In pregnant women quickening means the perception of fetal movements. This "feeling of life" appears in the form of intermittent, fluttering movements in the lower abdomen near the fourth month of pregnancy—occasionally as early as two and one-half to three months. Many patients describe it as "butterflies in the stomach." This is by no means a definite sign of pregnancy, since it has been known to be experienced by women who were never pregnant (false pregnancy). If a mother notes a sudden cessation of fetal movement, it should be brought to the OB's attention promptly.

RH FACTOR AND RH SENSITIZATION
In addition to the major blood groups (A, B, O), each person's red cells are characterized by the presence or absence of a specific substance, or antigen, the Rh antigen (referred to also as the Rh factor). This antigen is present in approximately 85 percent of Caucasian people, who are then designated as Rh-positive (Rh+), and it is absent in about 15 percent, who are designated as Rh-negative (Rh−). Among Negroes Rh-negative blood is found in only 7 to 8 percent, while among the Japanese in only 1 to 2 percent.

This substance becomes of particular significance mainly under two sets of circumstances: in blood transfusions, where transfusion of Rh-positive blood to Rh-negative persons may cause complications, ranging from a mild sensitivity reaction to severe hemolysis (destruction of red cells); and in pregnancy, where through an identical mechanism the baby may be exposed to serious damage or even fetal death. The danger arises when an Rh-negative wife gets pregnant by an Rh-positive husband and the baby's blood happens to be Rh-positive. It should be noted that an Rh-positive husband does not always produce Rh-positive children. This

will depend on whether he is Rh-positive homozygous (in this case all his children will be Rh-positive), or Rh-positive heterozygous (here the possibilities are fifty-fifty). Through special blood tests one can tell whether an Rh-positive person is homozygous or heterozygous.

The Rh disease of the fetus or the newborn is known as erythroblastosis fetalis or hemolytic disease of the newborn. An Rh-negative mother does not have to worry about erythroblastosis if she is carrying her first baby. The first baby is almost never affected unless the mother has had blood transfusions or a miscarriage in the past, so that she has been sensitized. Very often, however, she does become sensitized during her first pregnancy if the baby she is carrying happens to be Rh-positive, and this means trouble with the second and subsequent pregnancies.

Briefly, what is taking place is this: Rh-positive cells from the baby get into the mother's circulation and create antibodies. This occurs mostly during labor and delivery, but there is not enough time for harm to come to this first baby. With a subsequent pregnancy and another Rh-positive baby, more Rh-positive blood cells get into the mother's blood, and more antibodies are produced. These antibodies now go back to the baby, passing through the placenta, and they destroy the baby's red cells, resulting in hemolysis. Depending on the amount of antibodies, and therefore on the degree of hemolysis, the baby becomes icteric (yellow) and suffers from severe anemia, which to a considerable extent affects his brain. If the disease is too severe, the baby dies inside the mother's womb. These antibodies may, however, be measured in the mother's blood through special tests, and when large amounts are detected and the baby is big enough to be born, then the obstetrician will usually advise interruption of pregnancy and will induce labor before term in order to prevent irrepairable damage to the baby. All such babies need to have special blood tests right after birth and, if the degree of anemia and hemolysis is considerable, their blood is replaced through exchange transfusion, that is, through gradual removal of their blood and replacement with normal, fresh, non-hemolyzed blood. This is usually effective in arresting the disease process.

The Rh problem is not really a serious one for the Rh-negative woman who is married to a heterozygous Rh-positive husband. But it often becomes desperate when the Rh-negative wife of a homozygous Rh-positive husband gives birth to a baby with severe erythroblastosis fetalis or fetal death inside the uterus. In these cases, subsequent pregnancies are affected more severely and earlier, as compared with previous ones. Erythroblastosis can be prevented once testing of husband and wife indicates its possibility. This is done by giving the wife an injection of high-titer antibody globulin at 28 weeks or within 72 hours of delivery.

Neither Rh-positive women married to Rh-negative men nor Rh-negative wives of Rh-negative husbands have any problem with Rh disease in their children. The problem arises only when an Rh-negative woman marries an Rh-positive man, especially a homozygous one.

SALPINGITIS Salpingitis is an acute or chronic infection of the fallopian tubes. It is common during the reproductive span of the woman and is often due to gonorrhea or to a chlamydia infection. If not treated early and thoroughly, this type of infection advances to the chronic stage and then causes obstruction of the tubes and secondary sterility. Chronic salpingitis is also a frequent cause of irregular vaginal bleeding because of the spread of infection to the ovaries. The infection may also end in multiple adhesions in the pelvis, with a variety of painful symptoms. Occasionally, large abscesses may form in the pelvis which rupture and cause severe peritonitis; an emergency operation and removal of the womb, tubes, and ovaries may then be necessary for the survival of the patient.

This disease is also known as Pelvic Inflammatory Disease (PID). (*See also* the section AIDS AND OTHER SEXUALLY TRANSMITTED DISEASES.)

SEXUAL ACT Sexual intercourse consists basically of contact between the male and female genitalia, the male organ (penis) being inserted into the vagina through a series of rhythmic motions. Sperm (semen) is ejaculated through the male urethra and deposited in the female vagina at the neck of the uterus (cervix). The climax of the sexual act is accompanied by an all-consuming sensation of ecstasy known as orgasm. Orgasm is usually felt by both the man and the woman, but may not coincide in the partners. Normally the woman is slower to reach climax and requires a longer period of preparation (foreplay). Unless measures are taken to prevent conception, the sperm passes into the uterus, and can meet the ovum in the fallopian tube. This process is known as conception, and if it is successful the fertilized ovum is implanted in the wall of the uterus, where it then grows. (For conception to occur, however, intercourse must take place during the woman's fertile period, at a time close to ovulation. This period is generally about mid-way between successive menstrual periods.)

Many fears and taboos surround the sexual act, and it is quite common—especially on the wedding night—for either partner to be unable to complete the act successfully. Usually, however, with patience and understanding the husband and wife are able to achieve a mutually satisfactory relationship. Persistently incomplete sexual intercourse may result in tensions and anxiety. Counseling should definitely be considered.

STERILITY AND INFERTILITY The term sterility implies the inability to conceive because of abnormalities in the male, the female, or both; while the term infertility means the inability to produce a viable fetus—either because of sterility, or because of factors operating after a pregnancy has taken place. In order to use the terms correctly, then, we should speak of a sterile person or an infertile couple.

A popular misconception has existed over the years that the wife is usually the one responsible for the infertility. This is certainly not true. Since in almost 50 percent of the cases the husbands are sterile, therefore, the investigation of an infertile couple should concentrate on both husband and wife. Strangely enough, the male is often resistant to this approach, yet investigation of the husband is much easier, and may save many long and unnecessary tests on the wife.

In the woman, there may be either primary difficulties in ovulation (discharge of the egg from the surface of the ovary), or blockage in the passage through the fallopian tubes due to adhesions or infections; there may also be abnormalities in the uterus. Often an imbalance of hormone-regulation prevents proper implantation of the egg (ovum) in the cavity of the uterus. In some instances, lack of adequate supplies of thyroid hormone is responsible.

In the male, sterility may be the result of three general classes of misfunction: inability of the testes to produce live or efficient sperm—which in turn may be due to such factors as injury, age, thyroid or pituitary hormone deficiency, mumps, nutritional deficiencies, or exposure to radiation; blockage of the tract through which the sperm move, resulting from infection or after surgery performed relating to the vas deferens, the seminal vesicles, the urethra, the prostate gland, or the epididymis; and defective depositing of sperm within the female genital tract—which may be caused either by impotence or by anatomical abnormalities of the male organ.

In general, before a viable baby is born to a couple the following prerequisites must be fulfilled: A woman must have ovaries that are able to produce eggs (ova); and a husband must have sperm sufficient in quality and quantity, and must be able to ejaculate without difficulty at relatively frequent intervals—depositing the ejaculate through normal sexual intercourse in the vagina. From here, the sperm should be able to travel through the uterus, meet the egg, and fertilize it. Severe abnormalities in the structure and the number of spermatozoa (this latter usually runs as high as the billions in each ejaculated specimen) will result in infertility. As far as the female is concerned, in addition to being able to ovulate regularly she should have a normal vagina and possess normal secretions from the glands of the cervix which will allow the sperm to penetrate and ascend to the uterus itself. The uterus must be normal and the fallopian tubes open, so that the sperm can meet the egg for conception.

After conception, the female should manufacture adequate hormones (ovarian and other) to support the pregnancy. The fetus and the afterbirth (placenta) should develop without any major congenital abnormalities, and the pregnancy should be closely traced by an experienced specialist. Finally, the mother should be well-attended throughout the labor and delivery. If all these requisites are met, the couple can usually expect to be rewarded with the happy arrival of the newborn.

In short, the miracle of reproduction is far from being a simple process. The best witnesses of this are those unfortunate couples who go through months and years of medical tests and financial sacrifices for a dream that often never materializes.

Treatment. Since the causes of infertility are so numerous, the methods of treatment are proportionately varied. Existing medical complications should be treated accordingly; deficiencies in hormones of one or more glands should be rectified; infections should be treated with antibiotics; and anatomical anomalies in either the male or female should be corrected surgically. The investigation, diagnosis, and treatment of an infertile couple usually requires the cooperation of several specialists: the gynecologist, urologist, internist, surgeon, radiologist, the laboratory technicians specializing in endocrinological tests, and so forth.

STERILIZATION, SURGICAL An operation for the sterilization of a couple may be done either on the male or on the female. A man can be easily sterilized through a vasectomy, an outpatient procedure during which the spermatic cord is severed. Sterilization of the female is done either by tying (ligation) of the fallopian tubes, or if other indications merit it—such as fibroids—by hysterectomy (removal of the uterus). Either of these procedures can be done vaginally or abdominally, and the choice will depend on the individual case. Surgical tying of the tubes is easily performed in the postpartum period. Done with the instrument known as the laparoscope, ligation is generally feasible through a small abdominal incision. One of the advantages of surgical sterilization of the female is that it may be combined with plastic repair of the vagina, which undergoes relaxation after repeated childbirth.

STILLBORN Under a variety of pathological circumstances, some of them known and some unknown, a fetus of considerable size may die inside the mother's uterus. It is then called stillborn. If the baby remains dead inside the uterus for more than five or six weeks, it is liable to cause certain defects in the clotting mechanism of the mother's blood (hypofibrinogenemia). Special blood tests should be frequently performed for the early detection of such abnormality; in such cases the uterus should be evacuated before severe bleeding complications appear.

"STRETCHMARKS" (STRIAE OF PREGNANCY) These are pinkish or silvery lines over the skin of the abdomen and the upper thighs and breasts and are probably due to overstretching of the skin. The lubricants and other measures sometimes advocated are probably of no value. The "stretchmarks" gradually pale and become less obvious after the pregnancy but may be permanent.

TEMPERATURE CHARTS In the investigation of sterility in the female, a record of body temperature, taken daily immediately upon awakening, and carefully studied, will give valuable information on whether the patient is ovulating or not. (*See also* OVULATION in this section.)

TOXEMIAS OF PREGNANCY Under the general heading of toxemia are included a whole group of related complications, characteristically occurring during the last few months of pregnancy and disappearing spontaneously after delivery. These diseases have several symptoms in common and vary in severity from relatively benign abnormalities to very serious complications affecting several vital organs and jeopardizing the life of the mother. The cause of toxemia of pregnancy is not known. Accumulations of salt and water often are a part of the toxemic picture, but what causes the retention of salt is unknown. Approximately 10 percent of all pregnancies are complicated by toxemia, and this, together with hemorrhage and infection, are the three main causes of maternal deaths throughout the world.

Symptoms. The general common denominator of all the symptoms of toxemias of pregnancy are the following abnormalities: hypertension, swelling of the tissues, and presence of proteins in the urine.

Possibly the earliest sign of impending toxemia of pregnancy is excessive weight gain within a short period of time in a patient who is in the last two to three months of pregnancy. This weight gain is mostly in the form of extra water held by salt, infiltrating the tissues and appearing as generalized swelling (edema). The mother presents a "puffy" appearance and the legs and ankles become swollen. Depending on the severity of the condition, her urine will start to show the presence of variable amounts of albumin, and blood pressure may begin rising above normal. Constant headaches follow in more severe cases, and the patient begins to see spots in front of her eyes. The load that the heart has to carry increases suddenly, and the patient may experience shortness of breath.

The worst toxemia of pregnancy, and probably the most serious of all diseases that may complicate pregnancy, is eclampsia. The patient who develops eclampsia may exhibit part or all of the above-mentioned symptoms of preeclampsia, but in addition suddenly goes into convulsions and loses consciousness.

Treatment. Since the cause of toxemias of pregnancy is not known, their appearance cannot be prevented. We are able, however, to keep them under control and avoid serious injuries to the mother and the baby.

Self-restriction and sometimes salt-free diet will be necessary during the last few months of pregnancy. Diuretic drugs are usually used for excretion of excessive fluids and salts by the kidneys. Antihypertensive and sedative drugs are used to bring the patient's blood pressure down to normal limits. In more severe cases, the patient will have to be put in the hospital for complete bed rest and for frequent analysis of blood and urine, which will help guide the therapy.

The definite treatment of toxemias of pregnancy is accomplished by delivery of the baby. Sometimes the obstetrician may have to terminate the pregnancy, even prematurely, if all other methods fail to produce the desired goal.

TOXIC SHOCK SYNDROME (TSS) This syndrome is believed to be caused by the bacterium called staphylococcus aureus. The condition most often occurs in tampon users, but it has also been associated with contraceptive diaphragms and sponges when they have been left in the vagina for extended periods of time.

Symptoms. Sudden fever (usually 102° or more) and vomiting, diarrhea, fainting or near fainting when standing up, dizziness, or a rash that looks like a sunburn.

IF THESE OR OTHER SIGNS OF TSS APPEAR, YOU SHOULD REMOVE THE TAMPON, DIAPHRAGM, OR SPONGE AT ONCE, DISCONTINUE USE, AND SEE YOUR DOCTOR IMMEDIATELY.

There is a risk of TSS to all women using tampons during their menstrual period. TSS is a rare but serious disease that may cause death. The reported risks are higher to women under 30 years of age and teenage girls. The incidence of TSS is estimated to be between six and seventeen cases of TSS per 100,000 menstruating women and girls per year.

You can avoid any possible risk of getting tampon-associated TSS by not using tampons, by leaving diaphrams or sponges in the vagina no more than twenty-four hours, and avoiding their use during menstruation. You can possibly reduce the risk of getting TSS during your menstrual period by alternating tampon use with sanitary napkin use and by using tampons with the minimum absorbency.

TUBAL (ECTOPIC) PREGNANCY This is the most common type of pregnancy outside the uterus, also known as ectopic pregnancy. Because the tube is a small and thin-walled structure, the pregnancy cannot be maintained for long (rarely for more than three to four months).

Symptoms. The patient usually misses a period or two and has the usual early symptoms of pregnancy. A few days or weeks later, irregular vaginal bleeding and occasional "crampy" lower abdominal pains begin. (This latter is due to stretching of the thin wall of the fallopian tube by the enlarging fetus.) Depending on the site of the pregnancy within the tube, the fetus will eventually either be pushed into the abdomen or will rupture the tube. At this time the patient feels a sudden, staggering pain in the lower abdomen, which gradually becomes milder while the patient feels weak and fainty. This is due to internal hemorrhage from the ruptured tube. The

patient may collapse if bleeding is severe enough.

Treatment. The patient should be taken to the nearest hospital where an emergency operation can be performed in order to stop the bleeding; blood transfusions may be necessary and recovery is quite satisfactory once the lost blood has been properly replaced.

TUBAL LIGATION *See* STERILIZATION, SURGICAL in this section.

TWINS Twin births occur approximately once in 90 births, triplets once in 8,000, quadruplets once in 750,000. The role of inheritance in the production of twins is still being studied.

Twins may be the result of fertilization of one egg (identical twins), or of two separate eggs (fraternal twins). In the second case, the twins may or may not be of the same sex, and will bear no more resemblance to one another than other children of the same parents. Identical twins, on the other hand, are always of the same sex and resemble one another very closely.

Triplets, quadruplets, and quintuplets, may also be the result of fertilization of one, two, or more eggs, and they may be identical, fraternal, or of assorted variety.

From the obstetrical point of view, a mother who is known to carry twins should have very careful prenatal care, for nutrition should be specially planned to include extra iron and other minerals and vitamins, and she should get more rest than the average pregnant woman. Twin pregnancies usually terminate two to four weeks earlier than single ones, and the babies' weight is proportionately lower. There is also a high incidence of prematurity among twins.

ULTRASOUND By bouncing sound waves through a pregnant woman's abdomen, an image of the fetus can be produced on a screen. The technique can provide a variety of information, including the existence of twins, gestational age, location of the placenta, and fetal activity, and breathing. There is no evidence that the procedure harms the fetus.

UMBILICAL CORD A glistening cord-like structure connecting the baby's navel with the afterbirth (placenta), this organ serves for the transfer of blood from the placenta to the fetus, and vice versa, during pregnancy. The cord contains two small arteries and one large vein; its average length is twenty inches, although it may vary from a few inches to several feet in length. It is vital for the normal development of the baby in the uterus, and severe congenital or acquired abnormalities of the cord may result in early or late fetal death. A few days after birth, the cord dries up and falls off, leaving a button-like formation—the navel, or umbilicus—at the site of its juncture with the baby's body.

The most common complications involving the cord during pregnancy and endangering the life of the baby are prolapse, or expulsion, of the cord before delivery of the baby; this usually requires immediate delivery by caesarean section in order to prevent compression of the cord between the baby and the mother's bones, which may obstruct the flow of blood to the baby; fetal deaths from this complication are not unusual; knots of the cord; looping of the cord tightly around the baby's neck; and congenital anomalies of the vessels of the cord. In most of these conditions, the baby can be saved through caesarean birth, provided that the abnormality is detected early enough by the doctor.

UTERINE BLEEDING, ABNORMAL
Some forms of abnormal bleeding from the vagina are classified as menorrhagia or metrorrhagia. Menorrhagia is excessive menstruation, either in amount or duration, without intermenstrual bleeding. The extent of bleeding varies but is sometimes profuse enough to produce anemia. Menorrhagia in a teen-ager after onset of menstruation is not uncommon and may be severe and intractable. Metrorrhagia is intermenstrual bleeding. It has numerous causes among which are various kinds of tumors.

Many nongynecological conditions may be accompanied by abnormal uterine bleeding. Among these are certain acute infections, anemia, hemophilia, leukemia, gout, scurvy, malaria, emotional conditions, and diseases of the lungs, heart, and liver.

Gynecological conditions that are marked by irregular and/or abnormal uterine bleeding are abortion, miscarriage, fibroids of the uterus, chronic inflammatory conditions of the uterus, cancer of the uterus, tubal pregnancy (ectopic pregnancy), the menopause, placenta previa (heavy bleeding that may occur during labor), malposition of the uterus, inflammation of the tubes and/or the ovaries, hardening of the arteries, prolapse of the uterus, cervical polyp, and laceration of the uterine cervix.

Less common causes include vaginal ulceration, cervical ulceration, hyperthyroidism, overactivity of the pituitary, alcoholism, cirrhosis of the liver, scurvy, and tuberculosis.

UTERUS, SUBINVOLUTION OF THE
This represents the failure of the uterus gradually to return to normal size after delivery of the child. It is often accompanied by prolonged vaginal bleeding, and sometimes low-grade fever and backache.

Treatment. Treatment consists of special drugs (oxytocics) that make the uterus contract; quite often, scraping of the uterus is also necessary. This condition should be examined postpartum.

UTERUS (WOMB)
The uterus is located at the bottom of the female pelvis, between the bladder and the rectum, and consists of several layers of strong muscle surrounding the cavity of the uterus. In its nonpregnant state, the uterus is the shape and size of a flattened pear, and sits on top of the vagina. Its cavity connects with the vagina through the cervix (neck of the uterus) and with the ovaries through the two fallopian tubes. With the onset of puberty, the lining of the cavity of the uterus responds to the changing levels of hormones produced by the ovaries and undergoes hypertrophy and eventual shedding; these changes are manifested monthly in the form of menstrual periods. The muscle of the uterus has tremendous adaptability and, when pregnancy does occur, hypertrophies and stretches to huge dimensions, still maintaining its ability to contract strongly for expulsion of the baby and the afterbirth (placenta).

A variety of diseases can affect the uterus, ranging from infections to tumors, both benign and malignant. Abnormal uterine bleeding may be the result of diseases primarily involving the uterus, but more often is the reflection of ovarian problems and abnormal hormone production; the uterus is only the final "target organ" through which these latter abnormalities are manifested.

VAGINA (BIRTH CANAL) This structure, resembling a collapsed tube, serves to connect the vulva with the mouth of the uterus. On the average, it is four inches long and is surrounded by strong layers of muscular and connective tissues which allow it to stretch and permit the delivery of a full-term baby, with subsequent return to almost the original dimensions. After repeated childbirth the walls of the vagina undergo relaxation and the bladder and rectum may herniate into the vagina. This can be corrected with plastic surgery of the vagina, almost always combined with sterilization of the patient through tubal ligation or hysterectomy.

VAGINAL DISCHARGE Discharges from the vagina occur normally in a majority of young girls—even babies. They will frequently be noted on diapers and underpants. During adolescence especially, it may become quite noticeable and yet be entirely normal: there are great differences between individual normal girls. If, however, the discharge becomes sufficiently profuse to be bothersome— especially to the child herself; or if the color turns from grayish to yellow; some attention besides cleanliness may need to be given to it. This is especially true if the discharge is blood-tinged (except where menstruation is expected), if it seems to cause irritation about the orifice (vulvar irritation), or if the condition defies simple cleanliness. In such cases the doctor should be consulted. Adolescence often brings on an increase in a normal discharge of this sort. Except for cleanliness, this too can be disregarded.

Infections, generally mild in nature, are often responsible for the more exaggerated and stubborn types of vaginitis causing discharge. Until recently, gonorrhea was not uncommon as a cause. Nowaday it is rare in children—although more common in teenagers. Its results in children are almost never serious, as they may be in adults. There may be some danger of transmitting the infection to adults or infecting the child's eyes, but this is remote with ordinary cleanliness and if the doctor's instructions are carried out.

Occasionally a vaginal discharge is due to a small object (or tampons or parts of them) inserted by the child and retained in the vagina. This generally causes a discharge with a distinct odor and later some blood.

Treatment. Treatment consists in applying antiseptics, either local or general, but unless there is serious resultant irritation of the vulva the situation is seldom, if ever, serious. Foreign bodies must of course be removed.

VAGINITIS Infection of the vagina may occur at any age, from childhood to postmenopausal years. It is more common during the reproductive period, and is usually produced by microorganisms such as trichomas, monilia, gonococcus. In childhood it is often the result of insertion of foreign bodies, or contamination from the rectum through improper wiping. In postmenopausal women it is primarily the result of atrophy of the tissue lining the vagina.

Symptoms. Abnormal whitish, yellowish, greenish, or purulent discharge is the main symptom for infection of the vagina. Burning and itching, and local swelling and soreness are also frequent symptoms of vaginitis.

Treatment. Depending on the cause, treatment will consist of vaginal antibiotic suppositories, oral or injectable drugs, douches, hormonal therapy (if atrophy is present), etc. The results are generally good and only 5 percent of the cases will present difficulties with treatment.

VULVA The vulva surrounds the entrance to the vagina (birth canal) and consists of several structures. On the outside there are two folds of skin (labia majora) and within these two smaller folds (labia minora). At the upper end is the clitoris, and under it, the urethra (opening of the bladder). The hymen separates the vulva from the vagina.

A variety of diseases can involve the structures of the vulva, such as infections, irritations of the labia, and infections or cysts of Bartholin's glands and cancer.

INFANT AND CHILD CARE

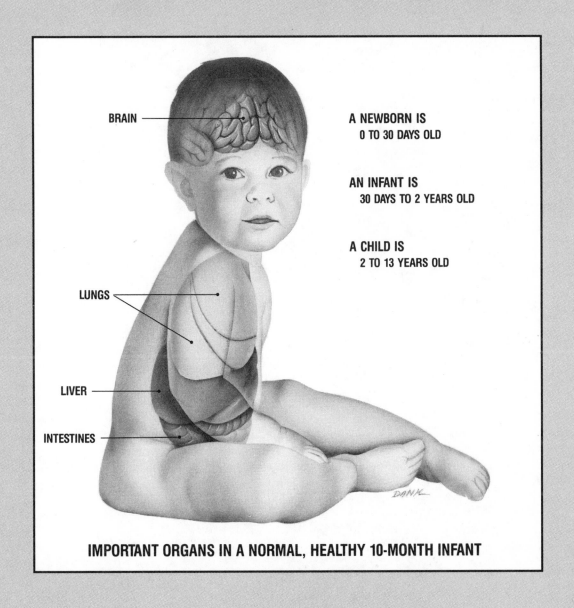

BRAIN

A NEWBORN IS
0 TO 30 DAYS OLD

AN INFANT IS
30 DAYS TO 2 YEARS OLD

A CHILD IS
2 TO 13 YEARS OLD

LUNGS

LIVER

INTESTINES

IMPORTANT ORGANS IN A NORMAL, HEALTHY 10-MONTH INFANT

The human infant comes into the world dependent on others for his care. The child's physiological and anatomical changes are rapid, as he or she matures and responds to the environment. Although born immunologically and otherwise immature, the basic body functions usually operate consistently from birth. Growth is rapid comparatively speaking from birth to two years of age. A pediatrician is a physician who specializes in the care of infants and children.

This section examines the basic anatomy and physiology of infants, some warning signs of ailments, and some possible treatments for common conditions. Childhood illnesses can be difficult, but for the most part, children's systems function predictably. Because of great strides in immunization and advances in antibiotics, most childhood illnesses are manageable.

Many disorders seen in children are not specifically confined only to children; and therefore, the reader is advised to see also other topic headings in the INDEX. The following is a list of the topics discussed in this section:

ANAL FISSURE
BEDWETTING (ENURESIS)
BIRTH INJURIES
BOWLEGS
BREAST, THE IMMATURE FEMALE
CEREBRAL PALSY
CIRCUMCISION
CLEFT LIP (HARELIP)
CLEFT PALATE
CLUBFOOT
COLIC
COMMON COLD
CRADLE CAP
CROSS-EYE IN CHILDREN
CYSTIC FIBROSIS
DECIDUOUS TEETH (PRIMARY, "MILK,"
  "BABY," FIRST, TEMPORARY)
DEHYDRATION
DIAPER RASH
DIARRHEA IN CHILDREN
DIPHTHERIA
DYSPLASIA OF THE HIPS, CONGENITAL
EAR INFECTION (OTITIS MEDIA)
EATING PROBLEMS
ECZEMA
EMERGENCIES

FEVER
HIP DEFORMITIES IN CHILDHOOD
IMMUNIZATION
INCUBATOR
INFANT FEEDING
JAUNDICE OF THE NEWBORN
MALNUTRITION
METATARSUS ADDUCTUS
MOLDING
NAVEL (UMBILICUS)
PEDIATRICS
POISONING
PREMATURE INFANTS
PSYCHOLOGICAL DEVELOPMENT IN
  CHILDHOOD
SLEEP DISTURBANCES
SPEECH DISORDERS
SUDDEN INFANT DEATH SYNDROME
  (SIDS)
THERMOMETER
THUMB-SUCKING
TOILET TRAINING
VERNIX
VOMITING, CYCLIC
VOMITING (EMESIS) IN CHILDREN
VULVA-IRRITATION

ANAL FISSURE A slit or tear or crack beginning just inside the anal opening and extending to the outside is called an anal fissure. It produces slight-to-severe pain and spasm at stool, and there is often a drop or two of blood on the outside of the stool. This condition is usually caused by the passage of hard, dry stools. Diarrhea may also cause anal fissure.

Treatment. If the stools are hard, softening may be achieved by adding more fiber and liquids to the diet or by using Colace, a stool softener. Constipating foods such as bananas and applesauce should be avoided. Infants may be given prune juice, baby prunes, or the indicated dosage of Maltsupex added to each feeding bottle. A bit of petroleum jelly or other lubricant pushed gently into the anal opening will soothe and cover the fissure so that the next stool will pass without irritation. If the condition persists for more than a few days, medical attention should be sought.

BEDWETTING (ENURESIS)   Enuresis is a common condition of childhood. It is defined as the involuntary discharge of urine occurring after the age at which bladder control is usually established. In general, children are not labeled "enuretic" unless the symptom persists beyond the age of six years. Bedwetting occurs once a month in more than 8 percent of school-age children.

Bedwetting occurs more frequently in boys than in girls. It becomes less common as children approach puberty. There is often a family history of bedwetting. Most children who wet the bed at night are very heavy sleepers who are difficult to arouse; some physicians believe that bedwetting is a sleep disorder due to problems of resistance to waking.

Treatment. There are several known treatments for bedwetting, none of which are very effective. They include limiting liquids after dinner, rewarding the child for being dry at night, installing an alarm system (marketed especially for this purpose) which wakes the child when he wets, and use of Tofranil, an antidepressant medication for adults with the side effect of decreasing bedwetting in children. The best cure for bedwetting, however, is patience because the child will eventually outgrow the condition. (*See also* BEDWETTING [ENURESIS] in the section MENTAL HEALTH.)

BIRTH INJURIES   The most common birth injuries are those involving the largest part of the newborn—the head. Lumps noticed on the head at birth are most often caused by blood serum or superficial blood beneath the scalp; these are almost always harmless and disappear early.

Other injuries involve fractures, the most common being of the collarbone. The physician may treat the condition with approved methods or may decide to let it heal (as often happens) by itself. Stretching of nerves in the neck may cause paralysis, often temporary, of the upper arm muscles.

Oxygen deprivation to the brain at the time of delivery can cause motor problems and developmental delay. Premature infants are more sensitive to oxygen deprivation than are term infants. (*See also* CEREBRAL PALSY in this section.)

BOWLEGS   All infants have bowing of the legs. By the first twelve to eighteen months, the legs have straightened but continue to be mildly knock-kneed. By age six or seven the legs will have progressed to their adult shape and angle. If the legs appear extremely bowlegged, a pediatrician or orthopedic surgeon should be consulted.

BREAST, THE IMMATURE FEMALE   Often, immediately after birth, the doctor, mother, or nurse may notice a definite swelling of the female baby's tiny breasts. This is quite common—and almost never important. It is the result of the mother's hormones (probably the lactogenic, or milk, hormone) still being active in the infant's blood. The condition—also occasionally seen in boys—is generally self-limiting, lasting only two or three weeks.

Female breasts during childhood are unimportant and nonfunctional. They grow very little until the beginning of adolescence, at which time they will begin to enlarge, usually asymmetrically by developing a "lump" underneath the nipple. Boys may also develop nubbins of breast tissue during early adolescence.

CEREBRAL PALSY   Cerebral palsy includes a wide variety of conditions affecting the control of the muscular (motor) system due to lesions in various parts of the brain. The defects in brain function may occur before birth or as a result of birth injury. Almost all cerebral palsy is due to lack of oxygen around the time of birth. Recent studies have shown that more than one-third of children with cerebral palsy weighed less than five pounds at birth. Premature infants are much more sensitive to lack of oxygen than are term babies.

Symptoms. Cerebral palsy produces weakness, paralysis, lack of coordination, tremor, rigidity, or spasticity which is usually noted within the first year of life and which is related to defects in those structures in the brain which control motor functions. The condition may or may not be associated with mental retardation, epilepsy, and other developmental abnormalities in the body.

Treatment. Severely handicapped children, who are frequently mentally subnormal, require hospitalization for adequate care. Children who are less handicapped may be cared for at home and may attend special schools where facilities for their needs are available; these individuals need vocational guidance and training in order to develop specific skills and become productive members of society. Children with mild motor defects and normal intelligence attend regular schools. They may have limitations in motor function which prevent full participation in athletic programs; however, it is important that all of their intellectual and motor skills be developed in a productive manner. If epilepsy is associated with cerebral palsy, anticonvulsant medicines are taken daily to prevent attacks.

CIRCUMCISION   The surgical removal of the foreskin (prepuce) from the head of the penis is known as circumcision. This procedure, routine for all Jewish male infants as a religious ceremony, has become a fairly frequent practice in the United States before the boy is brought home from the hospital. When performed for nonreligious reasons, it is done for the sake of cleanliness. The fact is that the circumcised penis is easier to clean, and there seems to be no record of cancer of the circumcised penis.

Immediately after circumcision, the head of the penis is quite raw, so that some type of ointment should be applied to prevent the wound from sticking to the diaper. Petroleum jelly is satisfactory. Urine should be forthcoming at regular intervals, and the size and trajectory of the stream carefully noted; this information is then passed on to the doctor.

CLEFT LIP (HARELIP)   This congenital anomaly is obvious at birth, a slit or gap being present from the nostril to the mouth on one or both sides of the upper lip. It is usually associated with a cleft palate. If the gum and palate are cleft, the baby has trouble creating any suction; the surgeon therefore tries to correct the lip as early in life as possible. Modern surgical techniques have been so perfected that some of these defects defy detection. (*See also* CLEFT PALATE in this section.)

CLEFT PALATE   Cleft palate and cleft lip are parts of the same congenital defect. All or part of the bony roof of the mouth may be absent, thus exposing the nasal passages and sinuses. The cleft may extend forward through the gum and the upper lip, producing the cleft lip.

Treatment. The only cure is surgery. The lip is usually repaired first, so that the baby may suck. The palate is done at a time when the surgeon feels he has enough tissue with which to work so as to cover the repaired bony palate; this is best done before speech habits are established, usually between the ages of eighteen and twenty-four months. Sometimes several operations are necessary in order to free the tissues in such a way that the defect may be corrected without undue tension. The cosmetic result is not always perfect, but more often than not it is very good indeed. (*See also* CLEFT LIP (HARELIP) in this section.)

CLUBFOOT   Clubfoot is a developmental condition in which the child is born with a foot twisted both upon itself and in relation to the leg. The forepart of the foot is inverted and twisted inward, and the heel is turned downward. Treatment of this deformity is properly begun shortly after birth. By means of multiple plaster-cast changes, the foot is gradually untwisted and held in plaster casts so that, with growth, it may develop properly. In highly resistant situations, operative procedures may be necessary to release contractures or lengthen and reposition tight tendons. A properly treated clubfoot should result in a stable, supple foot which is both functionally and cosmetically excellent.

Metatarsus adductus is a condition in which the forefoot turns in but it is not as severe as clubfoot, nor as difficult to treat. The forefoot is turned inward so that the child walks in a pigeon-toed manner, but the rest of the foot is usually normal. A child whose feet turn inward should receive medical attention as soon as the parents recognize this situation. There are many causes of in-turning of the feet in childhood and careful diagnosis is important. Treatment of the child with metatarsus adductus ranges from simple exercises performed by the parents to plaster casting if severe.

COLIC   The term "colic" is used to describe a group of symptoms which include intermittent abdominal pain and severe crying. It is most common in infants under three months of age.

An onset of colic is usually sudden; the cry is loud and continuous and may go on for hours. The baby's face may be flushed, the abdomen tense, the legs either drawn up or extended out, and the feet often cold. This may occur any time of day or night but classically occurs in early evening.

No one knows what causes colic. Holding the baby upright, using a swing, going for a walk, all have been tried with varying success. Changing the formula sometimes helps.

Breast-fed babies may develop cramps and colic if their mothers eat foods to which babies are sensitive: garlic, onions, cabbage, beans, chocolate, caffeine and cow's milk, to name a few.

Treatment. Therapy for colic is finding the cause and eliminating it. If all other methods fail, most doctors recommend a sedative solution which can be given with the feeding just prior to the worst time of outbreak. Patience in the knowledge by the parents that the condition is temporary and not serious, may help to ease the baby and parents through this trying time.

COMMON COLD   The common cold is a virus inflammation of the mucous membranes lining the nose, throat, and eyes. It begins suddenly with watery discharge from the nose, a few sneezes, a scratchy throat; and infants and children may run fever with the cold.

A common cold is not serious and should not last more than a week. If a condition lasts longer than this, it is not simply a cold and is either a secondary bacterial infection or an allergy. It is necessary to call the pediatrician.

Thus, if a child sneezes and has a watery discharge from the nose and eyes for more than a week, an inhalation allergy is a possibility and a search must be made for the offending substance.

Symptoms. A typical picture of the bacterial complication of a cold in childhood may be something like the following: A two-year-old child has had a cold for five days; just as it is about to go away, he begins to cry and develop an earache, the temperature rises to 102° F, and the discharge from his nose (which has been clear and watery) turns purulent with thick green or yellow matter. This is usually the time when the parent will seek medical advice, because now the child appears to have a treatable condition—a bacterial secondary invasion. The child may have developed pneumonia, an ear infection, bronchitis, or tonsillitis; or the infectious material from the nose may have caused an impetigo on the upper lip.

Treatment. The so-called "cold" is actually due to any one of a number of viruses, and at the present time we do not have precise treatments for virus-caused ailments. Tylenol® for fever, nosedrops, decongestants, antihistaminics, rest, and fluids are the time-honored remedies for the common cold.

CRADLE CAP   *See* SEBORRHEIC DERMATITIS in the section SKIN CONDITIONS.

CROSS-EYE IN CHILDREN   The medical term for this condition is strabismus. It is also called "squint." The condition is usually due to a weakness or imbalance of eye muscles resulting in either the turning in or out of one or both eyes.

In the first six months of life most babies do not always use their eyes together, but at six to eight months the eyes should be working together at all times. If this is not so, the baby should be examined by an eye specialist (ophthalmologist).

If a baby is using one eye to the exclusion of the other, the brain "suppresses" the image it gets from the little-used one and a condition of disuse atrophy occurs. If this situation is not corrected, the eye never regains its ability to see clearly (although the squint may be cosmetically corrected by surgery). A squint should never be ignored beyond the first eight to ten months of life on the assumption the baby will outgrow it. (*See also* CROSS-EYE [SQUINT OR STRABISMUS] in the section EYE AND VISION CONDITIONS.)

CYSTIC FIBROSIS Cystic fibrosis is essentially an inborn error of metabolism involving glands, such as the mucous, salivary, and sweat glands, which secrete an extremely tenacious mucus. This mucus produces changes in the lungs, liver, and pancreas by obstructing the flow of air or fluids to these organs. It is familial in nature and carries a strong hereditary factor. It is the principal cause of pancreatic enzyme deficiency in children, many of the cases of cirrhosis of the liver in children, and of most of the nontuberculous chest diseases. Every two and one-half hours a child with cystic fibrosis is born. Not too long ago these infants did not survive the first year of life; with modern treatment some patients are living into adulthood. The cause of the disease is not known.

Symptoms. Pulmonary and digestive symptoms are first noted; four out of five patients present such features before the twelfth month of life. They are often misdiagnosed as suffering asthma or primary lung disease. In 5 to 10 percent of babies with cystic fibrosis the first indication is intestinal obstruction. Rarely, infants may have prolapse of the rectum or portal hypertension (in the liver) as the initial sign. The most prominent feature is chronic respiratory disorder. Bronchial mucous obstruction makes the patient particularly vulnerable to respiratory infections that recur, each time leaving the breathing apparatus with more damaged lung tissue. Among common complications are lung collapse, lung abscess, coughing up of blood, and cor pulmonale. Sinusitis and nasal polyps are also common. Insufficiency of pancreatic enzyme production causes malabsorption, so that the affected child produces malodorous stools that are bulky and greasy. Even though his appetite remains good, he becomes malnourished. In the summer the cystic fibrosis victim suffers with abnormal perspiration which results in salt depletion of the body.

Cystic fibrosis is suspected in an infant or young child who fails to thrive despite a good appetite and normal food intake; has a chronic cough; foul, bulky, greasy stools; rectal prolapse; intestinal obstruction at birth; a sibling or first cousin with cystic fibrosis; recurrent respiratory infections; nasal polyps; excessive perspiration; stunted growth with pot belly; emphysema; and clubbing of fingers. Specific tests for salt content of sweat are extremely helpful in establishing the diagnosis.

Treatment. Therapy is aimed at thinning glandular secretions, and by providing frequent postural drainage. A spray of acetyleysteine two or three times a day has proved to be most helpful. Mechanical suction of excessive bronchial secretions is also beneficial. Postural drainage, exercise, and other physical methods are used. The child is taught how to increase lung intake of air by exercises that bring the diaphragm into prominent play in respiration. Diet is fortified with pancreatic enzymes, vitamins A, D, E, and K, while infants are fed a low-fat high-protein formula. Older children usually can take a normal diet. Salt loss is overcome by salt tablets and additional salt in the food. Antibiotics are prescribed freely with any evidence of lung infection and may be used on a prophylactic basis. Some children are treated at specialized cystic fibrosis centers. Although the underlying defect cannot be reversed, the outlook has improved considerably for survival into adulthood.

DECIDUOUS   TEETH   (PRIMARY, "MILK," "BABY," FIRST, TEMPORARY) These are the twenty teeth of the first dentition, and are usually erupted by the time a child is two years old. It is usual for the first tooth to appear at around six months of age, but this is familialy determined. The last of the deciduous teeth are shed (exfoliated) by about the age of eleven or twelve. (*See also* the section DENTAL HEALTH.)

DEHYDRATION This term, meaning drying out, describes a condition in which the body loses too much of its normal fluids and salts and fails to retain enough for maintenance of adequate circulation, proper excretion of waste products through the kidneys, and individual cell function. Small babies show poor tolerance to dehydration, and may go into coma and die if the condition is not quickly corrected.

Symptoms. The mildly dehydrated infant will have a dry mouth and scanty wet diapers. The severely dehydrated infant becomes listless and breathes shallowly, the eyes are half-closed and appear sunken, the fontanelle or soft spot is sunken in. Such an infant may excrete urine which is scanty, infrequent, and very concentrated. This usually is the result of gastroenteritis—often called intestinal flu—which produces vomiting and diarrhea.

Treatment. The treatment of dehydration involves replacement of fluids and salts such as potassium and sodium (electrolytes). If the dehydration is very mild, these may be replaced by giving the infant oral electrolyte solutions. If the dehydration is moderate to severe, it will necessitate hospitalization for slow intravenous replacement of lost fluid and electrolytes. Any child who loses large amounts of fluids by vomiting or diarrhea, or both, must be seen by a doctor without delay.

DIAPER RASH The term diaper rash is usually reserved for eruptions of the diaper area thought to be due to contact of the skin with urine and feces. Diaper rash is quite similar to heat rash and is the result of the macerative effect of the moisture (both urinary and sweat), the presence of a great number of potentially infective organisms from the urine and feces, and the susceptibility of the thin and vulnerable infant skin to the damaging effects of both these factors.

Symptoms. The buttocks and groin are the site of redness, small papules, occasional pustules, and in aggravated cases, peeling of the skin. Small boils can appear on the labia or on the penis.

Treatment. Thorough drying of the skin after each diaper removal and frequent change of diapers are essential for both prevention and treatment. Zinc oxide and other preparations which keep moisture off the skin are also frequently used.

DIARRHEA IN CHILDREN Diarrhea is the frequent passage of loose and/or watery stools. The form of diarrhea most common in children is due to a virus.

Symptoms. Diarrhea may or may not be accompanied by fever, cramps, and blood in the stool. (The presence of blood often characterizes dysentery, a more serious, bacteria-caused condition.) If the condition is severe enough, the patient may dehydrate.

Treatment. The mainstay of treatment is to give plenty of fluids to guard against dehydration. After twenty-four hours of only clear fluids, the diet may be slowly advanced to a low-fat, low roughage diet. Typically, it would consist of rice, toast, tea, banana, and applesauce. Most doctors advise stopping milk for several days and substituting only clear liquids; then, after two or three days, the milk is restored gradually in diluted form.

DIPHTHERIA Diphtheria is an acute infectious disease to which children are particularly susceptible and whose main focus is in the nose, throat, and larynx. The specific agent is a bacterium called *Corynebacterium diphtheriae*, isolated by Loeffler in 1884. This bacillus cannot survive outside the human body; hence, the human host is the only significant reservoir of the germ and the one responsible for its transmission, usually through cough. Not every person infected by the Loeffler bacillus contracts the disease; this will depend on the germ's virulence and the victim's susceptibility. Those in whom examination of the throat does reveal the presence of bacilli, but who do not exhibit clinical signs of illness, are called carriers. This condition is dangerous and such individuals should be isolated and intensively treated to prevent them from spreading the germ to receptive persons. The diphtheria organism is responsive to such common antibiotics as penicillin and erythromycin.

Virulent diphtheria bacilli have the property of secreting a specific poisonous substance (diphtheria toxin) which is responsible for the local damage characteristic of the disease, as well as for distant complications in the body.

Symptoms. The incubation period is short, ranging from one to four days. The clinical manifestations depend on the anatomical site of the primary infection (throat, nose, larynx) and the severity of the infection. Throat diphtheria is described here as a typical form. Onset of the disease is abrupt, with chills, moderate fever, malaise, and sore throat. On examination the throat is dull red in color, this stage being followed by formation of a grayish, gelatinous pseudomembrane which first appears over one tonsil, then spreads to the other. The neck glands are slightly painful. When the disease is mild, these are the only manifestations. The disease may, however, continue to spread upward to the back of the nose and downward toward the larynx, creating a particularly dangerous situation. (*See also* LARYNGITIS in the section RESPIRATORY CONDITIONS.)

If the disease is not promptly and vigorously treated, diphtheria toxin may give rise to serious complications, the most important being involvement of the heart (myocarditis) and of the nervous system (in the form of muscular paralysis). These complications usually appear during the third to fifth week of the improperly treated disease, when convalescence has been erroneously assumed.

Treatment. The most important step is prompt administration of diphtheria antitoxin in adequate amounts. The role of antitoxin is to bind and neutralize the diphtheria toxin and prevent further damage. Hence late administration may be ineffective if serious cellular damage has already occurred. Since the antitoxin is a foreign substance (horse serum), precautions should be taken if the patient has previously received other similar serums because of the possibility of an allergic reaction which may be extremely severe. Antibiotics may also be used if secondary bacteria are present. Bed rest is mandatory and the usual hygienic measures are helpful. A careful watch for the development of complications should be maintained.

Prevention by active immunization is feasible and practiced widely today, especially in combination with tetanus and whooping cough vaccination during infancy. Still, it should be remembered that booster doses are necessary at intervals because immunity decreases with time. If a person has been exposed to diphtheria and there is reliable evidence that he has been adequately vaccinated in the past, all that is required is a new booster dose of vaccine. If such assurance is not forthcoming, antitoxin serum should be administered.

DYSPLASIA OF THE HIPS, CONGENITAL This is a developmental disorder in which the hip joint is underdeveloped and the femoral head is either partly or completely out of place. It is usually recognized in infancy by apparent shortening of the involved leg, or asymmetric skin-folds over the thighs. The cause is unknown, but these are clearly genetic factors. Females are more commonly affected than males.

Treatment. The treatment of dysplasia of the hip depends on the age of the child at the time of diagnosis and the severity of the abnormality. It usually involves using a splint or harness and may involve casting and/or traction.

EAR INFECTION (OTITIS MEDIA) In the typical case of otitis media, the child has suffered with an upper respiratory infection for several days and suddenly develops fever, ear pain, or decreased hearing. Other occasions in which the parents should suspect an ear infection include a cold which persists longer than a week, irritability and inability to suck a bottle, persistent cough, and runny nose with a yellow or greenish color rather than white or clear.

Treatment. The treatment for otitis media is antibiotic therapy for ten days as well as an analgesic for pain. It is important that the physician recheck the affected ear at the end of treatment. (*See also* OTITIS MEDIA in the section EAR, NOSE AND THROAT CONDITIONS.)

EATING PROBLEMS It is very common for infants between the ages of one and three years to markedly decrease their appetite and become "picky" eaters. There is no such thing as anorexia or bulimia in children this young.

In most cases, difficulties stem from the fact that the parent's idea of what the child should eat and the child's idea are different. The parents are accustomed to the big appetite that the child had at four months old (and gaining two to three pounds a month), but the child is now growing and eating less.

Treatment. A healthy, happy, and up-and-around child is obviously not starving; accordingly, the parents must stop worrying and forcing the child to eat unless they want a neurotic child. The best way to feed the two-to-four-year-olds is to put small amounts of food in front of them on a plate; then if they want more, they will ask for it. If a child does not eat a well-balanced diet, supplemental vitamins should be given. It is important not to fight with a child during mealtimes, for a lifetime attitude toward food is being formed. Children should associate eating with pleasure, not controversy.

ECZEMA   In eczema the affected skin is dry, scaly, itchy, and sometimes reddened. It may also become crusty or "weepy." Common sites of the eruption are the cheeks, the inner areas of the elbows, and the backs of the knees, but it can be found on any part of the body. There is a genetic predisposition to eczema, and it is often found in people with a family history of asthma and allergic rhinitis (hay fever) as well as eczema.

Eczema in infants is frequently associated with the introduction of certain foods, particularly cow's milk, wheat and eggs. In older children and adults, it appears to be much less related to dietary factors, but rather to emotional factors, or contact with some irritants (soap, wool, etc.).

Treatment. The treatment of eczema involves removing the offending agent if identified, such as food; minimal bathing as soaps dry out the skin; the use of bath oils and creams to seal moisture in the skin; the use of topical corticosteroid creams; and oral use of antihistaminic drugs such as diplenhydramine (Benadryl®) or hydroxyzine (Atarax®.) (*See also* INFANTILE ECZEMA in the section SKIN CONDITIONS.)

EMERGENCIES   *See* the section FIRST AID AND EMERGENCIES. *See also* the EMERGENCY SURVIVAL GUIDE on the endsheets.

FEVER   The body's average temperature is 98.6° F, but it can fluctuate during the day, with mild elevations caused by exercise, warm clothing, hot weather, or warm food. Fever is defined as rectal temperature over 100.4° F, oral temperature over 100° F, and axillary (arm pit) temperature over 99° F. Physicians accept a rectal temperature as the most accurate. Temperature strips which are applied to the forehead have been found to be inaccurate.

Fever is the body's normal response to infections. Indeed, it may be helpful in fighting infections. The usual fevers that all children get are not harmful—most are due to viral illnesses. Most fevers with viral illnesses range between 101° F and 104° F and last for two-four days. The way the child acts is more important than the height of the fever in determining how serious the illness is. Fever causes no permanent harm until it reaches 107° F. While all children get fever, only 4 percent develop febrile convulsions. This type of seizure is almost always harmless.

Treatment. It is important to call the pediatrician immediately when a child with fever is less than two months old, and in all instances if the fever is over 105° F or if the child with fever is irritable or difficult to rouse. Acetaminophen (an aspirin-free substance) is the drug of choice for control of fever. It should be given in the correct dose by body weight (as specified on the package label) if the fever is higher than 102° F, or if the child is uncomfortable. The drug will need repeating every four-six hours since the fever will fluctuate until the disease runs its course.

The American Academy of Pediatrics has recommended that children not receive aspirin if they have chickenpox or influenza (any cough, cold or sore throat). This is because several studies have linked aspirin to Reye's syndrome, a severe encephalitis-type illness.

Sponging with lukewarm water will bring the fever down if acetaminophen doesn't work. A child with fever should receive extra fluids and should be dressed as lightly as possible. (For taking the temperature, *see* THERMOMETER in this section.)

HIP DEFORMITIES IN CHILDHOOD
Any child who walks with a limp or states that he has a pain in the hip or knee should be suspected of having disease of the hips and needs immediate medical attention. Likewise, any infant who has limited motion of one hip or who cries when his or her legs are spread in diapering should also be suspected of having hip involvement and should be examined by a physician. (*See also* DYSPLASIA OF THE HIPS, CONGENITAL in this section.)

IMMUNIZATION   Immunization is a major procedure in preventing disease. All children should receive immunization during the first year of life against diphtheria, pertussis (whooping cough), tetanus, and poliomyelitis. Vaccines against measles, mumps, and rubella (German measles) are currently given at fifteen months of age. Smallpox vaccination is currently not indicated in most areas of the world. A vaccine called HIB vaccine, usually given at eighteen months of age, protects against blood-bone infections caused by H. influenza B, a bacterium which can cause meningitis, epiglottitis and other serious infections in young children. Throughout the childhood years care should be taken to keep immunizations and booster shots current. A schedule of recommended immunizations is available at the pediatrician's office or at the local health department. Certain immunizations may be required for school and/or day care.

INCUBATOR Used for the maintenance of life in premature infants or those who are congenitally debilitated or severely ill, an incubator is a glass-enclosed chamber with mechanical means for the control of oxygen supply, temperature, and humidity.

INFANT FEEDING Successful infant feeding requires that a cooperative bond be formed between infant and parent (or other caregiver). Feeding time should be pleasurable for both parent and child. The emptying time of the infant's stomach may vary between one and four hours depending on the time of day and whether the food is breast milk or formula.

Breast milk is the natural food for infants during the first months of life. It is more easily digested than any of the formulas. "Spitting up," colic, and eczema are less common in breast-fed than in bottle-fed infants. Human milk contains antibodies from the mother which are helpful in decreasing infections in the baby during the first six months of life. The iron content of breast milk is lower than in formula, but it is more easily utilized by the infant. Except for vitamin D and fluoride, breast milk from an adequately nourished mother provides all the necessary nutrients for the baby. Vitamin D and fluoride (if the community water is not fluoridated) must be provided as supplements. There are few contraindications to breast feeding. These include active tuberculosis, malaria, chronic

poor nutrition, and a mother taking drugs not suitable for the baby's ingestion.

If the breast-fed infant seems satisfied at the end of nursing, has many wet diapers per day, and is gaining weight adequately (as measured by the physician, not the parents), then breast feeding may be considered a success. Two to four weeks after birth, when nursing is well established, it may be desirable to substitute some feedings with formula, in order to give the mother greater freedom and to get the baby accustomed to a bottle.

Cow's milk in a modified form is the basis for most commercial formulas. The cow's milk is heated so the protein is broken-down and sodium and potassium content reduced to levels near human milk; vitamins and minerals are added. Formula stays in the infant's stomach longer than breast milk, so the average bottle-fed baby will feed every three to four hours as opposed to two to three hours for the breast-fed infant.

In addition to cow's milk-based formulas, there are soy-based formulas, "elemental" formulas (formulas in which the proteins are very much broken-down), and formulas for prematures, very low birth weight prematures, and for children with metabolic diseases such as PKU (phenylketonuria).

It is currently recommended that solid foods not be introduced prior to five or six months of age unless a bottle-fed infant is drinking considerably more than a quart of milk per day or a breast-fed infant begins to decrease the time between feedings. The usual first food is cereal, because of its high iron content.

JAUNDICE OF THE NEWBORN More than half of term newborn infants and around 80 percent of premature infants are jaundiced during the first week of life. The yellow color of the baby's skin is due to accumulation of a pigment called bilirubin, which is a waste-product of the breakdown of hemoglobin, a protein found in red-blood cells.

During fetal life, the placenta eliminates bilirubin from the infant's body. In the mature infant, child and adult, bilirubin is excreted by the liver into the biliary system. During the first few days of life the baby's liver is immature and thus not able to excrete all the bilirubin with which it is presented. Thus it builds up in the blood and ultimately in the skin of the baby and causes a yellow cast to develop.

There are additional factors which may exacerbate the usual jaundice of the newborn. These include excessive bruising due to a traumatic delivery, Rh or ABO differences between the mother's and baby's blood types, transfusion, infection, and hypothyroidism.

Treatment. All jaundiced babies require medical monitoring by having periodic blood tests to make sure that the level of bilirubin doesn't rise too fast or get too high. If the bilirubin level gets to 14 or 15 (mgm/dl), the baby is placed under special lights (phototherapy) which cause the bilirubin level to decrease. If light therapy doesn't work or the bilirubin is very high (around 20 in a term baby) when first detected, the baby must have an exchange blood transfusion.

MALNUTRITION   An infant may receive insufficient food because of poverty or neglect, and malnutrition may result. Malnutrition may also result from organic conditions such as blockage in the digestive tract (by a tumor, pyloric stenosis, or intestinal obstruction), chronic diarrhea, colitis, liver disease, gastritis, osteoporosis (cystic degeneration of the bones), and tuberculosis. In a child it may also be caused by sheer refusal to eat brought on by emotional or mental conditions.

In the training of an infant, underfeeding may arise when a mother adheres rigidly to a schedule. She may ignore the infant's screams, adamant in her determination not to "spoil" the child. The baby may simply be hungry and the diet should be increased (after consultation with the physician). Psychological factors to which varying importance has been attached also color the clinical picture. (*See also* INFANT FEEDING in this section.)

METATARSUS ADDUCTUS *See* CLUBFOOT in this section.

MOLDING   During the course of the birth process the infant's skull may undergo a variable amount of reshaping (molding). The extent of this will be dependent on the size relationship of the infant's head to the mother's pelvis and pelvic outlet and the duration of labor. Also an area of swelling within the baby's scalp results from pressure on it by the gradually opening mouth of the uterus. The outcome is a somewhat elongated head with a puffy scalp, technically known as the caput succedaneum. All of this is reversible over the course of a few days and the molding disappears. The final size and shape of the head is determined by genetic factors.

NAVEL (UMBILICUS)   The navel, often called the belly button, is the mid-abdominal depression which is actually a scar indicating that point where blood vessels from and to the mother entered and left the unborn child's body. (For ruptured navel *see* HERNIA in the section GASTROINTESTINAL CONDITIONS.)

PEDIATRICS   Pediatrics is the branch of medicine that deals specifically with the health care of children from birth through adolescence. The pediatrician is especially concerned with aspects of proper growth, the prevention and treatment of common childhood diseases, and advising parents concerning a wide range of physiological and psychological factors in child development.

POISONING   *See* the section FIRST AID AND EMERGENCIES.

PREMATURE INFANTS   Infants delivered before thirty-seven weeks from the first day of the last menstrual period are considered to have a shortened gestational period and are termed preterm or premature. Prematurity is not defined by birth weight. A baby weighing five pounds or less but physically and neurologically mature and having gestational age of more than thirty-seven weeks is called a "small for gestational age" baby. True prematurity is more common among teenage mothers. Premature infants are more prone than term infants to respiratory distress syndrome, congenital malformations, brain hemorrhage, SIDS (sudden infant death syndrome), jaundice and other problems.

Tremendous strides have been made in the past twenty years in dealing with the many problems of low-birth-weight and very-low-birth-weight infants. More and more infants born as early as twenty-eight weeks gestation may now survive. The technology which keeps these babies alive is constantly being improved and changed. The incidence of premature births may also be reduced by drugs which are currently used to stop premature labor and allow the unborn infant to develop in its natural environment until it is fully mature.

PSYCHOLOGICAL DEVELOPMENT IN CHILDHOOD

Research indicates that the average human brain does not achieve complete maturity of function until about fourteen years of age. During the course of life, every person passes through standard phases of development: prenatal life, infancy, childhood, adolescence, early adulthood, adulthood, change of life (the climacteric), old age, and senility.

Maturation of the central nervous system, including the higher brain functions, is ordinarily measured by observation of different types of behavior. The infant, for example, should be sitting up at six months, standing alone at twelve months, walking at twelve to eighteen months, talking at fifteen to eighteen months, and becoming toilet trained by twenty-four months. The average child learns to count at age four or five, to read at age six, and to master increasingly more difficult subjects at the times when ordinarily presented in the regular school grades. (Similar patterns of development occur in relation to emotional maturation, to socialization, self-control, and ability to maintain personality integration under increasingly stressful life situations.)

Psychologists now recognize that wide individual differences normally exist in the rates of development of different mental functions. Children of high intelligence and superior native endowment tend to show precocious patterns of development, and schooling and other developmental experiences should be adjusted to their needs. Conversely, delayed patterns of development may result from many factors, emotional instability in particular. The child burdened with emotional conflict may show all kinds of developmental retardation, starting with late talking and toilet training in infancy, reading disabilities and other forms of educational difficulties in school, and a variety of conduct disorders in community life. Where extreme disorders of personality development are evident, the child should be seen by a child-guidance counselor, psychologist or psychiatrist. (*See also* the section MENTAL HEALTH.)

SLEEP DISTURBANCES

Disturbances in sleeping are usually more upsetting to the parents than to the children. The average infant will begin to sleep through the night by age two or three months. However, there are perfectly normal infants who will not sleep through the night until much later in the first year. This seems to be more common in breast-fed than in bottle-fed infants.

Some children will sleep through the night at the expected age but begin to wake at night in the second half of the first year. This may be perpetuated if the parent continually gives the child attention when he cries at night. Thus, it is suggested to let the infant cry for at least fifteen or twenty minutes to see if he will go back to sleep without parental intervention.

Nightmares characteristically begin around three years of age and are of two types: the common "bad dream" and the rare "night terror" dream. "Bad dreams" occur during REM (rapid eye-muscle movements) sleep. A child awakening during a REM phase usually remembers the dream and can be easily comforted and reassured. In the "night terror" dream the child is disoriented and very frightened and often appears to be sleeping with the eyes open and also may be perspiring and the pupils may be dilated. The child is often very difficult to awaken and usually cannot recall the dream.

Sleepwalking, sleep talking, teeth grinding and bedwetting are other common sleep disorders in children.

Treatment. Many children will have difficulty falling asleep and when they finally do, experience nighttime waking induced by separation anxiety (from their parents). As children become more aware of death, they may resist going to sleep for fear they may die. Parents should adopt a calm, understanding but firm attitude in dealing with their children's sleep problems. Bedtimes should be regular with variations minimal. A night light and allowing the child to leave the door open to the bedroom are often reassuring. The time before bedtime should be quiet, restful, and without stimulating television programs. (*See also* BEDWETTING [ENURESIS] in this section.)

SPEECH DISORDERS   There are three categories of speech disorder. The most common is the "functional" type; here the child appears to be quite normal in mentality and in structure, but the speech is abnormal. The stutterer, the stammerer, and the lisper are examples. The second type of speech problem is seen in the child whose speech defect is due to some anatomical defect: a cleft or short palate, enlarged tonsils and adenoids, etc. In the third type there is some abnormality of the nervous system, such as mental retardation, or some forms of epilepsy; the speech may be slurred, garbled, or otherwise distorted. Then too, the deaf child may be unable to speak, since he or she has been unable to hear spoken words and imitate them. "Tongue-tie" may also be a cause—if, however, a child can touch the tip of the tongue to the lips the tongue is not tied and the frenulum (the membrane attached under the tongue to the floor of the mouth) need not be clipped.

If the child does not have a vocabulary of at least five understandable words by the age of two years, an effort should be made to determine in which category the speech problem lies. Much progress has been made in recent years in diagnosing and treating these children. One very common speech anomaly will disappear if parents recognize it for what it is: stammering in the three-to-four-year-old, as "I—I—I—I—go—go—go—go—out." If wise parents realize this is a normal part of maturing, they will pay no attention, and the trouble will disappear within a few months. If they draw attention to it by making the child repeat the remarks correctly, the child may become so upset that an otherwise insignificant deviation may become a permanent speech problem.

SUDDEN INFANT DEATH SYNDROME (SIDS)   Each year thousands of infants in the United States die of a mysterious disorder known as Sudden Infant Death Syndrome (SIDS), also sometimes called "crib death." In such cases an infant, usually between two and six months of age, is placed in a crib or bed to sleep, usually with no noticeable signs of ill health, and then is found dead sometime later. A post-mortem examination indicates no known cause for death. SIDS is more common in premature and low-birth weight infants, in males, in babies from socio-economically deprived families, and in siblings of infants who have died of SIDS.

A condition termed ALTE (Apparent Life-Threatening Event) or "near miss SIDS" describes babies who have stopped breathing but have not died. To prevent SIDS these babies, as well as siblings of SIDS victims and premature infants who are considered at risk for SIDS, are placed on apnea devices which set off an alarm in case breathing stops. Life-saving measures can be initiated without delay. Portable devices are available for the home.

THERMOMETER   The clinical thermometer is a glass tube with graduated markings ranging from 94° F to 108° F (most foreign countries use the centigrade scale). The encased fluid—capable of expanding and contracting with temperature changes—is usually mercury. In clinical practice and in the home oral or rectal thermometers are used. The terminal of the oral thermometer is thin and about three-fourths of an inch long to facilitate placement under the tongue. The rectal thermometer has a short, spherical end for ease of rectal insertion.

Thermometers should be shaken before using until the fluid is at least as low as 96° F. The tips of rectal thermometers should be greased with petroleum jelly before insertion. A thermometer should be left in the mouth or rectum for three minutes before removing it for reading. For both types of thermometers the manufacturer's package instructions should always be followed. (*See also* FEVER in this section.)

THUMB-SUCKING   This is an infantile habit which usually begins in the first three months of life. Some authorities feel that it comes from an unsatisfied sucking drive. Others feel that it comes from hunger or colic pains and that the sucking action seems to quiet the baby. Still others feel that it is an inborn trait, as it is often familial.

As a substitute for the thumb some parents encourage their babies to suck on a pacifier. Most avid thumb-suckers continue until three years or so and will still be sucking their thumbs at age five or six when falling asleep at night.

Treatment. Placing obstacles to the sucking just seems to set a challenge for the child, who will pursue the habit even more aggressively. Applying bandages or tapes to the thumb seems to make no difference until the child is over five years of age. Most children give up the habit by age five or six. If not, the advice of a physician might be sought.

TOILET TRAINING As with other developmental milestones there is considerable variation about the time when children achieve sphincter control. Generally, bowel control occurs before bladder control. It is probably best to delay attempts at bowel training until eighteen to twenty-four months of age. By age three, about 90 percent of children are trained.

Control over urination is acquired later. Daytime control precedes nighttime control by several months to years. By age four, 90 percent of children have control over urination. It can be normal to wet the bed at night up to age five or six. (*See also* BEDWETTING [ENURESIS] in this section.)

VERNIX This is a whitish, cheesy material covering the body of the baby at birth. It does not reappear after having been removed by washing the baby.

VOMITING, CYCLIC Some young children have periodic recurrent vomiting, often accompanied by abdominal pain, migraine headaches, and diarrhea. The nausea and vomiting appear suddenly, may last one or two days, then disappear spontaneously. (*See also* VOMITING [EMESIS] IN CHILDREN in this section.)

VOMITING (EMESIS) IN CHILDREN Vomiting is the forceful emptying of the stomach via the mouth. It is a sign of a number of conditions, depending on the frequency, amount, color, and projectile of the attack. The simple "spit-up or wet burp" so often seen in babies is not serious; the gas bubble in the stomach simply pushes up a little bit of milk.

Although infrequent, vomiting may be a sign of milk allergy in an infant or older child. Forceful, projectile vomiting without associated fever or other symptoms may be a sign of intestinal obstruction and should be taken seriously.

Many children vomit once or twice when coming down with any illness, but the most common illness which produces vomiting is intestinal flu (viral gastroenteritis): there are great spasms of stomach cramps terminating in forceful emptying of the stomach. Often there are intermittent episodes of vomiting for a day or two with diarrhea following.

Nervous-system disease, especially if there is increased intracranial pressure as in concussion, blood clots, tumors, or meningitis will give rise to vomiting.

Treatment. It's prudent to seek the attention of a physician if vomiting continues. Besides doctor prescribed medications, the treatment for the vomiting of gastroenteritis includes clear liquids sipped slowly over time with progression to dry toast and crackers once the vomiting stops.

VULVA-IRRITATION (Irritations of the outer female genitals are discussed under VAGINITIS in the section FEMALE HEALTH CARE.) In female children and babies irritations are common in the vulvar area where the child's skin is exceedingly vulnerable. In girls older than babies, the most common cause of redness, soreness, and itching in this area is an irritating or infective vaginal discharge. Indeed, the vulvar condition may often be the most difficult aspect of vaginal discharges.

In severe conditions, a child is apt to scratch or manipulate the vulva locally, causing excoriations (raw lesions). For this reason these irritations, whether mild or severe, must have early medical attention. In stubborn cases, the cause may be sugar in the urine (perhaps from diabetes) and the physician will test for the presence of sugar because sugar encourages the development of local bacteria and yeast. The urine should also be frequently rechecked.

Because numerous skin conditions occurring in adults may also be found occasionally in children, any outbreak of pimples, rashes, or any unusual skin condition should be always called to the attention of a doctor. Allergic reactions to soaps and bubble baths should also be kept in mind.

Treatment. The rectal area may be similarly involved, and at the same time as the genital area. The physician will, of course, prescribe and direct the treatment of any disease which may lie behind vulvar irritation, which itself is more a symptom than a disease. Topical corticosteroid ointments may ease the discomfort and itching. Antihistamines by mouth may be of value.

AIDS AND OTHER SEXUALLY TRANSMITTED DISEASES

BACTERIAL DISEASES:
SYPHILIS
GONORRHEA
CHANCROID
SHIGELLOSIS
STREP INFECTIONS
URETHRITIS
(MYCOPLASMA)

FUNGAL DISEASES:
CANDIDIASIS
(MONILIA)

PROTOZOAN DISEASE:
TRICHOMONIASIS

VIRAL DISEASES:
AIDS
GENITAL HERPES
GENITAL WARTS
HEPATITIS B
CYTOMEGALOVIRUS

The current publicity surrounding acquired immune deficiency syndrome (AIDS) has focused attention on other sexually transmitted diseases (STDs). These diseases occur in young and old, in homosexual and heterosexual individuals. Some are caused by bacteria and virus and can only be transmitted by sexual contact. The conditions can be annoying or cause permanent disability or death.

The consequences can be deadly, and it is important for all to know the signs, symptoms, side effects, and treatments of STDs. Early diagnosis and treatment can eliminate or control the severe consequences of many of these infections. Responsible actions can determine the chances of transmitting or becoming infected.

The following is a list of terms identified in this section:

AIDS
CHLAMYDIA
GONORRHEA
HERPES, GENITAL AND ORAL

NGU
PID
SYPHILIS
WOMEN AND STDs

AIDS Acquired Immune Deficiency Syndrome (AIDS) is characterized by a defect in natural immunity against disease. People who have AIDS are vulnerable to serious illnesses which would not be a threat to anyone whose immune system was functioning normally. These illnesses are referred to as "opportunistic" infections or diseases.

Many individuals infected with the AIDS virus have no symptoms and feel well. Some develop symptoms which may include tiredness, fever, loss of appetite and weight, diarrhea, night sweats, and swollen glands (lymph nodes)—usually in the neck, armpits, or groin.

AIDS is spread by sexual contact, needle sharing, or less commonly, through transfused blood or its components. The risk of infection with the virus is increased by having multiple sexual partners, either homosexual or heterosexual, and sharing of needles among those using illicit drugs. The occurrence of the syndrome in hemophilia patients and persons receiving transfusions provides evidence of transmission of the virus through blood. The virus may be transmitted also from infected mother to infant before, during, or shortly after birth.

Most cases of AIDS have occurred in the following groups of people:

- Sexually active homosexual and bisexual men;
- Present or past abusers of intravenous drugs;
- Persons with hemophilia or other coagulation disorders;
- Heterosexual contacts of someone with AIDS or at risk for AIDS;
- Persons who have had transfusions with blood or blood products;
- Infants born to infected mothers.

AIDS is difficult to catch, even among people at highest risk for the disease. The risk of transmitting AIDS from daily contact at work, school, or at home apparently is practically nonexistent. Direct sexual contact or the sharing of IV drug needles remains the main transmitter of the virus.

Blood banks and other blood collection centers use sterile equipment and disposable needles. The need for blood is great, and people who are not at increased risk for getting AIDS are urged to continue to donate blood as they have in the past.

Casual contact with AIDS patients or infected persons does *not* place others at risk for getting the illness. No cases have been found where the virus has been transmitted by casual household contact with AIDS patients or infected persons. Infants with AIDS have not transmitted the infection to family members living in the same household.

Ambulance drivers, police, and firefighters who have assisted AIDS patients have not become ill. Nurses, doctors, and health care personnel have not developed AIDS from routine caring for AIDS patients. A few cases have been reported in health care personnel following accidental needle stick injuries, or the splashing of infected blood on an open or abraded area of skin.

The U.S. Public Health Service recommends the following steps to reduce the chances of contracting infection with HIV— the virus that causes AIDS:
- Don't have sex with multiple partners, or with persons who have had multiple partners (including prostitutes). The more partners you have, the greater your risk of contracting AIDS.
- Obviously, avoiding sex with persons with AIDS would eliminate the risk of sexually transmitted infection by the virus. However, if you do have sex with a person you think could be infected, protect yourself by taking appropriate precautions to prevent contact with the person's body fluids. ("Body fluids" includes blood, semen, urine, feces, saliva, and women's genital secretions.)
  —Use condoms, which will reduce the possibility of transmitting the virus.
  —Avoid practices that may injure body tissues (for example, anal intercourse).
  —Avoid oral-genital contact.
  —Avoid open-mouthed, intimate kissing.
- Don't use intravenous drugs. If you do, don't share needles or syringes.

Cases of AIDS related to medical use of blood or blood products can be prevented by use of HIV antibody screening tests at blood donor sites and by members of high risk groups voluntarily not donating blood.

There is no vaccine for AIDS itself. However, there is good reason to believe that individuals can reduce their risk of contracting AIDS by following existing recommendations. Communities can help prevent AIDS by vigorous efforts to educate and inform their populations about the illness, with special emphasis on educational activities for members of high risk groups. Meanwhile, the effort to produce vaccines and drugs against AIDS continues.

While there is no cure for AIDS, several medications have been used to successfully treat many of the opportunistic infections that those with HIV infection may contract. Several preliminary studies have shown that the use of certain medications may slow the HIV replication in those patients whose immune system is still functioning. It is because of these medications that HIV infection is becoming more of a chronic disease. The United States Public Health Service has urged all those who might be at risk for HIV infection to be tested. Those whose test results are positive should see a physician and seek advice about available treatments.

Further information about AIDS may be obtained from your local or state health department or your physician. The National AIDS hotline number is 1-800-342-AIDS or 1-800-221-7044.

For further information on drug treatment call 1-800-662-HELP.

CHLAMYDIA Chlamydia (pronounced *kla-mid-e-uh*) are widespread sexually transmitted microorganisms that are causing a national epidemic. An estimated three million Americans get chlamydial infections each year, making it three times more common than gonorrhea and thirty times more common than syphilis. Chlamydia may infect both men and women. It is thought to be a major cause of nongonococcal urethritis (NGU), cervicitis and Pelvic Inflammatory Disease (PID). These infections can cause infertility.

Tests that give accurate, quick results are now available to diagnose chlamydial infections. These tests can be taken even when there are no symptoms and are not painful.

Chlamydial infections can be treated with several different drugs. Because it is often present with other venereal diseases, such as gonorrhea, a doctor may prescribe a drug that can cure a number of infections at the same time.

GONORRHEA This is the most common of the venereal diseases, both of the male and female. With the advent of antibiotics, incidence of gonorrhea has been greatly reduced, but it is by no means eradicated. The infection is due to the gonococcus organism, and is con-

EXCERPTS FROM THE FOREWORD TO THE AIDS REPORT BY THE U.S. SURGEON GENERAL, C. EVERETT KOOP, M.D., Sc.D. May 1988

Acquired Immune Deficiency Syndrome is an epidemic that has already killed thousands of people, mostly young, productive Americans. In addition to illness, disability, and death, AIDS has brought fear to the hearts of most Americans—fear of disease and fear of the unknown. Initial reporting of AIDS occurred in the United States, but AIDS and the spread of the AIDS virus is an international problem.

The vast majority of Americans are against illicit drugs. As a health officer I am opposed to the use of illicit drugs. As a practicing physician for more than forty years, I have seen the devastation that follows the use of illicit drugs—addiction, poor health, family disruption, emotional disturbances and death. I applaud the President's initiative to rid this nation of the curse of illicit drug use and addiction. The success of his initiative is critical to the health of the American people and will also help reduce the number of persons exposed to the AIDS virus.

Education about AIDS should start in early elementary school and at home so that children can grow up knowing the behavior to avoid to protect themselves from exposure to the AIDS virus. The threat of AIDS can provide an opportunity for parents to instill in their children their own moral and ethical standards.

Those of us who are parents, educators and community leaders, indeed all adults, cannot disregard this responsibility to educate our young. The need is critical and the price of neglect is high. The lives of our young people depend on our fulfilling our responsibility.

AIDS is an infectious disease. It is contagious, but it cannot be spread in the same manner as a common cold or measles or chicken pox. It is contagious in the same way that sexually transmitted diseases, such as syphilis and gonorrhea, are contagious. AIDS can also be spread through the sharing of intravenous drug needles and syringes used for injecting illicit drugs.

At the beginning of the AIDS epidemic many Americans had little sympathy for people with AIDS. The feeling was that somehow people from certain groups "deserved" their illness. Let us put those feelings behind us. We are fighting a disease, not people. Those who are already afflicted are sick people and need our care as do all sick patients. The country must face this epidemic as a unified society. We must prevent the spread of AIDS while at the same time preserving our humanity and intimacy.

AIDS is a life-threatening disease and a major public health issue. Its impact on our society is and will continue to be devastating. By the end of 1991, an estimated 270,000 cases of AIDS will have occurred with 179,000 deaths within the decade since the disease was first recognized. In the year 1991, an estimated 145,000 patients with AIDS will need health and supportive services at a total cost of between $8 and $16 billion. However, AIDS is preventable. It can be controlled by changes in personal behavior. It is the responsibility of every citizen to be informed about AIDS and to exercise the appropriate preventive measures.

The spread of AIDS can and must be stopped.

tracted almost exclusively through intercourse. It is one of the most common causes of infertility, because if left untreated it obstructs the tubes (male epididymis and female fallopian tubes).

Symptoms. The symptoms of gonorrhea will depend on the organ involved. The first symptoms usually appear a week after exposure and consist of burning during urination, difficulty in emptying the bladder, and excessive urethral discharge, with pus. In the male the testicles may become swollen and tender; in the female the same thing happens to the glands at the entrance of the vagina (Bartholin's glands). If the infection spreads through the uterus to the fallopian tubes and ovaries, the woman will complain of severe lower abdominal pains and fever, and the whole picture will often be difficult to differentiate from acute appendicitis. Occasionally the joints can become involved, becoming warm, swollen, and tender (gonococcal arthritis).

Treatment. After proper diagnosis, treatment is relatively simple. Most cases can be cured with penicillin. It is important to find the original host of the infection and treat him or her, otherwise a cycle of reinfection is very likely to occur.

HERPES, GENITAL AND ORAL Herpes is a common viral infection. It causes cold sores or fever blisters (oral herpes), and it also causes genital sores (genital herpes). In the United States, oral herpes affects more than

50 million people, and genital herpes affects about 20 million. Herpes Simplex Virus Type II is the cause of genital herpes which is characterized by blisters in the genital regions of both males and females. It is primarily seen in adults and rarely seen before adolescence. Transmission occurs during sexual contact and can be present with or without symptoms. The virus may cause a type of meningitis and pregnant women with active disease are often advised against vaginal delivery because of the danger to the newborn. It is also thought that genital infection with this virus puts females at higher risk for cancer of the cervix. The virus can be transmitted to other body sites during heterosexual or homosexual activity. Reactivation of the virus commonly occurs, with or without visible blisters.

When the virus gets into skin cells, it starts to multiply. As your immune system fights the virus, the skin becomes red and sensitive. Soon after, one or more blisters or bumps appear. The blisters open, and sores that sometimes look like cuts in the skin remain. These heal as new skin tissue forms. During the first outbreak the area is usually painful and may itch, burn or tingle. You may also have swollen glands, headache, muscle aches or fever—similar to flu symptoms. Some people notice itching, or other sensations before they see anything on their skin. These are called "prodromal symptoms," and they warn that virus may be present on the skin. Herpes can be transmitted from the time these first symptoms are noticed until the area is completely healed and the skin looks normal again.

Condoms help to prevent transmission of sexually transmitted diseases (STDs). It is not known how effective they are in preventing transmission of genital herpes. Although laboratory studies have shown that the virus does not pass through condoms, they should not be relied on if you have any symptoms or signs of infection (sores, discharge, painful urination, itching, etc.).

It is important to see the doctor as soon as sores appear and before they begin to heal. A blood test cannot diagnose herpes. Another reason to see a doctor is for treatment. The recent antiviral drug (Zovirax) taken by mouth apparently shortens the duration of attacks, especially first attacks. Your doctor knows what medications are available and

can talk to you about them. Before using over-the-counter (drug store) medications or home remedies, check with a doctor.

Patients with oral and genital herpes can be treated but, at present, not cured. Here are some positive things patients can do:

- Take good care of your general health—eat well, get enough rest and exercise. Avoid physical and emotional stress as much as possible—don't let yourself get "run down."
- Keep the infected area as clean and dry as possible during an outbreak. This will help your natural healing process.
- Preventing self-spread is simple: do not touch the area during an outbreak. If you do, wash your hands as soon as possible. The herpes virus is easily killed with soap and water.
- Get the information you need so you aren't worrying unnecessarily. Understanding herpes gives you a positive way to deal with your concerns and fears.

NGU NGU stands for nongonococcal urethritis which means an inflammation or infection of the urethra (the tube that carries urine from the bladder) caused by something other than the germ that is responsible for gonorrhea.

NGU is one of the most common forms of sexually transmitted disease (STD). It is estimated that 2.5 million Americans are infected each year. NGU is treated with antibiotics, although not the same drugs used to treat gonorrhea.

PID Pelvic Inflammatory Disease, also called PID or salpingitis, is the most common serious infection involving a woman's reproductive system. Although PID may be caused by a variety of organisms and conditions, certain sexually transmitted diseases (STDs) and the use of an intrauterine device (IUD) for birth control are known to be especially important factors.

If not promptly diagnosed and treated, PID can damage the reproductive system. Scar tissue can form inside the fallopian tubes. This can result in infertility by partially or totally blocking the tubes, thus not allowing the egg to enter the uterus.

Formation of scar tissue can also increase

the risk of tubal pregnancy. Tubal pregnancy, which can be life threatening, is the result of a fertilized egg becoming implanted inside the fallopian tube rather than in the uterus.

PID should never be dismissed as insignificant or without consequences. Research has shown that women who have had PID once are at greater risk of developing this condition again. This may further the possibility of infertility and tubal pregnancy.

Diagnosis of PID is based on an in-depth medical and social history, a pelvic examination and laboratory tests. Treatment consists of any number of antibiotics, depending on the cause of the infection. PID can usually be treated on an out-patient basis, although in severe cases hospitalization may be recommended. (*See also* GONORRHEA, SYPHILIS, and AIDS in this section.)

In the treatment of all STDs, physician instructions should be followed carefully and all of the medication must be taken as directed. After treatment, it is important to be rechecked to make sure the infection is completely cured.

Sex partners should be treated for two reasons: to avoid your re-infection and to prevent them from suffering possible complications.

Avoid sex throughout the time of treatment since, until you're re-tested and proven cured, you might still be infectious.

How can I avoid getting an STD?

- Limit your number of sexual partners. Your risk of infection increases with the number of partners you have. If you and your sexual partner have no other partners, and neither of you has an STD—neither of you will be exposed. If you have one sexual partner, but that person has other partners, your risk of getting an STD is increased.
- Practice and encourage open and honest communication with your partner(s). Remember, some STDs aren't obvious in women. A woman may not know she needs to see a doctor unless her partner tells her she has been exposed to a disease.
- Use condoms. If properly used, they provide good (though not perfect) protection. Various foams and creams intended for vaginal use as contraceptives have been found to have some ability to kill STD germs.

- If either partner has an STD, *both* partners must be treated in order to avoid re-infection.
- If you or your partner have other sexual contacts, you should get regular STD checkups, at least four times a year.

If you need more information about STD, or if you need the name of a private doctor or a public health clinic, call the STD National Hotline, toll-free:

National 1-800-227-8922

In California 1-800-982-5883

SYPHILIS   Known as the great imitator, syphilis can affect every organ of the body and has produced almost every observed medical symptom. The range of the intensity and duration of this disease varies from "early" syphilis, with its primary ulcerated tumor mass (chancre) and secondary lesions of several types of appearance, distribution, and duration, to "late" syphilis, with its destructive lesions of the skin (gumma), heart and blood vessels, bones and joints, nerves and brain (paresis). So versatile are the manifestations of syphilis that it is even known to produce no significant damage in a relatively small percentage of patients who have remained untreated because of lack of medical facilities.

In addition to the types of syphilis with overt lesions of the skin and mucous membranes, the disease can exist for many years without signs or symptoms except for changes in the blood serology in congenital and in latent syphilis. Some forms of congenital syphilis, acquired from the mother during the course of pregnancy, and latent syphilis in which there are no signs of the disease other than a persistently positive blood test, constitute situations in which the diagnosis is established on the basis of the patient's history, repeated and varied blood tests, and the absence of other diseases capable of producing similar blood serologic changes (lupus erythematosus, vaccination).

The causative organism, a spirochete, *Treponema pallidum,* can be obtained for diagnosis from early lesions, and almost not at all from late (tertiary) lesions—an indication of the immune changes resulting from the infection. Infection takes place in so high a percentage of persons exposed to the organism (usually in the primary and secondary highly infectious lesions) that for practical and preventive purposes it can be assumed that sexual contact with a known "active" syphilitic will result in infection in the non-syphilitic partner. Approximately 10 percent of exposures result in infection with the syphilis organism. Males have a higher prevalence than females; there is also a higher prevalence among homosexuals. Because of this high contagiosity, it is well to treat all known "contacts" of a diagnosed syphilitic with immediate doses of antibiotic (usually penicillin), both to avoid spread of the disease in the community and to attempt to provide adequate treatment of the individual.

The advent of antibiotics has vastly altered the incidence of syphilitic infection wherever treatment is available. Antibiotic therapy has also altered the course of the disease because of the rapidity of the cure. Since antibiotic therapy, evidence of cure (ability to be re-infected) is usual enough to have resulted in the invention of the term "ping-pong syphilis" to designate the back and forth transfer of the disease by the presently affected sexual partner to the presently cured partner, with a reversal of the situation on treatment of the affected one.

Antibiotic therapy has had another profound effect on the management of this disease, that of the urgency of adequate treatment. It has long been known that in order to effect a cure, or at least improvement, in a disease of so many changes to so many organs, treatment must be sufficiently complete to ensure at least immunologic (serologic) evidence of change to normal, that is a negative test of the blood and of the spinal fluid. If remedies are given in insufficient amounts or for too short a time, and the treatment is inadequate for cure, the immune responses of the body are interfered with. Under these circumstances, a spontaneous cure effected by the body's own protective mechanisms is rendered impossible of completion, and a treatment cure is impossible to achieve. Since antibiotic therapy is so effective in curing syphilis, it is essential that medication be given early and adequately. The taking of antibiotics in lesser doses for shorter periods of time for concurrent "minor" ailments, such as boils, infected teeth, respiratory infections, is so commonplace that if the existence of a

syphilitic infection is suspected, the patient should be investigated quickly and thoroughly; and if a diagnosis of syphilis is made, adequate treatment should be administered to prevent the serious consequences attending the usually lesser dosage of antibiotics given for other conditions.

Treatment. Although antibiotics are of singular merit in the treatment of syphilis, the method of administration, the dosage and the duration of treatment depend on the stage of the disease and the age, sex, and general medical condition of the patient, and include considerations of prevention (as in pregnancy).

WOMEN AND STDs   If a pregnant woman has an STD and neglects immediate medical care, her unborn baby can be infected too. An estimated 300,000 infants die or suffer birth defects every year because of STDs they get from their mothers.

In addition, untreated STDs can lead to PID (pelvic inflammatory disease). PID can permanently hinder a woman's ability to have children.

STDs are the leading cause of infertility in the United States. Chlamydia and gonorrhea are the chief culprits.

Of the women now under 30 years old, at least 100,000 this year will suffer painful permanent damage to their reproductive organs as a consequence of untreated, or inadequately treated, gonorrhea. Many of these women will never be able to bear children.

While scientists have yet to establish a firm link between genital herpes and cancer, women infected with genital herpes are eight times more likely to develop cancer of the cervix as non-infected women. There is similar evidence that chronic trichomonal infection may predispose the cervix to cancer.

Many babies die each year as a result of infection with genital herpes transmitted to them at birth by their infected mothers. A few pregnant women with primary genital herpes infection in early pregnancy will suffer miscarriages due to this disease.

Twenty-five percent of all serious infant retardation is caused by congenital cytomegalovirus, a little understood sexually transmissible disease that produces virtually no symptoms in adults who harbor it.

PREVALENT SEXUALLY TRANSMITTED DISEASES (STDs)

Developed from American Social Health Association Information

DISEASES	SIGNS IN A WOMAN	SIGNS IN A MAN	CONSEQUENCES OF PROLONGED INFECTION	SPECIAL CONSIDERATIONS
GENITAL HERPES	Painful, blister-like, fluid-filled lesion (or cluster of lesions) on, in or around vagina. Often accompanied by swollen glands in groin area.	Same as in women, only on or around penis.	Under study at this time. Genital herpes has been implicated with a form of meningitis and associated with cervical cancer. Consequences to babies: Damage to internal organs, blindness, retardation, death. Acquired during birth.	Genital herpes is caused by a virus and cannot be cured. The initial infection will lapse into a latent state with periodic flareups often triggered by stress or fatigue. Genital herpes may be passed from an infected pregnant woman to her newborn during birth. A series of tests (cultures) taken from the cervix will help your doctor determine whether a cesarean section is required to protect the baby at time of birth.
GONORRHEA	Pus-like vaginal discharge, vaginal soreness, lower abdominal pain, painful urination.	Pus-like urethral discharge.	Pelvic Inflammatory Disease (PID)—tubal damage, pelvic adhesions and tubo-ovarian abscesses, tubal pregnancy which can lead to pathological sterility. Consequences to babies: Eye infection. Acquired during birth.	Even if the original gonococcal infection is cured, PID may predispose the body to repeated episodes of pelvic inflammation caused by a variety of organisms. Untreated gonorrhea and chlamydia are major causes of PID in women. PID can lead to infertility or ectopic (tubal) pregnancy. Symptoms of these two infections are similar, but chlamydia, unlike gonorrhea, cannot be cured with penicillin. It requires other antibiotics.
CHLAMYDIA	Symptoms similar to those caused by gonorrhea, but sometimes milder. Symptoms often take weeks or even months to develop.	Discharge from the penis and/or burning when urinating. Burning and itching around the opening of the penis. Symptoms may be present early in the day and go away, but they will come back. Many men will have no noticeable symptoms, or symptoms so mild that they go unnoticed.	For both men and women, a painful infection can develop requiring hospitalization. Can cause permanent damage to the reproductive organs and sterility. For women, the infection can complicate pregnancy resulting in the death of the unborn baby and, occasionally, the mother.	(See GONORRHEA.)
Sexually Transmitted NONGONOCOCCAL URETHRITIS (NGU) CERVICITIS	Symptoms similar to those caused by gonorrhea.	Occasionally, heavy pus-like discharge. More frequently, a mild watery discharge.	Pelvic Inflammatory Disease. (See GONORRHEA in this section.) Consequences to babies: Eye infections and pneumonia in newborn babies if their mothers have NGU.	Like gonococcal PID, non-gonococcal PID could lead to repeated episodes.
SYPHILIS	Rashes appearing almost anywhere on the body, including palms of hands and soles of feet. Chancre (lesion) on or in vagina, anus or mouth. Loss of facial or scalp hair in patches.	Rashes or hair loss in the same pattern as in women. Chancre on or around penis.	Brain or heart damage. Consequences to babies: An infected pregnant woman may pass syphilis to a developing fetus, which could lead to a variety of birth defects. Blindness, brain damage, heart defect, bone deformities, death. A baby may seem healthy at birth and develop symptoms later in childhood. Acquired in the uterus before birth.	Syphilis is particularly dangerous because symptoms will go away by themselves without treatment, but the disease remains in the body and can ultimately cause severe damage and even death. It can remain in the body for years. It can be cured at any time, but damage done cannot be repaired.

As AIDS spreads through the population, an increasing number of infants are born with the disease, transmitted to them from the pregnant mother transplacentally. The symptomatology is much as in the adult form, the course more rapid and always fatal.

Because of these and other similarly grave consequences, the growing epidemic of sexually transmitted disease (STD) is of concern. STD is almost as common as the common cold; but, unlike a cold, it will not go away without treatment, and its aftermath may be lifelong illness and disability or premature death.

Babies born to mothers with untreated STDs can suffer severe health consequences and even death. Gonorrhea in the birth canal during delivery can cause eye infections lead-

ing to blindness. Because of this all babies born in hospitals are treated promptly with medicated eye drops. Similarly, chlamydia and venereal warts can cause eye, ear, and potentially fatal lung infections. A woman with active genital herpes at the time of delivery can infect her baby. Infants who survive a severe herpes infection usually suffer physical or mental damage. If an unborn child is infected with syphilis, it will be born with congenital (present at birth) syphilis. The baby may appear healthy at first, but can later develop a number of consequences of the disease, including a heart defect, bone deformities, or brain damage. (*See also* HERPES, GENITAL, IN THE FEMALE in the section FEMALE HEALTH CARE.)

INFECTIOUS DISEASES

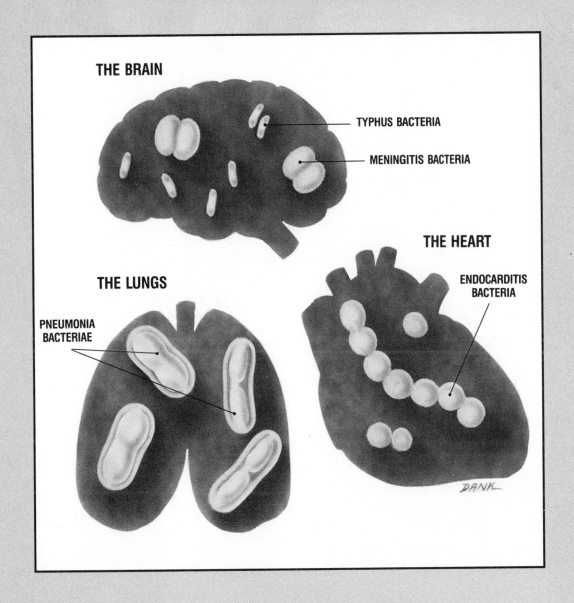

THE BRAIN

TYPHUS BACTERIA

MENINGITIS BACTERIA

THE HEART

THE LUNGS

ENDOCARDITIS BACTERIA

PNEUMONIA BACTERIAE

$\mathbf{T}$hroughout history mankind has experienced at times the devastating effect of infectious diseases. Whether spread by virus or bacteria, diseases can be passed from one to another quite rapidly. Man has fought the "black plague of medieval times," the "great white plague" (tuberculosis) in the early twentieth century, and currently battles the AIDS virus in major proportions.

This section focuses on the infectious diseases other than sexually transmitted ones. Examination of common symptoms and possible sources of treatment are also given.

The following is a list of terms identified in this section:

ANTITOXIN
ASEPSIS
ATHLETE'S FOOT
BCG VACCINE
BLASTOMYCOSIS
CHICKENPOX (VARICELLA)
CHOLERA
COCCIDIOIDOMYCOSIS
COLD SORES
COMMON COLD, THE
COMMUNICABLE DISEASE
CONJUNCTIVITIS, ACUTE BACTERIAL
   ("PINK-EYE")
CONTAGION
DYSENTERY
DYSENTERY, BACILLARY
ENCEPHALITIS
ENDOCARDITIS
EPSTEIN-BARR SYNDROME (EBS)
FOOD POISONING (BOTULISM)
GLANDULAR FEVER (INFECTIOUS
   MONONUCLEOSIS)
HEPATITIS
HEPATITIS B
HERPES, GENITAL
HERPES SIMPLEX
HERPES ZOSTER
HISTOPLASMOSIS
IMMUNIZATIONS
IMPETIGO
INFANTILE PARALYSIS (POLIOMYELITIS)
INFECTION
INFESTATION
INFLUENZA

LEGIONNAIRE'S DISEASE
LOCKJAW (TETANUS)
LYME DISEASE
MALARIA
MASTITIS
MEASLES (RED MEASLES)
MENINGITIS
MONONUCLEOSIS
MORBIDITY RATE
MUMPS
OSTEOMYELITIS
PELVIC INFLAMMATORY DISEASE
PHARYNGITIS
PHARYNGITIS, STREPTOCOCCAL
PITYRIASIS ROSEA
POLIO
PUS
RABIES (HYDROPHOBIA)
REYE'S SYNDROME
RHEUMATIC FEVER
ROSEOLA
RUBELLA (GERMAN MEASLES)
SABIN VACCINE
SALK VACCINE
SCARLET FEVER
SEPTICEMIA
SLEEPING SICKNESS
SMALLPOX
SPOROTRICHOSIS
STAPHYLOCOCCUS
THRUSH
TONSILLITIS
TOXOPLASMOSIS
TRICHINOSIS

TUBERCULOSIS
TYPHOID FEVER
UNDULANT FEVER (BRUCELLOSIS)

VENEREAL DISEASE
WHOOPING COUGH (PERTUSSIS)
YELLOW FEVER

ANTITOXIN Literally "against poison," an antitoxin is a substance which forms within the human body when certain toxins from without gain entrance into the organism. The toxins may come from germs, plants, or other animals. The antitoxin, therefore, is an antibody. Many of them are secured by introducing toxins in gradually increasing doses into horses. Then serum is taken from these animals and used (as hypodermically injected medication) to provide immunization in humans against specific toxins.

Some of the bacterias the human body may encounter pose their greatest threat by manufacturing a substance that may be poisonous to a distant bodily tissue. The organism of tetanus, as an example, produces a substance that binds to the nerve cells, hence it is a neurotoxin. This becomes manifest by spasm and rigidity of many muscles. In the face there is elevation of the eyebrows and the mouth is pulled into a smile; in the back, muscle spasm produces arching. The rigidity of jaw muscles gave the disease its old name of lockjaw. Once the toxin binds to the nerve cells it cannot be displaced, hence the importance of prevention in the approach to tetanus. This is produced by immunization in which the injection of tetanus toxoid produces antitoxin.

A comparable situation exists with diphtheria. Here the bacteria produce a toxin which weakens or paralyzes throat muscles and may be similarly toxic to the heart muscle. Still another toxin is that found in food poisoning, botulinus toxin.

ASEPSIS Asepsis is the absence of bacteria and other disease-producing microorganisms or germs. The care of the sick and modern surgical techniques are based in good measure on aseptic methods of avoiding infection. The meaning of asepsis is summed up in one word: *sterile*.

ATHLETE'S FOOT This common ailment is caused by fungi in persons who have the type of skin (sweaty) which is conducive to the abundant growth of the fungus and who also have inadequate local immunity to the effects of that fungal growth. The common location of the eruption between the toes is due largely to the persistence of moisture in these warm and occluded areas. While sweat is almost always available for fungal growth, moisture from inadequate drying of the feet after swimming and bathing is probably a more frequent precipitating factor in the occurrence of acute attacks of athlete's foot. The communicability of this disease is largely overstated as is evidenced by the fact that bedmates do not often contract the disease from exposure to each other; and more importantly, the eruption is not uncommonly seen on only one foot, the other apparently not affording identical opportunity for the growth of the fungus. It is apparent that compulsory foot baths in public pools accomplish little as compared with what compulsory drying of the feet would do for the protection of the individual.

Several species of fungi are capable of producing this disease. A few cause widespread fungus disease of the soles of the feet, palms of the hands, nails and other parts of the skin, and that only in an infinitely smaller number of people.

Symptoms. The eruption ranges from a slight scaling between the fourth and fifth toes to redness, oozing, and cracking of the spaces between all the toes and extension of the eruption to the adjacent areas of the feet. Secondary infection and bleeding of the cracked and fissured areas result from inattention to the earlier lesions.

Treatment. It is essential that the feet be kept dry. It may be necessary to institute a regime of frequent change of socks and shoes, and sometimes it may become necessary to wear sandals or perforated shoes to permit both the lessening of sweat production and the evaporation of the irreducible amount of sweat present. Minor attacks can be controlled by sponging the feet with rubbing alcohol to ensure final drying. The application of foot powders, while theoretically sound, nevertheless often induces further skin breakdown by the swelling of the powder on mixing with sweat and the forming of irritating masses. Antifungal ointments should be applied at night, when the foot is not encased in occlusive footgear. For more severe involvement and for oozing eruptions, cold wet soaks will relieve the subjective symptoms and reduce irritation and swelling. Plain cold water is both available and satisfactory, although the well-known potassium permanganate, boric acid, Burow's solution compresses, or soaks can be used if not too inconvenient.

The fungal antibiotic griseofulvin is a very effective remedy. Because of both the recurrences and the persistence of this disease, the use of an antibiotic should be reserved for either acute and disabling attacks, or for cases in which more simple remedies fail. A number of agents active when applied to the skin are available in cream, ointment and lotion form. They include miconazole, clotrimazole and ketoconazole. They should be applied for a time after the skin has seemingly cleared.

BCG VACCINE *See* TUBERCULOSIS in this section.

BLASTOMYCOSIS Caused by the fungus *Blastomyces dermatitidis* in the United States (few reported cases in Canada) and by the fungus *Blastomyces brasiliensis* in South America, this "deep" mycosis affects the skin and other organs, most notably the lungs. North American blastomycosis differs substantially from South American and is most characteristically located on the face, hands, arms, and feet.

Symptoms. The initial small ulcers or lesions enlarge, become pustular, ulcerate, and become crusted. On enlarging peripherally, the central portion heals and leaves thick scars. Multiple lesions can coalesce forming arc-shaped lesions. Concomitant lung involvement is usual. Diagnosis can be confirmed by biopsy examination of the skin lesion and by culture of the fungus.

Treatment. Small early lesions can be excised surgically to avoid extension of the disease and consequent disfigurement. Treatment with iodide has been largely displaced by stilbamidine injections. Although somewhat difficult to administer and with toxic properties largely attributable to degradation of the drug, stilbamidine is effective in the treatment of blastomycosis. More recently ketoconazole and amphotericin have been found of value.

CHICKENPOX (VARICELLA) Chickenpox is an acute communicable viral disease seen almost exclusively in children. It is so contagious that almost all have had it by the age of nine or ten.

Symptoms. Chickenpox is characterized by the gradual onset of red, discrete, small bumps on the skin, initially of the trunk, then of the extremities. On the first day there is usually a mild headache and a fever of about 100°. The following day there are new bumps, and the old ones have become water blisters. On the third day the blisters have become pustules, and on the fourth they begin to crust over.

The only condition with which chickenpox may be confused is flea bites; but the fact that the lesions in chickenpox come out in crops, and that there are lesions in the scalp (humans almost never get bitten there), makes this a fairly easy disease to diagnose. An occasional child will be very sick with a fever of 104° to 105°F. for four or five days; in this situation he will invariably have lesions in his mouth and down the throat.

The virus causing chickenpox is identical to that causing shingles. Shingles is almost exclusively a disease of the elderly. Rarely an exposure to one form of the viral disease may produce the other.

Once the blisters become dry the patient is no longer considered contagious.

Treatment. Treatment should include keeping the child away from susceptible children, making him comfortable, reducing high fever, and preventing secondary infection. The newer antihistamines will relieve the itching, and antibiotic ointments control skin infections. The itch may be alleviated by baths of tepid water to which bicarbonate of soda or oatmeal has been added (Aveeno®). With either, the water is allowed to dry on the skin and leave a residue. Aspirin should not be given: rare cases of Reye's syndrome may be produced by it. The antiviral drug, Zovirax®, has some impact on the virus of chickenpox but is rarely prescribed, except for cases of shingles. VZIG (Varicella Zoster Immune Globulin) may prevent or lessen the severity of chickenpox if administered within ninety-six hours of exposure to those who are not immune.

CHOLERA   This is an intestinal infection caused by a comma-shaped organism also called a vibrio, which is notorious for causing epidemics of severe dysentery. Cholera rapidly produces massive dehydration as pints of intestinal fluid literally gush out of the victim. Fluid therapy, by vein and by mouth, is life-saving, with antibiotics of secondary importance. Vaccination is a valuable preventive measure, although it is not recommended often, even for U.S. citizens traveling abroad. Risk is very small, negligible in fact.

COCCIDIOIDOMYCOSIS   This fungus infection (mycosis) is caused by the fungus *Coccidioides immitis* resident in the soil of hot dry areas and carried by dust storms. Infection of the lungs results from inhalation of the spores of the fungus, and the patient may be unaware of the infection or suffer a short febrile illness. San Joaquin or Valley fever, a progressive form of the disease involving almost all of the organs, including the skin, occurs infrequently in persons of low resistance. The progressive disseminated form can involve not only the lung but various organs, bone, meninges and brain.

Symptoms. The patient exhibits fever, weight loss, and weakness. The skin can be the organ of primary infection under rare circumstances of invasion of the organism at the site of injury. The skin modules enlarge and ulcerate; the local lymph glands also enlarge, and spontaneous healing occurs in a few weeks or months with residual scarring.

Treatment. Progressive coccidioidomycosis is treated with supportive measures and available antifungal antibiotics including amphotericin B and Ketoconazole.

COLD SORES   This common name for the disease herpes simplex is curious in the light of the fact that a high percentage of the afflicted have recurrent attacks on exposure to the summer sun. Of course cold sores do often accompany the common cold and other infections of the upper respiratory tract, but the disease is primarily due to activation of the causative resident virus by a "triggering" fac-

tor. In addition to the triggering agents already mentioned (infection, physical agents including ultraviolet light), both foods and drugs are frequent offenders. Although no food can be considered exempt from suspicion in patients in whom the triggering cause is obscure, the most commonly indicted ones are chocolate, nuts and fish. It should also be pointed out that in patients in whom the cause appears to be a preceding infection (common cold), the possibility that the medication taken for the infection has in fact triggered the cold sore must be considered. Everyday observation indicates the degree of transmissibility to others, such as family members, is low which emphasizes the importance of individual factors.

Symptoms. The cold sores consist of a small group of thick-walled blisters with very faint or no surrounding redness. In one or two days, yellowish crusting occurs, the result of some seepage of the blister serum. There is often accompanying itching, and sometimes a smarting or burning sensation.

Treatment. The antiviral drug acyclovir taken by mouth appears to diminish the severity of an attack. It is also available as an ointment. Local antibiotics (bacitracin and Neosporin®) are used for control of secondary infection.

COMMON COLD, THE   To the virus of the common cold and other respiratory viruses the target organ is the nose. The function of the nose is not primarily to perceive odors, but to warm, humidify, and filter the air so that when it reaches the bronchi and lungs it is at the proper temperature, is clean, and contains the correct amount of moisture. The secondary function of the nose is to perceive odor, which also contributes heavily to the sense of taste.

As the air enters the nose, it is warmed and humidified by the turbinates. The mucous blanket picks up tiny inhaled particles and carries them away. If the air is very cold and dry, the nose has to work very hard to bring inhaled air to the correct temperature and humidity; this may cause excess mucous secretion and a "runny nose." It may be so hot and dry that the continuous mucous blanket leaves a gap of exposed mucosa. The blanket is now no longer continuous; there is a chink in its armor; viruses (tiny, submicroscopic particles which are not affected by antibiotics) can now gain a foothold. If the exposed area is in the pharynx, a scratchy throat may develop. Then the common virus gains access to the bloodstream.

In such instances, the cold virus multiplies and causes some swelling of the mucosa. The virus spreads, and the nose, sinuses, throat, and ears become affected. The mucosal lining reacts to the stimuli by producing mucus and by swelling. The temperature rises and the tissues become red—even painful. (These are all classic signs of inflammation.) Swelling of the tissues makes breathing through the nose difficult. Excess mucus causes nasal dripping; the head feels "full"; body temperature is elevated.

Treatment. Since antibiotics do not help, what then should the patient with a cold do? The following steps might help relieve the discomfort of the cold:

- Bed rest. Time is saved in the long run by a few days of bed rest so that the body can fight off the virus and heal itself. If everyday activities are continued while the patient "heroically" pretends the cold does not exist, bacterial invasion of the weakened tissues can more easily occur. Bacterial complications are unpleasant and dangerous; they include pneumonia, sinusitis, and otitis media (ear inflammation). Thus, it pays to avoid the complications of the common cold by getting plenty of rest.
- Fluids. In addition to maintaining nutrition by adequate food intake, drinking more than the usual amount of juices, water, and other fluids will make a cold more bearable.
- Aspirin or aspirin substitutes. Aspirin, one of man's most versatile drugs, is effective in relieving the minor aches of a cold and in lowering an elevated temperature. Acetaminophen compounds (Tylenol) will also help to relieve aches and pains of a cold and reduce the fever. Reye's syndrome has not been associated with this compound. Aspirin should not be used if the viral infection is in fact flu or chicken pox; it has been associated with an apparently increased incidence of Reye's syndrome.
- Humidity. If a leg is broken, we set it in

proper alignment and put it at rest by using a cast. When the upper respiratory system is infected, we should help make its functioning easier by providing humidity in the inhaled air (one of the functions of the nose is humidifying). Some use cold vapor and some, steam vapor; as long as sufficient humidity is provided, either of them may be used.

- Nosedrops. Nosedrops shrink the swollen nasal lining and make breathing through the nose easier. These should, however, be used only on a physician's advice.
- Antibiotics. Antibiotics have no effect on the viruses causing the common cold and should not be used unless the physician feels there are definite indications. (Subsequent bacterial infection, for example, may respond to antibiotic medication.)
- The celebrated Nobelist Linus Pauling created a stir in 1970 with the publication of a book asserting that large doses of vitamin C had prophylactic and therapeutic benefits for the common cold. Most of the medical profession and experts on the viruses remained unconvinced, and trials with student populations did not substantiate the benefits claimed for vitamin C. It is yet to be proved that the many viruses producing the common cold can be warded off by vitamin C.
- "Cold tablets." These nonprescription medications may be helpful and probably cause no harm. They are usually composed of aspirin or aspirin-like compounds, together with an antihistamine and a drug that acts to make the breathing easier. Most of these drugs, however, should not be taken if you have high blood pressure and certain other health problems. It is a prudent idea to phone your doctor to make sure that it is all right to take this kind of medication.

COMMUNICABLE DISEASE *See* CONTAGION; INFECTION in this section.

CONJUNCTIVITIS, ACUTE BACTERIAL ("PINK-EYE") This common bacterial infection of the eye or eyes produces tearing, itching and redness of the affected eye. It is transmitted very easily from person to person in areas where poor hygiene is practiced. The disease is very common in small children and rarely seen in adults. In certain areas of the world, it is responsible for loss of eyesight among children.

Contact with the discharge from the eye should be avoided. Sharing of eye makeup and multiple eye dose medications should also be avoided.

Quarantine of the infected person is not necessary, but medical consultation may be advisable. Good hygiene and handwashing practices are very important in the prevention of epidemics. (*See also* CONJUNCTIVITIS in the section EYE AND VISION CONDITIONS).

CONTAGION   Contagion is the spread of disease from one individual to another by direct or indirect human contact or by an intermediate agent. In the latter, for example, the anopheles mosquito, which transmits malaria to man, is an intermediate agent. A disease may be both infectious and contagious.

DYSENTERY   Dysentery, a serious type of diarrhea, is the passage of very loose and watery, often bloody, stools seen in patients with an intestinal infection due to a variety of bacteria and parasites such as amoebas. The disease is more often contracted in foreign countries, especially in warmer climates. There are two kinds of dysentery: amoebic, caused by parasites, and bacillary, caused primarily by Shigella. (*See* DYSENTERY, BACILLARY in this section.)

Symptoms. Dysentery is usually accompanied by fever and extreme prostration; the patient may become rapidly dehydrated and go into a state of shock. The onset of the symptoms is rather rapid. Epidemics may occur, and on a lesser scale, whole families may suffer simultaneously after drinking from a common, contaminated source, such as a well. In carefully traced epidemics, one person will be found as the source of infection. This person may have no knowledge that he is a carrier (his system being immune to the effects of the germ), but his stools nevertheless contain the bacteria. Several germs are involved in dysentery, their identification depending upon their effect on different sugars when they are incubated: these include the typhoid, paratyphoid, *Salmonella,* and *Shigella.* In spite of good sanitation, these organisms are still found spo-

radically in the United States and, of course, are rampant in tropical and low-income areas. Travelers learn not to drink unboiled water in those countries and are usually warned against salads, raw foods, shellfish, etc.

Treatment. Treatment for dysentery depends on the severity of the symptoms, but if the patient is severely ill he should be hospitalized, since intravenous fluids and perhaps blood may be needed. Usually a sample is taken of the stool and a drug or two started immediately; once the organism is identified, the most effective antibiotic is continued. Results are often dramatic within twenty-four to forty-eight hours if the patient has not been dehydrated or is not too seriously sick.

DYSENTERY, BACILLARY   Bacillary dysentery is an acute infection of the bowel caused by bacteria (bacilli) of the *Shigella* group, and characterized by frequent passage of stools containing blood, pus, and mucus, accompanied by abdominal cramps and fever.

The *Shigella* are worldwide in distribution. The infection is spread from person to person. It is contracted by eating contaminated food and other objects. Human waste matter also spreads the disease, and flies may also be occasional carriers. Dysentery epidemics occur among overcrowded populations having inadequate sanitation; the disease is particularly common in younger children living in areas where the disease is prevalent.

The dysentery bacilli ingested with food and drink pass into the intestines. There they produce an inflammatory disease characterized by ulcers. In the adult, the disorder is usually limited to the lower half of the large intestine.

Symptoms. In children, the disease may develop suddenly with fever, irritability, loss of appetite, nausea, diarrhea, and abdominal pain. Within a few days the characteristic stool findings will be noted. The patient loses weight and becomes dehydrated, and the disease may end fatally.

In adults, most of the infections are not accompanied by fever and there may be blood or mucus in the diarrhea. Attacks of abdominal pain, vomiting, and diarrhea recur, mixed with episodes of apparent recovery. Mild cases last about a week, severe cases perhaps a month. A chronic form is recognized in tropical areas.

The finding of pus in the stool is strongly suggestive of bacillary dysentery. The diagnosis is proven by the isolation of *Shigella* from the stools.

Treatment. Fluid and salt-solution (electrolyte) administration is essential, particularly in young children. A number of antibiotics have recently been shown to be quite effective. The nutritional state must be carefully maintained. The diarrhea is also treated symptomatically.

Good sanitation—the elimination of flies and protection of food from contamination—is of primary importance in the prevention of this disease. Proper hygiene is the basic protective measure; there are no satisfactory methods of immunization.

ENCEPHALITIS Encephalitis is an inflammatory reaction of the brain, usually involving both the cerebral hemispheres and the brainstem. It is frequently associated with inflammation of the meninges, and is then referred to as meningoencephalitis. A wide variety of disorders produce encephalitis, including various infections and intoxications. Infections, in turn, may be due to viruses, rickettsiae, fungi, and a few bacteria such as the bacilli which produce tuberculosis. Some forms of encephalitis occur in epidemics and others occur sporadically. Birds are the reservoir of the virus of equine encephalitis, which is transmitted by mosquitoes to horses and man and occasionally results in epidemics of encephalitis. Other viral diseases produce similar epidemic spread. Rarely, encephalitis is also a complication of measles, chickenpox, and mumps, as well as vaccination against rabies and smallpox. Encephalitis may also occur with lead poisoning.

Symptoms. The patient is either drowsy or stuporous. The neck may be stiff and there may be headache and fever. Localized weakness, visual disturbances, disorders of speech and swallowing may be present. The patient may be irritable. In extreme cases, loss of consciousness and convulsions may indicate early demise. Examination of the cerebrospinal fluid usually reveals a slight increase in the number of white blood cells. The organism responsible for some types of encephalitis can be cultured from the cerebrospinal fluid. In other types of infections, studies of the blood serum during the acute and convalescent phases of the illness may determine the cause. Skin lesions associated with some of these infections may be characteristic.

Treatment. Specific antibiotic and chemical agents are used in the treatment of rickettsial infections such as Rocky Mountain spotted fever, tuberculous meningoencephalitis, and cryptococcal meningoencephalitis. A few specific drugs are available for the treatment of viral infections producing encephalitis. The patient with severe encephalitis requires constant nursing care and attention, with careful check of blood pressure and respiration. If there is severe difficulty in swallowing, the patient may require an opening into the windpipe (tracheotomy). If the patient is unable to breathe adequately because of weakness of the respiratory muscles, respiratory aids are required. Intravenous fluids are often needed to prevent dehydration in patients who are stuporous or who vomit frequently. Physical therapy and, subsequently, occupational therapy are essential for those who develop motor weakness or paralysis.

ENDOCARDITIS The endocardium is the smooth and glistening membrane that covers the entire inner surface of the heart walls and valves. Invasion of an area of the endocardium by bacterial organisms is called bacterial endocarditis.

When "blood-poisoning" is present from peritonitis, childbirth fever, or from an overwhelming infection due to almost any type of bacteria, the heart may be infected secondarily to the disease. The acute bacterial endocarditis that may be present in any case of "blood-poisoning" is not primarily an affliction of the heart, and is rarely discussed in association with the circulatory diseases.

Subacute bacterial endocarditis (SBE) is a distinct heart disease. It is due to bacteria of rather low toxicity that have colonized an area of the inner heart surface which has usually already been damaged by rheumatic fever or congenital deformity. This damage focuses a harsh stream of blood on a small bit of surface within the heart and causes the formation of a surface erosion that is vulnerable to bacterial implantation.

The organism involved is usually the so-called "non-hemolytic streptococcus" that can ordinarily be found in the mouth of even healthy subjects. A tooth extraction or sore throat may cause escape of these bacteria into the bloodstream where they freely travel to the heart and may attach themselves to endocardial spots roughened by stress changes or prior disease.

Symptoms. The symptoms of subacute bacterial endocarditis are usually those of a low grade fever and weakness. If these occur in a rheumatic patient or one with congenital heart disease, subacute bacterial endocarditis (SBE) must always be suspected. Diagnosis is based on a specimen of blood which shows the offending organism. Anemia is often present as a complication.

Treatment. Vigorous antibiotic therapy and bed rest have brought down the mortality-rate to a figure below 30 percent in the active phase of the infection. Those who recover usually show marked damage to the valves that were involved in the process.

Adequate surgical correction of congenital heart defects will prevent most bacterial endocarditis. Sometimes the only indication for surgery in a patient with no symptoms related to congenital deformity may be the prevention of bacterial endocarditis.

EPSTEIN-BARR SYNDROME (EBS)

Epstein-Barr syndrome is a disease caused by the Epstein-Barr virus, the same agent that causes infectious mononucleosis. Most patients are young women.

Symptoms. Frequent fatigue, headache and malaise are the most common symptoms. Other symptoms include sore throat, enlarged lymph nodes, cramping and vomiting.

Treatment. Treatment consists of relieving the patient's discomfort and pain. Antibiotics have not been effective in treating EBS. Chronic fatigue syndromes have followed EBS and are currently the object of much research and debate.

FOOD POISONING (BOTULISM)

Botulism is a serious form of acute poisoning following the ingestion of food containing a toxin produced by the bacterium *Clostridium botulinum*. The disease is almost always caused by the eating of improperly preserved food. The toxin produced by the bacteria may be found in such foods as string beans, corn, spinach, olives, beets, seafood, pork products, and beef. Cooking food at a temperature of at least 176°F. for thirty minutes before eating is a safeguard against botulism.

Symptoms. Symptoms develop within a day or two after eating contaminated food. The patient feels weak and tired and develops such visual disturbances as double vision, followed by difficulty in speaking and swallowing. The muscles of the extremities and trunk become weak; however, the mental faculties remain clear. There is no significant fever, and blood and urine tests are normal.

Mortality in botulism may be as high as 15 percent. Most fatalities occur between the second and ninth day and result from respiratory paralysis or bronchial pneumonia. Recovery is slow in those who survive.

It may be difficult to diagnose a single case of botulism, but the simultaneous occurrence of several cases following consumption of the same meal makes the diagnosis more likely. Bacteriologic tests often indicate the guilty organism.

Prevention depends on proper home canning and adequate heating of food before serving. Food showing any evidence of spoilage should be discarded.

Treatment. Treatment usually requires hospitalization. Antitoxin may be used, particularly in those who were exposed to contaminated food, but who have not yet developed symptoms of poisoning. For those with active botulism, treatment is largely supportive; that is, sedation, fluids by vein, antibiotics for respiratory infection, and so forth.

GLANDULAR FEVER (INFECTIOUS MONONUCLEOSIS)

This is a contagious disease (not common in small children), manifested by fever, swollen glands, and general malaise. It is usually accompanied by a sore throat and there may be a headache and stiff neck, a measle-like rash, and/or jaundice. The majority of the patients have an enlarged spleen. Some complain of fatigue for weeks and months. The diagnosis is based on the finding of typical white cells in the blood and by the special Paul-Bunnell test. Since infectious mononucleosis is more likely to be found in young adults or in older children, it is commonly called "the kissing disease." It can be confused with hepatitis.

Treatment. Recent studies have implicated a specific virus, the Epstein-Barr (E-B) virus, as the cause of the disease. There is no specific treatment, although cortisone drugs may be of symptomatic value. The patient should rest adequately; associated fatigue states are common and chronic forms of the disease producing chronic fatigue do occur.

HEPATITIS The commonly seen infections of the liver are caused by viruses. Infectious hepatitis or catarrhal jaundice is the result of ingesting food or water contaminated by fecal material containing the virus. It is referred to as hepatitis A.

Serum hepatitis B is caused by a virus which gains access to the body through injections. Contamination of needles, syringes, tubing, ampoules, or the injected material itself may be present. To combat this hazard great care is taken by pharmaceutical manufacturers to produce absolutely sterile injectable medications. Blood and plasma may contain the virus, and the patient who is given several transfusions is thereby increasingly exposed to the risk of hepatitis. Improved methods of processing blood and plasma have greatly diminished this risk. The grossly unsterile techniques of drug addicts using homemade syringes and needles (or discarded hypodermic needles) is a troublesome source of serum hepatitis. A vaccine against hepatitis B is available; it is advocated especially for health care workers.

Symptoms. The symptoms of the two types are similar, as is the treatment. The incubation period in serum hepatitis is usually longer, and the infection may not be apparent until three to six months after introduction of the offending agent to the bloodstream.

The symptoms in both forms of hepatitis often begin abruptly and include loss of appetite, nausea and vomiting, fever, and tenderness over the liver area. Often for smokers the taste for tobacco is lost. Jaundice usually becomes evident in four to five days and is due to an inability of the diseased liver to handle the pigment from the broken-down red blood cells. In epidemics of infectious hepatitis, however, jaundice may not be noticeable.

Recovery is usually uneventful after six to eight weeks of illness. Relapses are common and are often due to too quick a resumption of activity. In a small percentage of cases severe liver damage may occur and treatment is difficult. Therapy is nonspecific and bed rest is mandatory. The diet should be rich in protein, carbohydrates, and vitamins. Proper nutrition is often difficult because of continued nausea. Rarely, after severe cases of hepatitis, the liver may become cirrhotic.

HEPATITIS B *See* HEPATITIS in this section.

HERPES, GENITAL *See* HERPES, GENITAL AND ORAL in the section AIDS AND OTHER SEXUALLY TRANSMITTED DISEASES.

HERPES SIMPLEX Of the more than seventy herpes viruses identified, five are known to infect humans. Of these five, herpes simplex Type I and herpes simplex Type II are the most common.

Herpes simplex Type I produces cold sores and fever blisters, usually on the lips or on the mouth. On rare occasions Type I can erupt in the genital area. The disease can be transmitted by direct contact with active lesions. (*See also* COLD SORES in this section.)

Herpes simplex Type II causes genital herpes, perhaps the fastest spreading sexually transmitted disease in the United States. It is highly contagious whenever the characteristic blisters appear. The first attack of Type II, accompanied by burning and itching sensations, may last as long as a month.

The first symptoms of Type II would occur about six days after contact with an infected person. Prior to the appearance of the blisters, the individual may have fever, headache, or a generalized discomfort.

Often Type II infections occur again; for some individuals repeated attacks of the active phase have been reported. Usually the severity of the recurrence lessens over time, but they may continue for years at sporadic intervals.

Women with herpes simplex Type II antibodies have a much greater risk of developing cervical cancer. Pregnant women with Type II risk miscarriage, early delivery, and possible birth defects, especially if the baby is exposed to the virus during birth. Delivery by caesarean section may be recommended to reduce the risk of infecting the baby.

It is possible for the herpes virus to spread into the bloodstream and infect other organs in certain individuals, such as cancer patients or persons with kidney, lung, or blood diseases. These people have difficulty in fighting most infections.

There is no cure as yet for Type II herpes, although testing for vaccines is now underway. Some relief from symptoms can be obtained with medications such as Domeboro and Zovirax. Sexual contact during the active phase of Type II should be avoided.

Current information about herpes can be obtained by sending a self-addressed, stamped envelope to Herpes Resource Center, Box 100, Palo Alto, CA, 94302.

HERPES ZOSTER *See* Shingles in the section Skin Conditions.

HISTOPLASMOSIS   Caused by the fungus *Histoplasma capsulatum*, this deep mycotic infection usually results from inhalation of the spores, which reside in the soil and have been found most frequently in the Mississippi and Ohio River valleys. The infection varies from a disease with practically no symptoms to overwhelming infection, and the condition is often difficult to differentiate from tuberculosis. Active infection is probably the result of a general depletion of immunity as is evidenced by the high susceptibility of infants to the progressive form of the disease. It is not transmitted from person to person.

Symptoms. Aside from the skin involvement in the overwhelming progressive form, primary infection of the skin is rare and usually self-limiting. The red, nodular lesions of the skin occur more frequently on the penis, around the mouth, and on the buccal mucous membranes.

Bed rest and supportive measures are useful, and may alone be curative. For more serious cases a drug called amphotericin B is given in intravenous solution, and the drug ketoconazole taken by mouth has also proved of value.

IMMUNIZATIONS   The practice of giving live or dead cell material to a person in an effort to create an immunity or resistance to a particular disease is common today. Dead bacteria are given in shots to ward off whooping cough; toxoids are given to help the body resist diphtheria and tetanus; dead viruses "teach" the body to fight off poliomyelitis and measles; and finally, live viruses are used to build an immunity against smallpox, poliomyelitis, and measles. Special immunizations against rabies, mumps, Rocky Mountain spotted fever, and cholera are available, but are used only in unusual situations.

Diphtheria, whooping cough, and lock jaw (tetanus) shots are now universally given as a combined "DPT shot" beginning at two months of life; two more of these are used, at ages 4 and 6 months. Simultaneously, or following soon thereafter, the poliomyelitis vaccines (live and/or dead) are given. Measles vaccine is given anytime after the tenth month.

A booster shot of the DPT is usually given in the second year, again at age five before school, and approximately every three to seven years subsequently.

A number of recent studies show that the immunity conferred by tetanus immunization lasts longer than had been earlier supposed. The immunity titers run high for five to ten years and are easily boosted by another shot over this interval if the need arises. A booster every ten years is now recommended. In 1971 the Public Health Service, taking note of findings that the need for routine smallpox vaccination for travelers appeared obsolescent because of the disappearance of the disease in modern countries, modified its former policies. Later when smallpox officially disappeared, the vaccines were withdrawn and smallpox vaccination came to an end.

Rarely, are there reactions to the vaccines. Older individuals are advised to receive flu immunization every year, and a once only pneumonia shot and may occasionally have mild reactions. But there is no doubt that as with children, they save lives.

IMPETIGO   *See* Impetigo in the section Skin Conditions.

INFANTILE PARALYSIS (POLIOMYELITIS)   "Polio" is an acute viral disease characterized by fever, headache, stiff neck and back, and sore muscles, which often leads to paralysis. Until recently there were widespread epidemics of this disease, but thanks to the polio shots and drops the disease is now rarely seen.

The poliomyelitis virus invades the nervous system, killing the nerve cells that activate muscles. Once these cells are killed, no more messages are sent to the afflicted muscle so that it stops working, shrinks, and becomes useless (atrophies): hence the paralysis. When the virus involves the nerves leading to the throat and diaphragm muscles, the victim has bulbar polio. Here a respirator may be needed, because these are the muscles which control breathing; and without an adequate supply of air into the lungs the patient will die.

Treatment. Since polio is virus-caused, there is no specific treatment once the disease is established. Aspirin and hot packs are useful in easing the severe pain of the muscle spasms, and after the acute attack is over (in two to three weeks) a great deal is accomplished by the use of various physiotherapy devices to encourage weak muscles to regain strength and to reeducate good muscles to do the work of those whose use is permanently lost. Some authorities feel that at least two years are required for complete recovery, since muscle function may be returning all this time. Later, orthopedic surgery may help a great deal to transplant good muscles for bad, and to restore function.

The best treatment would be prevention. There are two methods of protection, the Salk vaccine and the Sabin vaccine. The Salk shots contain all three polio viruses which have been killed; a basic immunizing series consists of three monthly shots with a booster several months later. The Sabin vaccine is the live virus but it has been weakened to the extent that it will not produce the disease but still allows the body to develop protective antibodies, with three types administered separately at monthly intervals; it is given orally by dropper or on a sugar cube. It is best to administer a booster of the Sabin vaccine several months later.

Both vaccines are safe and highly effective. One or both methods should be begun in the first few months of life, but all ages should be immunized. The oral type lends itself better to mass or community wide immunization methods and is, of course, not painful as the shots are.

INFECTION Infection is a disease process that is due to a specific organism, such as a germ, virus or fungus. The term is sometimes erroneously used to indicate invasion of the body by organisms of higher orders, such as worms, which is called infestation. A disease may be both infectious and contagious, such as gonorrhea. Infection also means the communication of disease from one part of the body to another; this is autoinfection. Thus, bacteria from one site may spread through the blood stream and lodge elsewhere, for example in bone (osteomyelitis) or the heart (endocarditis).

INFESTATION Infestation is the invasion of the body by organisms higher in order than germs, viruses, fungi, and similar organisms. The most common type of infestation is that by worms.

INFLUENZA Also called the flu, or catarrhal fever, this condition is a specific infectious disease of man. Acute and self-limiting in its course, the disease occurs in epidemic attacks which have sometimes acquired pandemic proportions. While epidemics recur at frequent intervals, the pandemics do so only every twenty to thirty years—the most recent having taken place in 1968 ("Hong Kong" Influenza).

The disease is a viral infection. The first influenza virus (at present called Influenza A virus) was isolated in 1933; this was followed by the discovery of Influenza B in 1940 and C in 1949. (The three viruses have characteristics in common, but important differences do exist—particularly the fact that infection by one type of virus does not confer immunity against infection by another.) Each of these viruses can be further subdivided into strains.

Although epidemics tend to appear in the winter months, they may also occur in the summer and tend to show some cyclic tendency; thus, Influenza A occurs at about two to three year intervals and B at four to five year intervals. Occasionally both epidemics may run concurrently. Infection is transmitted through inhalation and all persons are susceptible regardless of age, sex, or race.

Symptoms. Symptoms may vary widely in severity and duration. The incubation period is short (one to two days) and the onset is abruptly announced by fever, chills, headache, lassitude, and diffuse pains, particularly in the back and limbs. Respiratory symptoms are similar to those of a "cold" or upper respiratory infection, but are characteristically of much lesser magnitude than in these conditions; on the other hand, the general symptom of being "sick all over" is more prominent. Patients are usually acutely ill for no more than three to five days, the fever then subsiding gradually over several more days. Most characteristic is the feeling of prostration which follows the acute symptoms and may prolong convalescence for several weeks, particularly in debilitated patients. The disease usually runs an uneventful course and complications are rare. When the epidemic is severe, fatalities have, however, occurred—mainly because of superimposed bacterial pneumonia, which especially affects individuals suffering from pulmonary or heart diseases.

Treatment. There is no specific treatment presently available. Supportive hygienic measures and alleviation of troublesome symptoms are the same as described for other respiratory infections. In debilitated persons, a careful watch should be kept for the development of pneumonia in order to institute early antibiotic treatment.

As regards prevention, the currently available vaccines contain a certain number of strains of both Influenza A and B virus. About two weeks after administration, some defense substances (antibodies) appear. The protection afforded is almost complete, but only against the specific strains used, and only for a period ranging from two to eight months. Thus, booster injections should usually be administered every year before the winter season.

For influenza A infection (and only for the A strain) the anti-Parkinsonian drug, amantadine, has been shown to be of value. Amantadine interferes with replication of the 'A' virus and thus shortens the duration and severity of the flu.

LEGIONNAIRE'S DISEASE   This disease came to national attention at an American Legion convention in Philadelphia in 1976 when over 180 people contracted this hitherto unidentified bacterial form of pneumonia. The middle-aged, elderly, and people with a weakened immune system tend to be affected the most. Transmission of the illness is by inhalation of aerosols contaminated with the specific bacterium. There are no known cases of direct person-to-person transmission.

Symptoms. The disease may manifest itself as a mild upper respiratory illness progressing to pneumonia. Delayed diagnosis of serious cases can prove fatal. Initially the symptoms include cough, high fever, and chest pain, especially when breathing deeply. Some patients may also experience severe pain in the cardiac, kidney, neurological and gastrointestinal systems.

Treatment. Many cases respond to oral antibiotics. Severe cases require hospitalization and administration of intravenous antibiotics.

LOCKJAW (TETANUS)   Lockjaw is a fatal disease caused by the toxin produced by bacteria introduced into the body through a break in the skin, usually a deep wound (like a nail-puncture). Although it is now rare, as compared with the early part of this century, it can still be fatal unless treated promptly and efficiently. It is relatively more frequent in children because they are more prone to puncture wounds. A newborn baby may acquire this disease if the umbilical cord is tied off with unsterile or dirty material.

Symptoms. Within a few days after tetanus germs have lodged in the body through a puncture wound, some muscle stiffness appears, especially about the neck. Soon the patient cannot open his mouth, is apt to develop localized muscle spasms, and may then go into convulsions or coma.

Treatment. Treatment of lockjaw must be prevention. Once the active disease is contracted it is difficult to treat—in spite of antitoxin which neutralizes the unbound but not cell-bound toxin. When treatment is started late, the death-rate is high.

It is simple to have basic tetanus shots in

the first year of life; later on, all that is necessary at the time of a wound or cut is to give a "booster" of tetanus toxoid.

If a child has not been immunized, a doctor should always decide—even in minor injuries—whether antitoxin should be given. (*See* IMMUNIZATIONS in this section and in the section INFANT AND CHILD CARE.)

LYME DISEASE   A bite from a deer tick infected with a spirochete bacterium produces Lyme disease, the most common tick-borne disease in the United States. The illness was first recognized in children in 1975 in Lyme, Connecticut. The deer tick, active during the spring and summer in Minnesota, Wisconsin, and the New England states, is found in heavily wooded areas as well as in well-groomed lawns. It is not transmitted from person to person.

Symptoms. Lyme disease occurs in three stages, which may appear singly or overlap each other. Symptoms may not be apparent or recognized for weeks after the tick bite. The initial stage is characterized by flu-like symptoms and an expanding red rash with a clear center. The second stage is marked by neurological and cardiac problems usually weeks to months after the appearance of the rash. The third-stage symptoms include chronic arthritic and neurological symptoms. Cases are often misdiagnosed as being rheumatoid arthritis or meningitis.

Treatment. Lyme disease, regardless of the stage, responds successfully to antibiotics. The sooner the treatment, the less the likelihood of the disease will develop severe stages.

MALARIA   Malaria (Italian *mala aria,* meaning bad air) is an acute, often recurrent, sometimes chronic parasitic disorder marked by paroxysms of chills followed by a high fever, presence of the parasites in the red blood cells, profuse sweats, often with enlargement of the spleen, and, at times, jaundice.

Cause. The cause of malaria is a protozoan, the plasmodium. Man is infected by the bite of the malaria-infected anopheles mosquito, or (among drug addicts) by the use of a common hypodermic syringe and needle, or by receiving blood in a transfusion from an infected donor. Malaria has become a very rare disease

in the United States. However, due to the frequency with which military personnel and tourists visit tropical countries, this cause of hemolytic anemia continues to be important.

Symptoms. Within ten to thirty-five days after exposure, symptoms appear as a relatively mild fever, chilliness, headache, and malaise which last for about a week and usually are regarded as and treated as influenza. Suddenly the patient is seized with a violent chill followed by profuse perspiration and fever that is extremely high. The fever lasts from one to eight hours, subsides, and the patient now states that he feels well. Then, every two days (or more, depending on the type of plasmodium with which he is infected) he is stricken by an attack of chill-fever-sweats. The high fever may be accompanied by severe headache, drowsiness, delirium, confusion, and even convulsions. In the chronic form, the fever is not as high, attacks are milder and shorter, and the patient is fatigued, listless, lacks appetite, and complains of headache. If malaria persists long enough, jaundice may develop, the spleen may become enlarged, and less frequently, the liver may enlarge.

Treatment. Treatment is most successful with quinine (obtained from the cinchona bark) and several synthetic antimalarial preparations such as quinacrine, pyrimethamine, primaquine, and chlorguanide.

Persons who contemplate travel in malarial countries can prevent malarial infection if any of the above mentioned antimalarial agents are taken in prophylactic dosage before, during, and for two weeks after such a journey.

MASTITIS   Mastitis is acute bacterial infection of the breast, and may occur in breast-feeding mothers a week or more after delivery. It is characterized by swelling, redness, and tenderness of the breast, accompanied by high fever and general malaise. Treatment consists of interruption of lactation, antibiotics, breast-support, and ice bags. Very often a breast abscess will form which will require incision and drainage of the pus.

MEASLES (RED MEASLES)   Measles (rubeola) is an acute communicable disease which runs a characteristic course. It spreads from child to child by droplet infection and is highly contagious.

Symptoms. On the tenth day after exposure, a susceptible child will develop a fever; then each day for the next four days the patient becomes progressively sicker, with increasing fever and dry, hard cough, bleary eyes, and lethargy. Finally, on the fourteenth day, a rash begins to break out around the hair line which takes about twenty-four hours to spread from the face to the feet. The rash is intensely pink, flat and solid on the face, and more scattered and spotted further down the body.

The patient does not feel any improvement until the day after the rash has appeared on the feet. At this point, the cough loosens up and diminishes, the fever subsides and the rash begins to fade from the face. Should the fever climb again, the cough get worse, or an earache develop, this usually means that a germ-caused complication has occurred, in which case an antibiotic may be prescribed by the physician.

Treatment. Since measles is caused by a virus, there are no specific measures against it except aspirin or aspirin-substitute, fluids, rest, and comfortable baths. There is no truth to the old wives' tale that light will injure the eyes of a measles patient. The disease itself might cause a nerve injury in a susceptible person, but not the light itself: light may irritate the eyes, but cannot damage them.

If parents are aware that their unimmunized child has been exposed to measles, they should have their doctor administer a modifying dose of gamma globulin. If given at the proper time and in the right amount, this substance will reduce the infected child's measles to a mild, yet immunizing, case.

Both the live and dead types of measles vaccine furnish good immunity for the uninfected child. (If a mother has had the measles, her baby is immune until the fourth to fifth month of life.)

As mentioned before, failure of the measles to improve on the day following complete appearance of the rash means that some complication has set in. If it is bronchitis or otitis media, the child should be seen by a physician. If the child develops measles encephalitis, the symptoms may be severe headache,

coma, convulsions, or other signs of nervous-system irritation. Measles encephalitis is a particularly distressing complication because it may leave the child with some neurological damage. However, this possibility should no longer be a threat because modern measles vaccination is so effective in preventing the original disease. Every parent therefore owes it to the child to make certain that measles immunization is carried out.

Note: Measles should not be confused with German measles (rubella). Despite the similarity in names, the two diseases are entirely different in many important respects, particularly in the fact that German measles during the first trimester of pregnancy constitutes a specifically grave threat to the fetus. (See RU-BELLA in this section.)

MENINGITIS Meningitis is an acute infection of the meninges (the covering membranes of the brain). It is caused by a wide variety of infecting organisms, including bacteria and viruses. Meningococcic meningitis occurs in epidemic form; other types of meningitis usually occur as isolated cases. The chief mode of spread appears to be by droplets.

Symptoms. The acute onset of headache, fever, and stiff neck are characteristic findings in meningitis. The patient may become drowsy or stuporous and may have nausea and vomiting. With progression of the infection, the cranial nerves may be involved and result in double vision, facial weakness, deafness, or other findings. Some types of infection are associated with skin rash. Convulsions and coma may develop.

Treatment. Bacterial infections producing meningitis are treated with antibiotics such as penicillin, sulfadiazine, chloromycetin, and tetracyclines. If the causative organism can be isolated from the cerebrospinal fluid (spinal tap) the drug or drugs which are most effective in treating this bacterial infection are administered; if the causative organism cannot be immediately identified and if a purulent infection is present, drug therapy is immediately instituted. Early treatment of bacterial infections is of the greatest importance in lowering the mortality rate and the incidence of complications. Prior to the discovery of the drugs which are currently available for treatment of meningitis, most forms of bacterial meningitis were almost uniformly fatal.

No specific drugs are available for the treatment of viral infections producing meningitis. In all patients with meningitis, hospitalization and expert nursing care are mandatory. Intravenous fluids are usually required.

MONONUCLEOSIS *See* GLANDULAR FEVER (INFECTIOUS MONONUCLEOSIS) in this section.

MORBIDITY RATE This is the ratio of the number of cases of a disease to the number of well people in a given population during a specified period of time, such as a year.

MUMPS An acute, communicable viral disease, mumps is manifested by swelling and tenderness of the salivary glands, the parotid (cheek) glands being the most commonly affected.

Symptoms. The patient will complain of a headache and/or an earache and run a fever of 100° to 101°, but will not be too sick. A youngster is usually given an aspirin-substitute and sent off to school, for the characteristic swelling of the face does not develop for several hours. This is the reason that such diseases as mumps keep circulating throughout the community; no one realizes the child has a communicable illness at the very time he is highly contagious.

Usually the swelling of the parotid glands is immediately below the earlobes. It feels like hard gelatin, is tender, and fills in the "pocket" at the earlobe, going back over the tip of the mastoid bone and then straight forward to swell the cheek, like that of a chipmunk. The only condition mumps is sometimes mistaken for is swollen lymph glands of the neck caused by infected tonsils.

Mumps virus may invade the submaxillary glands and the sublingual glands producing a double-chin effect. These swellings may occur simultaneously or one after the other, so that the disease may last for two to three weeks. In four to five days the swelling reaches maximum size and in about the same length of

time disappears. Once subsided the swelling cannot be seen but is still felt, and the patient is no longer contagious.

Two rare but distressing complications are possible in children's mumps. These are pancreatitis, which causes severe stomachache and often vomiting, and encephalitis with extreme headache, stiff neck and back, and lethargy. In the adult male and in older boys the sex glands (testes) may also be involved and fertility may be jeopardized. Because of these complications, it is of some importance that children be immunized with mumps vaccine before maturity. Mumps vaccine should not be administered during pregnancy and pregnant women should avoid a child who has mumps if they have never had the disease themselves.

Treatment. There is no specific medication for mumps. Acetaminophen alone is often recommended and may prove helpful. If the patient feels poorly, he or she should stay in bed. However, if the child feels well enough to move about the house, this can be permitted, for it will not affect the likelihood of complications. Consultation with a physician concerning a vaccination schedule for childhood disease is advised.

OSTEOMYELITIS Osteomyelitis is an infection of the bone or bone marrow. In children it most commonly occurs when an infection from another part of the body is spread to the bone. In adults any number of ailments including diabetes mellitus may be a background to osteomyelitis. A compound fracture may be the precursor.

Symptoms. A sudden onset of bone pain accompanied by fever are the common symptoms. In less severe cases the symptoms may be confused with arthritis or sprains.

Treatment. Intravenous antibiotics are effective. In rare cases surgical intervention may be required; the infected area is cleaned out. The disease may become chronic and recurrent and long courses of antibiotics may become necessary.

PELVIC INFLAMMATORY DISEASE
See PID in the section AIDS AND OTHER SEXUALLY TRANSMITTED DISEASES.

PHARYNGITIS   Because of its location at the back of the mouth, the pharynx (throat) is subject to "bombardment" by many bacteria and viruses from environmental air and the nose. If the host is susceptible and the bacteria are numerous enough, germs will establish a foothold and multiply to a point where symptoms of infection (pharyngitis) are noted: malaise, difficulty in swallowing, headache, and perhaps fever and swollen glands. If the tonsils are present, they will also become infected; even though other areas are also involved, the resulting condition is usually referred to as tonsillitis, because the tonsils appear most dramatically inflamed.

Treatment. When the illness is due to bacteria—which can be determined by a throat culture—improvement with an appropriate antibiotic is generally prompt. In the case of the streptococcus organism this may mean a ten-day course of the antibiotic. In viral pharyngitis antibiotics have no impact and only supportive measures (heat, gargles, analgesics) are applicable.

PHARYNGITIS,   STREPTOCOCCAL
Streptococcal pharyngitis or septic sore throat is inflammation of the pharynx (throat) due to the streptococcus germ. It is a common ailment easily spread by droplets, and there are asymptomatic carriers. If the disease occurs with a body rash, it is scarlet fever. While bacterial pharyngitis is most often caused by the streptococcus, it also occurs with pneumococcal and diphtherial infections.

Symptoms. The dominant complaint is a sore, burning, dry throat. Often a patient complains that he feels a "lump" in his throat. In addition, there are chills and fever, difficulty in swallowing, swelling of lymph nodes of the neck, and difficulty in speaking. The mucous membrane of the throat is red and swollen; there may be an obvious exudate (secretion). The pharyngitis may involve lymph nodes of the throat to the point where abscesses (singly or in a group) may form, or these may follow inflammation of the tonsils and sinuses. Usually there is swelling on one side of the neck.

Treatment. Antibiotic therapy is the treatment of choice. If a pharyngeal abscess does not rupture spontaneously, surgical intervention is required. Other measures include palliation of the sore throat (chipped ice, analgesics, ice collar, chilled fluids, etc). Fluids, fortified with vitamins, are given during the period the patient is unable to swallow solids. For treatment of diphtheritic pharyngitis, *see* DIPHTHERIA in the section INFANT AND CHILD CARE.

PITYRIASIS ROSEA   The causative agent has recently been isolated, and as suspected, this disease is of viral origin.

Symptoms. The initial or "mother" plaque is red, scaly, oval or round, and about the size of a half-dollar. It has been known to occur on almost any part of the body and is followed in two or three weeks by a generalized eruption of similar but smaller lesions distributed on the trunk, upper arms and thighs—the face, neck, and legs being infrequently affected. It is a common observation that lesions are less likely to appear on portions of the body with recent tanning from the sun. The lesions continue to appear for a period of from two to four weeks, after which they begin to fade. The disease has a total course of from six to ten weeks, with occasional instances of much shorter or much longer duration. There is almost always a lifetime immunity to subsequent attacks. The disease recurs rarely, and even more rarely a patient may have an attack every few years. There are usually no symptoms other than itching. The patient is able to pursue normal activities, especially since the disease is most often confined to the covered portions of the body.

Treatment. No treatment is usually necessary in this spontaneously involuting disease. However, it may be necessary to control itching and hasten the clearing up of lesions with oral antihistaminic drugs, emollient baths, drying (plain calamine) lotion, and exposure to sun (when possible) or sunlamp (with great precaution against burn).

POLIO   *See* INFANTILE PARALYSIS in this section.

PUS   The formation of pus is known as suppuration. Pus is the waste product of inflammation which includes fluid, dead white blood cells, fibrin (the threadlike, insoluble protein formed by the interaction of thrombin, a clotting element of the blood), and fibrinogen (a protein derivative found in the watery part of the blood, the plasma or serum). A discrete collection of pus is referred to as an abscess. Antibiotics may fail to penetrate an abscess so that surgical drainage may become necessary.

RABIES (HYDROPHOBIA) This virus-caused condition may be one of the most widespread sources of potential infection known, although public attention is focused on it only during sporadic outbreaks of alarm when one or more cases are reported in a community. Although the so-called "mad" dog is popularly believed to be the carrier, plentiful evidence would seem to show that many wild animals, such as foxes, wolves, skunks, and bears, also harbor the virus. Indeed, one of the most important carriers (vectors) has been shown to be the bat; infection from bat excrement and/or urine ejected during the creature's flight may be a possibility, and occasional instances of attack by a "mad" bat have also been reported.

Rabies is produced by a virus with a specific affinity for tissue of the nervous system. The virus migrates from the entry-point (scratch or bite-mark) along the peripheral (outlying) nerves until it reaches the spinal cord and the brain. Within the brain it multiplies, and some of the "descendant particles" migrate to the salivary glands. It is this migration which makes the bite of an infected animal so potentially dangerous.

Symptoms. In human beings, rabies has a flexible incubation period ranging from about ten days to as much as two years; the average is perhaps less than two months. Since the appearance of symptoms depends on the length of time it takes the virus to move from the site of entry to the brain, the closer the wound is to the head, the shorter the incubation period.

In man, rabies is generally marked by symptoms of moodiness, restlessness, a feeling of unease, and fever; this phase, however, lasts only a short while. As time goes on, the restlessness changes to frenzy and excitement which cannot be controlled. There is increased output of saliva, together with muscular spasms of the throat. These spasms are unbelievably painful, and since they are the result of the virus's infection of brain centers control-

ling breathing and swallowing, they can easily be triggered by such simple actions as attempting to swallow water. This phenomenon is what has given the disease its name, hydrophobia (Greek for water-fear) although a term meaning water-hatred might be more descriptive.

Since the patient discovers that drinking can be painful, dehydration is a factor often encountered: he simply refuses to drink liquids. There is, in addition, a progressive weakening which stems from increased difficulty in breathing, paralysis, and general exhaustion. Once overt symptoms appear, death usually occurs within a week.

Treatment. Aside from making the patient as comfortable as possible, there is no effective curative treatment of rabies once symptoms have made their appearance. Therefore, if there is any evidence that the attacking animal may be rabid, treatment must be started immediately—that is, before symptoms have a chance to develop. If at all possible, the animal should be caught and kept a week for observation, in order to learn whether or not it is rabid; if there is the slightest doubt or if the animal is not available, a program of injection of rabies vaccine should be instituted immediately. (An initial dose of "antiserum" may be given before the vaccine, to "buy time" while the animal is being observed.)

The most effective rabies vaccine is produced by special cells in culture-human diploid cell rabies vaccine (HDCV). HDCV is given in a course of five injections, occasionally with a follow-up booster.

Since, as was already mentioned, little can be done for the patient who has developed symptomatic rabies except to make him comfortable, the care indicated is that which would be given to any sufferer from convulsive disorders.

REYE'S SYNDROME Reye's syndrome is a disease of the brain that usually follows an acute viral infection. Children and adolescents are affected most commonly. It is a rare complication.

Symptoms. The symptoms, including repeated vomiting for one or two days, may appear as the patient is recovering from a short-lived illness. There may be signs of unusual rigidity and posturing and hyperventilation. In serious cases there may be kidney and liver problems. However, recovery is usually rapid and with little residual disability in patients who get Reye's after the age of one. Mortality in infants under one year of age is possible.

Treatment. There is no direct treatment for Reye's. Supportive measures including supplemental oxygen, intravenous fluids, and occasionally attempts to restrict brain swelling have been employed. Aspirin should *not* be used, as it appears that use of aspirin for such common illnesses as flu or chickenpox has statistically raised the incidence of Reye's syndrome.

RHEUMATIC FEVER   Generally thought of as heart disease, rheumatic fever is really a general disease of the connective tissue of the body (the more serious manifestations, however, center in the heart valves). The disease is due to an overreaction or supersensitivity to the effects of toxins produced by the same variety of streptococcus bacteria which usually causes strep throat or scarlet fever. It is known that rheumatic fever will develop in 3 percent of patients who receive no treatment for an exudative strep throat; however, if treatment is early and adequate, the incidence of subsequent rheumatic fever is only a fraction of 1 percent. A single attack of rheumatic fever does not seem to cause heart damage, but each subsequent attack may scar the valves of the heart.

Symptoms. The diagnosis may be difficult, or it may be all too obvious. It must be made by the doctor, but important suggestive signs include: painful joints, purposeless movements (St. Vitus' dance), and recurrent fever. A number of laboratory tests, including electrocardiograms, are usually used to confirm the diagnosis.

Treatment. Once the diagnosis has been firmly established, treatment is designed to eliminate (by antibiotics) any residual streptococcus in the system and to give the heart as much rest as possible, so that it may heal with a minimum of damage. Aspirin is of great help in alleviating the pain and fever of this disease, and some believe that large doses shorten its course. Some patients require oxygen and special heart stimulants because of the severe damage. Certain authorities claim to have speeded the healing process by the use of cortisone-like drugs. Sedatives may be necessary for treatment of restlessness. Activity must be kept down to a minimum through complete rest until the heart has recuperated and laboratory tests indicate that the disease is less active.

The most important part of treatment is prevention of subsequent attacks. Rheumatic patients are susceptible to recurrence of the disease once they have had it, and since each attack creates further heart damage, the solution is prevention of the strep throat which triggers the disease. Daily oral penicillin tablets or once-a-month injections of long-acting penicillin are the methods of choice. The "sulfas" or "mycins" given daily by mouth are a poor second to penicillin and are used only if the patient has become allergic to penicillin. Fortunately, this disease is not as common nor as devastating as it was twenty to thirty years ago.

Joint and Heart Complications

Symptoms. Characteristic tissue changes are seen in joint membranes, often accompanied by an outpouring of fluid into the cavity of the joint—knees, ankles, elbows, and even fingers.

All structures of the heart can be involved. The muscle fibers can show rheumatic changes, as can the valve leaflets and the membranes that cover the heart (the pericardium). With healing after an acute attack, scar tissue is deposited in the muscle, reducing its efficient contraction. Along the valves, scar tissue can cause a distortion in shape, and proper closure of the valve can be rendered impossible because the now-diseased valve is so malformed that it will not close tightly. Leakage of blood through the valve opening causes inefficient pumping of blood through the heart into the arterial system. Blood can even dam back into the lungs and cause an overfilling of the pulmonary vessels, with congestive changes and severely diminished space for the accommodation of breathed air.

Symptoms of rheumatic fever range from mild growing-pains in the muscles of the legs to a profoundly incapacitating general illness with high fever, sweating, and swollen and painful joints (especially in the ankles, knees, wrists, and fingers).

On examination there may be a heart murmur, and even enlargement of the heart. Characteristic findings may be seen in laboratory analysis of the blood (sedimentation rate and white-cell count). Although the electrocardiogram sometimes shows very little at first, before the disease has run its course many changes are usually apparent.

Treatment. Rheumatic heart patients need to have their condition followed for life by their physician. Medical treatment includes general care as well as specific and constant antibiotic attack on the bacteria that can cause and complicate further heart trouble.

Surgical relief (open heart surgery or balloon valvuloplasty) may be needed to correct damaged heart valves. A tightly scarred mitral valve (mitral stenosis) may require opening to a nearly normal size; while a leaking mitral valve (mitral regurgitation) may require open-heart surgical repair, with insertion of an artificial valve to replace the malfunctioning valve. Aortic valves deformed by rheumatic fever may also be repaired during open-heart surgery or an artificial valve replacement provided.

ROSEOLA   Roseola is an acute viral disease usually seen in children between the ages of six months and two years. It does not appear to be contagious even though it bears a superficial resemblance to the measles.

Symptoms. There often seems to be a triggering mechanism, in the development of roseola, such as cutting a tooth. The child suddenly develops a high fever (and may even have a convulsion) without any other sign of symptoms. The eyes may be a little red-rimmed, and there may be a trace of nasal stuffiness. The fever lasts seventy-two hours, disappears just as suddenly as it started, and is then replaced by a rash over the trunk, neck, and face, but almost never on the arms and legs. (If however, the fever recurs once the rash has made its appearance, the illness is not roseola.)

Roseola rash is pink, often slightly raised, and each spot is one-eighth to one-fourth of an inch in diameter. There are one-fourth to one-half-inch swollen lymph nodes on the back of the head on either side, directly above the neck.

Treatment. Roseola is a viral disease and treatment is only for relief of the fever. In contrast to measles, there are virtually no complications. Because the fever is so high and because the throat may be a little pink, some have mistaken roseola for strep throat and given the child penicillin for the disease. When the rash broke out, it was assumed the child was allergic to penicillin. Since roseola is the only disease in which a rash follows the fever, there should really be no confusion.

RUBELLA (GERMAN MEASLES)   German measles is a highly communicable viral disease characterized by the appearance of a generalized fine pink rash, swollen glands behind the ears, slight fever (no more than 101°F.), and red-rimmed eyes. The incubation period is fourteen days.

Symptoms. The symptoms of rubella usually last three days and the majority of patients are only slightly ill. The disease may be confused with a drug rash or scarlatina, but the swollen glands behind the ears indicate that it is rubella. Complications are almost unheard of, but if a woman in the first three months of a pregnancy contracts this disease, there is a marked possibility of producing a deformed or deaf baby; it is therefore important to expose female children to this disease early in life. Families and doctors should keep complete and available records so that girl children who have had rubella and are immune will have this knowledge later if they are pregnant and become exposed. The disease leaves permanent immunity, so the diagnosis should be confirmed.

Treatment. Once the rubella is contracted there is no effective treatment, and none is needed. In the first trimester of pregnancy, however, rubella poses a serious threat to the fetus; the virus is capable of passing through the placenta to infect and damage the developing fetus. An effective rubella vaccine has been developed and is particularly desirable as part of the immunization program of all young girls.

SABIN VACCINE *See* INFANTILE PARALY-SIS (POLIOMYELITIS) in this section.

SALK VACCINE *See* INFANTILE PARALYSIS (POLIOMYELITIS) in this section.

SCARLET FEVER The illness known as scarlet fever, scarlatina, and streptococcus sore throat with rash are all the same disease-process: a streptococcal sore throat—pharyngitis and/or tonsillitis—due to a bacterium with the ability to produce a toxin which makes the capillaries expand and cause a rash. Only a few strains of the strep organism can produce this rash. With most streptococcal illnesses there is no rash.

Symptoms. It is only two to four days from exposure to the onset of symptoms, which may be sudden and severe: chill, vomiting and fever to 103°F or even higher. A headache and prostration are usual, and there is almost always the complaint of a severe sore throat. Recently, the streptococcus infection has not been as debilitating as it once was; some patients today complain only mildly about their symptoms, and the temperature may climb no higher than 101°.

The throat is usually deep red and the tonsils blood-red often with white spots of exudate on them. The soft palate (the back part of the roof of the mouth) is usually red, and if there seems to be bleeding areas on it, the diagnosis of strep throat is most likely. The neck glands usually are swollen and can be felt on the second day of sickness just under the corner of the jaw bone. A culture is sometimes taken to confirm the diagnosis.

Treatment. Standard treatment is ten days of adequate doses of penicillin, which acts specifically against the streptococcus. As yet this bacterium has not become resistant to penicillin, as has staphylococcus. If a patient has become allergic to penicillin, one of the "mycins" is substituted with equally good results. It is important to treat the condition during the whole ten days, since complications (rheumatic fever, nephritis, abscess-formation) are virtually unheard of if this is done.

SEPTICEMIA Septicemia, a serious illness, occurs when the entrance of bacteria into the blood produces systemic symptoms. It can be a complication in those who have just undergone surgery or who have been inadequately treated for a serious infection. But it may follow as trivial a procedure as a catheterization.

Symptoms. Shaking, chills, fevers, and very low blood pressure are the common symptoms.

Treatment. Intravenous antibiotic treatment in addition to other therapies in a hospital environment are indicated.

SLEEPING SICKNESS *See* ENCEPHALITIS in this section.

SMALLPOX Smallpox is not seen in the U.S. today because of widespread smallpox vaccination. Indeed in recent years, it has not been reported from other parts of the world. It is possible therefore that the disease has really been wiped out. Until this is known to be a certainty, a description of the disease is given in the following paragraph.

The incubation period of smallpox is seven days. The disease will appear suddenly with a high fever, backache, and prostration. After two or three days the fever abates and numerous pustules appear over the whole body, especially the face. The disease lasts for days, the patients are usually very sick, and the death-rate can be high. There is usually scarring of the face.

Most public health officials believe that smallpox has disappeared and because of this, they no longer require mandatory vaccination.

SPOROTRICHOSIS Caused by the fungus *Sporotichum schenckii*, this mycosis is usually produced by infection at the site of skin injury which has been in contact with the fungus infested soil or wood. The fungal spores are found all over the world but enjoy their most active growth on timber.

Symptoms. The infection is most commonly present on the hands because of their availability for the trauma necessary for the organism's entry into the skin. The lesions are usually multiple, hard, nodular, and ulcerated. The regional lymph nodes can become enlarged, and in rare instances the disease can become disseminated. When the site of the infection is the face, the disease can be mistaken for an ordinary pustular infection except for its persistence and progression.

Treatment. Iodides taken by mouth in appropriate dosage are specifically effective. If laboratory facilities are not readily available for examination of the fungus, a trial course of iodide medication can be given. If the treatment results in a cure, the diagnosis can be presumed to have been correct even without laboratory confirmation. In severe cases the drug amphotericin may be given intravenously. Not transmitted from person to person.

STAPHYLOCOCCUS The staphylococcus is a bacterium which in recent decades has become resistant to some antibiotics, making it difficult to control—especially in hospitals, where it is known as "hospital staph." In some families where this germ has been introduced, it will pass from one member to another, producing a variety of infections over the course of months or even years. Thus, one individual may have boils, another, a furuncle, and a third, a paronychia (infection about the nail). Still another will have a sty, then impetigo; while a staphylococcus pneumonia, with abscess-formation, may put yet a fifth member into the hospital. The germ may also cause tonsillitis and middle-ear infection.

It is now thought that one particular member of the family harbors the "staph" in his nose (where it is warm and wet) and every time he exhales, blows out germs to infect someone else. In hospitals it has been known to float about in the air, invade even clean surgical wounds and, despite careful technique, cause wound infection and abscess formation.

Treatment. More than routine home cleanliness is necessary to eradicate "staph" infection. The family must bathe with special surgical soaps (showers are better than bathing in the tub); and an antibiotic ointment must be used on every cut, scratch, and sore, as well as put into every member's nose daily to kill whatever germs are harbored there. These rigid measures are taken for a month, then relaxed. Treatment of the individual infections is determined by the physician, on the basis of their nature and severity. Fortunately in the battle against "staph" newer and more potent antibiotics appear from time to time.

THRUSH This is a fairly common fungus infection of the mouth, occurring in babies during the first few weeks of life. It almost always stems from the same fungus infection (*Monilia*) as that found in the mother's birth canal (vagina); hence the mother and the baby should be treated simultaneously.

Symptoms. Thrush appears as white, slightly raised areas inside the cheeks, along the gums, and the edges of the tongue. These look like small milk-curds, but if rubbed off leave a raw area. The condition is usually harmless, but can be rather persistent.

Treatment. Certain new and very effective antifungal remedies can be prescribed by the physician to clear up the condition rather rapidly.

TONSILLITIS An acute bacterial infection of the tonsils, most often due to streptococcus, tonsillitis develops suddenly.

Symptoms. The tonsils are on either side of the throat near the back of the tongue, and when acutely inflamed are red and swollen, and usually have white spots (follicular exudate) on the surfaces. Tonsillitis is one of the most common diseases of childhood and causes fever, vomiting, headache, malaise, sore throat, and sometimes ear pain. The most common organism causing tonsillitis is the streptococcus. Viruses may produce a similar picture, and one cannot be sure in some instances whether it is a bacterium or a viral infection from the patient's complaints and the examination alone.

In some instances it is necessary to find out which specific organism is responsible for the infection. When this happens, a swab is used to take some bacteria from the infected tonsils. These germs are then grown in an incubator, identified, and perhaps even tested against different drugs to determine the most effective treatment for that particular case. Chronic tonsillitis implies that what started as a case of acute onset has subsided, but that some redness or dilated blood vessels remain on the tonsillar surfaces. There is usually some low-grade fever (up to 100°) and some swollen lymph glands under the corners of the jawbone.

Treatment. Baths or sponging to reduce the fever and acetaminophen for the relief of discomfort are the principal methods of home care. However, the doctor should decide when to treat, with what medicine, and for how long. A good general rule to follow is that if a comfortable warm bath and the acetaminophen significantly reduce a fever within two hours, the cause of the fever is not too serious and a delay of twenty-four to forty-eight hours is justified before seeking medical assistance.

If the doctor decides to start antibiotic treatment, it is important that the antibiotic drug chosen be continued for several days—usually ten—even though the patient may feel completely well by the fourth day. A significant number of complications (rheumatic fever, nephritis) may develop as a result of inadequate therapy. Some bacteria may even become resistant to the usual drugs because of early cessation of treatment.

TONSILLITIS

INFECTED TONSIL

Cases of chronic tonsillitis are often difficult to treat medically, and it is for this reason that tonsillectomy (surgical removal of tonsils) may be done. The size of the tonsils is not the sole criterion for removal; the frequency of attacks of tonsillitis and swollen glands is a better criterion for surgery. If a peritonsillar abscess has occurred, then tonsillectomy is mandatory. Before a decision can be made, there should be careful balancing of the risks of surgery against the risks of repeated infection. It should be kept in mind that many cases of repetitive tonsillitis are of viral ori-

gin, and viral sore throats will recur at the same rate post-tonsillectomy.

TOXOPLASMOSIS   A disease varying from the unnoticed to the lethal (especially to the fetus) is now recognized as being very widespread. It is produced by a minute intracellular parasite, the toxoplasma organism. In most instances the disease may be passed off as a mild flu-like infection. Surveys indicate that a third or more of the inhabitants of cities in the United States have had the illness and give positive skin tests. A first episode of toxoplasmosis in the pregnant woman, like rubella, can produce severe brain and retinal damage in the fetus (congenital toxoplasmosis). The disease can be acquired by eating raw beef, and there is evidence that cats may be household carriers. Infected cats are asymptomatic and shed the organisms in their stools.

In addition to the mild lymphatic form of the disease which resembles infectious mononucleosis, there is a rare chronic form with retinal damage, weight loss and diarrhea.

Treatment. Treatment with sulfa drugs and pyrimethamine (Daraprim®) is of value but does not assure removal of encysted organisms.

TRICHINOSIS   Trichinosis (also called trichiniasis) is a disease caused by a parasite, the roundworm *Trichinella spiralis*. Infection occurs when raw or inadequately cooked pork containing the encysted larvae is eaten. The larvae spread through the body, and those that reach muscle tissue survive.

Symptoms. Many people are believed to have trichinosis and not know it because they have no symptoms. Usually within a week or two after ingestion of poorly cooked pork, there is a bout of fever, severe muscle aches and cramps, and a characteristic swelling of the upper eyelids. Muscles of speech, breathing, swallowing, and chewing are frequently involved. The blood typically shows a high percentage of a reddish-staining white blood cell (eosinophilia). The illness may last for weeks or even a few months. Often it is disabling, but rarely is it fatal or does it produce permanent damage.

Treatment. Trichinosis is treated with the

drug thiobendazole. Steroid drugs are also of value. The disease may be prevented by the thorough cooking of all fresh pork. Farmers should not feed raw garbage to hogs for it may contain infected pork wastes.

TUBERCULOSIS Tuberculosis is one of the oldest diseases in recorded history. The earliest medical description called it consumption or phthisis because of its conspicuous feature: wasting-away. The disease is not unique to humans, affecting many animal species as well. No branch of the human race has been known to be immune to it, but the severity or prevalence of tuberculosis varies widely in different communities in relation to multiple factors: genetic (inherited resistance); rate of successive exposure (acquired resistance); changes in the virulence of the bacilli; and socio-economic factors (which affect both the nutritional state and the degree of exposure of individuals to the infected persons spreading the disease). Although great strides have been made in the fight against tuberculosis, it still remains one of the world's greatest killers.

Despite the impressive accomplishments in the fight against this disease, eradication of tuberculosis is not yet in sight. Furthermore, there have been shifts in the pattern of the disease and its distribution. For instance, formerly tuberculosis was predominantly a disease of young adults with comparatively low incidence in older individuals. As treatment became more effective and diagnosis more adequate, we witnessed an increased incidence of this disease in the elderly. Furthermore, from time to time, significant increase in the number of new cases has been reported in the general population. Whether this represents a true numerical increase or only reflects more intensive case finding and improvement in diagnosis remains to be seen.

The disease is caused by the tubercle bacillus, identified by Koch in 1882. Different strains of the germ affect man or animals preferentially, but crossover is possible. Man is affected by the human or bovine variety, seldom by the avian (bird) form. The bacillus is a rod-shaped organism which is identified by its characteristic staining properties and which grows only in the presence of oxygen.

As explained above, the bacillus will have different pathogenic effects (illness potential) according to its variety and the degree of resistance exhibited by the host. As a matter of fact, most first attacks are quickly overcome and the bacilli establish themselves in the body without causing actual damage. Occasionally, when the body defenses are weakened, the bacilli become virulent, multiply, and the clinical disease is established. In most cases tuberculosis is directly transmitted from person to person via droplets in the cough. The most common initial site of disease is therefore the lung. Occasionally it may enter the body through contaminated milk from a tuberculous cow, and the initial site will then be the bowel. Tuberculosis is not a hereditary disease. Infants are infected after birth.

In recent years, new strains of tubercle bacilli have been identified. These are generically called anonymous mycobacteria. They differ from the classic Koch bacilli in the biological properties, the nature of the disease they produce in man, and particularly in their apparent resistance to the conventional antituberculous drugs.

Symptoms. The tubercle bacillus may produce disease in almost any organ of the body, and the symptomatology will vary according to the location. Still, tuberculosis of the lungs is by far the most common form and the one from which most of the spread to other organs will originate. Tuberculosis of the lung is an insidious disease. The first attack, also called primary infection, is characterized by a nodular lesion in the lung which tends to heal spontaneously through the formation of a scar and the deposit of layers of calcium. This primary infection, which may attack at any age but preferentially in childhood or adolescence, commonly runs the course of a simple "cold" or "grippe," and usually goes by undetected. Nevertheless, at this time an important phenomenon occurs in the form of an allergic reaction. The person has been sensitized by the tubercle bacilli, a fact which can be detected by the appearance of a positive tuberculin skin test. Subsequently, although the lesion is cured, it continues to harbor live tubercle bacilli which may, under certain propitious conditions, become reactivated and generate the full-blown disease. Thus the disease may be continuous with the primary infection, or a period of many years may elapse before reappearance.

The symptoms of tuberculosis are insidious and appear only after the anatomical lung lesion has been active for weeks or months. As the bronchopneumonic focus sloughs its way into the bronchial tubes, cough and expectoration make their appearance—first as clear mucus, and later as blood-streaking if breakdown of a small blood vessel has taken place (hemoptysis). Slight toxic symptoms are present, such as moderate evening rise in temperature, easy fatigability, decreased appetite, weight loss, night sweats, vague digestive symptoms, etc.

Unfortunately tuberculosis symptoms can be deceptively inconspicuous. The disease may alternately progress and subside until both lungs are widely involved by successive discharge of the bacilli through the bronchi into hitherto healthy areas. By the same token, the lesion may extend and gain access to the blood circulation and establish itself in the brain coverings (meningitis), the bones, kidneys, genitals, etc. The disease is discovered at the time of an exacerbation or through routine physical examination.

From the above description it becomes obvious that the course of pulmonary tuberculosis for any given individual is unpredictable. The susceptible, weakened patient may show extensive lung cavities (cavern) or tuberculosis pneumonia when he first seeks medical attention, while in the less susceptible patient, the disease runs a less stormy course.

The natural defense mechanisms of the body against the tuberculosis lesion are manifested by the formation of fibrous (scar) tissue which tends to circumscribe the disease while certain cells called macrophages fight the bacilli. This sort of "cure" is at best a compromise toward arresting the spread of the disease. The bacilli are not killed and may erupt again, and the mutilated tissue—if large enough—will eventually produce either large, suppurating bronchial dilatations (bronchiectasis) or symptoms of respiratory insufficiency manifested by crippling shortness of breath.

The most common complication is an extension of the disease to the contiguous pleura

(pleurisy) with the common formation of fluid. The most dreadful complication (particularly in small children) is meningitis because of its difficult diagnosis at an early stage. Otherwise the disease may spread to practically every organ in the body. As previously mentioned, although such localizations usually follow in the wake of an original pulmonary lesion, tuberculosis in other organs may continue to be active while the pulmonary lesion has already been arrested.

Absolutely necessary for diagnosis is the presence of the tubercle bacillus. In the course of the disease, the bacillus is usually isolated from the patient's sputum, by examining the pleural fluid, or from the urine or cerebrospinal fluid. In the absence of sputum or because the patient swallows it, an alternate useful procedure is to examine the sucked-out (aspirated) gastric fluid. Occasionally a biopsy (surgical excision) of a small piece of gland tissue or bone marrow may be necessary.

The tuberculin test is a useful diagnostic tool. The purpose of this test is to detect the presence of past or present tuberculin infection. Tuberculin is a material extracted from cultures (growths) of tubercle bacilli and is administered by several ways: as an injection under the skin (Mantoux test); by slightly scratching the skin (scratch test); or by applying an adhesive band (Volmer patch). The result is read after forty-eight hours and is called positive when a little lump and redness develop in the injected area.

A positive result in a tuberculin test only means that the person has been exposed to tuberculosis, and that he harbors some tuberculous lesions; it does not imply that the lesion is presently active. Only in infants and small children is a positive reaction interpreted as actual disease. Many adults will exhibit a positive reaction although most of them were never aware of having had tuberculosis. On the other hand, a negative reaction proves quite conclusively that tubercle bacilli never entered the body. The test has diagnostic value in medical practice, but its greatest usefulness is as a screening tool for determining the prevalence of tuberculosis infection in a community, tracing sources of infection, and planning the necessary public-health measures accordingly.

Treatment. The need for treatment is self-evident when the patient has overt symptoms of active disease, but there is a large group of individuals in whom the indications are not so clear-cut. Most of the latter have been brought to notice only by findings during routine chest X-ray, and the present activity of the disease cannot be adequately ascertained. This is a rather common medical dilemma because of the relatively large number of individuals who are infected but in whom the disease has been spontaneously arrested, leaving only a lung scar. Still another dilemma is posed by the person with a positive skin test and negative chest X-ray. The decision may well be to treat anyway.

It is obvious that the yield of cure is far superior in new infections with lesions of smaller size, than in the far-advanced. Any treatment for tuberculosis, however, represents a long-term commitment with all its implications and should not be used indiscriminately merely because a suspicious pulmonary lesion has been detected by X-ray. The final decision must rest on a clinical evaluation of the history, physical examination, tuberculin test, repeated examinations of the sputum or gastric aspiration, and especially chest X-rays repeated at regular intervals to detect any changes in the appearance or extent of a lesion.

Treatment is presently based on specific antituberculous drugs, which include rifampin, streptomycin, isonicotinic hydrazide (INH), and para-amino salicylic acid (PAS), used most frequently in some combination. The drugs should be administered for prolonged periods of time, until the disease-process has been arrested and the bacilli are no longer recoverable. Sometimes, in advanced cases complete control of the disease is impossible, and the patient must be medicated indefinitely. Rifampin has been shown to have marked antituberculous activity, producing negative sputums in cases where other combinations of drugs have failed.

More advanced cases which cannot be resolved by drug treatment are considered for surgical procedures, particularly the selective removal of limited areas of lung tissue (segmentectomy, lobectomy) or sometimes of a whole lung (pneumonectomy). Old surgical procedures such as pneumothorax (collapse of the lung by injection of air) or thoracoplasty (collapse of the lung by removal of several ribs) are rare today.

Extraordinary advances in treatment have unfortunately created some new problems, mainly the emergence of drug-resistant strains of bacilli. Tuberculosis is essentially a chronic disease, prone to exacerbations and remissions. Even under the best conditions, when the disease is limited and in an early stage, intensive treatment is necessary for at least several months, followed by several years of anti-tuberculous drug coverage and periodic medical examinations. Since the advent of the "miracle" anti-tuberculous drugs, modern treatment has emphasized the need for early rehabilitation and return to normal activities while continuing active treatment. All this has lured many patients into a false sense of "short cures" with the unfortunate consequence that treatment may not be followed adequately and the disease may relapse. Erratic or insufficient intake of anti-tuberculous drugs carries the serious hazard of allowing the bacilli to become resistant to these drugs. Furthermore, dissemination of such drug-resistant bacilli to other individuals will in turn preclude from the new victim the possibility of being effectively treated.

The obvious aim in the fight against tuberculosis today is not to discover still newer, more effective drugs, but to prevent the spread of the disease by early detection of new cases which can be effectively treated before they in turn continue to spread the disease. Because of their relative simplicity, in this fight, the most important medical tools are the widespread use of routine chest X-rays and the tuberculin test. These have been successfully tested in the canvassing of entire communities.

In the last twenty years a great controversy has centered about the usefulness of the anti-tuberculous BCG (Bacillus Calmette-Guerin) vaccine. This vaccine is made of an attenuated type of tubercle bacilli which, upon injection into tuberculin-negative persons, transforms them into tuberculin-positive skin reactors. Under such conditions, it is postulated that the individual will develop defenses against future tuberculous infection similar to the relative immunity of individuals who have had a minimal tuberculous infection some time in the past and have thus become tuberculin-positive. The effectiveness of this vaccine is still under discussion, and its use in the United States is limited largely to crowded, poverty-stricken communities with a high incidence of tuberculosis, where other methods of preventing the spread of this disease are not feasible. In such cases, the children in particular should be vaccinated, preferably immediately after birth.

TYPHOID FEVER Typhoid (or enteric) fever is an acute, severe infection caused by the bacteria *Salmonella typhosa* with involvement of lymphatic tissue, and characterized by an abnormally slow pulse, high fever, a skin eruption, digestive disorder, and enlargement of the spleen. Improved hygiene has made the disease rare in North America. Likewise, prevention is easily obtained through vaccination (see below).

Symptoms. The patient first suffers chilliness, headache, loss of appetite, malaise, nosebleed, backache, and possibly diarrhea and/or constipation. If treatment is not instituted, the temperature rises in steplike progression over the next several days, reaches its peak in the third week, and gradually returns to normal in the fourth. The pulse is abnormally slow, and an eruption described as rose spots occurs. The spleen is enlarged and the patient may become delirious and fall into stupor. Sometimes there are sore throat, extreme nausea and vomiting, bronchitis, pneumonia, kidney infection, and even emotional upsets to the point of a frank psychosis.

Complications include intestinal hemorrhage, intestinal perforation, pneumonia, infection and clotting of veins (especially of the lower limbs), mumps, meningitis, inflammatory involvement of the heart, complete or patchy loss of hair, and inflammations of the kidneys, bladder, bones, joints, and gallbladder. Very common are miscarriages in pregnant women.

Treatment. Specific treatment, especially if promptly instituted, will abort the illness and result in prompt and complete recovery. The antibiotic, chloramphenicol, is the agent of choice. Symptoms are individually cared for, such as analgesics for pain (aspirin, codeine, etc.) and tranquilizers for emotional up-

sets. Supportive treatment is also prescribed.

Prevention and prophylaxis are accomplished by typhoid vaccine inoculations, usually given simultaneously with paratyphoid A and B vaccine. All persons who have come in contact with a typhoid patient or carrier, or those who contemplate travel to foreign countries should be immunized at least two months prior to taking a voyage to allow time for immunity to develop.

UNDULANT FEVER (BRUCELLOSIS)
Undulant fever is an infectious, febrile disease contracted by humans from animals; it is not transmitted from person to person.

The causative organisms belong to the brucella group. They are found in cattle, hogs, and goats from whose skin, excreta, or milk man contracts the disease.

Symptoms. Within five to twenty-one days after brucella enter the body, the disease begins insidiously (although some cases have been reported as occurring months after exposure to the organism) with influenza-like symptoms. A sudden onset with chills, fever, and extreme weakness sometimes occurs. The spleen is usually enlarged and tender to the touch. Inflammation of the testicles or ovaries may occur. There may be nerve and spinal cord pains, swollen and aching joints, and very rarely, bacterial endocarditis.

A myth has developed over the years that undulant fever is apt to be a long, drawn-out, disabling disorder. To the contrary, it is self-limiting, and, with the advent of antibiotics, the outlook is generally favorable. Relapses and recurrences are possible, however.

Treatment. The antibiotics, streptomycin or dihydrostreptomycin, combined with tetracycline comprise the treatment of choice. The sulfa drugs and Rifampin® may also be used. If the patient appears to be toxic, adrenocortical therapy is employed.

VENEREAL DISEASE A sexually transmitted disease or infection is referred to as venereal disease (VD). Examples include gonorrhea, syphilis, genital herpes, and acquired immune deficiency syndrome (AIDS). Infestations of pubic lice and scabies (a type of mite) are sometimes included in this category because they too are transmitted during sexual contact. (*See also* AIDS, GONORRHEA, HER-

PES, and SYPHILIS in the section AIDS AND OTHER SEXUALLY TRANSMITTED DISEASES.)

WHOOPING COUGH (PERTUSSIS)

Whooping cough, a contagious disease caused by a bacterium, may be mild or severe and may occur at any age—even under one month.

Symptoms. There is a gradual increase of a dry night-cough. At the end of two weeks the cough is very severe and comes in spasms, followed by a "whoop" during inhaling. The patient may vomit, turn blue, develop hemorrhages into the whites of the eyes, become dehydrated, and even interrupt breathing. Typically, this period lasts two weeks and is followed by two weeks of improvement. Altogether, the disease generally lasts six weeks. If the typical whoop is not present, blood counts and cultures are necessary to establish diagnosis. Early "baby shots" (DPT) are designed to prevent this disease, and while the well-immunized child may still contract the disease, it will be less serious.

Treatment. Steam inhalations, sedative cough syrups, small feedings, and oxygen may all be necessary. Antibiotics do not effect a cure; they are, however, necessary if secondary infection develops. There is a serum which is effective in reducing the severity of the spasms, if given early enough in the disease. A doctor should be called in for *all* stubborn chronic coughs.

YELLOW FEVER   Yellow fever is caused by a virus and is seen exclusively in subtropical and tropical climates; it is marked by an acute onset with fever, slow pulse, and, in its severe form, by albumin in the urine, vomiting of blood, jaundice, extreme weakness, and, perhaps, hemorrhage. The virus is brought to man through the bite of the infected *Aedes aegypti* mosquito. There has been no severe outbreak in this country in years.

Symptoms. The disease begins suddenly with a relatively high fever that may be preceded by a chill. The pulse becomes slow and the face, gums, and eyes take on a marked redness. There are various digestive manifestations. Within a week to ten days after onset three characteristic indications appear: "black vomit" (blood in the vomitus), albumin in the urine, and jaundice. Nosebleed, signs of hemorrhage in the skin, passage of blood in the stool, and other evidence of bleeding are common. In some countries the prognosis is grave (more than eight out of ten patients die in an epidemic); in others it is quite good. Prevention by good public hygiene is the best cure. Immunization is indicated for those who will be traveling to areas where the risk is high. Treatment consists of good nursing care and supportive care aimed at individual symptoms.

CANCER

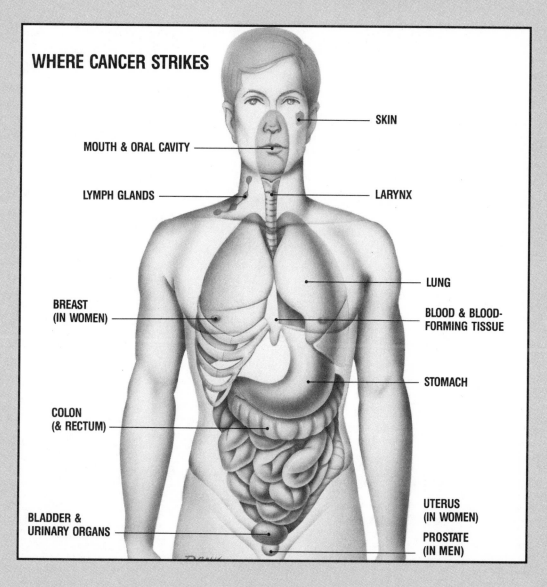

WHERE CANCER STRIKES

SKIN

MOUTH & ORAL CAVITY

LYMPH GLANDS

LARYNX

LUNG

BREAST
(IN WOMEN)

BLOOD & BLOOD-
FORMING TISSUE

STOMACH

COLON
(& RECTUM)

UTERUS
(IN WOMEN)

BLADDER &
URINARY ORGANS

PROSTATE
(IN MEN)

C ancer comprises a group of diseases in which abnormal growth and behavior of cells takes place. The process can be life-threatening and cancer continues to be the second major cause of death in the U.S. Despite the many advances in our knowledge of the disease some cancers such as cancer of the lung are on the increase. Prevention, early detection and diagnosis are of the utmost importance in achieving successful therapies in the struggle against cancer. General information on cancer and cancer treatments are presented in the first part of this section. The latter part addresses specific types of cancers.

CANCER Cancer is today the second leading cause of death in the United States. (The first is heart disease.) Estimates for 1989 indicate that 502,000 Americans have died of some form of cancer. If national trends continue, some 76 million Americans now alive will contract cancer sometime during their lifetime. Of this immense number, approximately one-half will die of cancer, despite a medical effort to cure and prevent cancer amounting to the greatest scientific assault on a single disease in history.

Since the turn of this century the problem of cancer has increased. In 1900, the disease accounted for only one death in every twenty-five. Today it is the cause of one death in five. Some of this increase is simply due to the fact that people today live longer. The longer a person lives, the more likely some form of cancer will manifest itself. In addition, some medical authorities believe the increased rate is due, in part, to an increased exposure of Americans to cancer-causing agents (carcinogens) in the home and in the work place.

This upward climb in the rate of deaths due to cancer has not been uniform for all types of cancer. Some varieties have remained more or less constant, while other varieties, such as cancer of the stomach, have actually shown a decline. In contrast, cancer of the lungs has literally skyrocketed due to cigarette smoking.

Perhaps the saddest aspect of all in the figures that document the rise of deaths due to cancer is the realization that a large portion of these deaths could have been prevented.

Cigarette smoking alone has been estimated to be a contributing factor in approximately 30 percent of all cancer deaths. Early detection procedures, such as the "Pap smear" test, if made use of by larger numbers, could also help prevent death, reducing the total fatalities due to cancer of the uterine cervix.

Many other types of cancer could be improved by detection and treatment at an early stage, before "regional involvement" occurs; that is, before the disease spreads to the lymph-node system in the area of the original tumor. After cancerous cells have dispersed into other regions of the body, the control of the cancer is made more difficult, if not impossible.

ESTIMATED PERCENTAGE INCIDENCE OF CANCERS FOR 1989, BASED ON AMERICAN CANCER SOCIETY FIGURES		
	Males %	Females %
Lung	20	11
Colon/Rectum	14	15
Urinary	10	4
Leukemia and Lymphomas	8	7
Prostate	21	—
Ovary	—	4
Uterus and Cervix	—	9
Breast	—	28
All other	27	22

The Nature of Cancer. Cancer has been aptly described as the growth of cells gone wild.

To understand what cancer is, we must first consider the complex nature of growth as it normally occurs in our tissues. The many and varied biochemical reactions that produce and control normal growth are so delicately balanced that it is a wonder any of us escape the abnormal growth process called cancer.

To understand the mystery of growth, we must begin with a single microscopic unit of life, the cell, for it is from the single cell that each and every form of plant and animal life, including man, originates. Once formed, the cells multiply and a living organism grows. An estimated ten trillion cells must be formed to make the fully grown human body.

Not all cells are identical. Beginning with the single cell at conception, there ensues a process called differentiation, which ensures that different types of cells are formed for the multitude of different tasks required for the proper functioning of a living organism. Thus, for example, as a human embryo develops, the cells that come together to form the liver have different traits from those that form the brain or the lungs.

Furthermore, growth does not end when the body reaches adult size. There must be additional, and continuous, production of fresh cells for repair and maintenance, because the wear and tear of everyday life destroys many cells. The skin, for example, would be worn away entirely in a very short time if there were not a constant supply of new cells replacing those rubbed or sloughed off.

A study of the regulated production and replacement of cells leads quite naturally to some very important questions:

How do cells multiply?

How do they differentiate to form harmoniously organized tissues and organs?

How do cells know when to stop making more of their own kind?

Exactly what mechanisms trigger the *unregulated* production of cells, which produces abnormal tissue?

When we are able to answer such questions thoroughly, we will be at the threshold of solving the biological riddle that is cancer, for cancer is simply the name given to a family of diseases marked by the failure of coordinated cell growth. In cancer it is as if the cells and tissues decide to go their own way, growing without restraint, at the expense of neighboring healthy tissue, which ultimately may end in the destruction of the organism.

The term tumor has come to denote any abnormal new growth (neoplasm). Some tumors are benign, which means they do not usually spread into adjacent healthy tissue. Benign tumors are often surrounded by a covering of fibrous tissue. In contrast, malignant tumors possess the capacity to spread and affect the functioning of other healthy organs.

Cancerous growths are particularly dangerous because each new cancer cell retains the capacity for disorderly growth, even if it breaks off and becomes separated from the parent mass of cancerous tissue.

Such a spreading—the medical term for it is metastasis—results in the establishment of "colonies" of related cancerous cells. These colonies continue to multiply at a site distant from the original formation of the disease. A pathologist can usually determine the original site of a cancerous growth by examining cancer cells in distant sites. For example, a "malignant tumor" of the thyroid that has metastasized into the bone may not only look like thyroid tissue under the microscope, but may even produce thyroid hormone as well.

The ability to metastasize, that is, to spread and establish new cancerous growth at a distance, makes cancer very difficult to treat. If the cancerous tissue has already metastasized at the time of diagnosis, a cure becomes harder to achieve.

Because treatment is so much more effective before metastasis has occurred, much stress is placed on early detection.

Cancer and Cell Mechanisms. Because cancer is essentially a derangement that affects the reproduction of cells, it seems certain that whatever produces cancer must act by upsetting the cellular mechanism that controls division into new cells. This mechanism lies concentrated within a small body of matter at the center of the cell, the nucleus. Within this nucleus there are curled a number of elongated structures, the chromosomes,

---

RISK FACTORS: WHAT INCREASES YOUR CHANCES OF CONTRACTING CANCER?

TOBACCO: Cigarette smoking causes approximately 83% of lung cancer. Pipe and cigar smokers, and snuff users, have an increased risk of lip, mouth, and larynx cancers.

SUNSHINE: Sun exposure is a major factor in the development of melanoma, and almost all of the over one-half million cases of non-melanoma skin cancer in the U.S. each year are related to exposure to the sun.

RADIATION: Excessive exposure to radiation can increase cancer risk. Radon in homes is also a potential cancer-causing agent.

WORKPLACE: Exposure to industrial agents (nickel, asbestos, radioactive wastes, chromate, vinyl chloride) increases cancer risk, particularly among smokers.

ALCOHOL: Cancers of the larynx, throat, esophagus, and liver occur more frequently in heavy drinkers, as do oral cancers. When alcohol is combined with cigarette smoking, the risk factor greatly increases.

HORMONES: Those women who undergo estrogen treatment during menopause are at greater risk for endometrial cancer.

NUTRITION: Obese persons are at greater risk for colon, breast, and uterine cancers. A high-fat diet is linked to the development of breast, colon, and prostate cancer. Salt-cured, smoked and nitrite cured foods pose greater risk for developing cancer of the esophagus and stomach.

Certain foods appear to help reduce cancer risk. High fiber foods may be beneficial in preventing colon cancer. Foods with vitamin A and D may protect against cancers of the esophagus, stomach, and lung.

which are responsible for each cell's capacity to divide into new cells. Chromosomes also determine what function and activity the cell has within the larger organism.

The carcinogenic (cancer producing) properties of such radiation as X-rays and ultraviolet rays, as well as of certain chemical substances—such as coal tar derivatives and some constituents of tobacco—appear to rise from the effects produced on the chromosomes. The precise ways carcinogens work their damaging effect is still imperfectly understood. The study of how carcinogenic agents influence chromosome development is a major area of medical research today.

Only a few decades old is the major discovery of the chemical composition and structure of chromosomes themselves. Through research conducted by biologists Francis Crick and James Watson, chromosomes were found to consist largely of DNA (deoxyribonucleic acid), which is coiled in a pattern similar to a circular staircase, or what is now called a "double helix" structure. It is now certain that the arrangement of four basic amino acids—adenine, cytosine, guanine, and tyrosine—constitutes a code that spells out the reproductive details and functional destiny of the cell. Apparently, then, carcinogens can bring about cancer by disrupting or changing the instructions of the DNA code. Carcinogens might also alter the DNA itself, or influence the way coded "messages" are carried about within the cell.

Causes of Cancer. The process by which a normal cell becomes a cancer cell is not well understood. Several different factors which, when combined, may interact to produce a change in the cell structure.

There are over 200 different kinds of cancer, and each may be related to a different cancer-causing process. However, most of these processes can be organized into genetic, viral, and environmental theories.

Genetics plays a role in some cancers—especially breast and colon. This may mean that a predisposition towards a certain cancer can be inherited.

Because it has been shown that viruses are composed of nucleic acids that can invade cells, it is quite possible that viruses may cause human cancer. Viruses become a permanent part of the cell's genes by becoming incorporated into the chromosomal structure. These changes in the cell's structure are not passed "horizontally," like cold viruses are passed person to person, but are passed "vertically" to subsequent generations of cells. This may in part explain the genetic theory described above. Viruses have been linked to lymphoma, cervical cancer, and liver cancer.

Environmental exposure to cancer-causing agents may be related to radiation exposure, alcohol and tobacco usage, dietary factors, hazardous materials in the workplace, and some medications. In general, one exposure to these environmental factors will not cause cancer, but repeated or prolonged exposure may.

It is also interesting to compare the incidence of various cancers throughout the world. It is evident that in countries, such as the United States, where cigarette smoking is widespread, the frequency of lung cancer is high. Stomach cancer is more common in Japan and Scandinavia than in the United States—but breast cancer is more of a problem in Europe and North America than in Japan. Environmental factors may play a significant role in explaining these differences.

Types of Cancer. Cancer is most broadly divided into three classifications: carcinoma, sarcoma, and blood and lymph malignancies. Carcinomas are those types of cancer that develop from the epithelium—the bodily tissues that make up the skin and the membranes lining the body cavities and hollow organs. Sarcomas, in contrast, evolve from nonepithelial tissues—bone, muscle, and nervous-system structures are examples.

Sarcomas are rare as compared with carcinomas. Their most common points of origin include fatty tissue (liposarcoma), muscle (rhabdomyosarcoma), cartilage (chondrosarcoma), bone (osteosarcoma), and lymph nodes (lymphosarcoma).

Carcinomas are by far the most common forms of cancer and within this class there are two subdivisions: squamous-cell carcinoma, which originates from surface epithelium such as the skin, and adenocarcinoma, arising from the ducts of glands such as the breast. Of the more than a hundred subtypes of these two forms of carcinoma that may occur, a scant six account for more than half the cases of cancer recorded annually. These main six subtypes originate at the following sites: lungs, large intestine and rectum, breast, stomach, prostate gland, and uterus.

Malignancies of the blood are called leukemia and those that originate in the lymph tissue are called lymphoma. There are many subtypes of each of these types of cancer, some of which are highly curable.

The Seven Danger Signals. Because the public must be alerted to the first symptoms that may mean cancer, the National Cancer Institute has placed great emphasis on its "Seven Danger Signals."

The most common warning signs of cancer are the following:

- **C**hange in bowel or bladder habits;
- **A** sore that does not heal;
- **U**nusual bleeding or discharge;
- **T**hickening or lump in the breast or elsewhere;
- **I**ndigestion or difficulty swallowing;
- **O**bvious change in a wart or mole;
- **N**agging cough or hoarseness.

These signs and symptoms can be caused by cancer or by a number of other problems. They are *not* a sure sign of cancer. However, it is important to see a doctor if any problem lasts as long as 2 weeks. Don't wait for symptoms to become painful; pain is not an early sign of cancer. (Note that these signs spell **CAUTION**.)

Unusual bleeding or discharge is one of the major symptoms of cancer of the uterus, especially when it occurs after menopause. A lump or thickening is one of the classic signs of cancer in general, not only in the breast but in other parts of the body as well. A sore that does not heal, or a change in warts and moles, may mark the onset of skin cancer. A change in bowel habits may be a sign of cancer of the intestinal tract, whereas a change in bladder habits may relate to cancer of the bladder itself, the prostate gland, or the kidneys. Persistent hoarseness frequently indicates cancer of the larynx (voice box), and a cough that lasts for any extended time without being related to some already-identified respiratory complaint, may signal the presence of lung cancer.

Preventive Measures. Sometimes an individual can actually prevent the onset of cancer by his or her own efforts. Many lifestyle choices can increase or decrease a person's risk for getting certain types of cancer.

Not all cancers have defined risk factors however, so preventive measures are not identified for all malignancies. We do know that cigarette smoking is probably the biggest cancer risk factor of all and may play a role in the development of many cancers, including lung. Parents should realize the special influence their own smoking habits have upon their children. Because studies have shown that the earlier smoking begins, the greater the hazard to health becomes, all family members should avoid or break the smoking habit.

Protecting the skin from sunlight's ultraviolet rays can decrease the risk of skin cancer. Sunbathing should be practiced in moderation with the use of sunscreen (at least SPF 15). Protective clothing should also be worn by those whose occupations require prolonged periods of work in the sun.

Choosing a diet that is low in fat and high in fiber with adequate amounts of Vitamins A and C can protect against cancer in multiple sites including colon, breast, and esophagus. Avoiding salt-cured, smoked, and nitrite-cured foods will lessen the risk of stomach cancer.

These and other good health measures are relatively easy to incorporate into an individual's and family's lifestyles.

Screening and Early Detection. Because the chance of cure increases with early evaluation and treatment, great emphasis is placed on detecting cancers before they have enlarged or spread to other organs. Early detection utilizes a three pronged approach—the individual, the health care provider, and screening tests.

The individual is responsible for self examination and recognition of warning signals (see "The Seven Danger Signals"). Breast self examination (BSE) allows a woman to become familiar with her breasts and therefore, she is able to note when a change occurs. BSE should be performed on a regular basis, usually once a month, by examining the breasts with the fingers to detect the presence of lumps, masses, or discharge. The American Cancer Society distributes free brochures describing this technique.

Self examination also includes checking the skin for changes in warts or moles; checking the mouth for persistent ulcers or thickened areas; and, in men, checking the scrotum for abnormalities of the testicles.

The health care provider is often able to detect cancer at an early stage by physical examination. The medical history may offer important clues for further investigation. Background information concerning the incidence of cancer in one's family may be of particular help.

There are also a battery of screening tests that enable the examination of many parts of the body where a cancerous growth might otherwise go undetected. Lab work and X-rays may be indicated in individual cases, but there are three screening tests recommended for all persons—the stool occult blood test for men and women, and the Pap smear and mammogram for women.

The stool occult blood test is performed by an individual at home. A small amount of stool is smeared onto a piece of treated cardboard. It is then sent back to the health care provider where it is tested for the presence of occult (hidden) blood. If blood is found, further evaluation is necessary to rule out colon or rectal cancer.

The Pap smear is a technique used to detect the presence of cervical cancer. A small spatula gently removes cells from the cervix for microscopic examination. The great value of the Pap smear is that abnormalities of the cervix can be detected long before cancer develops. By treating these early abnormalities (called cervical dysplasia), cervical cancer can be avoided. This is the perfect screening test for it allows a *precancerous* condition to be identified and treated, thereby saving lives.

Pap smears should be obtained yearly beginning at the age a woman becomes sexually active, or by age 20. Because vaginal cancers can also be detected with the Pap smear, it is recommended that women who have had a hysterectomy continue to get smears, although not as frequently.

Mammograms are low dose X-rays that can detect small breast cancers long before they can be felt. The smaller the cancer at diagnosis, the less likely a woman's breast will have to be removed. The American Cancer Society recommends one mammogram between the ages of 35 and 39; between the ages of 40 and 49, every 1–2 years; after age 50, every year.

As with any major medical procedure, patients should seek a second opinion from another qualified physician, and today more insurance companies require them. These are some questions patients should ask their doctors:

1. If a tumor, lump, growth, or cyst has been found, is it benign or malignant?

2. If it is malignant, has the cancer spread to other areas of the body?

3. What type of treatment is recommended? What are the risks involved?

4. Should this type of cancer be treated by a cancer specialist?

5. What is the cure rate of cancer cases similar in nature? Have new methods of treatment proven effective?

6. If drugs or radiation is used in treatment, what are the side effects?

7. What agencies, institutions, and support groups are available in the community that offer emotional, material, or financial assistance?

8. What kind of physical restrictions, if any, should be followed during and immediately after treatment? Will work activities be affected?

Treatment of Cancer. A sure diagnosis of cancer must be established before treatment is begun. No one should be subjected to the radical, extensive operations, or heavy radiation, or doses of drugs unless the diagnosis is proven. Fortunately, there are means available that provide the necessary proof. One such method is the biopsy.

A biopsy is the removal of a piece of suspected tumor tissue for microscopic inspection. A negative biopsy report does not always mean that no cancer exists, because the cells removed may not be the deranged cancer cells. A positive report, however, justifies the initiation of cancer treatment. It is, of course, essential to begin treatment as soon as cancer is detected. Any delay gives the cancer opportunity to grow and possibly metastasize into vital areas of the body.

The three major methods of cancer treatment are surgery, radiation therapy, and chemotherapy. Treatment is usually highly individualized and may utilize one or more methods.

Surgery for cancer is somewhat different from that for noncancerous conditions. A number of special operations have been devised for the solution of surgical problems associated with cancer. One of these is the removal of lymph nodes from sites adjacent to the cancer. These nodes, the cancer itself, and a wide margin of surrounding tissue, are removed when possible. The removal of the nodes is often an important procedure because metastasizing cancer cells often are transported through the lymphatic system.

Surgery may be used to remove the tumor in its entirety, to determine the extent of spread of the tumor, to remove as much tumor as possible to allow other therapies to work more effectively, or to assess the results of therapy.

Radiation therapy is largely restricted to the treatment of cancer. Although uncontrolled radiation has been found to produce various cancers, radiation in controlled and focused exposures provides a powerful weapon against cancer.

There are three general sources of radiation used in therapy, two being known before the turn of the century, the third being a product of the atomic age:

1. Naturally radioactive elements, such as radium
2. Machine-produced radiation such as that generated by X-ray machines and linear accelerators
3. Artificially radioactive isotopes, produced by exposure of nonradioactive elements to atomic reactions

The effect of these three radiation sources is the same: destruction of the cancer cell through penetration and interference with its chemical components.

A crucial problem inherent in irradiation of cancer is the difficulty of destroying all cancerous cells without causing irreparable damage to adjacent healthy tissues. The use of multiple paths of entry, or of rotation of the radiation sources around the patient, are techniques utilized to minimize this undesired damage. Thus, the cells in front of and behind the tumor receive less radiation. By carefully moving the source so that the tumor is at the intersection point of distinct beams, or so that the tumor lies at the center of a circle traced out by the source, the cancerous growth receives more radiation than does the surrounding tissues.

Radiation is delivered either externally or internally. External radiation means that a radioactive beam is directed at the tumor in an exact path. The patient is placed on a table and a machine delivers the radiation. There is no pain or any sensation associated with the treatment. Side effects are related to the area of the body in which the radiation is penetrating and to the amount of radiation received.

The use of internally placed radiation sources is another method of concentrating the power of radiation where needed. By taking radioactive substances and implanting them within body cavities, tissues, or the tumor itself, the full force of the radiation is directed at the cancer and damage to neighboring healthy tissue is reduced.

Radioactive isotopes have made the concentration of radiation far more flexible than formerly possible. The isotopes are simply variations of normal chemical elements, differing from their nonradioactive counterparts only in weight and in their ability to emit radiation. Some radioactive isotopes, such as iodine-131 and phosphorus-32, have special characteristics. These isotopes can be used to treat thyroid and bone cancers respectively, because these elements naturally gravitate to these sites, rather than circulate throughout the body.

When different sources of radiation are utilized, variations in the degree of penetration into tissue and the localization of the radiation can be accomplished by adjusting voltage. The higher the voltage, the deeper into the tissue the radiation can go.

Although radioactive cobalt was used for many years, many new supervoltage sources have been developed. The linear accelerator is able to deliver higher energy to the tumor while protecting the skin from the radiation "burns" seen in the past with lower dose machines.

Chemotherapy, the treatment of cancer with chemicals and drugs, is largely a development of the post-World War II era. The past thirty years have produced enormous progress in this area of cancer treatment. There are many cancers that are now curable with chemotherapy alone or in combination with other therapies. Choriocarcinoma (cancer of the placenta), Hodgkin's disease, testicular cancer, and some forms of leukemia are all examples of cancers cured by chemotherapy.

Other chemotherapy treatments, applied to other types of cancer, have been used to control and decrease tumor growth, but they are not expected to be cures. In this setting, chemotherapy may either ease pain or temporarily reverse cancer cell activity. Unfortunately, cancer cells often become accustomed to a given chemical and a new one must be substituted. By a systematic changing of drugs, it is sometimes possible to maintain the patient's life for extended periods.

There are at least fifty different chemotherapeutic drugs, and each one has its own set of side effects. These side effects can range from mild fatigue to intense nausea, loss of hair, lowered blood counts and general weakness. Most drugs come in intravenous form, but there are oral forms also available. While most chemotherapy used to be administered in the hospital setting, safer drugs make outpatient or home administration a possibility today.

One variety of chemotherapy consists of administering steroid sex hormones. As might be expected, this type of treatment is generally used in cases of cancer of organs related to the sex of the patient. Thus, for cancer of the female breast, an anti-estrogen hormone may be given, and for cancer of the male sex organs or the prostate, a female hormone is sometimes used.

The search for new and more powerful chemotherapeutic agents continues. One problem in the development of chemotherapy is extremely troublesome, discovering chemicals that will attack cancerous cells more readily than normal tissue. With our growing knowledge of synthetic compounds, the future is promising.

Unproven Cancer Remedies. One of the reasons that cancer causes so many deaths is that patients have delayed treatment. This delay may be caused by ignorance of symptoms, reluctance to face the facts, or putting off regular physical examinations. Another cause for delay is a particularly distressing one, placing one's trust in unproven cancer remedies and programs of treatment.

Why patients reach for unproven or experimental drugs and treatments stems in part from their perception, whether justified or not, that conventional methods are ineffective. In 1975 the drug Laetrile (amygdalin) was termed "worthless" by the Food and Drug Administration, yet many cancer patients spent money and valuable time using this drug. Some even believed they benefited from the drug. Not until definitive research is completed should excessive hope be placed in unproven methods. What is claimed a "cure" may only be a means to separate patients from their money. The "cancer cure" offered may be something as primitive as an amulet or a poultice. But then again, the explanation may be deceptively "scientific," a matter of mysterious serums, chemicals, or machinery.

False "healers" can sometimes be recognized by the following characteristics:

- They guarantee a cure for every case, or they ignore serious, potentially fatal consequences.
- They explain their status by saying that the established medical profession is jealous of, or plotting against, them.
- Their "cures" are secret and are based on some "natural" principle overlooked by everyone else.
- They are frequently overly interested in the patient's ability to pay for treatment and may offer elaborate payment plans.
- They can present "testimonials" from "satisfied customers."

How is it that the self-announced "miracle man" can produce testimonials to his treatment's effectiveness? There are three answers: the testimonial-writing patient may never have had cancer in the first place, for not all tumors or swellings are cancerous; many cancers are slow growing and may even undergo temporary improvement as a natural part of their development; the delayed effects of previous treatment with X-rays or with useful drugs may be the actual explanation for an apparent improvement.

Perhaps it is the fear that the very word "cancer" inspires, or the still-mysterious details of its origin, that cause some cancer patients to seek out treatment that has exaggerated claims of success. Whatever the reason, the treatment of cancer seems to attract an unusual number of fraudulent and deluded "healers." Medical societies, governmental health agencies, and the American Cancer Society attempt to protect the public by distributing information and monitoring medical practices. However, too many people are still misled; too much money is wasted; and precious time is lost all because of the cure that never came true.

The Family Faces Cancer. When a definite diagnosis of cancer has been made, both the patient and the family are immediately confronted with a host of problems. Unfortunately, the mere word "cancer" produces in some persons an overwhelming shock. This response may be due to the erroneous assumption that cancer is an automatic death sentence. If the realization that a family member has cancer only gives rise to despair or panic, there may be a delay of treatment, a delay that jeopardizes the health and life of the person with cancer.

Once cancer has been discovered, two temptations must be resisted: to pretend that the diagnosis is incorrect; or to fall prey to useless, "unorthodox," or unproven cancer remedies.

Another problem families must often face with loved ones who have cancer is whether "to tell or not to tell" the patient the nature of the disease. In most cases the patient already has an idea concerning the true nature of his or her condition. Whether to tell or not depends largely upon psychological and economic factors, such as the state of the patient's morale and mental stamina, and practical considerations for the future with regard to business and provisions for dependents.

Physicians differ in their opinions concerning this subject. Some doctors offer candid appraisals of a patient's condition only if directly asked to do so. Others feel obligated to speak frankly about the course of a patient's illness, even if the report will be very difficult for the patient to accept.

In most cases, of course, it is best to tell the patient the nature of the disease. When a person genuinely wants to know the possible consequences of his or her condition, facing and sharing the problem among family members, physicians, and friends may increase the solidarity and morale of all concerned.

The question of concealment is a particularly delicate and poignant problem in childhood cancer. Regrettably, many of the forms of cancer prevalent among the young are very severe. Their personal response to their illness may be fraught with confusion, in addition to the pain and discomfort of the disease itself. The child may pass through a stage in which the parent is blamed for not stopping the painful symptoms. However, annoyance directed at parents generally passes and is succeeded by curiosity in treatment procedures. Because children are highly sensitive to the behavior of their parents, it is important for parents not to unduly fuss over or spoil a child with cancer.

Family roles may change when the diagnosis of cancer is made. It can become a time of great upheaval but the opportunity for communication and support may strengthen family bonds. Allowing others (friends, church groups, and others) to assist with transportation, meals, and errands takes some of the burden off the family while increasing the base of support.

Practical Problems in the Home. One of the chief difficulties associated with cancer is that treatment is often long and expensive. Family income may be drastically reduced and the life-style of the family may be changed due to the details and requirements of cancer treatments.

There are, however, means of reducing the hardship that accompanies a family's fight against cancer. Almost every community offers help through agencies, private and governmental, that can cushion the blow. Certain hospitals throughout the country are able to supply treatment at greatly reduced rates, or free in cases of dire need. The cancer stricken family should acquaint itself thoroughly with the resources available through official agencies. Inquiries may be directed to health and welfare departments on the state or local level.

The one voluntary agency that deals with the total problem of cancer is the American Cancer Society which, in addition to its widespread programs of education and research, provides various services in many communities. The Society is largely decentralized, operating in state and community units. Many of these units make available assistance in the form of sickroom supplies, dressings, and transport facilities. Some units may sponsor support groups for persons with cancer and their families. Oftentimes, contact with a person who has had a similar diagnosis and treatment can be arranged to provide a personal level of information and support. A letter or telephone call to the nearest unit office will not only supply details, but will also set in motion provision of whatever services are locally available.

In the event of terminal illness, many communities now have access to hospice care. Hospice care is the provision of nursing care, pain management, emotional and spiritual counseling, and a variety of other services necessary for the dying. Care is usually provided in the home although some communities may have a facility designated for this purpose.

Future Prospects. The search for a substance or treatment method that can zero in on cancer cells, destroy all of them, yet cause little or no damage to adjacent healthy tissue is the objective of most cancer research. Such a hypothetical drug or program of treatment is often referred to as a "magic bullet" capable of hitting only cancerous cells.

One example of a promising field of inquiry is immunotherapy, using biological response modifiers (BRM's). These agents change the relationship between the tumor and the host by changing the way the body responds to tumor cells. Two areas that are undergoing intense research are interferon and monoclonal antibodies.

Interferon is produced naturally by the body and appears to exert an antitumor effect by stimulating the immune system to kill cancer cells.

Monoclonal antibodies are produced in the laboratory, but they may be able to be used to carry toxins or chemotherapy drugs directly to the tumor. This may decrease the generalized side effects usually produced by those drugs.

Summary. In conclusion, the specific biological mechanisms that cause cancerous growth are still not completely understood. However, the scientific investigation for cancer cures continues, emphasizing areas such as research into roles played by viruses, genetics, and carcinogenic substances. Improved surgical techniques, new anti-cancer drug therapies, and safer radiation technologies are being sought out, tested, and implemented. The proportion of curable cancers will undoubtedly increase, just as it has over the last half-century. Yet, although the treatment of cancer is the responsibility of the medical profession, much of the anti-cancer effort depends on prevention and early detection and these are dependent upon an informed and concerned public.

WHERE TO GET MORE INFORMATION ABOUT CANCER

1. The National Cancer Institute can be a source for free pamphlets about various cancers and cancer treatments. Write:

    Office of Communications
    National Cancer Institute
    9000 Rockville Pike
    Bethesda, MD 20205

2. The American Cancer Society has local units in many communities, which offer educational materials. One can also write for information. Write:

    American Cancer Society, Inc.
    1599 Clifton Road, N.E.
    Atlanta, GA 30329

3. The Cancer Information Service maintains a toll-free, national telephone number, which can be used to obtain information about cancer and related sources. The number is: 1(800)4CANCER (1-800-422-6237).

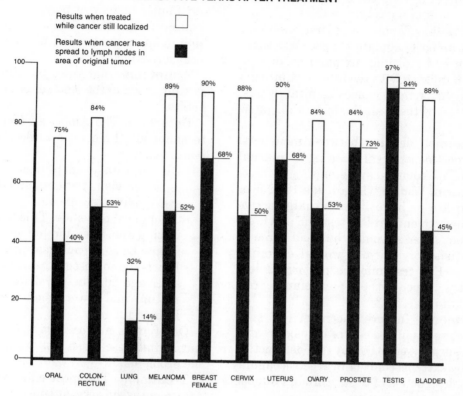

PERCENTAGE OF PATIENTS FREE OF CANCER FOR AT
LEAST FIVE YEARS AFTER TREATMENT

Results when treated
while cancer still localized

Results when cancer has
spread to lymph nodes in
area of original tumor

*Adjusted for normal life expectancy.
This chart is based on cases diagnosed in 1979-1984.

Source: Surveillance and Operations Research Branch,
National Cancer Institute

CANCERS BY SITE

CANCERS BY SITE   Listed below are the most common cancer sites. General information is given on each, including the rate of occurrence, risk factors, symptoms, diagnosis and treatment. If certain factors have been found to be important in the prevention of that type of cancer, information is given as well.

BREAST

Incidence. In 1989 approximately 142,900 new cases occurred in the United States.

Risk Factors. At risk are women over 50; those having a family history of breast cancer; those who never had children or who had a first child after age 30.

Symptoms. These include a lump in a breast that does not go away; thickening, swelling, dimpling, skin irritation, retraction or scaliness of the nipple, nipple discharge, pain or tenderness.

Diagnosis. Mammography is a valuable diagnostic technique. Biopsy is recommended for all suspicious lumps. The American Cancer Society recommends monthly breast self-examination for women over age 20. Physical examination of the breast by a physician should be done every three years from ages 20–40 and then every year. It is also recommended that women ages 35–39 have a baseline mammogram. Women 40–49 should have a mammogram every 1–2 years and women over 50 with no symptoms should have one every year.

Treatment. Various methods may be used depending on the woman's preferences and medical situation. Surgery can vary from local removal of a tumor to mastectomy, radiation therapy, chemotherapy or hormone manipulation. Many times two or more methods may be used in combination. Patients should discuss with their physicians all options available.

CERVIX

Incidence. In 1989 there were 13,000 new cases of cancer of the cervix in the U.S.

Risk Factors. Women who first had intercourse at an early age are at risk. Also those who have had multiple sex partners or who have been infected with the human papilloma virus (a virus that causes genital warts, transmitted by the male during sexual intercourse).

Symptoms. Bleeding between menstrual periods, postmenopausal bleeding or unusual discharge are common symptoms.

Detection. Women who are age 18 or over and who are or have been sexually active should have an annual Pap test and pelvic examination. After a woman has had three or more satisfactory normal annual examinations, the Pap test may be performed less frequently upon the physician's recommendation.

Treatment. In precancerous (in situ) stages, changes in the cervix may be treated by local surgery, cryotherapy (the destruction of cells by extreme cold), or by electrocoagulation (the destruction of tissue through intense heat by electric current).

COLON/RECTUM

Incidence. In 1989 there were 107,000 new cases of colon cancer and 44,000 new cases of rectum cancer. Their combined incidence (151,000) is second only to that of lung cancer.

Risk Factors. Persons at risk are those with a family history of colon and rectum cancer; family history of polyps in the colon or rectum; inflammatory bowel disease. A diet high in fat and/or low in fiber content may be a causative factor also.

Symptoms. Signs are bleeding from the rectum, blood in the stool, or change in bowel habits.

Detection. The American Cancer Society recommends three tests to detect colon and rectum cancer:

- Digital rectal exam by a physician during an office visit. Patients should have one every year after age 40.
- Stool blood test slide. This is a method of testing the feces for hidden blood. This should be done each year after 50.
- Proctosigmoidoscopy every 3–5 years after age 50. The physician inspects the rectum and lower colon with a hollow lighted tube.

Other tests and/or X-rays may be recommended if these three tests reveal any possible problems.

Treatment. The most effective method of treatment is surgery, at times combined with radiation. In cases of colon cancer, a permanent colostomy, the creation of an opening in the abdomen for elimination of body wastes, is seldom needed. (*See also* ILEOSTOMY AND COLOSTOMY in the section GASTROINTESTINAL CONDITIONS.)

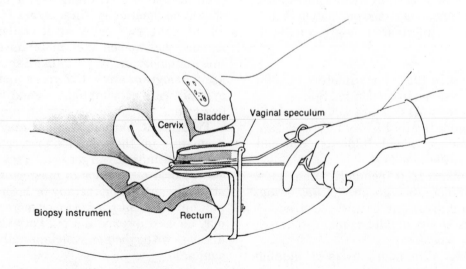

Biopsy of the cervix. The doctor uses an instrument to perform a biopsy or remove a small piece of tissue from the cervix.

LEUKEMIA

Incidence. In 1989 there were 27,300 new cases. About 25,000 cases were in adults and 2300 in children.

Risk Factors. This cancer is found in the bloodforming tissues and occurs in both sexes and all ages. Causes of most cases are unknown. It has been linked to excessive exposure to radiation and certain chemicals, such as benzene.

Symptoms. Early signs of acute leukemia in children appear suddenly. This may include fatigue, paleness, weight loss, repeated infections, easy bruising, nose bleeds or other hemorrhages. Chronic leukemia can progress slowly and with few symptoms. Diagnosis can be made through blood tests and an examination of the bone marrow.

Treatment. Chemotherapy is the most effective method of treatment. Anticancer drugs may be useful as well as bone marrow transplantation.

LUNG

Incidence. In 1989, 155,000 new cases occurred.

Risk Factors. Factors include cigarette smoking; history of smoking 20 or more years; or exposure to certain industrial substances such as asbestos. Exposure to radiation may contribute to lung cancer.

Symptoms. Lung cancer is difficult to detect early; symptoms often do not appear until the disease is in advanced stages. Warning signals include a persistent cough; sputum streaked with blood; chest pain; recurring attacks of pneumonia or bronchitis.

Diagnosis. Procedures used to diagnose cancer of the lung are chest X-ray, sputum cytology test, and fiberoptic bronchoscopy.

Treatment. Options include (depending on the type and stage) surgery, radiation therapy, and chemotherapy. Often a combination of the above is used.

Prevention. Cigarette smoking is responsible for 85 percent of lung cancer cases among men and 75 percent of cases among women. Smoking accounts for about 30 percent of all cancer deaths. Those who smoke two or more packs of cigarettes a day have lung cancer mortality rates 15 to 25 times greater than nonsmokers. If you smoke, quit. If you don't smoke, don't start.

OVARY

Incidence. In 1989 there were 20,000 new cases in the United States. This type of cancer causes more deaths than any other cancer of the reproductive system.

Risk Factors. Risk increases with age, with the highest rates for women 65–84. Women who have never had children are twice as likely to develop ovarian cancer as those who have. Breast and endometrial cancer increases a woman's chances of developing ovarian cancer twofold.

Symptoms. Ovarian cancer often shows no signs or symptoms until late in its development. The most common sign is an enlarged abdomen caused by collection of fluid. Rarely will there be abnormal vaginal bleeding. Women over forty who have vague digestive disturbances (stomach discomfort, gas, distention) that persist and cannot be explained by any other cause may need a thorough checkup for ovarian cancer.

Detection. Thorough pelvic examinations are important. The Pap test, useful in detecting cervical cancer, does not reveal ovarian cancer. Women over 40 should have a cancer-related checkup every year.

Treatment. Options in treatment include surgery, radiation therapy, and drug therapy. Surgical treatment usually includes the removal of one or both ovaries, the uterus (hysterectomy), and the fallopian tubes.

PANCREAS

Incidence. In 1989 there were 27,000 new cases of cancer of the pancreas. This cancer is the fifth leading cancer killer.

Risk Factors. The highest frequency of incidence occurs between ages 65 and 75. The incidence is twice as high for smokers as nonsmokers. The disease is 30 percent more common in men and occurs about 50 percent more frequently in black than in white Americans. High fat diets may be a risk factor.

Symptoms. This is a "silent" cancer, one that occurs without symptoms until it is advanced. Thus far, only a biopsy yields a certain diagnosis.

Treatment. In 59 percent of the cases, diagnosis is so late that no treatment is used. Treatments used are surgery, radiation therapy, and anticancer drugs, but so far these have had little influence on the outcome.

PROSTATE

Incidence. In 1989 there were 103,000 new cases in the United States. About one out of eleven men will develop prostate cancer at some point during his lifetime. This is the third highest incidence of cancer in men, next to skin cancer and lung cancer.

Risk Factors. About 80 percent of all prostate cancers are diagnosed in men over age 65. Black Americans have the highest rate of incidence in the world for reasons not currently known. There is some familial association, and dietary fat may be a factor.

Symptoms. Signs and symptoms of this cancer are the same as benign conditions such as infection or prostate enlargement. These include weak or interrupted flow of urine; inability to urinate or difficulty in starting urination; need to urinate frequently, especially at night; blood in the urine; urine flow that is not easily stopped; painful or burning urination; continuing pain in lower back, pelvis or upper thighs.

Detection. Every man over 40 should have a rectal exam as a part of his annual physical checkup. Men over 40 should be alert to changes such as urinary difficulties, continuing pain in lower back, pelvis or upper thighs, and should contact their physician when these occur.

Treatment. Surgery or radiation therapy may be the treatment chosen to cure prostate cancer if found early in a localized state. Hormone treatment and anticancer drugs also may control prostate cancer for long periods by shrinking the size of the tumor and relieving much of the pain.

SKIN

Incidence. There are over 500,000 cases a year, the majority being highly curable basal or squamous cell cancers. The most serious is malignant melanoma, which strikes about 27,000 persons each year.

Risk Factors. Excessive exposure to the sun is a primary factor. Also at risk are those with a fair complexion, or who have an occupational exposure to coal tar, pitch, creosote, arsenic compounds or radium. There is very little skin cancer among blacks because of heavy skin pigmentation.

Symptoms. Note especially an unusual skin condition, especially a change in the size or color of a mole or other darkly pigmented growth or spot; scaliness, oozing, bleeding or the appearance of a bump or nodule, the spread of pigment beyond the border, a change in sensation, itchiness, tenderness or pain. These are all warning signs of melanoma.

Treatment. There are four methods of treatment for early skin cancer: surgery (used in most cases), radiation therapy, electrodesiccation (tissue destruction by heat) or cryosurgery (tissue destruction by freezing).

Prevention. Avoid the sun between 10 a.m. and 3 p.m. and use protective clothing. Use sunscreen preparations containing PABA (para-aminobenzoic acid). They come in varying strengths ranging from those that permit gradual tanning to those that allow almost no tanning at all; choose those with SPF of 15 or higher. Children, especially, should be protected from traumatic sunburns.

UTERUS

Incidence. In 1989 there were 34,000 new cases of cancer of the body of the uterus (endometrium). Cancer of the endometrium afflicts mostly mature women and the diagnosis usually is made between the ages of 55 and 69.

Risk Factors. Those with a history of infertility, failure of ovulation, prolonged estrogen therapy, obesity problems, and a family history of endometrial cancer are at risk.

Symptoms. Signs include bleeding between menstrual periods; excessive bleeding during periods; postmenopausal bleeding or unusual discharge.

Detection. About 90 percent of uterine cancer cases detected early can be cured. The Pap test is only 50 percent effective in detecting endometrial cancer. Women over 40 should have a pelvic exam every year. Women at high risk of developing uterine cancer should have an endometrial tissue sample taken at menopause.

Treatment. Precancerous endometrial changes may be treated with a hormone. Uterine cancers generally are treated by surgery or radiation, or by a combination of the two.

ALLERGIC CONDITIONS

MECHANISM OF ALLERGY

2. ANTIGENS ENTER THE BODY THROUGH THE SKIN, RESPIRATORY & GASTROINTESTINAL SYSTEMS

ANTIGEN

1. ANTIGENS OR ALLERGENS ARE PRODUCED BY A VARIETY OF EXTERNAL AGENTS

3. THE ANTIGENS PERMEATE THE TISSUES, ENTER THE BLOOD STREAM AND REACT WITH SPECIAL "MAST" CELLS

4. INTERACTION BETWEEN ANTIGENS AND ANTIBODIES ON THE SURFACE OF THE MAST CELLS CAUSES THE LIBERATION OF SEVERAL CHEMICALS

MAST CELL

BLOOD VESSEL

5. THE MAST CELL CHEMICALS PRODUCE THE ALLERGIC SYMPTOMS: ASTHMATIC ATTACKS, HIVES, SNEEZING, MUCUS SECRETION, ITCHING, ETC.

$\mathbf{A}$n allergic person may react in the presence of certain pollens, foods, and chemical agents. These allergens cause the body to react in a number of ways: by sneezing, coughing, itchy eyes, fatigue, or other manner. Allergies are thus inappropriate manifestations of bodily mechanisms. They may be a nuisance in some, while to others, these conditions can be quite debilitating. Although not always easily diagnosed, they are nonetheless quite common.

This section examines the forms of allergies, how they are diagnosed, and how treated. The following is a list of terms identified in this section:

ALLERGIC ECZEMA *See* CONTACT DERMATITIS and ATOPIC DERMATITIS in this section.

ALLERGIC REACTIONS IN CHILDREN Allergic reactions in children are somewhat different from those in the adult. Children will show symptoms more quickly but will recover sooner. Food allergies are most common during the first two years of life.

In early childhood, allergic states are usually caused by inhalants such as dust and animal furs. As the child gets older, pollens and molds play a bigger part. By contrast, an adult tends to remain allergic to the same thing or things.

Symptoms. While adults do not ordinarily change their symptom systems, those of an allergic child tend to change frequently. Eczema may be followed by a respiratory allergy. Rhinitis and hay fever can develop into asthma, and—conversely—asthma can turn into hay fever. Skin tests are more reliable in children than in adults.

Children do not "outgrow" their allergies but change their symptom system as they grow older. The major complications of allergy in children are sinusitis, emphysema, chronic bronchitis, bronchiectasis, deformed chests, and personality defects.

It is important to recognize an allergic disease as early as possible, because treatment will be much more effective if started at a younger age. One should suspect allergy in an infant when there are frequent vomiting, skin eruptions, excessive sniffling, diarrhea, and marked irritability. Diagnosis is based on the patient's history, physical examination, and skin tests. Continuous wheezing in an infant might indicate allergic asthma but could mean such disorders as cystic fibrosis, birth abnormalities, swollen neck glands, tuberculosis, tumors, and swallowed foreign objects.

When asthma begins under the age of two, the prognosis is poorer than if it starts at an older age. On the other hand, the earlier the skin manifestations of atopic dermatitis develop, the better the prognosis for complete recovery (of the skin eruption).

Most upper-respiratory allergies start between the ages of one and three years. Emotional upsets can trigger or aggravate an asthmatic attack, and such attacks may be precipitated by respiratory infections. The common inhalant causes are house dust, pollens, and molds. Some doctors feel that airborne algae may play a part in causing asthma. Food allergy can also bring on an attack.

Children with allergic rhinitis are subject to many colds. As they get older, they may develop chronic sinusitis and nasal polyps. Their hearing may be impaired and their behavior affected. In cases of recurrent nosebleeds (epistaxis) one should consider an allergic rhinitis as an important cause.

Allergic conjunctivitis may be atopic (due to pollen, dust, or foods), contact (due to drugs or chemicals), or infectious (due to bacterial products). Corneal ulcers and impaired vision are complications.

Treatment. Tonsillectomy should not be performed to cure asthma, especially since this operation will itself occasionally be followed by an asthma attack. Treatment consists of removing the cause, alleviating the symptoms, protecting against house dust, and (in selected cases) psychotherapy for both the child and the parents. Change of climate is sometimes beneficial. The child should be permitted normal activities, but not beyond the point where physical exertion begins to make breathing difficult.

The potentially allergic child is the child whose family has a strong history of allergies. Some medical authorities believe that such children should be prophylactically treated as infants. For the first nine months of life the infant should be breast fed or given heat-treated milk or milk substitutes. The earliest solid food should be barley, rice, corn, or oats. Eggs should be avoided for at least six months. Oranges, cocoa, fish, and nuts should be eliminated from the diet for at least one year. (*See also* CORYZA, ALLERGIC; FOOD ALLERGY in this section.)

ALLERGIES   An allergic person reacts abnormally to something that does not affect the normal person, allergy itself being an altered reactivity of the tissues in various organs, brought about by previous contact with a given substance. In other words, a person becomes allergic by first being exposed to a substance, then reacting to re-exposure to it. An allergic reaction is an "immune" (immunologic) phenomenon based on chemical interaction between a foreign-acting material (antigen) and a specific substance produced against it by the body (antibody).

How does a person become allergic? One either inherits an allergy (hay fever, asthma, allergic rhinitis, atopic dermatitis, urticaria, and migraine) or one acquires it (drug reactions, contact dermatitis, allergy to infection, and physical allergy).

When introduced into the body (by contact, ingestion, inhalation, or injection), simple chemicals and complicated proteins that will stimulate the production of a specific substance, or antibody, are called antigens. The antibody is a specific protein which is produced by certain body cells (found in the lymph nodes, spleen, liver, bloodstream, and skin) when stimulated by the presence of an antigen. Immunity, in turn, is a state in which the body is protected against the ill effects of a foreign agent.

The allergic reaction will occur almost immediately if the antibodies are circulating in the blood or will be delayed if they are confined to the tissue cells. The symptoms of allergy are due to the liberation of certain chemicals (histamine, serotonin, heparin, bradykinin, acetylcholine) when the antigen reacts with the antibody.

Symptoms. Allergic symptoms can involve any part of the body. The following list is an example of the types of symptoms that may be due to allergy:

Eye—Swelling and eczema of the lids, visual disturbances, increased tearing, conjunctivitis

Ear—Eczema, dizziness, hearing loss, Ménière's syndrome, inflammation of the middle ear

Nose—Sneezing, stuffiness, dripping, recurrent nosebleeds, nasal polyps, eczema

Mouth—Dry fissured lips, gingivitis, drooling, "stomach sores"

Respiratory System—Wheezing, coughing, croup, pneumonia

Digestive Tract—Colic, stomach-aches, vomiting, itching anus, constipation, diarrhea, swelling of the abdomen, bloody stool, mucous colitis, ulcerative colitis

Nervous System—Headache, malaise, irritability, restlessness, numbness of hands, tingling hands, tension, fatigue, dizziness, anxiety, fever, convulsions, encephalitis

Cardiovascular System—Extra heartbeats, flutter (atrial fibrillation), Buerger's disease, hemorrhage into the skin, anemia, low blood pressure, and rapid heartbeats

Genito-urinary System—Bedwetting, frequency of urination, painful urination, and inflammation of the vulva

Musculoskeletal System—Tremors, muscular aches and pains, backache, pain in neck and/or shoulders

Skin—Excessive sweating, pallor, circles under eyes, eczema (atopic and contact), hives, swelling of the face and lips, hemorrhage into the skin

Constant research is being done in the field of allergy. Certain diseases such as polyarteritis nodosa and ulcerative colitis are believed to be allergic in nature.

A new concept has developed over the last few years—"autoimmune diseases." These are conditions in which the individual becomes hypersensitive to his own body-substances. Some of these "autoimmune diseases" are rheumatoid arthritis, rheumatic fever, thyroiditis, atopic dermatitis, dermatomyositis, and systemic lupus erythematosus.

Allergic phenomena also occur with infections. Tuberculosis, leprosy, deep fungus disease, and syphilis produce a positive skin test only during or after the infection has taken place whereas diphtheria and typhoid will give a positive skin reaction only before infection occurs and then becomes negative. The PPD (purified protein derivative) test is an example of the hypersensitivity that develops in normal persons after a single exposure to TB. A minute amount of PPD injected into the skin then will produce an obvious inflammatory response. This response tends to close in and surround the tubercle-bacillus. This is why although many people are infected with the tuberculosis organism, only a few go on to have the significant disease. Here the allergic response to the bacteria is a good one with protection against the harmful effects. Those who develop active tuberculosis do so because of an overwhelming invasion of the bacteria or a lack of proper allergic response, in which case the PPD may be negative despite the clear evidence of TB. This state is sometimes referred to an anergy.

Diagnosis of Allergies

How does one know whether or not one is allergic to something, or is showing symptoms that are allergic in nature? Allergic symptoms can be the same as those of many other diseases. A doctor is best equipped to make this decision. He or she will come to a conclusion by using several diagnostic approaches. The doctor will ask for a detailed history, perform the appropriate physical examination, have whatever laboratory studies are necessary performed, and where indicated will use skin tests.

A patient's history is probably one of the most important helps in arriving at a diagnosis of allergic disorder. When did the symptoms start? Did they occur gradually or suddenly? At what age did they begin? Are the complaints affected by emotional disturbances, by physical activity, by the weather? Is there any seasonal variation? How frequently do the complaints come on? How long do they last? What previous treatment has the patient been given, and with what results? These and many more questions must be answered to obtain a good background for substantiating a diagnosis of allergy.

Physical examination of the patient will give the physician further valuable information. The general appearance is important. A darkish discoloration about the eyes, combined with mouth-breathing, may indicate a nasal allergy. The habit of rubbing the nose with an upward motion of the hand can mean hay fever or asthma. A pinched appearance of the face can mean asthma. An eruption in the folds of the elbows and knees may be indicative of atopic dermatitis. A breaking-out on the hands may indicate contact dermatitis. Examination of the eyes will reveal whether there is redness, excess tearing, inflammation, and itching (evidence of chronic rubbing). Examination of the nose will indicate the condition of the nasal membranes: whether they are swollen, red, or pale, and whether there are any polyps or evidence of recent bleeding. Examination of the mouth and throat will show inflammation, postnasal drip, enlarged tonsils, or adenoids. Examination of the chest will pick up wheezing or any difficulty in breathing. The shape of the chest can indicate the status of the breathing habits. A swollen, gaseous abdomen may be significant of food allergy.

Laboratory studies will consist of nasal smears, complete blood count, chest X-rays, and thyroid-function tests. In many cases of nasal allergy a smear from the nose will reveal a preponderance of the white blood cells called eosinophils. In some cases of asthma, hay fever, atopic dermatitis, and so forth, a blood count will reveal an increase in these same cells. The blood count will also reveal any anemia or other disturbances. A chest X-ray is necessary to rule out certain infectious diseases. A thyroid-function test is given, since certain thyroid disturbances can mimic allergic states. Other laboratory procedures may be employed, depending on the individual case.

After the physical examination and laboratory studies have indicated the presence of an allergy, skin tests are employed to confirm or deny any suspicions gained from the history. There are six main types of skin tests:

Scratch tests. Scratches are made on the forearm or back. A small drop of the material to be tested is placed on, and rubbed into, the scratch. A positive reaction consists of the formation of a wheal within twenty minutes. (This method is relatively safe and in most cases should be the first type of test done.)

Intradermal tests. A small amount of a specific dilution of the extract to be tested is injected just under the upper layers of the skin. The amount of redness and whealing produced within twenty minutes indicates the degree of allergy. (The chances of reaction in a very sensitive individual are greater with this method than with scratch tests.)

Conjunctival tests. A drop of aqueous extract is dropped within the lower eyelid. The test is read within five minutes by the amount of redness, itchiness, and tearing. (As only one test can be performed at any one time, this test is limited to those materials which are negative on scratch and intradermal tests, yet where the case history seems to indicate that this is the substance the person is allergic to.

Inhalation test. The extract is sniffed into the nose and, if positive, there ensues a great deal of sneezing and watery discharge. (Although an excellent test, this is often followed by a severe generalized reaction.)

Patch test. The suspected substance is applied to the skin, in a predetermined concentration. It is covered with an adhesive-tape dressing and left on for forty-eight hours. The reactions are read twenty minutes after removing the dressings. Positive reactions consist of redness and blistering. (This test is used where a contact-type allergy is suspected. It is useless if the allergy is to something inhaled or eaten.)

When it is not possible or practical to give a skin test directly to a patient because of severe apprehension, a marked allergic state, or insufficient normal skin, then one can use the technique of *passive transfer:* Blood is drawn from the patient and a serum prepared. A known nonallergic individual is injected with this serum in several sites. Forty-eight hours later the test materials are injected into the previously marked serum-sites. The results are read as in the intradermal method. This is called the PK method after the discoverers, Prausnitz and Küstner. A more recent away-from-the-body testing method utilizes the patient's serum to which the allergen is added and a product of the interaction is detected by a radioisotope method (RAST test).

Treatment of Allergies

The most important aspect of the treatment of any allergy is to find the cause and then avoid it. This is possible when contact dermatitis is due to chemicals, dyes, or metals; hives are due to medications or foods; headaches to foods, and so on. However, even when the allergic cause is known, it may be impossible completely to avoid the causative agent (inhalants, bacteria, physical agents).

Most therapeutic agents in allergic diseases are used for the benefit derived from the relief of specific symptoms. The chart on the next page lists, in a general way, the different types of medications that are used for symptomatic relief.

Other treatment consists of special breathing exercises in asthma and emphysema; oxygen for asthmatic attacks; surgery for intractable asthma and bronchiectasis; psychotherapy; change of climate; avoidance of cold air intake; intermittent positive pressure (artificial respiration); sucking-out of material from the lungs (bronchoscopic aspiration); and opening of the air-passage by incision (tracheostomy).

In the treatment of inhalant and certain other allergies (where one cannot very well avoid such substances as pollen, molds, or dust), the physician may employ a method known as desensitization or hyposensitization. The principle behind this procedure is to inject small diluted quantities of the offending substance at set intervals, in an attempt to decrease the incidence of clinical symptoms due to that substance. This method works best in inhalant sensitivity (ragweed pollen) and most poorly in food allergy. Insect hypersensitivity of the inhalant and sting types may also be treated by this method.

There are five general ways in which hyposensitization may be achieved with the injection treatment.

Co-seasonal. Treatment is started during the season of highest sensitivity. Small amounts of the diluted extracts are given every one to three days. If used properly, this can be a very effective way of treating hay fever. It does, however, carry a greater risk of reactions (sneezing, itchy eyes, itchy nose, itchy palms, hives, coughing, wheezing, and difficulty in breathing).

Pre-seasonal. Injections are given weekly up to the season during which the patient experiences greatest difficulty.

Perennial. Injections are given year round. Seasonal and nonseasonal allergies can be treated by this method.

Immediate. This occasionally-used method is one in which small doses of a solution of the

ALLERGY MEDICATIONS

SYMPTOMS	ORAL MEDICATION	INJECTED MEDICATION	TOPICAL MEDICATION
Nasal congestion, stuffed nose, sneezing	Antihistamines Sedatives	—————	Decongestants (Sprays and local injections)
Wheezing, coughing, and difficulty in breathing	Antihistamines Analgesics Antibiotics Arsenic Bronchodilators Ephedrine Expectorants Sedatives Steroids Tranquilizers	Antibiotics Bronchodilators Epinephrine Gamma globulin Steroids	Bronchodilators (atomizer or undertongue absorptive agent) Special detergents to loosen mucous plugs
Itchy, watery eyes	Antihistamines Ephedrine	—————	Epinephrine (eyedrops) Saline and boric acid eyewash Steroid eyedrops
Itchy skin	Antihistamines Analgesics Steroids Tranquilizers	Steroids	Steroids Wet compresses Drying lotions
Aches and pains	Analgesics Antihistamines Sedatives Vasoconstrictors	Analgesics Vasoconstrictors	Cold compresses
Nausea and vomiting	Antihistamines Sedatives	Antihistamines Sedatives	—————

offending material are injected every twenty or thirty minutes over a span of twenty-four hours. Bee and wasp venom immunity have been achieved by this method.

Repository. The offending substance is prepared as an emulsion or as a special alum-precipitated pyridine complex. (All other methods use extracts made in water solutions.) The advantage of this technique is that fewer injections (from one to eight) are necessary to achieve apparent immunity. A great many extracts prepared in this manner are still at an experimental stage.

ALLERGIST   This term or title refers to a physician whose practice is limited to the study, diagnosis, and treatment of those disorders believed to be allergic.

ANAPHYLAXIS   Anaphylaxis is an immediate, severe, and potentially fatal constitutional reaction with symptoms of difficulty in breathing, generalized hives, swelling of the face and neck, and complete collapse. This type of dangerous reaction may follow the taking of any drug, serum, vaccine, or extract to which a person may be severely allergic. Today penicillin is the most common drug causing anaphylaxis. Insect-sting reaction can also cause this condition. Because of anaphylaxis risk, persons allergic to eggs should not take any vaccine prepared in a chick embryo, and horse-sensitive individuals must avoid vaccine prepared from horse serum (tetanus antitoxin). Anaphylaxis is one of the distant risks to courses of allergy shots.

ANTIHISTAMINICS   Antihistaminics comprise a wide group of drugs designed to block the effects of histamine, a substance released by the tissues at the time of an allergic reaction. Theoretically, the antihistaminics are supposed to compete with histamine at the target-cell level—the skin in eczema or the nasal mucosa in hay fever—and prevent excessive outpouring of secretions. In actual practice, beneficial effects are limited and antihistaminics' usefulness is greater in diseases such as hives or hay fever than it is in asthma or eczema. Antihistaminics usually produce some side effects the most prominent of which includes sedation.

ATOPIC DERMATITIS   This is an allergic skin disorder belonging to the atopic group of diseases which are characterized by a high incidence in members of the same family; a tendency for the afflicted to have more than one form of the disease, occasionally simultaneously but not infrequently in succession (hay fever, asthma, migraine); and a persistent high "eosinophil" count (a greater than usual number of this type of white blood corpuscle), present also in other diseases and significant only as a diagnostic aid.

Symptoms. The disease begins in infancy with a reddened scaly eruption of the face and extremities, and often associated with cradle cap, a greasy scaling of the scalp. The condition improves with or without treatment. A great number of patients have no further indication of this condition but may develop the other forms later. In those in whom the condition persists the next attack occurs at about two or three years of age and usually takes the form of flexural eczema with some reddened thickening at the bends of the elbows and knees. The nape of the neck may also be the site of red papules, thickening, and crusting. At six years of age, recurrence is again noted, and at puberty the disease takes on the appearance and distribution commonly seen in the adult. Since the incidence of atopic dermatitis is so low in adults, and even in adolescents, as compared with its incidence in infancy and childhood, it is apparent that a very high percentage of the afflicted young undergo some immunologic or other alteration making them nonsusceptible to further dermatitis of this type. In the adult the disease may be confined to the elbows and knees, but is more often generalized and involves the body and the face as well. The skin becomes markedly thickened and ridged, with a grayish hue, and no matter how well treated, presents the scratch marks of persistent itching. Atopic dermatitis can persist through early adult life, but is extremely uncommon after forty years of age. In pregnant women the condition has been known to both worsen and improve during the period of gestation. If a remission is noted in early adult life, it is likely to be permanent.

In all the stages of the disease the lesions can become infected, and in young children this is almost the rule. In the young, too, the disease is more moist and the lesions consist of greasy crusts, easily removed with some resultant bleeding. The older patients have lesions that are dry, thick, leathery, and ridged.

The allergic responses in these patients are myriad, often fleeting and changing, but always persistent. Removal of an allergen (food) known to cause flare-up of the eruption or immunization to a known inhalant allergen (dust, pollen) does not often result in improvement—probably because still another allergen or group of allergens will constitute the provocative agents and sustain the disease. However, removal of known or suspected allergens can be useful, especially if these substances are not essential to a person's diet or environment. Attempts at desensitization are less useful but nevertheless worth trying in some selected cases. Change of environment can cause dramatic improvement. The change can be a small one (within the same city, for instance), or it can be one to a place which differs greatly in temperature, humidity, in grasses and trees, and in elevation (usually the higher the altitude, the better). For patients with relatively mild cases of this disease, seeking a "cure" by measures which are disruptive to their personal and family lives is unfortunate since no prediction can be made of either the place or the time of "cure." In patients with extensive involvement of the skin who cannot function in their usual activities, seeking relief by means of change of environment, by immunization procedures, or by psychotherapy may be rewarding if local and systemic treatment have failed. With the presently available drugs such as antihistamines, cortisones, and antibiotics, the need for such measures has lessened considerably.

Treatment. In addition to the elimination of, and immunization to, the usual causative allergenic substances, treatment consists largely of reducing the itching (soothing baths, lotions, oral antihistaminic drugs), sedation (aspirin, tranquilizers) and reducing the inflammatory process (one of the cortisone drugs locally applied or given in "courses" by mouth, or in aggravated cases, by injection). If the flare-ups are notably seasonal, and a pollen is the likely major causative allergen, temporary removal to an area known to be free of the pollen is obviously essential. In cases in which the attacks are related to the menstrual cycle, the nature of that relationship should be studied endocrinologically for the possibility of suitable treatment. Sympathetic understanding of the patient's distress and reassurance as to the ultimate outcome will permit the patient to seek available symptomatic relief.

CONTACT DERMATITIS   At first largely thought of as due to contact with plants (poison ivy), contact dermatitis is now recognized to be the result of an allergic response to literally hundreds of substances present in modern man's environment. There is no inherited tendency to this condition, and it is not associated with or related to other forms of allergy. (It would be more correct to consider this condition a contact-*type* dermatitis because some of the substances causing it can be encountered both in the external environment (causing dermatitis on contact with the skin) and on internal administration (causing dermatitis on reaching the skin through the bloodstream). Drugs like penicillin, quinine, and Benadryl® are examples of internally administered remedies capable of producing contact-type dermatitis.)

Although it is usual for the causative substances to come into direct contact with the skin, the contact may be unobserved when the substances are carried in volatile materials and are deposited on the skin in uniquely susceptible areas, such as the eyelids. Thus rotogravure (printing of comics and magazines) causes a dermatitis if exposure is experienced by placing the paper in front of the patient, who has no contact with the paper itself. The eyelids are affected by the volatile material emanating from the printed paper. So too, perfumes, insecticides in spray containers, room deodorizers, and the like can cause allergic contact dermatitis in the absence of obvious contact.

Some substances cause dermatitis in areas seemingly distant from application to the skin (nail polish on the eyelids and face, hand creams on the face and neck); or the dermatitis can surround the area of intended application (contact drug-allergy sparing the area treated for one of many reasons). But most commonly a substance causing an allergic contact dermatitis produces an eruption at the site of application of the substance and in the configuration in which the substance has been applied. It is for this reason that poison ivy or other plant dermatitis usually occurs in lines corresponding to the stroke of the leaf, root, or twig carrying the allergen of the causative oil. Hair dye causes an eruption around the face and neck where the hair touches, and only more rarely on the scalp, which is less susceptible to sensitization. Bubble gum causes an eruption (not always allergic) around the mouth, where the material lands after the bubble bursts; and nickel causes an eruption at the area of bra hooks and on the thighs of men who carry nickels in their pants pockets. One of the most common sites of poison ivy dermatitis in young boys is the penis, it being common for little boys to use the woods for their toilet and to not wash the allergen from their hands first.

The eruption caused by an allergy to substances applied to the skin does not "spread." The lesions continue to appear over a period of time depending on the amount of substance deposited on that particular site and on the degree of allergy present. The blisters occurring in severe eruptions do not contain the causative allergen and the serum oozing from them does not cause further lesions. Only previous contacts with longer periods of development, or further contact with the causative substance, are capable of continuing the eruption of new lesions.

Symptoms. The eruption consists of a reddening of the skin and the formation of papules and finally of blisters, depending on the severity. The location and extent of the eruption depend entirely on the areas of application of the causative agent. In prolonged instances crusting and secondary infection are not uncommon. If large body areas are involved, chilliness is usual and there may be a fever. Itching is moderate to intense. In some areas the eruption gives a sensation of burning. The course of the disease depends on the extent of involvement and on the degree of success in removing the patient from further exposure to the causative substance. Hence patients with a generalized eruption caused by an injection of a drug (penicillin, Thorazine®, dye for X-ray visualization) will continue to produce lesions until the substance is eliminated from the body. So too, patients sensitive to mangoes will continue to have a dermatitis in the anal area until the fruit is no longer present in the stool. Avoidance of continued exposure to the causative substance is sometimes made difficult by inability to determine the cause from the history or from the appearance of the eruption.

To establish a particular substance more certainly as the cause of the eruption, the patient can be deliberately exposed to the suspected allergen in a manner similar to the one causing the eruption. This is called the "use" test and is especially revealing in instances in which other testing has failed. More common in dermatologic practice is the "patch test." The suspected substances, properly prepared, are placed on the skin and covered with a patch in the center of which is an occlusive film (cellophane) to protect the substance from an admixture with the adhesive of the patch. This is allowed to remain in place for forty-eight hours (or less if the patient feels some itchiness due to an earlier response). The reaction consists of an eruption of redness, papules, and blistering similar to the original eruption. If the testing has been properly carried out, even faint redness can be significant of a positive result and means that there is a causative relationship between the substance and the eruption. A response to testing may be negative and yet not necessarily mean that the substance was not causative. The many reasons for the lack of significance of the negative reaction to a patch test are best exemplified by the finding that some substances require exposure to light (photoallergy) to produce a reaction, and when a truly occlusive patch test is applied, the substance will be absolved from blame because a reaction was not possible in the absence of light. There are instances of inadequate patch test results due to excessive dryness of the skin and an inability, therefore, for the substance applied actually to come in contact sufficiently to produce a reaction; or instances of too much moisture of the skin, with resultant masking of a reaction by another reaction due to moisture. As with all tests, an interpretation of both the method and of the result is essential for proper evaluation.

The duration of allergic sensitivity of the contact type is many years, in most instances for life. Patients tested as long as thirty years after their last possible exposure to substances to which they were then allergic give positive reactions to patch tests as before. It is clear from this that, except under extraordinary circumstances, avoidance of substances known to produce allergic contact dermatitis is essential to prevention of recurrence of an eruption.

Treatment. In addition to removal of the offending substance, treatment consists in allaying the inflammation with cold compresses (water); application of lotion (calamine); local or systemic administration of the cortisone drugs; use of antihistaminic drugs to reduce itching; and antibiotics, locally or systemically administered, for secondary infection.

Desensitization or immunization is not usually effective. While injectable material of extracts of many plants (poison ivy, poison oak) is available, only patients for whom further contact with the substances is unavoidable (farmers, florists, foresters) should avail themselves of this type of prevention, since successful immunization is usually limited.

CORYZA, ALLERGIC   Also called allergic or vasomotor rhinitis, this is a condition in which there is an inflammation of the mucous membranes of the nasal passages due to hypersensitivity to some substance. Animal danders (cat, dog, and others), food and house dust are among the culprits. There are two types: the seasonal (usually due to pollens and soil molds, with symptoms appearing mainly in the spring, late summer, and fall) and the perennial type, which occurs all year round (although worse in fall and winter and usually due to foods and the presence of animals).

Symptoms. Typical symptoms of allergic coryza are sneezing, nasal congestion, an itchy and/or drippy nose, constant sniffling, mouth-breathing, frequent throat-clearing, occasional dry coughing spells, red, itching and tearing eyes, swollen eyelids, and itchy ears.

Complications consist of nasal polyps, sinusitis, diseases of the ear, nosebleeds, loss of the sense of smell, and in some cases the development of asthma.

Treatment. The foods or animals to which the patient is allergic should be avoided. Antihistamines, eye drops where indicated, occasional use of nasal decongestants, steroids in severe cases, and hyposensitization in selected cases are also applicable.

FOOD ALLERGY   There is probably no food grown or processed to which someone is not allergic. To complicate the picture further, an allergic response to some foods may not be due to the food itself. There are today multiple food additives to which the individual may also be allergic: coloring agents, acids, alkalies, antioxidants, bleaches, maturing agents, flavors, emulsifiers, preservatives, stabilizers, thickeners, and nutritional supplements.

Food allergy may start at any age but most commonly first appears in infancy. The reaction to the food may occur immediately or be delayed for up to twelve hours after eating. Even if an individual is allergic to a certain food, exposure to it does not always cause a reaction; there seem to be external factors that control this. Infection, frequent consumption of the food, eating a great deal of it at one time, cold weather, emotional tension, and a general lowered physical resistance seem to increase the reaction to the offending food. Symptoms in a food-sensitive person can be provoked by eating the food, smelling it, or receiving blood from a donor who has eaten the suspicious food a few hours earlier. The most common foods to which people are allergic are cow's milk, wheat, eggs, seafood, chocolate, strawberries, and citrus fruits.

Symptoms. Food allergy in infants will manifest itself as colic, excessive "spitting up," chronic diarrhea, eczema, and a stuffy, runny nose. Some unexplained deaths in infancy may also be due to severe food allergy. It has been reported that some hypersensitive infants have gone into shock after eating milk and eggs. A positive skin test to egg white in a very young asthmatic child usually is a bad sign, indicating a severe course ahead.

Food allergy in children usually causes diarrhea, eczema, or hives. In adults the common symptoms are hives, diarrhea, rhinitis, headache, and asthma. Other symptoms reportedly attributable to food allergy in some cases are hand dermatitis, ulcerative colitis, indigestion, abdominal pain, earaches, inflammation of the mouth, canker sores, excessive sweating, bad breath, constipation, frequency of urination, bedwetting, contact dermatitis, conjunctivitis, personality changes, and so forth. An aromatic oil in coffee has been held responsible for the allergic symptoms of migraine, asthma, indigestion, malaise, rhinitis, and hives in those who drink the brew.

Diagnosis of food allergy is made by a careful and complete history. A "food diary" is helpful in recording the foods eaten and any reactions that may have developed. An elimination diet instituted by removing suspicious foods may help pin down the cause or causes of the difficulty. Skin tests may be used but have to be interpreted very carefully, as they are not too reliable in food allergy.

Treatment. Treatment consists of simple avoidance of the offending foodstuff. This is difficult and will require a great deal of label-reading—especially if a common food such as eggs, milk, corn, or wheat is involved. Special "allergy-free" recipes are available so that the remaining permissible foods can be prepared in an appetizing and attractive manner.

In the case of the potentially allergic child, one should delay introducing eggs, wheat, fish, corn, cocoa, and cow's milk into the diet. The nursery should be kept free of feathers, kapok, and wool. One should avoid unnecessary injections of horse-serum medications as well as antibiotics.

GRASS POLLEN ALLERGIES Grass pollen is produced in the late spring and during the summer. The common grasses causing "grass hay fever" are bluegrass, timothy, orchard, redtop, Bermuda, Johnson, sweet vernal, and rye.

The symptoms of pollen reaction (pollinosis) consist of red, teary eyes, stuffed and runny nose, and spasmodic sneezing.

HAY FEVER (POLLINOSIS) Hay fever is a very poor term for a disorder which involves neither hay allergy nor increased temperature. The disease is now more properly called pollinosis. It is more commonly found in individuals with an allergic background.

There are three types: tree hay fever, which occurs in the spring and early summer; grass hay fever, which occurs in the late spring and summer; and weed hay fever, which starts during the late summer and continues until the frost. The symptoms are due to an allergy to the pollen of one or more plants. The severity of the complaint depends on the amount of pollen present in the air. Thus symptoms may be many and severe, or few and mild.

Symptoms. The eyes become itchy, red, swollen, tearful, and begin to burn; the throat becomes swollen, with attendant itching and burning; and the nose itches, burns and feels full. There is a watery-to-thick nasal discharge, together with sudden attacks of severe sneezing. The sinus cavities may swell and become full of fluid. (These symptoms are seasonal, depending on the type of pollen to which the individual is allergic.) Nasal polyps, sinusitis, and asthma are the most common complications.

Diagnosis is made on the basis of a history of seasonal complaints plus positive skin tests. A smear made from the nasal membranes shows an abundance of a certain type of cell (eosinophil).

Treatment. Treatment consists of hypo-sensitization, nasal sprays for temporary relief, antihistamines, ephedrine, epinephrine, masks and nasal filters, installation of air conditioning, and—if necessary—change of climate during the pollen season.

HEADACHES, ALLERGIC Headaches may be due to an allergic reaction to a food, drink, or inhalant, or may be a secondary manifestation associated with an allergy. If unrelated to allergy, headaches may be due to emotional stress, various infectious diseases, tumors, or exposure to noxious fumes.

The primary allergic headache is caused by a hypersensitivity to a food (such as milk, chocolate, grains) or an inhalant (such as molds, dust). The headache pain is probably due to dilation of the blood vessels of the brain, which occurs upon exposure to the substance causing the allergy. Allergy symptoms such as dizziness, vision impairment, abdominal pain, nausea, and vomiting may accompany headache. Migraine headache, with its throbbing, recurrent one-sided pain, may be induced by sensitivity to certain foods and drugs.

Allergic rhinitis and sinusitis in which there is swelling, infection, and pressure will produce secondary allergic headache. In such a circumstance the headache is usually over the forehead or on the top of the head.

Treatment of allergic headaches consists of finding the cause of the allergy and removing it. Headache pain can be alleviated with antihistamines, analgesics such as aspirin, vasoconstrictors, and whenever possible, desensitization to the allergy-inducing substances.

HIVES (URTICARIA)

HIVES (URTICARIA) This common eruption consists of raised, reddened lesions often surrounded by a halo of unelevated redness, occurs at all ages and represents an allergic reaction of the "immediate" type. While a period of about ten days (but often more) is required for an allergy to develop the first time a patient shows evidence of having become allergic to a substance, the succeeding attacks will occur in from only a few minutes to several hours after exposure to the causative substance.

Symptoms. The eruption is usually generalized in distribution but may be confined to particular parts. Thus, only the arms and legs may be involved; or the eyelids, lips or face; or only portions of the body exposed to the sun (photoallergy). Each lesion goes through a cycle of redness, swelling, surrounding pink halo (flare), and gradual fading. The presence of lesions in different stages of development, and often joining with each other, gives the appearance of blotchiness. This eruption is accompanied by much itching, and when the palms and soles or the lips or eyelids are intensely swollen, there may be pain and burning sensation.

Depending on the type of hives and the nature of the causative agent, the eruption can be of short duration or last for many months; and it can occur as a single attack or be a recurrent disease.

Hives can occasionally be of such large size as to warrant the designation giant hives (angioneurotic edema). The lesions can reach the size of a lemon and completely involve areas like an eyelid or the lip. This type of lesion is not usually present over the entire skin but can nevertheless be of more serious nature than the eruption of more usual size. Not only does the involved part become distorted and incapable of function, but there is also not in-

frequent association of swelling of the throat and larynx with impairment of breathing. Neither the causes nor the treatment differ from the more usual type of hives; only the need for early, effective treatment is more immediate.

Still another type of hives is papular urticaria, seen mostly in young children. This disease tends to recur seasonally, usually in the spring. The eruption, which is usually confined to the outer sides of the arms and legs, consists of small, hard papules which feel like buckshot, slightly reddened and usually scratched. Often the scars and discolorations of lesions of previous attacks are mixed with the current ones. A very high percentage of cases of papular urticaria is caused by an allergy to insects, accounting for the seasonal occurrence. Treatment is the same as for hives of other appearance and causation, except that the use of insect repellents is effective in prevention. It should also be noted that, almost without exception, this type of reaction is seen in children only, and spontaneous cure even in severe and prolonged cases is the rule.

The most common cause of hives is medication taken by mouth or administered by injection. Contrary to general belief, drugs of such ordinary usage as to be considered standard remedies, no matter how frequently taken previously or in what dosage, can at any time in the patient's use of them cause an attack of hives which will be followed by like attacks each time the drug is taken thereafter. Aspirin is a common example. Some drugs are more likely to produce this type of allergic reaction, and it is necessary for this reason for patients with known previous reactions (hives) to be especially cautious not only in taking new remedies, but also in the use of previously tried remedies with a high incidence of allergic responses. Excretion of drugs is variable and the hives persist for as long as the drug remains in the body. It is obviously urgent to determine the cause of the eruption as quickly as possible in order to discontinue the taking of the offending agent.

Older than drugs, of course, among the known causes of hives is food. While patients often indict unusual foods as causative of an attack, neither the uncommonness, the "spiciness," nor any other taste-related characteristic of the food is a factor in its being constituted as an allergenic cause of hives. Why a person becomes allergic at one particular exposure to a food and remains allergic to that food from then on is not yet known. There is neither a common factor among the causative allergens nor among the persons affected.

Hives can also be caused by physical agents, such as light (including ultraviolet rays), heat, cold, stroking, and physical pressure of varying intensities. As in hives of other causation, the reason for the sudden onset is unknown.

Substances foreign to the body, as for instance serum from another animal species (horse serum) or from an incompatible human source (serum or blood), can cause hives without additional systemic involvement or can produce a more inclusive reaction, serum sickness. These instances are usually readily recognized because of the immediately preceding administration (but sometimes as long as ten days earlier) of the causative material.

Treatment. Removal and future avoidance of the causative substance is essential for cure. In patients in whom it is not possible to determine the cause (and in all cases before specific treatment was available) alleviation of this eruption results either from unknowing removal of the allergen or from a spontaneous immunization, the mechanism of which is also unknown.

The antihistaminic drugs and the cortisones are the most effective remedies, though each may be more effective than another in different circumstances. Local remedies include cold compresses and lotions. Administration of adrenalin, heretofore a frequently used remedy, is now reserved for relief of great swelling interfering with function (eyes, mouth, hands, and feet), and is followed by the previously-mentioned antihistaminics and cortisone drugs.

HOUSE-DUST ALLERGY   House dust is a conglomeration of many materials. It contains small amounts of kapok, cotton lint, feathers, wool, fragments of paper, orrisroot, silk, molds, tobacco, insects, pyrethrum, animal danders, flaxseed, and glue. It is found all over the house but mainly in mattresses, box springs, pillows, toys, upholstered furniture, comforters, heavy drapery, rugs, stored cloth-

ing, and in heating systems. The older the furnishings the more potent the house dust.

House-dust sensitivity is more common in people who have a family history of allergy. In springtime, housecleaning will bring on symptoms. In the fall, the use of a furnace that has been standing idle for several months will precipitate attacks—one reason why house-dust difficulties are more common in the colder northern climates.

Symptoms. Nasal congestion, spasmodic sneezing, postnasal drip, wheezing (asthma), and headaches are common symptoms of house-dust sensitivity.

Treatment. Reducing the dust exposure, decreasing clinical sensitivity, and relieving symptoms are the basic means of therapy.

Dust-control is difficult but very necessary—especially in the case of the highly allergic individual. There should be no upholstered furniture; no rugs and rug pads; no pillows containing kapok, down, or feathers; no stuffed toys; no heavy draperies; no comforters or quilts; no stored clothing in the bedroom; no dry sweeping; and no animals in the home. The mattress and box spring should be covered with special covers. Furniture should be cleaned with oiled cloths. If possible, steamheating units should be used rather than hot-air furnaces. If this is not possible, then all parts of the furnace system should be thoroughly cleaned (and not by the house-dust allergic person!) before turning the heat on for the winter season. Use commercially available dust-sealers on furniture and rugs. Wherever possible, use linoleum floor coverings. Bedcovers may be of cotton or rayon. Pillows should be made of Dacron or foam rubber. A filter mask should be worn when the house is being cleaned. An electrostatic precipitator or room water-filter will lower the dust-content in the circulating air.

The usual method of reducing clinical sensitivity is by hyposensitization, employing the perennial method. Some doctors hyposensitize by using the house-dust extract in special dilutions mixed with glycerin, then placed under the tongue and allowed to dissolve there.

The individual symptoms may be relieved by using the appropriate medications such as antihistamines, mild nasal decongestants, and analgesics.

IDENTIFICATION CARDS Because of the severe reactions that can occur when one is exposed to a substance to which one is strongly allergic, it has been recommended that allergic individuals carry identification cards. Such cards would give the person's name and address, and supply information on blood-type, dates of vaccination, and all immunization procedures. Any previous or known drug, serum, extract, or vaccine reaction would be listed in a special space on the card. Such a card would be invaluable in emergencies when the patient's medical background is unknown. This card could save lives.

INJECTION TREATMENT The injection treatment of allergies refers to those methods in which doctors attempt to decrease the allergic symptoms by injections of various concentrations of the allergenic substance. These methods are known as desensitization or, more properly, hyposensitization. One cannot completely eliminate the hypersensitive state, but one can decrease it to the point where no symptoms are manifested upon exposure.

Injections may be given during the season of greatest sensitivity (co-seasonal), before the season of most difficulty (pre-seasonal), or all year round (perennial). The number and frequency of desensitizing injections varies; they are usually given more frequently early on and less frequently after a year or two. Thus, they may vary from perhaps weekly to monthly. From time to time reports appear of attempts to produce long-acting "shots."

INSECT ALLERGIES Insects can affect certain persons in a variety of ways. Some will develop asthma or allergic rhinitis on inhaling the dust from the bodies of some insects (May fly, caddis fly, housefly, mushroom fly, aphid, moth, butterfly, beetle, water flea, silkworm). Certain moths and caterpillars can cause a blistering eruption on contact with the sensitive person's skin.

Symptoms. The most common reactions are produced by bites and stings. Most insects will cause a local wheal or hive at the site of the sting. Bee, mosquito, and yellow-jacket stings have caused acute urticaria. The bites of fleas, mites, and mosquitoes have caused a condition known as papular urticaria, in which there are many small, itchy, raised spots that develop long after the responsible insect is gone. Severe anaphylaxis and death are not uncommon immediately following the sting of bees, hornets, wasps, and yellow jackets. Nausea, vomiting, and diarrhea may occur after a bee sting. Although not actually an insect, the spider also has been involved. A brown-spider bite is followed by local inflammation; then ulceration and scarring. The black widow spider will cause agonizing cramps and (in children) some fatalities.

Treatment. The treatment of insect allergies consists of antihistamines, epinephrine, ephedrine, steroids, calcium, and drying antiseptic lotion. After a bee sting one should scrape or tease the stinger out of the skin since it may break on a pull and part will remain imbedded in the skin. As a preventative method, 5 percent DDT or other insect killer should be sprayed in the environmental area. Insect repellents may be used on the skin and clothing. Hyposensitization to bee, wasp, yellow jacket, and hornet venom may be necessary. Hyposensitization to insect inhalant antigens may help those asthmatics with this allergy.

Emergency treatment for an insect sting to which there is a known or suspect allergy consists of applying a tourniquet (if stung on an arm or leg) above the sting-area and applying cold packs to the site. The doctor will inject epinephrine, aminophylline, and cortisone, and will give oxygen. Some severely allergic persons carry the epinephrine with them in emergency doses for immediate administration in the event of a sting.

MOLDS AND ALLERGIES Molds and fungi belong to the plant world but do not contain chlorophyll. Many fungi live on decaying material, some are plant parasites, and a very few cause disease in man. They reproduce by spores and although they grow in the soil, their spores are air-borne like pollen.

The important molds causing allergic reactions are *Alternaria, Hormodendrum, Helminthosporium, Pullaria, Aspergillus, Penicillium, Chaetomium, Phoma, Fusarium, Rhizopus, Mucor,* dry rot fungus, smuts, and rusts. Allergy to molds is more common in adults than in children.

The mold-spore content of the air is lowest during a snowfall. It is highest during the dry weather that follows the first heavy frost. April through November is the "mold season."

Symptoms. Mold sensitivity will cause such allergic disorders as conjunctivitis, perennial and seasonal rhinitis, asthma, atopic dermatitis, and croup. Diagnosis is made by skin-testing.

Treatment. Avoiding such sites as damp basements and swampy areas is important. There should be frequent vacuum-cleaning of upholstery, rugs, draperies, bedding, etc., and moldy items should be exposed to sunlight. Air conditioning is also helpful. Hyposensitization is frequently beneficial.

NASAL POLYPS AND ALLERGIES

Polyps are pale pink (sometimes gray), soft growths in the nose. They are the most common growth of the nasal interior. Removal can give great relief from the symptoms of nasal blockage. Many, if not most, nasal polyps are the result of nasal allergy and they will quickly recur if the allergy factor is not controlled.

PATCH TESTS

This type of skin test is used extensively to determine the cause(s) of contact dermatitis, an eruption caused by the application of a substance to which the patient has become allergic. If the suspected substance is a liquid, a drop of the original solution or of a known nonirritating dilution of the solution is placed on the skin (back or arms). Over this is placed a bandage whose gauze surface has been previously covered with an impervious material (cellophane, wax paper). If the suspected substance is a solid (cloth, plastic, etc.), the material is moistened with a small amount of water and covered with a bandage as outlined above. If several substances are applied at the same time, each bandage will be numbered to make identification possible. The most useful and practical sites for application of patch tests are the inner sides of the upper arms, the upper chest, and the upper back.

The bandage patches are removed in forty-eight hours, unless itching or burning at the site indicates an early reaction and makes prompt removal of the bandage necessary. The reactions range from faint pinkness to blistering and are some indication of the degree of sensitivity that the patient has developed. False positive reactions are usually the result of application of an irritating (not sensitizing) substance and may require dilution of the material if further study is indicated. False negative responses are the result of a variety of factors and may mislead the patient in discarding the tested material as a possible cause of the dermatitis.

Only contact dermatitis can be studied with the patch test procedure. Drug eruptions (other than those producing contact dermatitis), hives, infantile eczema, and atopic dermatitis are, for varying reasons, not clarified by patch test studies. Patch tests are useless if the allergy is to something inhaled or eaten. It is essential that the substance be applied in a dilution not irritating to the skin and in a diluent not itself irritating or capable of altering the test substance. Interpretation of the result is often complicated by redness resulting from pressure of the bandage, or from slight heat rash due to the tight fit of the patch, or from irritation caused by the adhesive material.

Patch tests are of inestimable value to the dermatologist and the allergist. Although a negative result can usually be interpreted as an absence of allergy to the test substance, a negative result does not constitute evidence of the inability to develop an allergy to that substance at a later time.

PERSONALITY CHANGES IN ALLERGY

The personality changes that can occur in an allergic person may be due to the allergy itself; the symptoms present; or the treatment employed.

Confusion and unpleasant behavior may be due to edema of the brain, which in turn is caused by an allergy to some food (as in certain cases of migraine). An allergic response of the nervous system can cause symptoms such as irritability, depression, and restlessness.

An atopic child, because of all the attention his illness brings him, can become self-centered and selfish. Persons with severe allergies may be so afflicted that they avoid people and stay by themselves, becoming overwhelmed with self-pity in an almost schizophrenic manner.

Emotional disturbances, such as drowsiness, irrational behavior, hysteria, or confusion, can be caused by medications that are used in treating the allergic state. (*See also* EMOTIONS IN ALLERGY in the section MENTAL HEALTH: PSYCHIATRIC AND PSYCHOLOGICAL CONDITIONS.)

PHYSICAL ALLERGIES Some people are allergic to such natural phenomena as light, heat, cold, and pressure. This hypersensitivity is called physical allergy. Physical allergy can cause such diverse symptoms as asthma, rhinitis, urticaria, gastrointestinal upsets, tremors, weakness, headaches, convulsions, and shock.

Allergy to light is an interesting phenomenon. The combination of certain drugs plus exposure to sunlight will cause a marked sunburn reaction in susceptible persons. Exposure to the same amount of sunlight—but without the drugs—causes no reaction. Antibiotics, sulfonamides, tranquilizers, antidiabetic drugs, and sedatives are a few of the groups of drugs that may be involved.

In certain cases the presence of specific chemicals or plant-life in contact with the skin will produce an eczema only if sunlight is present; in the absence of one or the other there will be no reaction. This is known as a phytosolar reaction. Limes, figs, meadow grass, wild parsnips, lady-slippers, and gas plants are some of the plants involved.

Some individuals develop hives (urticaria) on exposure to sunlight, with or without drugs or chemicals; and—although not exactly an allergy—there are those in whom exposure to sunlight produces paroxysms of violent sneezing.

Heat, too, will cause small red wheals (hives) over the body in certain persons.

Cold allergy may be due to the presence of abnormal proteins in the body. The hives associated with this physical allergy are large and may be accompanied by swelling of the lips, tongue, and face. Exposure to cold may also flare up as an asthmatic attack. Cold allergy is especially dangerous in the summer, when the afflicted person goes swimming. The sudden change in temperature can cause the cold allergy to manifest itself, and the sufferer may even drown while undergoing the reactions.

Pressure urticaria occurs after prolonged intense pressure. The parts involved become swollen and sometimes painful. Dermographism (literally skin-writing) is a milder form in which wheals may be induced by stroking the skin.

Treatment of the physical allergies depends on the type and severity. Antihistamines and some form of hyposensitization may be employed.

POLLEN AND ALLERGIES Pollen is a dust-like, powdery material produced by seed-bearing plants. The important pollens in inhalant allergies are those that are air-borne. Hay fever, asthma, and allergic rhinitis are diseases that can be caused by inhaling pollen. There is also one form of contact dermatitis known as ragweed dermatitis in which the eruption is caused by exposure of the skin to ragweed pollen.

Trees pollinate in the spring and early summer, grasses in the late spring and summer, and weeds in the late summer and autumn. The amount of pollen in the air at any one time depends on a number of factors. The pollen count increases with heightened wind velocity or temperature, with sunshine, and at altitudes under 5,000 feet. It decreases with increased rainfall or atmospheric humidity, with decreased temperature, and at altitudes over 5,000 feet.

Pollen counts are taken by exposing a glass slide covered with a very thin layer of some sticky substance, such as petrolatum, to the atmosphere. The air to be sampled is permitted to flow over this surface, the pollen adhering to the slide. The number of pollen grains per square centimeter of slide, as counted under a microscope, is then defined as the pollen count.

The grasses whose pollens cause the most difficulty in the United States are bluegrass (June grass), timothy, orchard, redtop, Bermuda, Johnson, sweet vernal, rye, and corn.

There are eight groups of trees whose spring pollinations have caused symptoms: birches, alders, and hazels; beeches, oaks, and chestnuts; elms and hackberries; mulberries; walnuts, hickories, and pecans; poplars, aspens, cottonwoods, and willows; maples and box elders; and ashes, olives, and privets.

Many kinds of weeds cause trouble among

allergic persons. In the ragweed family are the short ragweed, giant ragweed, Western ragweed, Southern ragweed, cocklebur, rough marsh elder, and tall povertyweed. The wormwood and sage group consists of annual sage, biennial sage, sagebrush, pasture sage, sand sagebrush, prairie sage, and tall wormwood. In the pigweed family there are pigweed, spiny pigweed, and western waterhemp. The goosefoot group includes lambsquarter, sugar beet, shadscale, Russian thistle, and summer cypress. The English plaintain is the most important representative of the plantain family. Hemp and hop belong to the hemps, while sorrel and rhubarb are included under the docks.

When one is allergic to one of the grasses one is usually also allergic (in different degrees) to other members of the grass group. Timothy is often employed as the grass representative. (This type of cross-reactivity also occurs within the different groups of trees and weeds.) (*See also* ASTHMA in the section RESPIRATORY CONDITIONS and HAY FEVER in this section.)

RAGWEED POLLEN/ALLERGY Members of the ragweed family (short ragweed, giant ragweed, Western ragweed, Southern ragweed, cocklebur, rough marsh elder, and tall povertyweed) pollinate from summer until frost.

Persons allergic to ragweed pollen develop what is commonly called hay fever by inhaling the pollen.

The symptoms of hay fever or pollinosis (the more correct term) consist of itchy, red, tearful eyes with an itchy, burning nose. There occur multiple attacks of severe sneezing. (*See also* HAY FEVER (POLLINOSIS) in this section.)

SCRATCH TEST *See* ALLERGIES in this section.

SEASONAL ALLERGIES Seasonal allergies are those allergic disorders which occur only during certain seasons: ragweed hay fever in the fall, grass hay fever in the spring, and so on.

SKIN TESTS The skin and related organs of a person with suspected allergies may be used for testing various substances. If the allergen is a food or an inhalant (dust, dander, pollen) the scratch, intradermal, conjunctival, inhalation, or electrode tests may be used. If the allergen is of a contact nature (chemicals, cosmetics, toilet articles, jewelry) then patch testing is done. (*See also* ALLERGIES in this section.)

VASOMOTOR (AND ALLERGIC) RHINITIS *See* CORYZA, ALLERGIC in this section.

DENTAL HEALTH

FRONT VIEW OF MAXILLARY (UPPER) CENTRAL INCISORS

APEX OF ROOT

PERIODONTAL LIGAMENT

ROOT CANAL

CEMENTUM-COVERED ROOT

ALVEOLAR BONE

GINGIVA (GUM)

PULP CHAMBER

ENAMEL-COVERED CROWN

Teeth are important in speech, in appearance, in growth of the jaws, and overall physical health. The first step in the complex process of digestion is accomplished by the teeth. The condition and placement of the teeth may have an impact on other physiological discomforts as well.

Humans develop two sets of teeth over their lifetime, with the permanent teeth in place by the teenage years. This section examines the composition and development of teeth, proper dietary and cleaning regimens, and various dental disorders. Good dental health can benefit the functioning of the entire body. Dentists specialize in the examination and treatment of teeth; oral surgeons handle any extractions which prove difficult; orthodontistry is concerned with the proper positioning of teeth; and dental hygienists are responsible for cleaning routines.

The following is a list of topics identified in this section:

ABRASION
ABSCESS, DENTAL
AMALGAM, DENTAL
ANOMALY, DENTAL
ATTRITION
BAD HABITS AND DENTAL HEALTH
BASE
BICUSPIDS (PREMOLARS)
BRIDGE, DENTAL
BRUXISM
BRUXOMANIA
CALCULUS (TARTAR)
CANKER SORES
"CAPS"
CROWN, ARTIFICIAL
CROWN (NATURAL)
CUSPIDS (CANINES, EYETEETH)
DENTAL ANESTHETICS
DENTAL CARIES (CAVITIES)
DENTAL FLOSS
DENTIFRICE
DENTISTRY
DENTURES
DENTURES, CARE OF
EROSION, DENTAL
FLUORIDE (FLUORIDATION)
GINGIVITIS
HALITOSIS (MOUTH ODORS)
IMPACTED TOOTH (IMPACTION)
IMPLANTS, DENTAL

INCISORS
INLAY
MALOCCLUSION
MANDIBLE
MAXILLA
MOLARS
MOUTH
MOUTHWASH
PERICORONITIS
PERIODONTAL DISEASE
    (PERIODONTITIS, PYORRHEA)
PROPHYLACTIC ODONOTOMY
PROPHYLAXIS (ORAL)
RESTORATION
ROOT-CANAL TREATMENT
SALIVA
SALIVARY GLANDS
SILICATE
TARTAR
TEETH, FORMATION AND
    DEVELOPMENT OF
TEETH, FUNCTION AND POSITION OF
TEETH, INJURED
TEETH, PHYSIOLOGY OF
TEETHING
TOOTH SURFACES
TOOTHBRUSH
TOOTHBRUSHING
WISDOM TEETH

ABRASION Abrasion is the abnormal wearing-away of the surface of a tooth, usually due to some mechanical cause. This may occur on any exposed surface of the tooth, including a portion of the root, if it is not protected by the covering of the gingiva. Abnormal wearing-away of teeth should be distinguished from that which is normal (attrition).

When abrasion results from faulty brushing, the abraded region is usually located on the area of the necks of the teeth which face the lips or cheeks, and the area is wedge-shaped. It is interesting to note that abrasion due to overzealous brushing, or to the use of excessively abrasive cleaning agents, will be more severe on the left side of the arch for right handed "brushers" and on the right side for left handed ones.

Abrasion may also be caused by other factors:

- Toothpick, dental floss, and dental tape—the indiscriminate use of any of these may result in abrasion of the surfaces between the teeth at their neck.
- The repeated biting of thread; opening of bobby pins, holding of tacks, nails, needles, or a pipe in the teeth may result in an abraded area on the biting edge, which is notched.
- The habitual use of chewing tobacco, betel nuts, or the accidental ingestion of abrasive agents such as sand (sand-blasters) or other dust will result in the abrasion of the biting surfaces of the crowns.

Abrasion which results in a thinning or loss of the protective enamel may result in exposure of the more sensitive underlying dentin, resulting in pain which may require treatment by the dentist.

ABSCESS, DENTAL This term describes a localized collection of pus within the tissues which is surrounded by a "limiting" membrane. The symptoms of an abscess may be swelling, redness, pain, and heat. Two important types are periapical abscess—one occurring at the apical (apex) region of a tooth due to the death of the pulp tissue (*see* Root-canal Treatment in this section); and periodontal abscess—one occurring in the tissues immediately surrounding the tooth, such as gingiva, bone, or the periodontal membrane.

An abscess which breaks through its limiting membrane, burrowing through the surrounding bone to the external soft tissue, may result in a gum boil. As the contents accumulate, increased pressure will cause rupture of tissue and drainage of the pus into the oral cavity.

AMALGAM, DENTAL An amalgam combines mercury and other metals and is used for filling teeth. Because of its silver color, its use is usually confined to the posterior teeth.

ANOMALY, DENTAL Anything which, in the process of development, exceeds a permissible range of variation, produces an anomaly or malformation. Since the blueprint for the body is determined in the early weeks of development, most anomalies—including dental ones—have their origin at this time. Nonetheless, some anomalies are not predetermined, but result entirely from environmental influences in the postnatal period. Deciduous teeth begin developing at about six weeks, and the permanent dentition at about six months after conception—the process continuing after birth until the complete formation of the permanent third molars (at approximately twenty years). Below is a listing of some of the more important and/or common dental anomalies:

Anodontia—Complete lack of development of any or all of either the primary or the permanent teeth

Supernumerary teeth—The development of extra teeth

Mesiodens—The development of supernumerary teeth located between the central incisors of the upper jaw (maxilla)

Peg laterals—A peculiar shaping of the lateral incisor teeth, in which the crown resembles a peg

Mulberry molars—An anomaly of the biting (occlusal) surfaces of molar teeth, resulting in a mulberry-like appearance

Natal teeth—Prematurely erupted teeth present at birth. Occasionally an infant is born with erupted mandibular incisor teeth, either supernumerary or normal. In either case, it may be necessary to remove them if they interfere with nursing or if there is danger of their being sucked into the lungs.

Fusion of teeth—The fusion of the crowns alone, or the entire crowns and roots, of two teeth

Mottled enamel—The development (on the crowns) of spots which are originally white but later darken through staining

Micrognathia—Underdeveloped jaws

Macrognathia—Overdeveloped jaws

Microdontia—Teeth that are smaller than normal

Macrodontia—Teeth that are larger than normal

Ankyloglossia—("Tongue-tie") restricted movement of the tongue due to size or location of the frenular attachment

Tori—An excess growth of bone usually located in the midline of the hard palate and/or on the tongue side of the lower jaw. Tori are usually asymptomatic but may interfere with the wearing of dentures.

ATTRITION   Attrition is the normal wearing-down of the surfaces of teeth due to the mastication of food. This occurs primarily on the biting surfaces. It accounts for the worn-down appearance of the incisor teeth of some older people. It may be more marked and more widespread in societies where there is much chewing of hard objects. It may present both cosmetic problems or pain and sensitivity if the dentin is exposed.

BAD HABITS AND DENTAL HEALTH There are a number of physical habits which may be detrimental to dental health. Among these are thumb- or finger-sucking; tongue-thrust; excessive use of pacifers or teething rings; biting on pencils, hairpins, or other hard objects; lip-biting; resting of chin in hand ("thinker's pose"); sleeping on one side of the face with constant pressures exerted in one area of the dental arch; use of a pipe in one area of the mouth; abnormal and constant movements of the jaws (biting cuspid to cuspid); bruxism and bruxomania (persistent gritting of teeth); excessive use of toothpicks or other objects for cleaning the teeth; bone-chewing; cigar-chewing; cuticle- and nail-biting; excessive use of citrus juices; excessively hard or soft diet; mouth-breathing; nail- or needle-holding; cracking of nuts or opening of bottles with the teeth; and thread-biting.

The adverse effects of some habits upon the teeth or their supporting structures are too involved to mention here. Diagnosis and correction of these habits is often extremely involved and may require the advice of professional personnel in many fields. On the other hand, some—such as thumb-sucking and nail-biting—are quite easy to detect and (in some cases) simple to correct.

As with all habits, the individual will is the deciding factor in correction. In the very young, this is of course difficult to instill, but patience and competent advice will aid in the solution of this problem.

BASE   This is a layer of dental cementlike material placed in the deep parts of a cavity to serve as insulator and medication (sedative) for protection of the pulp.

BICUSPIDS (PREMOLARS)   These are the eight permanent posterior teeth, located behind the cuspids, which replace the eight deciduous molars.

BRIDGE, DENTAL   A bridge is an artificial appliance used to replace one or more missing teeth. The remaining teeth are utilized for support and retention, and the appliance is intended to restore the function and appearance of the lost teeth. A fixed bridge is one which usually is cemented in place by the dentist and which cannot readily be removed by the patient. A removable bridge is one which is designed to be easily removed by the patient. (It is sometimes referred to as a removable partial denture.) It is axiomatic that any artificial replacement of teeth or their parts requires continued and scrupulous care by both the patient and the dentist. (*See also* DENTURES in this section.)

BRUXISM   The gritting and grinding of the teeth while sleeping (medically referred to as bruxism) may cause excessive, premature, and abnormal wearing-away of the biting surfaces of the teeth. The unusual pressures created are generally injurious to the supporting structures. Not only is there excessive wear on the involved teeth but also changes in the bite. Sometimes a plastic dental plate to be slipped over the teeth before retiring is prescribed.

BRUXOMANIA   This is the unconscious habit of gritting and grinding of the teeth while awake, usually during times of nervous tension.

CALCULUS (TARTAR)   A hard deposit of calcified material usually found on the crowns or roots of teeth, calculus is believed to be precipitated from the saliva or other secretions and is usually found in greater amounts on teeth which are located nearest the opening of salivary glands. There are two main types: that which begins forming on the visible surfaces of teeth and is usually sand-colored (supragingival [above-the-gum] calculus); and that which begins forming beneath the gum line and is usually black (subgingival [below-the-gum] calculus).

Either type acts as an irritant to the supporting structures of teeth and should be periodically removed by the dentist or dental hygienist. Calculus is one of the major contributing factors in periodontal disease. Different individuals form calculus at varying rates. On average a cleaning at approximately six-month intervals is recommended. Dental flossing on a daily basis is recommended for removal of interdental calculus as well as food fragments.

CANKER SORES   The scientific name for canker sore is aphthous stomatitis or aphthous ulcer. Canker sores most commonly occur in the mouth and may be caused by such things as jagged teeth, ill-fitting dentures, or the irritation to mucous membrane caused by an improper "bite" of the jaw. Emotional stress, reactions to drugs, and foods such as chocolate, walnuts, and citrus fruit may trigger canker sores in some individuals. When canker sores appear on mucous membrane surfaces other than the mouth (e.g. vagina), menstrual difficulties and gastrointestinal disturbances should be looked into as possible causes.

A canker sore is usually between an eighth of an inch to as much as an inch in diameter. It is circular or oval, has a bright red circumference, and is greyish-white. The sore begins in the soft tissue of the mouth and within a few days may appear as a small punched-out hole. Often pain is felt before the sore appears.

Women are more susceptible to canker sores than men. Usually, if one member of the family has canker sores, other family members have them as well. Yet, unlike fever blisters, which are caused by the herpes simplex virus Type I, canker sores are not contagious.

Treatment of canker sores may include the administration of an antibiotic suspension held in the mouth to coat the ulcer. Steroid pastes or ointments may be applied. Keeping some chips of ice in their vicinity for a few minutes may also be helpful. Nonsevere cases usually heal in ten to fourteen days without treatment.

"CAPS"   This is a colloquial term to describe artificial crowns placed on individual teeth, which closely resemble the natural teeth in shape and color. (*See* CROWN, ARTIFICIAL in this section.)

CROWN, ARTIFICIAL   An appliance constructed of porcelain, gold, plastic, or other combination of substances, an artificial crown is designed to cover and form the top (coronal) part of a tooth, utilizing the natural root for attachment. A crown may restore normal appearance to the residuum of a decayed or badly damaged tooth. Crowns may also be used to correct bad bites and for cosmetic purposes.

CROWN (NATURAL)   The crown is that visible portion of a natural tooth which is covered with enamel.

CUSPIDS (CANINES, EYETEETH)   The cuspids are the four spear-shaped anterior teeth located at the corners of the mouth. A permanent set replace the deciduous cuspids.

DENTAL ANESTHETICS   Certain agents when injected, inhaled, applied, or otherwise administered, result in a loss of sensation in the affected area. Primary use of such anesthetics in dentistry is to prevent pain during certain procedures. There are two main types:

A local anesthetic. One which is injected or applied topically to anesthetize a specific area of the body.

A general anesthetic. One which may be inhaled, injected, or otherwise applied to render the entire body insensible: for example, pentothal sodium, which is injected into the bloodstream, or nitrous oxide ("laughing gas") which is inhaled.

DENTAL CARIES (CAVITIES)

Early detection and correction of dental caries (decay) by the dentist is of the utmost importance. Left untreated, dental caries will deepen through the enamel and dentin to the pulp, resulting in pain and possible loss of the tooth. Early treatment of caries is simplest, less expensive, and more likely to succeed than delayed treatment.

What you can do to break the chain of dental caries:

Theoretically microorganisms may be destroyed by the use of certain topical antibiotics, but the antibiotic will soon wash away.

The soft, white deposit—plaque—found on unclean areas of teeth may be prevented from forming, or may be removed by proper brushing and the inclusion of "cleansing" foods in the diet (apples, raw carrots, cabbage, celery, etc.).

There are many types of carbohydrates—sugars—but some are more readily converted into tooth-destructive acids than others. It has been shown that refined carbohydrates (such as those found in the majority of soft drinks, candies, pies, cakes, cookies, etc.) are most directly related to dental caries. The between-meal use of these foods should be discouraged, especially among children and adolescents, and the amount eaten at mealtime kept to a minimum.

The most obvious method of controlling the amount of acid formed is to keep the total intake of refined carbohydrates (sugars) to a minimum at all times. Sugars ingested, or acids formed, should be removed as soon as possible after eating (preferably by brushing the teeth within fifteen minutes).

The resistance of enamel and dentin to "leaching-out" of calcium (decalcification) and eventual decay may be enhanced by the ingestion or application of proper amounts of fluorides. This may be accomplished by the following methods:

- Inclusion of fluorides in drinking water
- Direct application of fluorides to the teeth by the dentist
- Use of some dentifrices containing fluoride
- A recent development, some resins are applied to deep pits of fissures in the teeth to prevent decay. There are some who advocate applying such sealants more extensively and replacing worn out resin on a regular basis.

DENTAL FLOSS

This is a waxed or unwaxed strand of cotton, silk, or synthetic fibers which is used to remove certain materials from between the teeth. The routine daily use of dental floss which removes interdental plaque not responsive to toothbrushing is a recommended anti-caries procedure.

A short piece of dental floss is carefully worked diagonally through the contact areas, without snapping the strand into the soft tissue (which may cause harm). The floss is then moved upward along the surface of each tooth and out through the contact area.

DENTIFRICE

Any preparation used to assist the toothbrush in cleansing the accessible surfaces of the teeth is known as a dentifrice. Such preparations may be in the form of flavored liquids, powders, or pastes which contain soap or detergents.

Powders and pastes usually contain some type of abrasive. A common constituent of pastes is a liquid, such as glycerin. The powders are generally more abrasive than the pastes and liquids, and thus might be more easily misused. The primary purpose of abrasives is to remove stains from teeth; if, therefore, teeth are not prone to staining, there is no real need for the abrasive agent. The occasional use of sodium bicarbonate (baking soda) with a wet toothbrush will usually prove very effective in the removal of stains.

It should be noted that the use of a toothbrush and a dentifrice should not only cleanse the teeth, but should also be beneficial to other oral structures, such as the gingiva. This involves both proper use of the brush itself and choosing a dentifrice which aids in the cleansing action. (The use of dentifrice containing fluoride compounds has proven to be effective in the reduction of caries, but the fact remains that this method alone is not the best one for applying fluorides; it is merely one technique of topical application.)

A mixture of equal parts of salt and sodium bicarbonate remains one of the best available cleansing agents; another is a mixture of sodium bicarbonate and hydrogen peroxide. But in all cases the choice of the dentifrice, the brush, and the technique of brushing should be determined by the dentist on the basis of individual needs.

DENTISTRY   In the art and science of dentistry this control includes two elements: prevention and treatment. To this end dentistry embraces various specialties concerned with these complex concepts:

Endodontics. A branch of dentistry which has to do with the diagnosis, treatment, and correction of diseases occurring within the pulp of teeth (root-canal fillings)

Oral Pathology. A branch of dentistry which has to do with the diagnosis of diseases of the mouth in relation to all changes from the normal (benign and malignant growths)

Oral Surgery. A branch of dentistry which has to do with surgical procedures related to all physical structures of the mouth (extracting teeth and treating fractures of the related bones)

Orthodontics. A branch of dentistry which has to do with the diagnosis, prevention, and correction of abnormal or irregular positioning of teeth and their related structures, so as to maintain proper function and aesthetics (straightening of teeth)

Pedodontics. A branch of dentistry which has to do with dental care in the treatment of children (children's dentistry)

Periodontics. A branch of dentistry which has to do with diagnosis, prevention, and treatment of abnormal conditions of the structures which support the teeth (gum problems and periodontal disease)

Prosthodontics. A branch of dentistry which has to do with the functional and aesthetic replacement of missing oral structures, so as to maintain proper function and pleasing appearance by artificial means (dentures and crowns)

Public Health Dentistry. A branch of dentistry which has to do with the total relationship of dental health to the community (fluoridation of drinking water).

DENTURES   This term is generally used to denote those removable appliances which are designed as the replacement for several or all of the missing teeth and their adjacent tissues. The artificial teeth are attached to a base which resembles the gingival tissue.

There are two main types of dentures: full (complete dentures), replacing all of the missing teeth in either the upper or lower jaw; and partial dentures, replacing some, but not all, of the missing teeth and depending upon remaining natural teeth and tissues for retention and support.

Any artificial appliance replacing a part of the body which has been gradually or suddenly lost (for example, an artificial limb or a crutch) is not readily tolerated by the rest of the body, especially the immediate area. The entire body must become accustomed to the changes necessary in its daily routine. The same is true to some degree in regard to persons adapting to full or partial dentures. This replacement (prosthetic) appliance cannot possibly be as efficient as the organ or organs it replaces, especially if these were functioning well when they were lost and replaced. Full dentures, for example, may be no more than 40 percent as efficient as the normal teeth which they replaced. If, however, only a few teeth existed at the time of replacement, or those that were replaced were not functioning completely, the prosthetic appliance may be more efficient than the natural teeth. The final success of any dental prosthesis depends primarily upon the patient's ability to adapt to it, assuming that it has been designed and constructed with the individual's particular requirements in mind. The factors that must be considered can only be ascertained and evaluated by a dentist who has given careful study to all facets of the patient's physical and psychological traits.

In some cases, it is possible to remove the remaining teeth and replace them immediately with previously constructed dentures (immediate dentures). In other instances, the remaining natural teeth must have been extracted some time prior to the initial phases in construction of dentures; this allows sufficient time for healing and for stabilization of the process of resorption which always follows the extraction of natural teeth.

Although the gingiva and bone eventually become more physically static, the process of resorption (and other changes) invariably continue throughout life, just as other physical characteristics change. These changes require that dentures be adjusted, readapted, or remade periodically, since although they themselves do not normally change, the living parts with which they are associated do. When the physical changes reach a certain point, the dentures must be remade or altered to fit the existing condition. This "remake" or alteration (reline, rebase) requires the utmost skill and training on the part of the dentist, who is able to diagnose and prescribe the exact changes necessary to ensure the proper design of the revised appliance.

The mere refilling of the dentures by the addition of material to replace the resorbed tissue is not necessarily enough to ensure the proper functioning of dentures. Other needs, such as occlusion of the denture with the opposing teeth, the restoration of profile and speech characteristics, and changes in jaw interrelationships and movements must be considered.

DENTURES, CARE OF Although dentures are inanimate objects which normally do not change, they must be cared for properly. Dentures should be stored in room-temperature water when not in the mouth. The dentist will usually inform the wearer as to whether or not dentures should be worn during sleep; in general, they are removed at night to provide rest for the tissues upon which they lie. The dentures themselves may be cleansed either with ordinary dentifrices and a brush, or with special denture-cleaners and brushes. Care of the gums (gingiva) and remaining teeth is of primary importance. These should be brushed to remove accumulated food particles and to provide needed stimulation. In many cases, warm salt water as a mouth wash is beneficial.

EROSION, DENTAL Dental erosion refers to the wedge-shaped loss of the hard substance of a tooth, usually on the surfaces of teeth next to the lips and cheeks near the gum line. The eroded area is usually highly polished, and the condition is believed to be caused by a combination of mechanical and chemical (acid) factors. Severe cases of erosion must be restored by filling.

FLUORIDE (FLUORIDATION) A fluoride is a compound of the element fluorine with another element (such as sodium or tin) which in solution "disassociates" to liberate the fluoride ion. When incorporated into the teeth in one manner or another in proper trace amounts, this ion tends to reduce the incidence of dental caries.

There are two methods of administering fluorides: topical application (directly to the teeth) and ingestion through the digestive tract. Topical application is best accomplished by particular procedures utilized by the dentist, although another method is the regular use of fluoridated dentifrice. (Topical application implies that the teeth have already erupted into the mouth and are accessible.) Ingestion of fluorides may be accomplished by including them in drinking water or taking them in prescribed liquid or tablet form. This ingestion of fluoride is most beneficial during the actual formation of the tooth.

The exact mechanism of the action of fluoride in increasing the resistance of teeth to dental caries is still unknown. However, the fact remains that in our lifetime few methods of disease control have been more completely researched or thoroughly proved than fluoridation.

In order to effectively reduce the incidence of dental caries, it is known that the fluoride compound must be in solution and actually deposited within the tooth in the form of the fluoride ion. This is accomplished much more thoroughly and readily when the ion is deposited in the tooth during its actual formation, although once a tooth has formed and erupted into the oral cavity, fluoride may be deposited into the teeth by means of topical application by the dentist. An ideal situation would be one in which the child received fluoride by ingestion during the ages in which teeth were forming (up to twelve to fifteen years), fluoride tooth pastes were used, and periodic topical applications were made by the dentist.

The effectiveness of fluoridation varies with the individual and is directly related to many other factors, such as diet, heredity, dental caries susceptibility, habits, arrangement of teeth, and oral hygiene. Fluoridation should therefore not be considered a panacea. It does not reduce the need for the competent advice of a dentist.

GINGIVITIS Inflammation of the soft tissue (gingiva) covering around the necks of the teeth is called gingivitis. It may be localized or generalized, depending upon the number of teeth involved. It may be caused by local irritation, overfunction of the related tooth, lack of stimulation to the tissues, the eruption of teeth, faulty restoration, viruses, bacteria, psychosomatic factors, and general body disturbances.

Symptoms. Gingivitis produces redness, swelling, tenderness, and possible bleeding of the gingival tissue.

Treatment. As with all diseases, primary treatment is removal of the cause. Generally the cause can be ascertained only by a dentist, but proper diet and oral hygiene are under the control of the patient. The vast majority of cases will respond to proper gingival stimulation, but untreated gingivitis may progress to more serious periodontal disease. Gingivitis and the periodontal disease may respond to long-term administration of the antibiotic tetracycline.

HALITOSIS (MOUTH ODORS) Unpleasant odors of the mouth may be due to a variety of causes: primarily, they arise from the decomposition of substances within the mouth which also create a bad taste. These decomposed products include both the dental tissues (teeth and gums) and accumulated food debris; oral hygiene, properly practiced, is the best defense against the problem. Basic to such hygiene is the rapid removal of debris from the teeth and the furrows of the tongue by brushing and flossing. Furthermore, it is evident that certain foods possess a characteristic odor which influence the breath. This can be corrected by a scented mouthwash.

In some cases odors may be related to infected tonsils, severe cirrhosis of the liver, and systemic problems of the lungs or digestive tract. The uncontrolled diabetic may have a "fruity breath" and a person with kidney problems may retain urea, giving rise to "ammonia breath." In a persistent "bad breath" problem, medical and dental examination is indicated.

IMPACTED TOOTH (IMPACTION) A tooth which fails to erupt normally and which does not assume its intended position in the dental arch may be considered to be partially or completely impacted. A partially impacted tooth is visible, to various degrees, in the oral cavity, whereas a completely impacted tooth is not visible, and its position can only be ascertained by radiographs (photographs depending upon X-rays instead of light). The completely impacted tooth may be covered only by the soft tissue of the mouth (mucosa), or it may be completely imbedded in the jawbone. The usual treatment is extraction.

IMPLANTS, DENTAL Dental implants are one recent approach to the replacement of missing teeth. A screw-like device made of a compatible metal or plastic is inserted into the jawbone. Although the initial models were sometimes rejected by the body, more recent versions based on experiences with various kinds of orthopedic implants into bone have been more successful. One model has minute perforations into which the cells of the jawbone can grow, thus producing stability for the device. One kind of implant is used to give stability to the problem of the usual denture, by anchoring what would otherwise be a full denture to several implants. Thus the denture can't slip around or come loose. Implants require the skill of an experienced dentist and are expensive.

INCISORS The incisors (literally cutters) are eight chisel-shaped front teeth, four in either arch, which are present in both the permanent and the deciduous sets of teeth. Those located nearest the middle of the face are termed the central incisors and those adjacent to these are the two lateral incisors.

INLAY An inlay is a filling consisting of gold, porcelain, or other materials which is constructed primarily outside the mouth and is then cemented into the prepared tooth. An inlay has superior strength as compared to the usual filling and is more applicable to a very large cavity.

MALOCCLUSION Abnormal positioning of the upper and lower teeth, so that they do not "mesh" properly when the jaws are closed, is known as malocclusion. The offending deviations from acceptable normal standards may result from malpositioned and misshapen individual teeth; improper size, shape, and relation of the jaws; congenital deformities; cleft palate; and fractures of either or both jaws.

MANDIBLE   The mandible is the horseshoe-shaped lower jaw which forms the movable part of the chewing mechanism and which supports the lower teeth.

MAXILLA   The maxilla is the upper jaw—the fixed part of the masticatory mechanism which supports the upper teeth in an arch-like arrangement.

MOLARS   The large posterior teeth having four or more cusps are the molars. There are eight in the deciduous dentition (replaced by the eight permanent bicuspids) and twelve in the permanent dentition which have no primary predecessors. The first adult tooth to erupt is the first permanent molar (six-year molar). The second permanent molar erupts at about age twelve and is referred to as the twelve-year molar. The permanent third molars are the wisdom teeth, usually the last teeth of all to erupt at about age twenty, and so named since this is presumed to be the age at which some wisdom is acquired.

MOUTH   The oral cavity is the main point of contact with the outside world in the newborn infant. While its importance diminishes as times goes by, the mouth continues to be the source of many pleasurable sensations. Because of the rich nerve supply, taste and the perception of texture are highly developed. The lips, tongue, teeth, palate, and salivary glands all help in the preliminary preparation of the food before swallowing. The extensive blood supply to the structures of the mouth aids in preventing most infections that might be expected from the constant minor burns and scratches to which the area is ordinarily subjected. Interestingly, a bite inflicted by another individual usually becomes severely infected, but one's own germs seldom cause trouble. Various difficulties peculiar to the mouth and its structures are discussed under their appropriate headings. (*See also* the section HOME NURSING CARE.)

MOUTHWASH   In general usage, this term implies a liquid with a pleasant taste or odor for rinsing the mouth. However, the council on Dental Therapeutics of the American Dental Association "does not accept mouthwashes for unsupervised use by the lay public." Routine rinsing of the mouth is not a substitute for proper toothbrushing, although at times a dentist may prescribe the practice in relation to individual needs.

PERICORONITIS   This condition is an inflammation of the soft tissue covering the crown portion of a partially erupted tooth. Most commonly it involves the permanent third molars (wisdom teeth).

Symptoms. The soft tissue may swell to the point that the jaws cannot be completely closed without striking this swollen area, which further injures the inflamed tissue. If untreated, the infection may spread into adjacent tissues, producing swelling which results in difficulty in opening the jaws (trismus) and swallowing.

Treatment. Treatment usually involves the use of antibiotics, irrigation of the area, and perhaps surgical removal of the soft-tissue covering (operculum) or the tooth itself.

PERIODONTAL DISEASE (PERIODONTITIS, PYORRHEA)   This is the term given to the progressive destruction of the periodontal structures (supporting structures of the teeth) which originates in the gingiva (gum) and involves the periodontal membrane, epithelial attachment, supporting bone, and the cementum.

The root of a tooth is surrounded by bone and attached to the bony socket (alveolus) by means of the fibers of the periodontal membrane which runs from the cementum of the root to surrounding bone. The gingiva is also attached to the tooth by means of a band of tissue, the epithelial attachment. Between the tooth and the gingiva is a normal space, called the gingival sulcus.

The healthy gingiva normally fits snugly around the tooth, but if for any reason the epithelial attachment is broken and moved down the root toward the tip (apex), the depth of the sulcus increases and a pocket is formed. This pocket provides an area for the accumulation of food, other debris, and calculus which further reduces the resistance and health of the adjacent tissue. The inflammatory process is progressive, and the periodontal membrane and bone surrounding the tooth are destroyed. This wave of destruction continues moving apically (tipward), the involved tooth eventually becoming loose and possibly assuming a slightly different position. Once the bone around the root has been destroyed, it cannot rebuild to its original height. The supporting structures may become so damaged that the teeth cannot be maintained and must be removed.

It is difficult to imagine, but a tooth which shows no evidence of dental caries can be lost as a result of this insidious process. In fact, periodontal disease is the major factor contributing to the loss of teeth in people past thirty years of age.

The major causative factors in periodontal disease may be classified as irritational, (dys)functional, and systemic. Some examples of local irritation are deposits on the teeth (calculus), packing of food between the teeth, malformed or malpositioned teeth, and mechanical irritation (cavity margins, damaged fillings, and improper tooth-brushing). Overfunction (excessive stress on the teeth, excessive muscular pressures), underfunction (lack of contact between opposing teeth), and abnormal habits (clenching or grinding of the teeth) are examples of dysfunctional factors. Among the systemic causes of periodontal disease are faulty nutrition, allergies, psychosomatic factors, and hormonal imbalance related to the menstrual cycle.

Treatment. The treatment of this disease, as of all other dental diseases, involves removal of the cause, restoration of normal function, increase of tissue-resistance, and stabilization of the health and integrity of the tissue. This may be accomplished by procedures performed primarily by the dentist or primarily by the patient.

Those accomplished by the dentist are scaling, which is the mechanical removal of calculus, diseased cementum, and soft tissue and conservative surgery, permitting the scaling to be done more thoroughly. (In more serious cases the affected bone and the soft tissue overlying it may be removed or reshaped.)

Those accomplished by the patient upon instruction from the dentist are mechanical in nature: stimulation of the soft tissue by various means, such as with toothbrush, rubber stimulators, and finger-massage.

PROPHYLACTIC ODONOTOMY This term refers to those procedures, whether mechanical or chemical, which have as their objective the prevention of dental decay. This particularly applies in areas of the teeth which appear to be likely sites of decay and also in those teeth with developmental faults. These areas may be reshaped or restored by fillings.

PROPHYLAXIS (ORAL) Oral prophylaxis describes those measures aimed at the prevention of oral and dental diseases—especially the mechanical cleaning of the teeth by the dentist or dental hygienist utilizing scaling and polishing techniques.

RESTORATION This is a general term in dentistry which usually refers to a filling or a bridge.

ROOT-CANAL TREATMENT Root-canal treatment encompasses those procedures which involve removal of the entire pulp from a tooth, so that the root canal and chamber can be cleaned, sterilized, filled, and sealed. The resulting tooth will be "non-vital," since there will be no nerves or blood supply within it; hence, it will not respond to such external stimuli as heat or cold. However, the treatment does not affect the supporting structures, and the tooth can remain in the arch and continue to give additional service. The tooth so treated will be subject to dental decay just as any tooth in the mouth. When the supporting structures are healthy and the pulp canal can be treated, root-canal therapy may be resorted to instead of extraction.

SALIVA Saliva is a mixture of clear fluids secreted into the mouth by certain glands (salivary glands). These fluids lubricate the mucosa and aid in preventing dehydration of all soft tissues of the mouth. During chewing (mastication), the saliva is mixed with food, aiding in swallowing and initiating digestion. Saliva is usually alkaline and possesses a great capacity for neutralizing acids; in addition, it contains materials which delay or halt bacterial growth; both of these characteristics reducing the possibility of dental caries. Saliva also helps certain fillings to remain moist and thus to maintain their color, stability, and durability.

The quantity and quality of saliva varies

with each individual. Its flow is stimulated by mastication or other stimuli capable of affecting the nervous system (such as the sight and smell of food). Breathing through the mouth for long periods of time may result in excessive evaporation, producing a reduction in the lubricating qualities of saliva.

SALIVARY GLANDS   These are specialized organs, associated with the oral cavity, whose function is the production and secretion of the watery fluid called saliva. The principal salivary glands are the parotid, the submaxillary, and the sublingual. These occur in pairs and empty their saliva into the mouth through the salivary ducts.

The parotids are the largest of the principal glands. They lie embedded on either side of the face, just below and in front of each ear; the ducts carrying the saliva of these glands into the mouth course through the cheeks and empty into the oral cavity opposite the maxillary second molars. The secretion is usually quite thin and watery. Epidemic parotitis is a viral infection of this pair of glands, its more common name being the mumps.

The submaxillary glands are located, one on either side, just in front of and below the angles of the lower jaw. The saliva from these glands is emptied into the mouth through the ducts which are located beneath the tongue, one on each side of the frenulum of the tongue.

The smallest pair of salivary glands are those located beneath the tongue, the sublingual glands. These, too, empty into the mouth beneath the tongue.

In addition to the three pairs of major salivary glands, there are a number of smaller accessory glands which also produce some saliva. These are located primarily in the roof of the mouth and on the inside of the lips.

Partial or complete blockage of the ducts of the major glands may result from swelling or the presence of salivary stones (sialolith). In these conditions the glands continue to secrete saliva, but since it cannot pass out of the glands and into the oral cavity, it backs up into the gland, causing it to swell. This swelling may be especially noticeable and painful when a hungry person with this obstruction sees or smells food, inasmuch as the glands are stimulated to produce still more saliva in preparation for the anticipated food. If this ob-

struction prevails for long periods, the glands may be damaged and begin to shrink (atrophy).

Treatment. The treatment of sialolithiasis involves locating the position, size, and nature of the stone or stones and removing this obstruction. Though this may occur spontaneously, frequently a dental consultation is necessary to determine if the salivary stones (calculi) should be removed surgically or expressed manually. In some stubborn cases of sialolithiasis, surgical removal of the salivary gland and its ducts is required.

SILICATE   A semi-permanent filling material, silicate is used primarily in the anterior teeth because of its color-matching qualities.

TARTAR   *See* CALCULUS in this section.

TEETH, FORMATION AND DEVELOPMENT OF   To develop an understanding of the oral cavity and its related structures, it is essential to consider all the influences which occur throughout life. Within the womb (uterus), the development of the oral structures is dependent upon such factors as heredity and environment. Hereditary influences include such factors as size, shape, color, and number of teeth; size and shape of facial bones; and similar characteristics.

During the formative period of the unborn child (fetus) the "within-womb" environment is directly related to the pregnant woman, since many factors affecting her health may in turn produce an effect upon the fetus itself, even though it is enclosed by a sac in the womb. In some cases prolonged treatment of the mother with certain antibiotics (tetracyclines) may cause the first teeth of the newborn to be more yellow-gray than normal.

At birth, certain structures of the oral cavity have already developed; however, no functional teeth are normally visible. The first teeth (variously known as primary, milk, temporary, or deciduous teeth) begin formation within the bones of the jaws of the unborn child and are in various stages of development beginning six weeks after conception and until they appear in the mouth.

After birth, the individual teeth continue to develop, and through the process of eruption they migrate toward the oral cavity from their

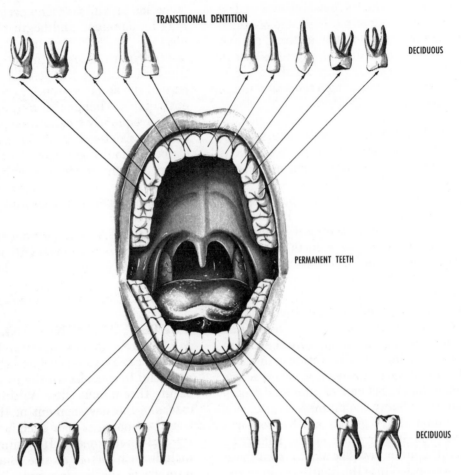

TRANSITIONAL DENTITION

DECIDUOUS

PERMANENT TEETH

DECIDUOUS

positions within the jaws. This process continues throughout life; however, once the teeth of one jaw contact the teeth of the opposite jaw, the rate of eruption decreases. The lower teeth usually precede the corresponding upper teeth in erupting, and teeth usually erupt earlier in girls and in slender individuals. The teeth emerge into the mouth in a pattern of eruption which follows a normal sequence, even though there is a time variable for each individual. This applies to both primary and permanent teeth. In fact, a time exists when some primary and some permanent teeth are simultaneously present in both arches, indicating a mixed or transitional phase of growth and development. During one phase in growth, more than forty teeth, primary and secondary, are in various stages of development.

When the primary teeth appear, they are twenty in number: ten in each jaw, arranged to form two horseshoe-like arches—an upper (maxillary) and a lower (mandibular). This primary set consists of teeth of various sizes and shapes, depending upon location and function, which match one another in both the upper and lower arches. For convenience, the ten teeth of the upper arch may be described in terms of the five on the right and the five on the left, using the midline of the face as a dividing point; the same principle applies to the ten teeth of the lower arch. The five corresponding teeth in each of their four quadrants have identical names in relation to their position and function in the arch. Beginning at the midline in the front of the mouth and progressing backward, the primary teeth are the central incisor, lateral incisor, cuspid, first molar, and second molar.

It is frequently thought that, since the primary teeth are shed at a relatively early age, their retention is not important since the permanent teeth will eventually replace them. Why expend time and effort retaining baby teeth when they are destined to be shed eventually? But it is a mistake to consider the premature loss of primary teeth unimportant. Usually, all of them are in place from the age of two until about age seven. Certain ones appear as early as six months of age while others remain as late as twelve. During this latter period, children undergo rapid mental and physical changes, and their teeth are essential for their proper development. Unless the primary dental arches remain intact until these teeth are destined to be shed normally, problems of adequate space and proper position for the succeeding permanent teeth can be created. Then too, if the primary dental arches do not remain intact until the proper time for shedding, it may be difficult (if not impossible) for nature to achieve the orderly transition from the primary to the permanent teeth.

Even though all the primary teeth are lost in a definite pattern, the permanent teeth may not occupy ideal positions in their respective arches. Every tooth has a specific reason for being in the dental arch, and thought must therefore be given to the complications which may result from the premature loss of any tooth for any reason. A definite knowledge of all factors related to growth and development is essential to proper alignment and function of either the primary or secondary teeth. It is therefore advised that children should be examined periodically, beginning at an early age (usually about four when a child is old enough to follow instructions), in order to diagnose, treat, and prevent minor dental deformities, thus minimizing the possibility of prolonged and expensive dental procedures later on. These early visits are also valuable in that the child begins his adjustment to dentists and dental treatment without fear.

Eventually the permanent (secondary, adult) teeth occupy positions in both arches in a normal sequence of growth and development for the individual. Primary teeth are normally shed as some of the permanent teeth assume their positions.

In addition to the twenty secondary teeth which assume the positions of the twenty shed primary teeth, the first permanent molars erupt and occupy positions behind the last primary molars (which will not be shed until about age twelve). In many cases parents may mistake these permanent first molars for pri-

mary teeth, since at this time all of the deciduous teeth are usually still present. The first permanent molars serve as "keystones" for the proper positioning of the adult teeth. If they are lost because of neglect, the child becomes a "dental cripple" at an early age (approximately six years).

It will be noted that more teeth are present in an adult than in a baby, for more than twenty permanent teeth will replace the twenty primary teeth which are shed. The second teeth (adult, or permanent) usually consist of three additional molar teeth in each quadrant. The completed permanent dentition therefore usually consists of thirty-two teeth: sixteen in the upper arch and sixteen in the lower.

As with the primaries, the sixteen teeth of either the mandibular or the maxillary arch may be divided into two groups—those on the right (eight) and those on the left (eight)—again using the midline as a dividing point. In each of the four quadrants there are thus eight teeth which have corresponding names. Beginning at the midline and progressing backward, the permanent teeth of each arch are the central incisor, lateral incisor, cuspid ("eye-tooth," canine) first bicuspid (first premolar), second bicuspid (second premolar), first molar (six-year molar), second molar (twelve-year molar), and third molar (wisdom tooth).

Thus, many events must follow in orderly sequence for adult dentition to function properly. These changes involve the formation and development of unobservable teeth in the jaws and the eruption of twenty primary teeth (by two years of age). These are in turn replaced by thirty-two adult teeth. Any disturbance in these events during this entire process of transition will result in the diminution of the functional efficiency and appearance of the entire dentition.

One may speak of a usual sequence in which individual teeth—primary or permanent—are replaced in normal individuals. Variations do exist from individual to individual, since "birthdate age" may differ from "dental age," depending upon hereditary and environmental influences. However, preceding, during, and following the eruption of teeth, their supporting structures are also developing.

THE PERMANENT DENTITION

THE DECIDUOUS DENTITION

ROOT

CROWN

* ERUPTION (YEARS)

7+
8
11
10
10
6+
12+
17

CENTRAL INCISOR
LATERAL INCISOR
CUSPID
FIRST BICUSPID
SECOND BICUSPID
FIRST MOLAR
SECOND MOLAR
THIRD MOLAR

** ERUPTION

UPPER
(MAXILLARY)

UPPER
(MAXILLARY)

MIDLINE

MIDLINE

LOWER
(MANDIBULAR)

LOWER
MANDIBULAR

17
12
6
11
10
9
9
6+

THIRD MOLAR
SECOND MOLAR
FIRST MOLAR
SECOND BICUSPID
FIRST BICUSPID
CUSPID
LATERAL INCISOR
CENTRAL INCISOR

CROWN
ROOT

* Plus or minus 1 year
**Plus or minus 1 month
All teeth are drawn to same magnification

TEETH, FUNCTION AND POSITION OF

In some cases it is possible to demonstrate that either the upper or the lower arch, or both, may not be sufficiently "long" to accommodate the teeth which must occupy positions within them; if an arch thus lacks sufficient room, the teeth will be twisted, rotated, crowded, and malpositioned. The same result may be observed if the teeth are excessively large or extra teeth are present.

Spacing between some of the teeth is normal and desirable in the primary dentition. Once all of the permanent teeth have erupted, however, spacing is detrimental both to the teeth and their supporting structures. Such spacing can occur either when the arch is large but the teeth are normal in size, or when there are fewer teeth present (for example, before all the permanent teeth have erupted or when some are lost). Either of the above situations may be evident in various proportions in the upper or lower jaws. Furthermore, certain habits may create problems related to the positioning and functioning of the teeth: thumb-sucking, tongue-thrusting, the biting of foreign objects, etc.

The premature loss of a primary tooth may create a problem of insufficient space, resulting in the malpositioning of the permanent tooth. An opposite possibility is that in which a primary tooth may be retained for a longer period than normal, preventing the proper sequence of eruption of permanent teeth. The premature loss of a primary tooth results in movement of the remaining adjacent teeth into the empty space, so that the permanent tooth which is in the process of developing does not have sufficient room to erupt. This is particularly serious if it is a primary molar which is lost before the first permanent molars erupt; since the latter are the first adult teeth to appear, any malpositioning of these keystones influences the positioning of all the permanent teeth. The teeth are designed to sustain themselves and their supporting structures, and any malpositioning hastens their loss.

In order to function properly during the process of chewing, the teeth of the upper arch must occupy positions which will allow them to "mesh" properly with the teeth of the lower arch, in a fashion similar to the meshing of gears. It is the lower jaw (mandible) which opens and closes, and provides the forces necessary for chewing; whereas the upper jaw (maxilla) acts as a fixed base. In the process of chewing, forces are created by the contraction of particular muscles which pull the lower jaw against the stationary upper jaw, pulverizing the food between the teeth. It is this repeated opening-and-closing action that reduces the size of the food particles between the upper and lower teeth, permitting the food to be intermixed with saliva, and swallowed. The efficiency of mastication depends upon the number of chewing strokes it takes to pulverize food particles to a particular size; if the teeth do not mesh (occlude) properly—that is, if teeth are missing, malpositioned, or badly broken-down—this efficiency is greatly decreased. More stresses and strains are placed upon those teeth present, and teeth that are so badly overworked and made to perform extra functions may thus be lost.

Though the primary function of the dental apparatus is mastication of food, it also functions in the production of sound and, needless to say, it is related to aesthetic appearance.

The individual teeth of both arches are designed to perform specific jobs related to their position and shape. The incisors, located in the front of both arches, are chisel-shaped and designed for cutting like the blades of scissors; the cuspids occupy a position at the corners of the arches and are spear-shaped for holding, tearing, and cutting. Collectively, these teeth are known as the front (anterior) teeth. The six front teeth in the upper arch are in a more forward position (overjet) and overlap the six corresponding lower teeth (overbite).

The bicuspids and molars are positioned at the back of the arch and are hence known as the back (posterior) teeth. These have pointed projections (pyramidal cusps) and broad biting surfaces like a potato masher, designed for crushing and grinding food. When the muscles contract and pull the lower jaw upward, the chewing surfaces of the lower back teeth make contact, in a meshing action, with large areas of the opposing surfaces of their upper counterparts. To prevent biting of the cheek and tongue, the upper posterior teeth are placed closer to the cheek than are the lower; these latter, in contrast, are placed closer to the tongue. The tops of the cheek surfaces of the lower posterior teeth thus fit into the middle of the biting surfaces of the upper posterior teeth.

The lower jaw (mandible) has two projections which rise in a more or less vertical direction from its horseshoe-shaped body. By means of these projections, the mandible is hinged on either side to the temporal bones of the skull, just in front of the ears. These temporomandibular joints, right and left, are so designed that the mandible can move from side to side and forward and backward, as well as up and down like a hinge. A cartilaginous disc between the bones of the joint permits smooth functioning during various movements. Malpositioned, lost, or badly broken-down teeth may produce problems related to the temporomandibular joints by not permitting smooth movements. Either of the joints, or both, may become painful; a clicking sound may develop; or dislocation can occur. In fact, any disease which can affect the joints of the body (rheumatism, arthritis, etc.) may produce problems in the temporomandibular joints. System-wide factors may also affect the muscles related to opening and closing the jaw. For example, "lockjaw" (tetanus) is produced by a bacterium (*Clostridium tetani*) commonly found in dirt; this bacillus can enter the body by contaminating a wound, and eventually cause spasms of the muscles of the jaw. (Tetanus shots are one of the routine immunizations given to children because, without protective measures, the percentage of fatalities is extremely high.)

TEETH, INJURED   Injuries to teeth are usually the result of a traumatic blow. The result of such damage may be displacement of the tooth from its normal position in the socket, fracture of any or all of the hard tissues of the tooth, or a combination of the two.

Displacement of a tooth may be complete—in which case the tooth is removed from its socket—or partial, the tooth being moved from its normal position but remaining attached.

Fractures of a tooth may involve the enamel; the enamel and dentin; the enamel, dentin, and pulp cavity; or the root and its pulp canal. Due to their location, front teeth (especially those which protrude) are most often involved.

There are other possibilities, however. In some cases there is neither displacement nor fracture, but rather a rupture of the blood vessels of the pulp, producing a "pink tooth." The pulp may degenerate because of pressure from the hemorrhage, producing a "darkened tooth." Displacement of the first teeth may result in injury to the underlying developing permanent teeth.

In some instances, teeth which have been completely displaced from their socket may be replanted by a dentist. Partial displacement may also be treated by the dentist, the tooth being manually returned to its original position and stabilized by some mechanical means.

Fractures involving only the enamel may be treated by smoothing the rough edges, or by restoring the missing part. Those involving the enamel and dentin may have more serious consequences since the dentin possesses the ability to transmit pain impulses to the pulp and may eventually result in pulp damage.

If the fracture involves the protective wall of the pulp and exposure of it to the external environment, immediate treatment is essential if the pulp is to be preserved. Fractures of the root always involve the pulp, but healing may occur if the broken parts are joined and stabilized. Any damaged tooth, regardless of the severity of the injury, may be loose for some time; eventually, however, it usually resumes its normal stability.

TEETH, PHYSIOLOGY OF   To withstand all the forces related to mastication, the individual teeth have certain things in common: their composition, supporting structures, and general formation and arrangement within the jaws. Though there are many individual differences between the primary and the permanent teeth, their basic composition is similar in that each consists of four tissues—enamel, cementum, dentin, and pulp. (The first three are hard tissues and the last is soft.)

Enamel, the hardest substance in the body, is composed primarily of inorganic calcium compounds arranged in rods. Between the rods are microscopic amounts of organic cementing material which binds the rods together. It is this protective cover which is initially penetrated by dental caries (dental decay). The bulk of the tooth under the enamel and cementum is dentin, which is bone-like. The dentin, in the form of tiny tubules, contains more organic material than the enamel and is rapidly destroyed once the decay process has penetrated the enamel. The dentin tubules transmit sensations of heat and cold from the exterior to the internal nerves of the tooth in the form of pain. Hence, repeated periodic pain in a tooth should be a warning that the protective coverings of the tooth are no longer intact. Early dental treatment can usually resolve this problem, alleviating the pain and preventing the possible loss of the tooth.

Each tooth is divided into a root and a crown. The root is usually longer than the crown and is that part which is embedded in the bone of the jaws; the crown is the part which is usually visible in the oral cavity and contacts the adjacent and opposing teeth. Since the crown is exposed to the oral environment, it is subject to destruction from wear and the process of decay. The dentin of the crown is covered by a hard mantle of enamel and the dentin of the root is covered by a thin layer of cementum.

There is a longitudinal canal in the center of the hard tissues of the crown and root which ends as a minute opening at the tip of the root (apex). The pulp occupies this canal and furnishes the blood and nerve supply. As long as the tooth is alive, it can form new dentin along the walls of the pulp canal or chamber to protect the pulp from external harm. (Enamel does not possess this ability.) If the blood supply is destroyed (either by a blow which ruptures the vessels, or by bacteria which enter the pulp via a deep cavity) the tissue will die; the tooth will not respond normally to external stimuli (heat and cold) and the pulp will be non-vital. Unless dental treatment is initiated, a health hazard exists, since bacteria can infect a local area of the jaw, and from there the whole body. The tooth may have to be removed unless the root canal is cleaned, sterilized, and sealed (root-canal filling).

It has been mentioned that the crowns of the teeth vary in shape according to function; this is also true of the roots. The upper and lower front teeth usually have one root apiece, the lower molars have two, the upper molars have three, and the bicuspids may have one or

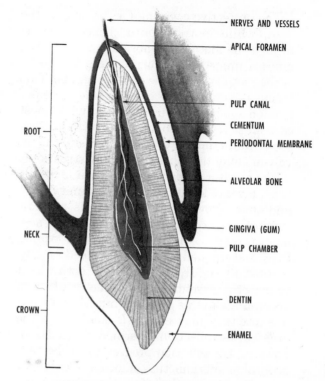

THE TOOTH AND ITS SURROUNDING STRUCTURES

two. (The cuspids, located at the corners of the arches, have the longest roots and should be retained as long as possible. These strong teeth may eventually serve as attachments for artificial appliances which replace other missing teeth.)

The supporting structures act mainly to hold the roots firmly fixed in the jaw. The portion of either jaw which provides this support is the alveolar bone, and the bony socket is called the alveolus. Fibers of a particular membrane (the periodontal) are dense and elastic, and attach the alveolar bone to the cementum of the root. This ligament not only serves as a means of attachment for the tooth but also acts as a shock absorber, cushioning the tooth and bone for the forces of mastication. Though the membrane occupies the small space between the root and the "socket," it consists of thousands of fibers which encompass the tooth from its apex to its neck. This allows the tooth to move very slightly without injuring the blood vessels and nerves which enter the tooth at its apex. If any disease or injury results in damage to the periodontal membrane, the tooth will no longer be anchored properly to the bone and will become loose.

The protective covering for the body is the skin, while in the mouth the covering is termed the mucous membrane (mucosa). The mucosa immediately surrounding the necks of the teeth is called the gingiva (gums). This tissue is subjected to considerable forces of friction and pressure during chewing. Utmost care must be taken to avoid injury to it, since such injury might eventually result in involvement of the other supporting structures.

The mucosa appears pink, since it lacks the thick layer of keratin found in ordinary skin, and thus allows the blood vessels to show through. The color of the gingiva serves as a measure of its health: normally it is pale pink, firm, and stippled, and does not bleed readily. It must fit tightly around each tooth like a collar, otherwise debris from the mouth will accumulate in this area and infection of varying intensity may ensue. If confined to the gingiva, the infection is termed gingivitis; if, however, the infection progresses to the periodontal membrane, the condition is known as periodontitis. If either of these conditions persist, the structures supporting the teeth are weakened, and even though the involved teeth may be free of caries they may eventually be lost because of insufficient support. Periodontal disease is the major cause of tooth-loss in people past thirty. (Before this age, the major cause is dental caries.)

A tooth develops beginning at the biting edge and proceeds gradually to the end of the root. The root is not actually fully formed until the tooth has been visible in the mouth for some time; this accounts (in some cases) for the mobility of newly erupted teeth, both deciduous and permanent. The life cycle of both sets of teeth is similar except for the fact that the deciduous teeth are naturally shed, whereas those of the permanent set are intended to remain in function throughout life.

A tooth actually begins forming from certain cells which line the fetal jaws. These cells begin to multiply and grow at the site of each future tooth. In this stage, the "tooth-buds" within the fetal jaw do not actually resemble a tooth but (as their name implies) are actually bud-shaped; later, the buds begin to resemble the shape of the teeth they are to form. This is the "blueprint" stage, and it is during this phase that damage to the bud may result in a badly shaped tooth.

The cells of the bud begin to specialize, each group assuming the role of forming a certain part of the tooth: some are delegated to form enamel, others dentin, and so forth. At this point the developing bud resembles only the outline, or soft framework, of the crown portion of the tooth it is destined to produce. This spider web-like framework is then gradually filled in and hardened by the deposition of certain inorganic salts, mainly calcium phosphate. This calcification process results in the formation of the familiar hard enamel and underlying dentin of the crown and—eventually—the root. These inorganic salts of calcium are derived from the bloodstream of the mother in the case of teeth developing in the unborn child and the bloodstream of the child itself after birth. Once teeth have been completely calcified, calcium salts can *not* revert to the bloodstream of the mother; calcium in the teeth of the mother therefore cannot be removed during pregnancy to be deposited in the forming teeth of the fetus. The apparent increase in dental caries and other oral diseases during pregnancy is generally due to neglect of oral hygiene, the acid products of vomitus, poor dietary habits, and hormonal changes in the oral tissues.

The source of bloodstream calcium and other necessary minerals for calcification should be assured by adequate intake of foods rich in calcium and vitamins. The role of vitamins A, B, C, and D in the development and calcification of teeth is well established, and these must be present in adequate amounts.

After the enamel and dentin of the crown have been calcified, the root begins to take shape through formation and calcification of the dentin and cementum that comprise it. At the time the root begins to grow, the tooth begins its movement toward final eruption into the mouth. As mentioned previously, however, the entire root is not completed for two to four years following the eruption of the tooth.

The eruptive process is essentially the same for deciduous and permanent teeth; but in the case of those permanent teeth which actually take the place of deciduous ones, the deciduous root must be resorbed or shortened before the erupting permanent tooth beneath can take its intended position in the mouth.

The precise mechanism of the forces which cause a tooth to erupt, or those factors responsible for the resorption of the deciduous roots, are not completely understood. Neither the eruption of all teeth nor the shedding of deciduous teeth can be explained by the mere fact that the root of the erupting permanent tooth is growing in such a way that its crown is causing pressure on the root of the deciduous tooth to be shed; in other words, the eruption of all teeth and the exfoliation of deciduous teeth cannot be explained solely on the basis of pressure. This is proven by the fact that occasionally a tooth without a root will still erupt, and a primary tooth may be shed that has no underlying permanent tooth to cause pressure. Deciduous teeth which do not shed, because of the lack of permanent teeth to replace them may remain in position.

Nature has been extremely lenient to man in providing him with two different sets of teeth. This doubling of organs does not occur in any other part of the body. The development and eruption of deciduous teeth, their shedding and replacement by permanent teeth, and their shape and arrangement so that they are self-sustaining, are all only a small part of the master plan and miracle of life.

TEETHING   The word teething refers to the problems associated with the eruption or "cutting" of the first teeth. Both the primary and secondary teeth must emerge into the mouth through the soft tissue that covers the bony crypt in which they develop. Although the exact process by which a tooth erupts and penetrates the covering mucosa is not known, it is understandable that more problems can be expected while this is occurring for the first time—in the primary dentition. Thus the gum at the site of cutting may become sensitive and inflamed.

In the past, many childhood illnesses (coughs, fevers, diarrhea) were attributed, without factual evidence, to the eruptive process. However, mild disturbances of the gums during this process can explain the child's slight fever, irritability, increased flow of saliva, and constant chewing of objects placed in the mouth.

Teething normally involves an orderly sequence of tooth eruption in which only a very few teeth are involved at any one time. An unrelated fever may accelerate the eruptive process, resulting in more than the usual number of cutting areas. Inflammation and pain may be increased (especially in the child who is already ill); however, once the tooth has erupted, the symptoms will diminish. Persistent problems require dental consultation.

Clean, soothing teething substances should be substituted for objects which can result in infection. The supervised use of ice placed in a clean towel can solve some problems related to teething, without recourse to other medication. A similar, though more complicated, series of events may follow the eruption of permanent third molars (wisdom teeth) of the adult. (*See also* Pericoronitis in this section.)

TOOTH SURFACES   Generally, each tooth has five surfaces, each related to the direction in which it faces. The biting surface is termed the occlusal surface; the surface which faces the midline of the face is termed the mesial surface; the surface which faces away from the midline is the distal surface; the surface which faces the tongue is the lingual surface; and the surface which faces the cheeks or lips is the facial surface. (In the posterior teeth, the facial surface is termed the buccal, whereas in anterior teeth it is termed the labial surface.)

Dental decay may involve any one or all of these five surfaces, and the design and type of the restoration depends upon the extent of destruction. Thus, an occlusal restoration involves only the biting surface, whereas a restoration of the mesial, occlusal, and distal surfaces (Mod) involves three sides of the tooth. Not until dental decay has been removed can the dentist determine the extent of the necessary restoration, which would depend upon the number of surfaces affected. Since there are thirty-two permanent teeth with a total of 160 surfaces (32 x 5), and twenty temporary teeth with one hundred surfaces (20 x 5), this makes 260 surfaces which, at one time or another, are potential areas of decay.

TOOTHBRUSH   A toothbrush is designed to facilitate cleansing not only of the teeth, but also of associated structures of the oral cavity. These include furrows of the tongue, the gums, and the inside of the cheeks. The brush may also serve as a means of stimulating the gums. It would therefore be better to consider a toothbrush as a "mouth-brush" or a "gum-brush."

An incorrectly used toothbrush can cause damage to the structures of the oral cavity. The dentist should therefore be consulted to assist in the proper selection of a brush, with due regard to individual differences, requirements, and needs. In general, the adult brush should consist of a long straight narrow handle (five to six inches long) and a working head of soft bristles which are arranged in two rows, six tufts to a row. The bristles, whether synthetic or natural, should be of even height (one-half inch). Each person should preferably have three brushes, so as to allow sufficient time for them to dry thoroughly between brushings; this will ensure that they are clean and maintain their stiffness. When the bristles are loose and become dislodged during use, the brush should be discarded and replaced. (A single toothbrush bristle forced into the gingiva can act as a foreign body, like a splinter, serving as a source of irritation and possible inflammation.) Toothbrushes should be discarded and replaced periodically, particularly after a cold or similar illness.

A child's brush should be of a similar design, except that it is necessarily smaller and should be somewhat softer. This type of brush is usually called a junior brush.

Electric toothbrushes of various styles are available. The brushing head itself is the same as that of a manual toothbrush; the main difference lies in the mechanical action involved. The final decision as to the type of brush needed should always be decided by the dentist on the basis of the individual's needs. There are, for example, specially constructed brushes for use on dentures, bridges, for patients wearing orthodontic appliances, or for those with certain periodontal problems.

TOOTHBRUSHING When properly manipulated, the toothbrush aids in cleaning the teeth and stimulating the gums. Improper toothbrushing includes inadequate as well as overzealous techniques. Since there are so many variations from individual to individual, the method of brushing should be determined by the dentist in order to make this procedure as effective as possible. In general, the teeth should be brushed for a period of three minutes, and this within fifteen minutes of eating. If this is done, the debris remaining after eating, as well as any by-products resulting from carbohydrate (sugar) conversion into acids, will be removed, thereby minimizing the possibility of dental caries. When brushing is done properly for three minutes, the gums will also be maintained in a healthy state, thus decreasing the possibility of periodontal disease.

Only the chewing surfaces of posterior teeth should be brushed with a scrubbing (back-and-forth) action. All other surfaces of the teeth and their adjacent gums should be brushed in the following manner: Place the bristles in line with the teeth, with the ends of the bristles pointing away from the teeth while resting on the gum; then rotate the brush in the hand, while pulling it toward the biting surface of the teeth. This enables the bristles to stimulate the gums and pass over and in between the teeth in a cleansing motion. In this manner, groups of teeth in each arch are brushed in the direction in which they "grow," by brushing down on the "uppers" and up on the "lowers."

WISDOM TEETH These are the permanent third molars, which usually erupt at age seventeen to twenty-four years.

Mental Health: Psychiatric and Psychological Conditions

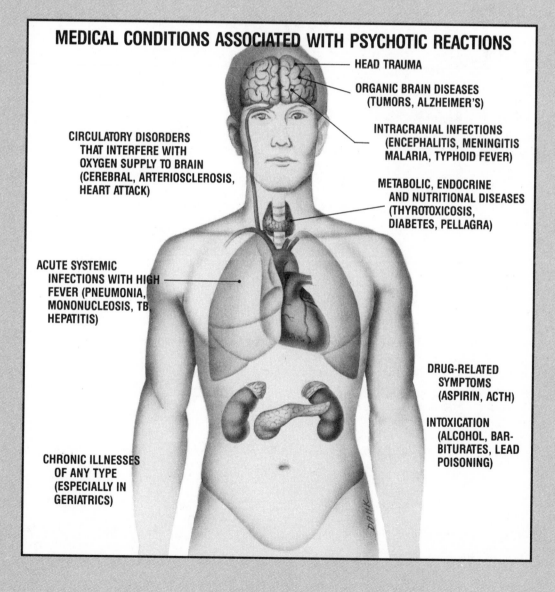

MEDICAL CONDITIONS ASSOCIATED WITH PSYCHOTIC REACTIONS

HEAD TRAUMA

ORGANIC BRAIN DISEASES (TUMORS, ALZHEIMER'S)

INTRACRANIAL INFECTIONS (ENCEPHALITIS, MENINGITIS MALARIA, TYPHOID FEVER)

CIRCULATORY DISORDERS THAT INTERFERE WITH OXYGEN SUPPLY TO BRAIN (CEREBRAL, ARTERIOSCLEROSIS, HEART ATTACK)

METABOLIC, ENDOCRINE AND NUTRITIONAL DISEASES (THYROTOXICOSIS, DIABETES, PELLAGRA)

ACUTE SYSTEMIC INFECTIONS WITH HIGH FEVER (PNEUMONIA, MONONUCLEOSIS, TB, HEPATITIS)

DRUG-RELATED SYMPTOMS (ASPIRIN, ACTH)

INTOXICATION (ALCOHOL, BAR-BITURATES, LEAD POISONING)

CHRONIC ILLNESSES OF ANY TYPE (ESPECIALLY IN GERIATRICS)

Understanding the function and impact our minds have on us is the concern of the mental health field. Health care professionals know that the mind can exert tremendous pressure on an individual and may in turn cause physiological disorders. Study of the mind has emerged in the last century as one of the fastest growing branches of medicine.

This section examines certain symptoms of emotionally and mentally disturbed patients and the possible treatments. Counseling and therapy have long been reliable sources; in recent years, however, interesting new drugs with powerful effects on the emotions such as anxiety, phobias, depression, and radical mood shifts have been developed.

The following is a list of the topics identified in this section:

ADDICTION Addiction is a state of periodic or chronic intoxication detrimental to the person and to society, produced by the repeated consumption of a drug, natural or synthetic. Its characteristics include an overpowering desire or need (compulsion) to continue taking the drug and to obtain it by any means; a tendency to increase the dose (tolerance); and a psychological and sometimes a physical dependence on the effects of the drug so that withdrawal of the drug is associated with anguishing symptoms and cravings.

Addiction always involves a state of physical and psychological dependence on some drug or chemical which a person comes to crave and cannot do without. The principal addiction-producing drugs are alcohol, morphine, heroin, crack, cocaine, the barbiturates, amphetamines, and other central nervous system depressants, including Valium®. Individuals may become psychologically dependent on hallucinogens and marijuana and its derivatives, but do not generally become physically dependent. There is considerable evidence that family dysfunction and relationships with peers who use drugs are important factors in escalating drug usage among adolescents. Drug abuse in adolescents is particularly problematic as important developmental tasks may not be accomplished and the teenager often develops few adaptive mechanisms to cope with stress —other than dissipating psychic pain through drug abuse.

ADLERIAN INDIVIDUAL PSYCHOLOGY Alfred Adler (1870-1937) was an early pupil of Sigmund Freud who broke away from his master's teachings to form his own school of individual psychology. Adler disagreed with Freud about the importance of sexual factors in neuroses and emphasized the study of ego-functioning. In his medical practice Adler had observed the remarkable ability of nature to compensate for losses of function. Adler developed the concept of the inferiority complex: feelings of negative self-regard which everyone experiences because of real or imagined inferiorities. Adler pointed out that persons with extreme feelings of inferiority may be severely handicapped in facing situations unless able to develop compensatory adjustments. Adler felt that a very important cause of inferiority feelings involves fears of castration or sexual impotence, called castration anxiety. (See also CASTRATION ANXIETY; FRIGIDITY, SEXUAL in this section.)

One of Adler's great contributions was his style-of-life theory, referring to each person's characteristic use of psychological mechanisms in developing a strategy for satisfying his personal needs. An example would be the pampered, spoiled style, in which an only child learns to control his environment by developing temper tantrums whenever thwarted. Adler gave marked attention to such situational factors in personality development as birth position in the family. He studied the special problems of the only child, the oldest child, the youngest child, and middle children, in relation to brother-and-sister rivalry and social development. It is now generally accepted that Adlerian Individual Psychology provides an important supplement to Freudian psychoanalytic theory.

ALCOHOLISM Modern psychiatry recognizes that alcoholism is just as much a disease as the common cold, and almost as common. Alcohol has always been one of man's antidotes for emotional stress and nervous tension.

Alcohol is one of the most potent and widely used drugs known to man. From ancient times, people have learned to distill grain in order to produce ethyl alcohol, which has a wide range of pharmacological effects. The ancients learned to use it as a pain killer, and it became widely used as an anesthetic. Until modern times, it was customary to perform amputations once a patient was completely intoxicated.

Even more potent is the ability of alcohol temporarily to reduce mental anguish, nervous tension, and anxiety. It is well known that mental stress increases in direct proportion to the ever-growing complexities of civilized life. Alcohol abuse may be understood as a means of coping with life stress, although the relief is temporary, since the abuse subsequently weakens the ability to cope, and feelings of tension, anxiety, or depression are heightened.

There is no single cause of alcoholism. Biomedical, psychological and social factors all play a role, and stressful events sometimes serve as catalysts for drinking behavior. Genetic factors are important and a family history of alcoholism is often found in the background of alcoholics.

Because of its anesthetic and initial anxiety-reducing effects, alcohol may quickly lead to dependence in genetically and psychologically vulnerable individuals. Most alcoholics initially drink quite innocently, at first in reasonable amounts at social gatherings or for periodic relief from feelings of nervous tension. Only gradually does there develop dependence on alcohol for the temporary relief of emotional distress.

The unfortunate fact is that increasing doses are required to produce these tension-relieving effects, so that the person has to drink larger and larger amounts, to the point that toxic effects begin to appear.

Recent research focuses on the predisposing genetic factors to alcoholism. Thus, some alcoholics are exceedingly sensitive to small amounts of alcohol which, while harmless to the non-alcoholic, may set the alcoholic off on a prolonged drinking spree. Each individual appears to have a characteristic threshold for development of toxic effects from heavy drinking. The heavy social drinker may become an alcoholic during times when increased amounts of alcohol are utilized to cope with emotional stress. When alcohol is taken in large amounts, it is a potent toxin. Alcohol is a depressant of the central nervous system and potentiates the effects of many other psychiatric drugs, including tranquilizers and sedatives.

Symptoms. In the typical pattern of developing alcoholism, a vicious cycle arises in which the alcoholic has to drink more in order to obtain temporary relief from anxiety and emotional distress. Some alcoholics develop a pattern of continuous drinking without adding food intake, so that serious nutritional and vitamin deficiencies may develop. The alcoholic typically denies his addiction to alcohol and shows no control in limiting his excesses.

Psychologically, alcoholism has many effects in common with other drug addictions. It interferes with many aspects of a person's life—causing deterioration in job performance, conflict and distress with spouses and children, progressive estrangement from other family members and friends, and deterioration in health. Sometimes the end result is the "skid row drunk" now deprived of all social and financial resources. As alcohol abuse progresses, there is often a subtle deterioration of personality as the alcoholic becomes progressively dependent upon the drug. The chronic alcoholic is gravely disabled but there is little hope for change until the individual openly acknowledges dependence upon alcohol.

Treatment. The first step in treatment is to recognize that alcoholism is a serious, relapsing disorder that typically causes depression, unemployment, and family dissolution, as well as being a symptom resulting from such events. Therapeutic approaches should be supportive, flexible, and non-judgmental. It will do no good to punish, criticize, or lecture the alcoholic for his misdeeds. The main goal of treatment is to repair the social and physical damage experienced by the alcoholic and to restore self-esteem through group membership and support that substitutes for dependency on alcohol.

Many alcoholics require hospitalization during the treatment process. Short-term hospitalization provides detoxification and medical stabilization. Drugs such as Antabuse may also be helpful in suppressing the urge to drink by providing painful reminders of its consequences. Alcoholics who drink while taking Antabuse become physically ill.

A critical treatment ingredient for alcoholism is to aid the alcoholic to feel less defensive, lonely, and rejected so that he or she can feel the acceptance and support of peer group membership. This principle accounts for much of the success of AA—Alcoholics Anonymous—in which the alcoholic is accepted unconditonally by other alcoholics who aid him through the difficult periods of relapse that characterize rehabilitation. For those alcoholics who can accept AA, the movement is a source of enormous help, group support, and acceptance. An initial step in the rehabilitation of an alcoholic often consists of taking him to an AA meeting and discovering whether he is able to accept the program and recognize his dependence on alcohol. Often an individual's acceptance of Alcoholics Anonymous takes considerable time. Many hospital treatment programs offer AA meetings on the hospital ward or maintain ties with AA programs in the surrounding community.

Other treatment interventions may be important. Family counseling is often needed to help family members cope with the stress of living with an alcoholic. Living with an alcoholic parent often takes a heavy toll upon children in the family who may have progressively assumed parental functions relinquished by the alcoholic. Groups like Al-Anon or Al-A-Teen provide support for the spouses and children who must cope with an alcoholic family member. Once an individual becomes dependent upon alcohol, psychotherapy alone is rarely helpful. Such treatment

approaches should be used in conjunction with other treatment modalities; i.e., Antabuse, AA attendance, family counseling, etc.

Finally, psychiatric experience teaches that before any alcoholic may be helped it is necessary for him to admit openly that he is an alcoholic and that alcohol is a poison for him. Sometimes alcoholics need to hit "rock bottom" before there is acceptance of the idea that the individual is physically and emotionally dependent upon alcohol. While some alcoholics recover and return to moderate social drinking, the vast majority must remain totally abstinent if they are to be rehabilitated.

AMBIVALENCE, EMOTIONAL Psychiatrically, ambivalence refers to the coexistence of opposed and contradictory emotions, attitudes or impulses directed toward a person or a situation. Ambivalence exerts important psychological effects both upon the person who expresses the ambivalent emotions and upon the person who is the object of the emotions themselves.

Ambivalence originates dynamically when a person has conflicting feelings or attitudes toward another. For example, a mother may alternatively display love and hatred toward her child, even to the point of feeling impulses to injure the child physically. The mother may not understand or appreciate the sources of her mixed emotions and may develop intense feelings of guilt, self-accusation, or inhibition in response. Psychiatric treatment is indicated in cases where a person develops intense ambivalence expressed by impulses to harm another person or to contemplate suicide because of powerful guilt feelings or the inability to integrate shifting feelings of love and anger toward important others. Psychiatric treatment of ambivalence is directed at helping the person to understand and accept the powerful and conflicting emotions and to develop more socially adaptive ways of expressing them.

In psychiatric terms, the person who is the object of such conflicting emotions is often confused and uncertain about the stability of relationships, feeling loved and valued when positive feelings are expressed, and rejected when anger suddenly erupts. A mother who simultaneously expresses love and hatred toward her child may confuse and frustrate the child who cannot know what is expected from him. The child often develops reactive feelings of guilt or confusion or may feel that he has done something bad or is unlikable, in an effort to understand the mother's puzzling reactions.

The best way to respond to ambivalent behavior on the part of another person is often to comment and describe the behavior and its accompanying confusing messages, rather than simply retaliating in kind.

AMNESIA   Amnesia is an inability to remember events occurring over a specific period of time. It accompanies a variety of organic brain disorders. These include the time intervals related to a convulsion or period of stupor or coma, a head injury, drug intoxication, dementias, severe chronic alcoholism, and other conditions.

ANGER AND AGGRESSION   Anger, fear, and love are the three instinctive emotions on which all affective life is based. The noted American psychologist John B. Watson showed that anger is expressed very early in life, as for instance if an infant's limbs are pinned down so that it cannot move. Such restriction instinctively stimulates a rage reaction: the child is thwarted and screams in anger.

Modern psychologists recognize the importance of anger in mental life in terms of the frustration-aggression-hostility theory. This hypothesis states that a person becomes frustrated (angry) whenever he is thwarted or blocked in life. Anger stimulates aggression toward the objects seen as being thwarting or frustrating, and thereby results in overt hostility.

The whole world is organized in terms of such opposites as hot-cold, life-death; and love and hate are opposite sides of the same coin. Every person should therefore expect to encounter his share of negative emotion both in himself and in others. All major social upheavals are inevitably associated with a great deal of frustration and anger expressed as hatred of those who are seen as thwarting or frustrating. Similarly we may expect underprivileged children and others to show a great amount of antisocial aggression in expressing their frustration.

Treatment.   Destructive and self-destructive expression of anger is an important sign of emotional distress in a child or an adult. Often, there may be accompanying problems in school, job performance or satisfying relationships with others and symptoms of some degree of antisocial behavior. Attention should be directed toward alleviating possible stress factors in the surrounding environment or within the family. When there is a history of long-standing, maladaptive expression of angry feelings or impulses, psychiatric evaluation and/or treatment is generally indicated.

ANOREXIA NERVOSA   This condition is a body image disorder involving significant weight loss, loss of appetite and endocrine changes. Occurring primarily in teenage girls, this disorder appears to operate symbolically to overcome feelings of helplessness associated with efforts to resolve personal and family problems.

Symptoms.   Anorexia nervosa is most common in young women who are fearful of growing up, enmeshed in overly involved family relationships, and cut off from their inner emotional life. Often the anorexic symptoms call attention to troubled and dysfunctional family circumstances. Adolescence appears to be a crucial developmental stage as the girl feels incapable of progressive emotional separation from the family. The girl becomes preoccupied with dieting and food fads, caloric intake may dramatically decline, the heart rate may slow, and menstruation ceases. Sometimes the patient may vomit after meals in an effort to maintain low body weight. (*See* BULIMIA in this section.) If the condition is left untreated, dramatic weight loss may follow, leading to progressive starvation, serious metabolic complications, even death.

Treatment.   Patient should receive psychiatric care as soon as self-induced starvation symptoms become apparent. Treatment should be directed at restoration of an appropriate body weight, correction of metabolic imbalances, and also involve psychiatric treatment directed toward uncovering both individual and family conflicts which perpetuate the disorder.

ANXIETY AND FEAR   Psychiatrists distinguish between fear, which is conscious, and anxiety, which is unconscious. The primitive cause of fear is withdrawal of support or security. All emotions have both psychological and physiological components. Under the stress of modern living, every person to some degree experiences reactions of fear and insecurity which may assume neurotic proportions; that is, reactions which are actually incapacitating.

Fear and anxiety reactions may be observed at all periods of life. Psychoanalytic evidence indicates that many infants begin to develop anxiety reactions as early as the first weeks of life if they are not fed and handled properly. The neurotic infant manifests anxiety by finicky eating habits, irregular bowel habits, sleep disorders, crying, and general irritability.

Many factors in early infancy and childhood can stimulate anxiety reactions. Anything which threatens the child's physical or emotional security tends to stimulate fear reactions revealed by a wide variety of behavior problems, including bed-wetting, eating and sleeping disorders, lying, stealing, masturbation, nervousness, and other symptoms of anxiety. In adults, symptoms may be even more diversified, it being widely understood among psychiatrists that anxiety states interfere with normal functioning of all the systems of the body.

Anxiety reactions are the commonest form of psychoneurotic states, almost as frequently met with in the general population as the common cold. Almost every person shows some degree of anxiety, and it has been estimated that at least twenty million people in the United States are more or less incapacitated by neurotic anxiety reactions. The commonest pattern of neurotic anxiety reactions is the anxiety tension state.

Symptoms. Among the common symptoms of the anxiety state are overall feelings of weakness, tension, and nervousness; band-like headache; muscular pain in the back of the neck; dryness of the mouth and difficulties in swallowing food, as though there were a lump in the throat; irregular "sighing" respiration, as though the individual could not take a deep breath; fast and irregular pulse (often with dropped heart beats and a feeling of faintness); cramps and "butterfly" feelings in the stomach; diarrhea or constipation, of-

ten with abdominal discomfort; menstrual irregularities; and feelings of generalized tension and shakiness throughout the body. The sufferer will often complain of peculiar, bizarre sensations, such as knife-like pains in the head, twitching of muscles of the scalp or face, crawling sensations underneath the skin, and atypical pains and aches. These symptoms vary widely from patient to patient, with no standard pattern, and with emotional instability as the only common element.

Where anxiety and fear become extreme, the symptoms become exaggerated in what is known as a panic reaction—an extreme state of anxiety in which the person feels that some terrible thing is about to happen. There are very frightening body sensations suggesting imminent death or insanity. Such panic states may occur in the form of horrible nightmares, in which the person dreams that some terrible tragedy is occurring. Patients commonly complain: "I feel I'm going to die. I feel I'm choking to death. My heart is pounding terribly. I have a feeling of impending doom, as if something terrible is going to happen to me."

Treatment. It is extremely important to recognize anxiety states as psychological reactions, which should be treated by a psychiatrist. A common diagnostic error consists in mistaking some of the physical signs of emotional upset for symptoms of organic disease.

Since the average patient is convinced of a physical cause for his symptoms, the first step in treatment is to teach the patient that emotional upsets can produce bodily disorders. The patient is taught to trace back to what caused the upset and so gain an understanding of the true causes of his trouble. A further part of treatment consists of training the patient to accept and cope with inevitable feelings of anxiety. No one can live completely anxiety-free, so it is necessary to teach children how to cope with inevitable, transient feelings of insecurity and inadequacy—through verbal communication of their feelings and turning to adults for support and guidance.

APHONIA   This form of aphasia is marked by loss of speech function. It may be organic in origin but often occurs as a phenomenon of conversion hysteria (a form of psychoneurosis), particularly when the conscious stimulus is a frightening one. In this instance, it is assumed that the speechlessness is a reaction to an unconscious emotional conflict.

Treatment. In the absence of organic factors, immediate restoration of speech can be obtained through hypnosis. However, this is not a "cure"; to avoid repetition of hysterical aphonic attacks or equivalent neurotic reactions, psychotherapy must be instituted.

ART THERAPY This is a form of occupational therapy in which patients are encouraged to express themselves through all kinds of artistic projects. Psychiatrists have discovered that patients should be encouraged to participate in a full program of work and recreational activities, as a means of encouraging social relationships and as a source of self-esteem. Artistic activities have great psychological value because many patients are able to express in their artwork hidden emotional conflicts or feelings, not otherwise revealed through verbal communication. Frequently the patient reveals his mood through the selection of colors to use in his drawings or paintings and may also express the content of his psychological problems in the artistic productions themselves. Psychiatrists may gain further understanding of an individual psychological problem by review and study of the patient's artistic efforts.

Art therapy is an important part of the rehabilitation programs of mental hospitals to encourage patients to be active, to decrease morbid self-preoccupation, and to develop new interests or hobbies. It is often a useful adjunct in treatment, particularly with individuals who have difficulty with verbal communication of feelings and thoughts.

AUTISM, INFANTILE Autism refers to phantasy thinking such as occurs in daydreaming. Freud early pointed out that most autistic thinking is wish-fulfilling, the person imagining pleasant events which do not ordinarily occur in real life. Daydreaming is a normal phenomenon during all periods of life and particularly in childhood when the child imagines all kinds of things which he could not realistically accomplish.

Autistic thinking and excessive daydreaming become abnormal when used to escape from real life and avoid unpleasant tasks. Withdrawal into autistic thinking may occur in children whose real-life situations are so unhappy or conflict-filled that the child seeks pleasure in daydreaming. Some authorities believe that excessive daydreaming may be an early symptom of schizophrenia, in which the person literally withdraws from an intolerable reality into a more satisfying world of make-believe. Diagnosis of schizophrenia, however, cannot be made on the basis of this symptom alone, because many gifted people spend long periods in daydreaming that may be completely normal. Daydreaming becomes abnormal in direct proportion to its delusional and completely unrealistic nature.

Infantile autism refers to a discrete psychiatric syndrome. Its essential features include a lack of responsiveness to others, gross impairment in communication skills, resistance to any change in the environment, and preoccupation with inanimate objects. These broad impairments become evident before 30 months of age.

AUTOEROTICISM According to the sex psychologists autoeroticism (rather than masturbation), is the preferred term to describe a normally secret practice. It can be defined as the practice of friction or vibration of erogenous areas (mostly the penis or clitoris) to produce pleasurable sensations. In older people, autoeroticism goes beyond this to an imitation of the sex act; but such is not often the case in very young children or even in adolescents. The practice is mainly carried out for the physical pleasure it generates. (*See also* MASTURBATION in this section.)

BEDWETTING (ENURESIS) Psychiatric theories that attempt to explain bedwetting view enuresis as a response to stress, particularly if the child has previously achieved bladder control. The focus is upon such stressful events as entry to school, birth of a sibling, or other sources of emotional stress or anxiety that affect the child. Many children experience reactive feelings of shame, embarrassment or self-consciousness as a result of bedwetting. While it is true that some emotionally disturbed children wet the bed, most enuretic children are not emotionally disturbed. Almost all children will eventually outgrow their enuresis.

Physiological causes for enuresis can be discovered by means of laboratory tests. Kidney or bladder disease may be uncovered by routine urinalysis or urine culture and (if necessary) by kidney X-rays. Sometimes an obstruction where the bladder joins the urethra may cause uncontrollable dripping during daytime and at night. If it is determined that the child has no problems holding urine and emptying the bladder while awake, then structural malformities or infectious diseases can usually be eliminated as causes.

For the chronic bedwetter, the best of all medicines is parental love and patience. Harsh punishments and ridicule always make the problem much worse. Parents should understand that the condition usually corrects itself over time, and that patience and a calm response are called for. Amitryptiline, an antidepressant drug, is often quite useful as part of the treatment program. (*See also* BEDWETTING [ENURESIS] in the section INFANT AND CHILD CARE.)

BULIMIA Recurrent binges of overeating characterize this condition though it may coexist with or alternate with anorexia nervosa. A particularly severe form, bulimia nervosa, is characterized by feelings of loss of control of overeating with attempted control by self-induced vomiting, the taking of laxatives and/ or diuretics. Alteration of bulimic episodes and rigid dieting may also occur.

Symptoms. In well-established bulimics, abrasive scarring of the knuckles from the dental trauma of the induced vomiting and erosion of the enamel of the inner surfaces of the teeth from the acidic gastric contents may be noted. The binging and vomiting often occur in secret and may go on without being suspected. Weakness and disturbances of the blood salts may be a tipoff to the disorder; both occur when the potassium or chloride content of the blood diminish too much. Weight may fluctuate up and down to an unusual degree, though the threat to the body which is seen in severe anorexia does not generally occur.

Treatment. It is generally apparent with most cases that some form of psychotherapy or counseling is needed. In severe cases hospitalization may be advised. A number of anorexia-bulimia or eating disorders clinics have sprung up over recent years to which a referral can be made. Antidepressants may be of value.

CASTRATION ANXIETY According to Alfred Adler, the primary cause for inferiority complexes in men was fear of sexual impotence or castration. Adler also believed that many young girls developed feelings of insecurity upon discovering sex differences in the external genitals. The term often refers to fears of deprivation or loss of power in either sex, or to the consequences of humiliating domination and retaliation by a more powerful person. Such fears sometimes occur in boys who are struggling with feelings and impulses related to the Oedipus complex. (*See* OEDIPUS COMPLEX in this section.)

Psychiatric studies show that among some impaired parents or caretakers, it may be common to punish a child, particularly a boy, by threatening to cut off or injure the external genitals. Children who have been so threatened are understandably likely to develop castration anxiety. As it is important for all children to feel positive and secure about their sexual identity and role, any threat of castration or injury is very threatening and a potential source of emotional conflict in later life. Therefore, punishment of a child should never be accompanied by threats, humorous or otherwise, to cut off or injure the genitals.

CLAUSTROPHOBIA Claustrophobia is defined as pathological fear of closed places. The claustrophobe experiences extreme fear and apprehension when required to enter a closed space—such as a closet, subway car, or elevator—from which there is no easy escape. Claustrophobia is not a disorder in itself, but rather a symptom of underlying unconscious conflict which may require psychoanalytic treatment to uncover. A claustrophobe should be discouraged from paying too much attention to the symptom, and induced to seek psychiatric help to discover its unconscious cause.

Many cases of claustrophobia are caused by childhood conditioning in which the child was inadvertently confined in a closed space. Such experiences may stimulate great anxiety and continue to produce symptoms for years. In other cases, claustrophobia may develop when the child observes an older person behaving hysterically in a closed place.

COMPULSIONS A compulsion is an irresistible impulse to repeat some senseless activity. Compulsions are not disorders in themselves, but only symptoms of underlying unconscious complexes. Almost all normal people are mildly compulsive in performance of such senseless acts as avoidance of cracks in the sidewalk, repeated return to the house to check the doors, or irrational and repetitive carrying-out of rituals. A classic example is the washing compulsion: the impulse to wash an inordinate number of times a day.

Psychoanalytic theory states that compulsive behavior is usually determined by an overly strict superego (conscience). The compulsive act is interpreted as a symbolic defense against some forbidden impulse; for example, in the washing compulsion it is interpreted that the person probably feels very guilty about some fancied misbehavior and is symbolically cleansing himself by endless washing. Compulsions become pathological when their performance seriously interferes with routine duties in life. There are a variety of treatments for severe compulsions including medication, behavior therapy, and psychotherapy.

CONDUCT DISORDERS As a result of studies in child psychiatry, it is now acknowledged that many children develop transient disturbances of conduct—lying, stealing, deceit, fighting, destructiveness, truancy, running away, cheating, and so on—in the course of normal development. Such disorders are not regarded as serious the first time they occur, as it is recognized that most children learn from experience, learn more adaptive ways of expressing their impulses, and pass through periods of instability as normal phases of development. Children tend to experiment with a number of social and asocial behaviors to discover the limits of what society and, in particular, what their family will tolerate. If the child is firmly and appropriately punished, required to make reparation where indicated, he soon learns to adapt to social limits and

accepts the values that the parents seek to transmit.

Symptoms. Habitual conduct disorders, repeated in spite of increasingly firm social limits, are regarded psychiatrically as evidence of both disturbed personality development and family dysfunction. Repeated lying, cheating, stealing, or running away are usually symptoms of significant emotional disturbance, and tend to persist until the child's needs for love, protection and firm limits are met and dysfunctional family patterns are altered. Fighting, cruelty, and undesirable aggressiveness are often symptomatic of underlying feelings of deprivation in the child, or may reflect the child's maladaptive identification with family members who are themselves aggressive and punitive.

Treatment. Where a child continues to demonstrate conduct disorders in spite of normal corrective influences, underlying psychological difficulties should be suspected and the child and family referred to a clinic for psychiatric evaluation. Experience indicates that symptoms of conduct disorder are not improved by endless punishment, no matter how severe, and may indeed make matters worse if parental punitiveness or rejection has a role in the child's disturbed behavior. In such instances, family counseling, as well as individual help with the child, is often indicated.

CONFLICT, MENTAL Modern psychiatry believes that some form of mental conflict underlies most functional (non-organic) mental disorders. The conflict may be between emotions, ideas, impulses, or any combination of these. In order to be mentally healthy, a person should be self-consistent and integrated in all the departments of his life. Conflict results in a house divided against itself, with the resultant toll of inefficiency and maladjustment, as the person struggles to resolve the inconsistent forces within himself.

This leads to an important rule for mental health, namely, that each person should strive to be self-consistent with what he considers to be the highest truths and the greatest good. Faced with many conflicting alternatives in life, every person must decide what is best for himself and strive to be consistent with this. Peace of mind depends largely on freedom from guilt, anxiety, and conflict. Antisocial behavior usually is simply not worth the cost which it entails in the form of anxiety and guilt.

It is now generally recognized that unconscious mental conflict underlies many functional psychiatric disorders, particularly the neuroses. A frequent cause of unconscious conflict is socially unacceptable impulses which are repressed from consciousness, only to appear in symptom formation; unexpressed hate toward a parent, for example, may cause psychosomatic symptoms of headache or high blood pressure. It usually requires psychoanalytic treatment to discover the underlying conflicts.

CONVERSION REACTION

A classical form of psychoneurotic disorder is that of conversion hysteria. In psychoanalytic terms, the symptoms of hysteria are interpreted as being converted from original socially unacceptable impulses into more socially accepted overt symptoms: physical (or somatic) symptoms which, on the surface, appear unrelated to their true cause. Neurotic hysterical symptoms are capable of imitating almost every known physical and mental symptom. Thus, hysterical vomiting during pregnancy may be interpreted as a symbolic rejection of pregnancy, while "phantom pregnancy" (pseudocyesis) may mimic symptoms of pregnancy even though conception has not taken place. Conversion reactions are very common in wartime, when fearful soldiers have high unconscious motivation to escape from military service by developing hysterical blindness, deafness, loss of sensation, or paralysis. In each of these conditions, high levels of emotional conflict express themselves in terms of symptoms of physical disease. Conversion reactions are best tested by psychoanalytic methods in the hands of a competent psychiatrist.

DEFENSE MECHANISMS

Every person develops a distinctive personal style of life, involving strategies for securing pleasure or goals and avoiding pain. The famous psychiatrist Sigmund Freud invented the concept of defense mechanisms to describe a variety of behavior patterns which people use unconsciously to avoid conflict. In general, the purpose of a defense mechanism is to defend the ego from critical attacks by others. A typical defense mechanism is escape, whereby a person avoids everything unpleasant; for example, a young girl who is afraid of speaking in public may, for instance, claim illness as an escape mechanism. The very insecure spend so much time escaping the things they fear that they accomplish little in life. Psychiatrists believe that the best defense is not to try to conceal fears, but to admit them frankly and learn how to cope with them.

DELIRIUM TREMENS

Delirium tremens is a clinical disorder producing an acute psychosis associated with marked tremors. It is usually associated with abstinence for a few days after prolonged excessive alcohol intake, but it may also appear during the course of other types of brain disorder. In rare cases this clinical picture may be associated with acute inflammatory disorder of the brain or with severe vascular disease of the brain.

Symptoms. Delirium is manifested by hallucinations together with extreme restlessness and hyperactivity. The patient may be dangerous to himself and to others. Marked tremors involving the face, tongue, arms, and legs occur. Characteristic visual hallucinations include animals (such as snakes and rats), peculiar faces, and similar images which the patient may freely describe during the acute state. There may also be auditory hallucinations of voices which usually defame the individual. The patient appears extremely fearful during periods of active hallucination. Convulsions frequently occur and memory is defective. Liver disease and involvement of the brainstem and peripheral nerves may be associated with this disorder.

Treatment. Hospital care is essential. Sedative drugs are used to calm the marked restlessness and overactivity. If the patient is extremely hyperactive, restraints are necessary until adequate sedation can be obtained. Due to the patient's lack of cooperation, it is usually necessary to give medication by injection until the delirium has been brought under control. Intravenous fluids are required to prevent dehydration. Subsequently, adequate caloric intake and supplementary vitamins are important to maintain nutrition.

After recovery from delirium tremens, appropriate treatment for the underlying alcohol dependence should be initiated.

DEPRESSION   Depression is an abnormal mental state characterized by severe feelings of melancholy, worthlessness, sadness, self-depreciation, and self-hate. Everyone has normal moodswings ranging from excitement at one extreme to depression at the other extreme. In a normal person these moodswings are usually of mild degree, oscillating between mild exhilaration and mild depression or melancholy. Such cycles of emotionality are entirely normal. Under certain conditions, however, they become abnormally exaggerated, resulting in pathological excitement and depression.

Symptoms. The depressed person feels that everything has gone wrong in the world. He tends to lose interest in life, nothing appeals to him any more, and he derives no enjoyment from normal things; instead, he tends to brood about all the evil in the world, particularly his own sins and shortcomings. Many depressed people cry constantly and express feelings of worthlessness and self-hate.

There are two important patterns of depression: reactive and endogenous. In reactive depressions, mood-disturbance is to some degree proportionate to some real event in the person's life. A widow may become depressed following the death of her husband, and in this case there is a valid reason for her reaction. Reactive depressions are relatively hopeful as to outcome and usually disappear within a matter of months, irrespective of treatment.

Endogenous depressions are apparently due to physical disorders of the brain centers controlling emotions. They tend to appear insidiously without any obvious cause. Psychoanalysts believe that some endogenous depressions may involve unconscious reactions of self-hate, in which the person is punishing himself for something very evil which he thinks he has done. Whatever the cause, endogenous depressions tend to show a pattern of increasing melancholy and depression until, at their height, the depressed person may feel that all is hopeless and suicide the only solution. At this point the person may lose interest even in eating and have to be force-fed.

Some depressed patients show a large hysterical component manifested by crying, agitation, and overt displays of anguish. This behavior represents an unconscious bid for sympathy and help from observers. Unfortunately, reassurance or solace does little good for those in an agitated state, since their verbalizations are largely irrational and unanswerable.

Treatment. All seriously depressed persons should be admitted immediately to a psychiatric hospital because of the ever-present danger of suicide. It is safest to consider the seriously depressed as potentially suicidal, to be kept hospitalized as long as any depressive trends remain. One of the worst mistakes is to accept reassurances on the part of a depressed person that he or she is not contemplating suicide.

Depressive states are often treatable through a variety of psychiatric interventions. While many cases of mild to moderate depression spontaneously recover within six or eight months, it is generally appropriate to institute psychotherapy and consider use of antidepressant medication. In severe depressive states, psychotherapy is generally not helpful as an initial intervention. Antidepressant medication is generally prescribed, and if not successful, a course of electroconvulsive therapy is indicated. With patients who seem to have a very high risk of suicide, electroconvulsive therapy (ECT) may be the treatment of first choice. The use of antidepressant drugs and/or ECT results in a very high percentage of remission of depressive symptoms, so the patient becomes more amenable to psychotherapy directed toward resolving underlying conflicts and stresses: guilt, feelings of worthlessness, unexpressed anger and relationship problems.

A competent psychiatrist should always be consulted concerning the seriousness of suicidal threats, which should never be dismissed as attention-getting devices or attempts to manipulate. Any severely depressed person is potentially suicidal and ironically may become more suicidal as the depression initially lifts, so that every effort must be made for the patient's safety.

EATING PROBLEMS IN CHILDREN
Problems with food usually develop because of insufficient knowledge on the parent's part, or because of emotional tensions that are brought to the table. The most common complaint is that the child (usually aged two to four years) will not eat.

It is possible that the "non-eating" child is sick or anemic and needs medicine or a tonic; in most cases, however, difficulties stem from the fact that the parent's idea of what the child should eat and the child's idea of what he will eat are two different things. The parent is used to the big appetite that the child had when he was four months old (and gaining two to three pounds in a month), but the child is now growing—and eating—less.

Treatment. If the child is healthy, happy, and up-and-around, he is obviously not starving. The best way to feed the two-to-four-year-old is to put small amounts of food (amounts he will be sure to eat) in front of him on a saucer; then if he wants more, he will ask for it. This is a far better situation than having the parent continually pleading with the child to eat.

The types of foods are important. In infancy milk was the baby's most important food. After one year of age it is probably the least important and, like all white foods, is merely a "bonus" of extra calories after the basic meat and fruit (vegetables if the child wants them) are consumed.

Too many parents have been falsely led to believe that if the child at least drinks his milk he will be all right, even if nothing else is eaten. This is a fallacy. Milk lacks iron, is often highly constipating, and some people are allergic to it, suffering embarrassing amounts of gas and stomach cramps. This is not to say milk should be neglected or avoided, however. Since it is a major source of calcium, it should unquestionably be part of the diet of all children.

Children in the two-to-four group do not chew easily, so they are apt to prefer ground meat. Frankfurters, hamburgers, and soft-cooked chicken are often the only foods that small children will eat willingly. Fruits and vegetables have the same nutritional elements in them, and are therefore quite interchangeable. Bread and dairy products round out the diet. Since vitamins are found in all these foods, supplements are not usually necessary.

Although a child can be taught most of the good and bad eating habits of the parents, there is very little truth to the rule that if the parents like or dislike a specific food, the child will also dislike or like it. It is simply not so. The best rule is keep mealtimes simple and keep them pleasant.

ELECTRA COMPLEX Sigmund Freud defined the Electra complex as an unhealthy emotional attachment of a daughter toward her father, in which the daughter was unable to adjust to men of her own age because of a morbid attachment to the father. According to psychoanalytic theory, each young girl's ideal conception of the opposite sex is based on the relationship with her father. Normally, she is able to break away from her over-idealized father-image and make a normal adjustment to some younger man; when the father fixation is unduly strong, however, the girl may never be able to break away from her father's influence, thus making satisfactory adjustment to a man of her own age impossible. Fathers would be wise to discourage undue dependence by daughters, who should be encouraged to make their own decisions in becoming acquainted with young men of their own age.

EMOTIONS Feelings and emotions constitute the affective life of a person and together are regarded as one of the major components of psychic life, the others being cognition and volition. Feelings and emotions are biologically more primitive than intellect, appearing earlier, both in the history of the race and the development of a person.

The basic feelings are pleasure-pain, excitement-relaxation, and like-dislike. Feelings and emotions may be understood as primitive evaluatory reactions which underlie intuition. The basic emotions are fear, anger, and love. All emotions involve a fusion of physiological and psychological components, and are true psychosomatic reactions. Every emotion involves not only a mental state, but also a physiological pattern; both are integrated and coordinated in a unified emotional experience.

In order to understand each emotion, it is necessary to understand not only the primitive, instinctive, conscious component, but also the physical changes occurring simultaneously. When one is angry, the heart beats faster, blood pressure goes up, blood is rapidly distributed to the body musculature, the face becomes flushed, and the adrenal glands pour extra adrenalin into the bloodstream—all these changes being physical preparation for fighting. Anger is thus a biologic emergency-state. If one becomes angry often enough, he may remain in a constant state of biologic preparedness, associated with high blood pressure (hypertension) and other unhealthy circulatory changes.

In contrast, fear is associated with an entirely different pattern of physical changes. A person may suddenly become pale, start to tremble and shake, feel general weakness, and even empty bladder and bowels involuntarily. There may be feelings of dizziness, fast or irregular pulse, abdominal faintness or quivering, and generalized muscular trembling. In chronic neurotic states, these fear symptoms may persist indefinitely, to the point of disabling the person.

Under the influence of love, a person feels happy and at ease. He may experience feelings of pleasurable excitement and tension, but ordinarily these do not interfere with his work. The person in love tends to be friendly, uncritical, and at peace with the world. His vital functions proceed normally and harmoniously.

The negative emotions of fear and anger are associated with disruptive physiological changes which can seriously interfere with healthy living. It is desirable to have a healthy and active emotional life, but excessive emotionalism almost inevitably results in a wide variety of psychosomatic symptoms and physiological disorders both in the person himself and in those who must react to him. The term neurotic refers to nonorganic disorders of emotional origin, and upset emotions are found in all neurotic disorders. Emotions provide the powerhouse of mental life and are healthy as long as they are kept under control, but they can be associated with all kinds of symptom formations if they get out of control. It is therefore important for the individual to understand what his emotions are and, also, how to control and modify them appropriately.

EMOTIONS IN ALLERGY Emotional disturbances can influence the course of an allergic disorder and, conversely, allergic problems can cause emotional disturbances. There are, however, only a few allergic-type diseases in which emotional problems are a true cause of the disorder (psychogenic urticaria, some cases of migraine headaches, and pseudoallergy). In general, psychosomatic states are a secondary factor, as emotional upsets will intensify and even trigger an allergic attack.

Psychological problems frequently arise where chronic allergic states are involved. For instance, there are overprotective parents who go to extremes in taking care of an allergic child with asthma or eczema. In this situation the family life revolves entirely around a self-centered, selfish child. The rest of the family become irritable and unhappy. The suddenness of asthmatic attacks keeps both the family and the sick person continually worried and anxious, and fear of suffocating often converts a mild asthmatic attack into a severe one.

Fully as bad as the overprotective parent is the direct opposite: the indifferent careless parent who neglects the basic cares of an allergic offspring. This rejection leads to severe psychological problems.

At school, teachers must contend with the sniffing, itching, coughing, restless, overactive, sensitive, and chronically ill child. Their reactions to the allergic child will in part affect the child's emotional response to his illness.

Persons with allergic rhinitis, with their constant noisy breathing and sniffing, constitute an annoyance to the people around them. This soon becomes obvious to afflicted individuals, who then tend to avoid human contact and keep to themselves.

Individuals with atopic dermatitis who are constantly scratching and reveal an unattractive eczema also avoid public exposure and try to lead a solitary, self-pitying type of existence. The emotional status of such people is affected by discomfort, sleeplessness, disfigurement, and the chronic quality of their skin disorders.

Allergic headaches may be accompanied by mental symptoms (confusion and personality changes) due to edema of the brain. Some migraine headaches of non-allergic origin are psychogenic; individuals suffering from these are usually perfectionists, tense, and have very rigid personalities.

There is a true allergy of the nervous system with such symptoms as overactivity, restlessness, clumsiness, irritability, insomnia, sluggishness or depression, unusual behavior, inability to concentrate and nervous tics or paleness, dark circles under the eyes, stuffy nose, swollen eyelids, excessive saliva, heavy sweating, abdominal pains, headaches, and bedwetting. Before considering allergy, a physician should rule out all other possible causes when confronted with such an array of symptoms.

Certain cases of chronic hives (psychogenic urticaria) occur as a response to emotional conflict. These are most common in middle-aged women and older children. The wheals usually develop with a burning sensation.

When a person escapes reality and responsibilities by laying the blame for an unpleasant situation onto an allergy, he is said to have a pseudoallergy. This type of individual can have all the classic symptoms of any truly allergic disorder.

Emotional disturbances may be symptoms of treatment-reaction, since such states as drowsiness, irrational behavior, hysteria, confusion, impotence, and nervous movements can be caused by the medications being used in treating the allergic patient. (*See also* the section ALLERGIC CONDITIONS.)

EXISTENTIAL PSYCHIATRY   This is a recent movement in psychiatry, involving application of forms of existentialism to problems of mental illness. Existentialism is concerned with the meanings of being and living. Psychiatrists are treating increasingly large numbers of patients who complain of a newly-recognized pattern which existential psychiatrists call the noögenic neurosis: doubts that life has any meaning, and despair about existence in general. A leading existential psychiatrist attributes this condition to an existential vacuum, caused by Man's loss of primitive security-in-instinct and loss of certain traditional values of the kind which governed life in earlier times. Modern man has lost his traditional belief in religion and established authority and has found nothing

to replace them, so that he is left bankrupt, in a spiritual vacuum. Existentialism is concerned with the search for life meanings and reasons for being. When faced with patients who complain that life no longer seems to have meaning, the existential psychiatrist attempts to teach more solid values to live by.

A major concern of existential psychiatrists is self-actualization, or helping the patient to become what he can become. Many persons become thwarted and feel stalemated by internal and external factors which block personal growth. (Psychologists believe that there are many psychic conflicts which can act as blocks and that personal growth tends to resume if negative factors are removed.) An important part of the problem consists in helping people to see themselves more positively and hopefully, so that their lives open up in new directions. Anything which stimulates positive growth resources tends to result in genuine self-actualization.

EXTROVERSION—INTROVERSION
The famous Austrian psychologist Carl G. Jung was the first to construct a psychological scheme based upon the outgoing or inward-looking nature of a person's whole approach to life. Extroversion is defined as the trait of being basically outgoing, interested in the outer world, and liking others. Introversion involves an inward-looking, sensitive, withdrawn, shy approach to life. At first it was believed the two types represented opposite and distinct forms of personality; later research has shown that pure forms of either are rare. Most people represent a balance of outgoing and introverted traits. An individual may be extroverted in social situations in which he feels at ease and introverted where he feels insecure. Except in extreme degrees, introversion and extroversion are both normal traits, apparently determined by inherited or constitutional factors.

The extremely introverted child may have some difficulty adjusting socially, because of shyness and self-consciousness. It does no good to force such a child to socialize; this may make the child more anxious and insecure. Best is the application of gentle but firm pressure on the child to relate to other children, providing opportunities for easy social relationships, yet not making the child feel conspicuous by calling attention to his shyness.

It should be clearly understood that both extroverts and introverts can succeed well in life, each in his own way. Much harm can be done by trying to force a child to be something he is not. The extroverted child usually has an easier time developing socially because of his outgoing interest in other people, but most introverts are able to make compensatory adjustments for getting ahead socially. This is a problem which each child must be allowed to work out in his own way.

FIXATION, DEVELOPMENTAL Studies have shown that young people normally pass through a series of developmental stages in more or less orderly patterns. The child's sex interests, for example, are first directed towards sensations from his or her own body (autoeroticism), then toward experiences with the same sex (homoeroticism), and finally (after puberty) towards relationships with the opposite sex. Freud was first to emphasize that developmental fixations may occur in which the person becomes "frozen" on one level, failing to mature towards higher levels. Developmental fixation has been suggested as one cause of homosexuality, the child becoming fixated on objects of the same sex, and failing to develop normal opposite-sex interests. Similarly, fixations may occur in eating or elimination habits, so that the person fails to mature beyond infantile levels because of emotional conflicts. Many adults show arrested emotional maturation caused by childhood fixations which impeded normal development.

FREUD, SIGMUND Freud is recognized as one of the major influence on developments in modern psychological and psychiatric science. Born in 1856, he studied medicine and showed an early interest in neurological and psychological disorders. While still studying in Paris under Charcot, he made the startling observation that seemingly physical disorders might be caused by psychological conflicts. Freud's greatest contribution was his theory of an unconscious mental life, in which ideas or impulses incompatible with the conscience (superego) are thrust back (repressed) into the unconscious—from which they can gain expression only in disguised form, such as for-

mation of symptoms, humor, or mistakes.

Before Freud, no attempt had been made to comprehend the symbolic meanings of the (apparently) incoherent and irrational ravings of the mentally disordered. Freud was the first to attempt to differentiate between the manifest and latent meanings of behavior. (Manifest signifies the obvious or apparent meaning of behavior, latent referring to its unconscious significance.) He first discovered the possible significance of latent meanings in his study of dreams, where he was able to show that—though apparently meaningless—dreams might actually be interpreted in terms of unconscious complexes. Freud applied this same method to the understanding of latent or unconscious motivation in many other types of psychological phenomena: neurotic symptoms, origins of wit and humor, and the small distresses (psychopathology) of everyday life.

Early in his investigations, Freud became convinced that unconscious sex-conflicts were a major factor in causing mental disorders. His development of the theory of psychoanalysis involved intensive study of the various stages of psychosexual development through which everyone passes. He gave special emphasis to disorders resulting from unhealthy resolutions of the Oedipus complex, which involves unconscious love of the male child for his mother (with corresponding hostility towards the father), or, conversely, the Electra complex if the child is a girl.

Psychoanalysis may be seen as an attempt to understand the psychology of unconscious complexes and their symbolic representations. An important offshoot of psychoanalysis has been the development of projective psychologies, which involve methods for discovering the unconscious significance of obvious behavior. Freud's greatest contribution was perhaps his insistence on understanding and studying the emotional-impulsive determiners of mental life. Though Freud died in 1939, many years of intensive research will be needed to determine the validity of many of his theories.

One of Freud's major contributions was his invention of an entirely new school of psychology: the topological psychology of the unconscious. This theory pictures mental life as dominated by the dynamic conflict of powerful forces, both instinctive and acquired. Freud termed the innate, instinctive, unlearned drives and energies the id—conceived to include socially unacceptable expressions of sex, hate, life- and death-instincts. Opposing the forces of the id (instinct), Freud postulated the ego (the "I"), incorporating all the training imposed by society. That part of the ego involving concepts of right-and-wrong was designated by Freud as the superego (the censor or conscience).

Freud postulated continuous conflict between the forces of the id seeking expression, and repressive control exerted by the superego. He explained certain mental disorders as occurring when the superego was no longer strong enough to repress impulses from the id, the imbalance gaining expression through symptom-formation. "Psychoanalysis" comprises methods devised by Freud for the investigation of unconscious conflict, and the bringing of them into consciousness under conditions where they can effectively be controlled and turned into socially acceptable channels. The general validity of the Freudian theory of the unconscious has now gained wide acceptance, though specific applications have not been proved scientific'

A cogent criticism of Freudian theory is that it places too much emphasis on the problems of psychosexual development to the exclusion of other factors known to influence behavior. Though psychosexual aberrations may underlie some types of mental disorder, these are only one of many potential causes. Historical evidence indicates that Freud was self-critical, modest, and self-effacing. He would have been the first to admit the limitations of his theories. Much of the controversy and criticism of psychoanalysis in recent years has arisen from efforts of his disciples to create an authoritarian and dogmatic psychoanalytic cult.

Even if many Freudian theories are eventually proved to be invalid, Freud's contribution will be that his discoveries opened up entire new areas for scientific investigation and forced a complete reappraisal of earlier theories.

FRIGIDITY, SEXUAL Sexual frigidity—indifference or aversion to sexual relations—among women is a complex psychiatric problem, and its many causes require inten-

sive study. There are large innate differences in sexual excitability which exist on a constitutional basis. Studies in both lower animals and man have shown wide individual differences in sex drive; some cases of apparent frigidity may therefore be understood simply in terms of constitutional lack of sex drive.

Psychoanalytical theory, however, stresses the presence of emotional conflict and ambivalence as the major factor in most nonorganic frigidity. Of the three primitive emotions of fear, anger, and (sexual) love, fear and anger are biologically overriding because of their survival-value; they thus tend to inhibit the sex drive. Strong fear or strong anger, therefore, typically inhibit sexuality, so that sexual frigidity may occur in any situation where emotions of fear or anger predominate. This means that for optimum sex performance a woman should be free of internal conflict, anger, or fear.

Psychological studies universally indicate that sex behavior in human beings is learned, not instinctive. Adult performance is largely determined by sexual experience in early life. Where the child has been conditioned by unpleasant, frightening, or painful experiences with sex, frigidity may occur in later life. Psychoanalytic studies place special emphasis on sexual trauma (shocking experience) in which the child has been conditioned to respond to sex in unhealthy patterns. The victim of rape or sexual attack, for example, may subsequently show neurotic aversion to sex experiences.

Much also depends on early sex-attitudes. Many young girls are taught by older women that men are brutes, that sex is disgusting, and that menstruation and childbearing are curses which must be (unwillingly) borne. Such teachings tend to produce fear and revulsion concerning sex later in life. It is far more healthy for mothers to teach young girls that love can be beautiful; that men and women naturally complement each other; that menstruation is to be welcomed as an event indicating preparation for motherhood. More adequate sex education would undoubtedly prevent much of the frigidity now produced by ignorance and lack of proper training in sex roles. Persistent frigidity usually requires psychiatric treatment to discover its causes, and no young person should be too embarrassed to seek such help.

FRUSTRATION TOLERANCE

Frustration tolerance is a psychiatric concept referring to a person's ability to tolerate normal amounts of frustration and thwarting without breaking down emotionally. Psychoanalytic theory points out that many very young children develop feelings of "infantile omnipotence" during the first weeks and months of life when they are more or less pampered and spoiled, the parents attempting to satisfy all their needs. Freud explained this phenomenon by pointing out that the behavior of young or immature people is largely determined by the Pleasure-Pain principle, whereby the child seeks only pleasures and avoids pain. He also pointed out that as the child grows older he begins to face the Reality principle, the demands and limitations exerted by the culture in which he lives. Each person must therefore learn to balance the Pleasure-Pain principle against the demands of Reality.

Very young children develop rage reactions and have temper tantrums whenever thwarted and not allowed to have their own way. In the course of normal development the child learns, however, to accept and tolerate a certain amount of interference and thwarting of his needs. The degree to which any person learns to tolerate frustration without breaking down emotionally is termed the frustration tolerance.

One of the goals of education and conduct training is to teach the child to face increasingly difficult problems in life while remaining psychologically whole and in control of the situation. School systems, athletic programs, and military training programs provide tasks of progressively increasing difficulty which the child is trained to master by developing all types of self-control. The adult who displays temper tantrums or a break-down in emotional behavior lacks that frustration tolerance which can be acquired only through emotional retraining under psychiatric supervision.

GROUP THERAPY

Practical psychiatric experience indicates that a number of patients with similar problems may be treated in group-therapy sessions. The earliest experiments with group therapy started with the Washingtonian Movement (an early association of alcoholics to help themselves) and with Alcoholics Anonymous, where it was discovered that a large number of individuals could help one another in many ways. Group therapy works best with patients of roughly the same age, education, and clinical type, who presumably have lived through similar experiences. Members of a therapy group lose their embarrassment over being mentally ill in the course of talking with others who have the same problems and who are also learning how to solve them. Those just entering a therapy group are comforted by the acceptance and friendship of people who have similar experiences.

If group therapy sessions are properly conducted, participants learn to be frank in discussing their problems, particularly things about which they have been oversensitive in the past. Frank group discussion encourages members to give their opinions and reactions in helping each other. Psychiatrically, group therapy is most effective and economical because it makes professional help available to a large number of people simultaneously.

GUILT

Feelings of guilt stem from self-hate and regret over transgression of the moral code. Every society tries to instill morality in children by rewarding good and punishing bad behavior, so that moral codes become second nature (are internalized) and operate as conscience (censor, superego). The whole question of right-and-wrong is complicated by great differences in standards between cultures. Some cultures (or parents) make a terrible fuss over relatively slight misbehavior, while others accept relatively serious transgressions without much punishment.

Psychiatrists try never to take a "laying down the law" (authoritarian) attitude towards misbehavior or to criticize the patient in any way for what he has done. Experience indicates that such attitudes simply result in further lowering of the patient's self-esteem; the psychiatrist seeks to understand the basis of disturbed behavior while aiding the patient to appreciate the self-destructive consequences of his actions.

HALLUCINATIONS Hallucinations involve the projection of inner experiences into states of clear consciousness so vividly that the individual cannot distinguish them from the real world and believes they actually exist. Most common are auditory hallucinations, in which the person thinks he hears voices talking or giving him commands, which he then frequently feels compelled to obey. In visual hallucinations, the patient sees people or things which are not truly present. (More rarely, there may be olfactory or tactual hallucinations, in which the patient smells or feels things which have no real existence.)

Hallucinations may be interpreted as expressions of unconscious mental life, which the patient is unable to distinguish from real events; or such phenomena may reflect altered biochemical processes in the brain, occurring in schizophrenia, manic depressive illness, or drug-induced psychosis.

HOMOSEXUALITY In this century great psychiatric progress has been made in understanding the causes and methods for dealing with homosexuality—sexual preference for a person of the same sex—an area in which superstition and misunderstanding have done much to confuse scientific study of sex deviations.

Prior to the studies of Freud, homosexuality was considered a form of degeneracy which was subjected to severe punishment. Freud's studies of psychosexual development showed that almost all young people normally pass through a period of interest in members of their own sex, and that such interest should be considered morbid homosexuality only when a person, on becoming an adult, sought sexual outlet with the same sex. Thus, because of the influence of psychoanalytic studies, homosexuality has come to be regarded as a variant development rather than as a separate mental disorder.

In actual practice, modern societies tend to leave homosexuals to their own devices so long as their activities do not become socially obnoxious or dangerous to the morals of the young. Scientific studies (such as the Kinsey report) show a high incidence of homosexual activity among both sexes. Although much of this might consist of mutual masturbation or minor petting practices among teen-agers, the Kinsey report helped to dilute the connotations of severe abnormality to at least some homosexual behavior.

Symptoms. A distinction should be made between the confirmed homosexual who shows no interest whatsoever in the opposite sex and heterosexual persons who have occasional homosexual feelings. It is entirely normal for an individual to feel sexually attracted to a person of the same sex; such feelings alone should not cause panic unless they are acted out in such ways as to interfere with relations with the opposite sex (heterosexuality). Studies of men in army or prison situations, where there is no possibility of contact with the opposite sex, indicate that many normal men and women have transient attachments to persons of their own sex which are broken off when normal heterosexual opportunities again return. Probably no man is 100 percent masculine, nor any woman 100 percent feminine; rather, everyone represents some combination of masculinity and femininity in such ratios as 90-10, 70-30, 50-50, etc. Some people are optionally (facultatively) bisexual; that is, attracted to both sexes and without a firm preference for either.

Homosexual tendencies may be either latent or manifest, depending on whether they are unconscious and unexpressed, or conscious and overt. Psychiatric experience indicates that many people have latent homosexual tendencies which may never be expressed in action unless the person is subjected to some form of sexual attack or seduction.

The causes of homosexuality have not been exactly established and are very complex. In a small number of cases there appears to be a physical basis, the person having many secondary sexual characteristics of the opposite sex. In other instances homosexual attack or seduction in early life may undoubtedly be a predisposing cause, particularly if occurring during crucial periods of psychosexual development. Another possible factor is failure of the child to achieve a healthy identification with the parent of the same sex. In boys, for example, it is desirable for the father to set a healthy pattern for masculine identification, so that the son learns early normal male sex roles.

Treatment. Homosexuality constitutes a difficult therapeutic problem, usually requiring intensive psychoanalytic treatment. This has been estimated to produce "cures" in about one-fourth of such patients. Others may show varying states of improvement including restoration of potency with members of the opposite sex, capacity for heterosexual marriage with occasional lapses, etc. Decreasing automatic disapproval of the homosexual, increasing militancy of the gay groups, and more open discussion of the problem are evidences of change toward less punitive attitudes in society at large.

HUNGER, UNUSUAL Hunger is a complicated sensation that has physiological as well as psychological origins. True hunger should not be confused with appetite, as appetite may continue long after hunger pangs have been satisfied by the first few mouthfuls of food. Hunger pangs result from actual contractions of the stomach, causing disagreeable sensations in the upper abdomen when expected food is not forthcoming.

The level of circulating blood-sugar (controlled by insulin from the pancreas) is thought to be important in the regulation of hunger sensations. Thus, pancreatic disturbances may cause unusual hunger if excessive amounts of insulin are being secreted. Where the food that is actually digested and absorbed is inadequate, continued hunger may result. At times of increased need for foods, such as during the heavy growth-periods of teenagers, hunger is also prominent. Because of the intimate psychological relationships between hunger and appetite, however, there are many instances of chronic disease when hunger is strangely not present. Persistent unusual hunger in an individual who is consuming adequate amounts of food should lead one to suspect the possibility of intestinal parasites, such as tape worms—which are more common than generally believed. (*See also* WORMS [ASCARIASIS] in the section GASTROINTESTINAL CONDITIONS.)

HYPNOSIS;   SUGGESTION Suggestibility underlies a wide range of phenomena including autosuggestion (self-hypnosis), hypnosis, posthypnotic suggestion, and similar trance states. It involves the establishment of a dominance-submission relationship in which the submitting (suggestible) member accepts and responds uncritically to suggestions or directions.

Suggestion effects can occur in all degrees of strength, from the casual influence of one person by another during conversation, to the deepest levels of hypnosis. Psychologically, it comprises a process of communication in which one person attempts by use of stimuli—usually verbal or symbolic in nature, but exclusive of argument or direct command—to induce an idea, feeling, decision, or action in another by circumventing the latter's critical and intellectual powers. The procedure consists basically in presentation of stimuli which build up or release attitudes, or heighten the release of responses—all with a minimum of reflective thinking on the part of the person to whom the suggestions are given.

Suggestion-effects and hypnotism have been known and practiced ever since the earliest days of tribal communities. They have been used by religious healers in all ages, from the primitive witch-doctors to the modern, faith-healing cultist. Hypnotism was first studied scientifically by Mesmer, who believed that suggestion-effects were caused by passage of a current ("animal magnetism") from one person to another. Later experiments proved that there was no such current and that the effects were due purely to psychological dominance of one person over another. There are countless methods for securing suggestion-effects and hypnosis, including fixation of the subject's eyes on a bright object held just above eye-level; giving of suggestions in a low, monotonous voice; or use of other paraphernalia which the subject has been led to believe can control him mentally. Once a subject has been hypnotized successfully, it becomes easier and easier to produce the hypnotic state with minimal stimuli.

Medical specialists have done extensive investigation of the possibility of using suggestion and hypnotism for such therapeutic purposes as pain removal. Hypnosis has been widely used during minor surgery, childbirth, and the extraction of teeth, to suggest to the patient that he will feel no pain. Such methods are effective only with subjects who are able to enter deep stages of hypnosis. There is currently considerable controversy over the value of hypnosis in psychiatric practice, and its most valuable use today is confined to the uncovering of unconscious material which had been repressed or forgotten.

Use of hypnosis for symptom-removal has been less successful, and is now generally discredited. It had been hoped that both mental and physical symptoms could be eliminated by giving hypnotic suggestions that they would disappear. Experience has shown that only those symptoms caused by suggestion can be made to disappear through suggestion. In some cases where a symptom has been caused to vanish by hypnosis, it has been found that another symptom quickly appears to take its place.

Posthypnotic suggestion involves a method for continuing the effects of suggestion after the hypnotic trance has been terminated. It was learned that, while hypnotized, patients could be instructed to carry out tasks after the trance was ended. Under the influence of such posthypnotic suggestion, the subject carries out instructions automatically, often without conscious awareness of their source. Posthypnotic suggestions have been utilized for purposes of symptom-removal by suggesting, under hypnosis, that the person no longer experience the symptom on awakening. Unfortunately, this method has proved effective only with minor symptoms caused by suggestion effects; it is totally ineffective with symptoms determined by organic causes. Posthypnotic suggestion effects can have little influence on deep emotional conflicts which underlie many psychoneurotic disorders.

Hypnosis has also been used to produce automatic writing, for the study of unconscious conflicts. While under hypnosis, the subject is given a pen and instructed to write either about anything which comes to mind, or on some particular topic. The person is told not to censor his material but to attempt to recover forgotten memories. Under hypnosis many persons can remember events which are completely beyond their recall while conscious; this seems to be evidence in support of the psychoanalytic contention that nothing in life is ever completely forgotten.

INFANTILISM Infantilism is an inhibition or blocking of emotional development, so that the child remains at, or regresses back to, infantile patterns of behavior; for example, when a young child passes through a very painful emotional experience, it is not unusual for him to regress to infantile eating, speech, motor, and toilet habits. The child may have to be toilet-trained and taught to take care of himself once more, until he feels emotionally secure enough to develop more mature habits. Regression to infantile behavior patterns typically indicates feelings of great insecurity on the part of the child, who is symbolically asking to be loved and nurtured like a baby again.

Infantile behavior patterns tend to be reinforced and perpetuated by parental overprotection, in which the parent spoils and pampers the child, thereby encouraging it to become neurotically dependent. Every child must learn to tolerate pain and adversity without breaking down emotionally, crying, or showing other infantile patterns; children develop their personality resources and become emotionally independent only by resolutely facing and solving difficult problems of life.

Infantile regressions often occur when a new child is born into a family, partially displacing older children from parental attention and affection which they have been accustomed to receive. Such older children may regress back to infantile behavior in an attempt to regain the attentions which they have lost.

"INSANITY" (MENTAL ILLNESS) Until the relatively recent development of Freudian psychoanalytic theory and modern psychopathology, little was known about the causes or nature of mental states. One of the most unfortunate historical beliefs related mental disorder to witchcraft; many of the early forms of psychiatric treatment in fact consisted of types of punishment supposed to drive out evil spirits. It is only within the last century that mental cases have been moved from prisons and into the healing atmosphere of hospitals.

With this revolution in psychiatric thinking there has occurred a change in terminology: lunatic, derived from a mistaken belief that a relationship existed between lunar phases and onset of mental symptoms; insane, from the Latin *insanus,* unhealthy; and crazy have been abandoned in modern psychiatry as not being properly descriptive.

The question may be raised whether many mental disorders are in fact diseases at all, rather than learned patterns of behavior from disturbed interpersonal relationships. We now know that many serious physical illnesses may have psychiatric symptoms as a manifestation of the disease process and that a variety of drugs can produce organic brain dysfunction. Current studies of so-called functional (non-organic) disorders have failed to demonstrate any biological or cellular changes that cause the abnormal processes. However, many research studies have demonstrated alterations in chemical processes in the brain associated with severe mental illness and there is growing evidence of genetic factors in psychotic illness. There remain, nevertheless, many less severe psychiatric disorders for which no organic basis can be demonstrated. These disorders must be regarded as resulting from disturbed social relationships and exposure to significant environmental stress. It has therefore become usual to speak of personality disorders, adjustment disorders, mood disorders, organic disorders, psychotic disorders, and so on, rather than using a vague or obsolete term such as insanity, lunacy, or mental disease.

INSECURITY Emotional insecurity is now recognized psychiatrically as an important cause of neurotic anxiety symptoms. A person may feel insecure or deprived concerning both material and psychological needs. Most obvious deprivations concern physical needs for food, shelter, and material possessions, and thus one may feel insecure if physical livelihood is threatened.

More subtle and important, however, are emotional insecurities relating to fears, threatening hostility, or loss of love. Psychoanalytic studies of early childhood indicate that each child must feel loved and wanted if he is to develop normal self-confidence and independence.

Another cause of feelings of insecurity is poor health or illness in early childhood which threaten existence. Children with delicate health tend to be insecure, fearful, and anxious. Lack of physical attractiveness, small size, or physical weakness or deformity may produce feelings of inferiority resulting in psychological insecurity. A wise parent might make it clear that many happy and successful adults do not have the physical attributes of the great athletes.

INTELLIGENCE, NATURE OF Theories concerning the nature of intelligence have recently undergone a revolutionary change and there is increasing recognition of the complexity of the problem of measuring human abilities. Earliest attempts to measure intelligence (around 1890) utilized memory tests since at that time intelligence was considered to be highly dependent upon memory. Within a short time it was discovered that memory comprises only a limited part of intelligence, and that memory tests cannot be used to predict intellectual level. The first modern intelligence test was devised shortly after 1900 by Alfred Binet, who designed age scales consisting of intelligence test items suitable for children of different ages. The Stanford-Binet, an American revision of the original Binet scales, was the first formal test constructed of items arranged at different mental age levels and scored by an Intelligence Quotient (IQ). The Intelligence Quotient (IQ) is obtained by dividing the child's mental age in months by his chronological age. (*See* INTELLIGENCE QUOTIENT in this section.)

From the 1920s to the 1940s, the Stanford-Binet was the most widely used intelligence test in America, until the advent of the Wechsler intelligence scales for adults and children, developed after World War II. Both the Stanford-Binet and the Wechsler scales consisted of verbal and performance test items derived from practical experience concerning what children of different ages were able to do. Since both the Stanford-Binet and Wechsler scales resulted in one averaged IQ or mental ability score, it was believed that intelligence involved a single ability occurring in all persons to a greater or lesser degree. It was believed that this intelligence matured progressively from birth to about fourteen, paralleling the maturing of the cerebral cortex.

A new era was introduced after World War II with the invention of highly complex statistical methods for analyzing the correlations of scores on various types of intelligence tests.

The new mathematical methods demonstrated that many different abilities are involved, rather than a single factor called intelligence. This newer system of classification recognizes general, group, and specific factors of intelligence. The general factor found in all measures of intelligence appears to be identical with the intelligence measured by the Stanford-Binet and Wechsler scales. Among the group factors—less broad than the general factor, but still flexible enough to cover certain broad types of intelligence—are verbal, mathematical, memory, and mechanical factors. (The mathematical factor for example, involves the ability to handle numbers and other symbols in all kinds of mathematical applications.) In addition, there have been discovered a large number of specific intelligence factors involving very special abilities which are important in such things as musical or artistic performance.

This new concept of intelligence, recognizing that human intelligence depends upon a large number of abilities, has resulted in the construction of entirely new types of tests, measuring all the factors of ability which have been shown to exist. Thus, the whole field of intelligence measurement is far more complicated than formerly believed and requires much more extensive testing programs to measure all the newly discovered factors. The whole problem has become even more complicated since the discovery that actual performance is influenced by many other personality factors in addition to innate ability. Success in life, for example, is a product of emotional stability, level of motivation, levels of self-control, and many other specific psychosocial factors. An emotionally stable, highly motivated child of relatively low intelligence may actually perform better than a child of very high intelligence who is emotionally unstable and poorly motivated. So it is that many personality factors in addition to innate ability determine the actual level of performance.

INTELLIGENCE QUOTIENT (IQ) The IQ was devised to provide a standard method of comparing levels of intelligence among different groups of people at all age levels. It is obtained by dividing the person's mental age (as determined by his intelligence test scores) by his calendar (chronological) age expressed in months, then multiplying by 100. Thus, if a child has a determined mental age of 96 months, and his chronological age is also 96 months, his IQ is 100. The higher the mental age in relation to the chronological age, the higher the child's IQ.

Based on the distribution of IQ scores over the whole population, psychologists have developed an arbitrary system for classifying IQ levels as follows:

Classification	IQ Range
Profound retardation	0–19
Severe retardation	20–34
Moderate retardation	35–49
Mild retardation	50–69
Borderline (low-average)	70–89
Average	90–109
Above average	110–139
Very superior	140–above

In recent years clinical psychologists have learned that the IQ should be evaluated with considerable caution in making predictions concerning a child's actual ability. Intelligence tests are highly weighted with items relating to verbal and symbol-handling abilities, so that children with high reading- and vocabulary-ability tend to get the best scores and may be overrated, while children lacking these abilities may be underrated. Though the IQ is one of the best predictors of academic success, it does not inevitably predict success in actual life situations. Clinical experience has shown that many people with very high IQ's have not been particularly successful in life, while many who are actually very successful never did well academically or on intelligence tests. Success in life is a most complex matter which is not necessarily predictable via intelligence tests.

School authorities sometimes place too much emphasis on IQ measurements when classifying children as to ability levels or predicting what they will do. Clinical psychologists have learned that success in later life may be more determined by a child's special abilities or talents, involving highly specific factors of intelligence, rather than by his average level of intelligence or IQ.

The whole field of intelligence testing is new, and many current tests are not valid for the purposes for which they are being used. They are often more valid for predicting what a child cannot do than what he can do. It is always necessary to test a child repeatedly in order to get a true estimate of his abilities, since he may not perform at his best on any one test. To get the most comprehensive measurement of a child's abilities, it is necessary to give dozens of tests measuring all known mental abilities in order to discover special talents on which later success may be based.

MANIC-DEPRESSIVE PSYCHOSIS

This psychosis typically involves a pattern of recurring disturbed mood: mania and depression. The illness may begin with either mania or depression followed by a period of normal mood. Typically, manic excitement lasts for several weeks or months and may be followed either by depression or a period of normal mood. These disturbances of mood tend to recur, although a few patients may have only one or two episodes during a lifetime. This disorder frequently begins relatively early in life between ages 15 and 35. There is often a family history of a mood disorder, and genetic factors play an important role in the transmission of manic depressive illness. Sometimes episodes of mania or depression begin insidiously; in other instances, the episode appears to be precipitated by environmental stress.

Symptoms. In the manic or excited phase, increased activity, heightened emotionality, feelings of grandiosity, and irritability are principal symptoms. Patient becomes overactive and excitable, talking excessively, singing, shouting, and engaging in frenzied activities—often reflecting impaired judgment. Flight of ideas, distractibility, disturbed thinking, hallucinations and delusions may all accompany heightened activity levels. The sexual drive tends to be heightened and the patient may be too agitated to eat or sleep properly. Hospitalization during the acute phase of mania is generally required.

During the depressive phase, the person tends to become melancholy, blue, and painfully withdrawn. Loss of interest in routine activities, crying episodes, and anguished feelings of guilt and inadequacy are common. As the depression deepens, the patient may show retardation in many areas of mental and physical functioning; thinking and speech slow down, there is difficulty falling asleep or midnight awakening, and hallucinations and delusions may occur. There is an increasing risk of suicide.

Treatment. The use of lithium carbonate, major tranquilizers, antidepressants, and electroconvulsive therapy (ECT) have completely revolutionized the treatment of manic depressive illness. It was previously necessary to hospitalize patients with manic depressive illness for prolonged periods; now hospitalization may be generally shortened as symptoms respond to medication or ECT. Patients who have either severe mania or depression should generally be hospitalized until the periods of excitement, disturbed thinking, grossly impaired judgment, and suicidal risk have lessened. Then appropriate psychotherapy interventions may be initiated and attention directed toward family members who often cope with considerable stress when dealing with a severely manic or depressed patient.

Fortunately, the outlook for manic depressive illness is now much more optimistic, particularly with the use of lithium carbonate and antidepressants to minimize or lessen the frequency of recurrent episodes. Frequently the patient may return to significant periods of normal functioning, and the severity of future episodes may be lessened by careful attention to early warning signs of disturbed mood.

Many manic depressive patients remain on treatment with lithium for years, apparently without any serious long-term side effects.

MASTURBATION Revolutionary changes have occurred during the last seventy-five years in medical-psychiatric attitudes toward many types of sex behavior formerly thought to be perverted and pathological. First, anthropological cross-cultural studies have shown the wide range of social and ethical attitudes towards various ways of expressing sexuality, demonstrating that there is no universal agreement on what a culture permits or considers pathological.

Secondly, Freudian discoveries concerning normal patterns of psycho-sexual development have greatly increased acceptance of behaviors formerly considered completely abnormal and perverted. Freud was the first to point out the facts about infantile sexuality and the various phases of interest in different sex-objects shown by normal children. He showed that erotic sensitivity usually appears early in infancy, young children first developing sexual gratification from the oral regions in feeding and sucking activity. Later, the child may be erotically stimulated by excretory functions and zones—a stage labeled by Freud as the anal-erotic phase of normal development. Still later, usually around puberty, sexual interests become fixated on genital areas as the child discovers normal heterosexuality.

Freud pointed out that every normal child usually experiments with many types of auto-erotic (self) sexual stimulation, and he insisted that many older terms such as masturbation or self-abuse were illogical and inexact, expressing moralistic religious taboos which are scientifically untrue. There is no scientific evidence of any causative relationship between autoeroticism and any form of mental disorder. Though mentally disturbed persons characteristically show poor judgment in expressing sexuality, this may be understood as a symptom rather than a cause. Each child must, however, learn the appropriate social and legal limitations relating to expressions of sexuality.

Treatment. In the past, overly strict taboos and superstitions concerning a supposed relationship between uncontrolled sexuality and mental disorder caused masturbation to be severely punished and suppressed. It is now understood that punishment or severe repressive measures simply create neurotic conflict and further exaggerate the problem. Parents should regard children's developing sexual interest as completely normal, to be channeled into socially acceptable directions rather than to be completely repressed. The child must learn not to become socially conspicuous or a public nuisance. Ordinarily, the child's sexual development takes place most smoothly when parents show a tolerant, accepting attitude, patiently helping in the channeling of impulses in socially acceptable directions without creating conflicts in the child by becoming over-anxious or openly disturbed by its behavior. In extreme cases, where a child has developed such conflicts over problems of sex

development that he expresses sexuality in socially unacceptable ways, it may be desirable for the parents and child to go to a child guidance clinic where the problems can be solved under psychiatric supervision.

MENTAL HYGIENE This is a branch of preventative psychiatry dedicated to the prevention of mental disorders and to the development of mental health. The founder of the modern mental hygiene movement was Clifford Beers who, early in the 1920s, wrote of his experiences as a mental hospital patient and led a movement for the establishment of child guidance clinics, adult psychiatric clinics, and improved mental hospital facilities.

It is now widely accepted that a person may be free of significant mental defects or disorders and still be relatively inefficient, unhappy, and unproductive unless he can live positively, establish close and gratifying relationships, and fulfill his potential.

Mental health research has proved that a large number of social, economic, and political factors determine mental health, and that such public welfare advances as higher wages, better living standards, more educational facilities, and more opportunity for rehabilitation and recreation are very important factors in mental health. Preventative social psychiatry has also made great progress in discovering interpersonal social factors causing epidemic ill health.

MENTAL ILLNESS As recently as the nineteenth century, mental illness was not well understood and was treated by superstitious, unscientific methods which in many cases only made the mental patient worse because of mishandling. The major breakthrough occurred with public recognition that mental disorder was a medical, not a criminal, problem. Formerly, mental patients were handled like criminals, often housed in prison-like institutions and punished, rather than treated. (Even the legal procedure for committing a mental patient usually required the assistance of a sheriff.)

Particularly since World War II, there has been more general acceptance of the idea that mental patients should be given the same type of sympathetic care customarily given patients with physical disease. With the advent of tranquilizing drugs and the understanding that a mental patient is ill rather than evil, there has been a progressive liberalization and improvement in community methods for dealing with psychiatric problems. Padded cells, straitjackets, locked wards, and lifetime custodial institutionalization have largely been abandoned in most mental hospitals.

In most states a mental patient can now be voluntarily admitted to a psychiatric ward without having to go through an embarrassing court procedure. In the best mental hospitals patients are handled with such understanding and tact that violent episodes are becoming less frequent and are controlled by tranquilizing drugs rather than by force. Patients are now kept largely in unlocked, open wards in pleasant, homelike surroundings and with a full daily program involving intensive psychotherapy, occupational therapy, recreation, and opportunities for gainful employment.

As a result of psychiatric advances, it is now no longer necessary for the milder cases even to be sent to a mental hospital, while a large percentage of first admissions to psychiatric hospitals are being routinely discharged as cured after a few months of intensive treatment. It can truthfully be said that now there is great hope, not only for cure, but also for prevention of many psychiatric conditions.

NAIL-BITING This is an early symptom of emotional conflict and anxiety. In young children it has significance only as a symptom of the underlying emotional stress. Nail-biting frequently develops during periods of increased tension and conflict when the child is under emotional pressure from the environment. Usually it is only one of a group of nervous symptoms including eating and sleeping disturbances, nose-picking, thumb-sucking, skin-picking, and tics.

Treatment. There is no specific treatment for nail-biting, which usually disappears spontaneously as the child becomes older and more mature. If this and other neurotic symptoms interfere too seriously with adjustment, the child should be referred to a child guid-

ance clinic for psychiatric treatment for deeper underlying causes.

NARCOANALYSIS Narcoanalysis is a method of analyzing unconscious conflicts, in which the patient is studied while under the influence of hypnotic drugs. In World War II it was discovered that psychiatric patients who had had severely disturbing war experiences (about which they were not able to talk while in a normal waking state) could be made more accessible under heavy sedation by hypnotic drugs which inhibited conscious defenses and brought repressed experiences to the surface. By this method, patients suspected of harboring repressed traumatic experiences in the unconscious are given heavy sedation and then asked about their deepest problems as they are about to fall asleep. Occasionally, this method is used as part of diagnostic assessment with psychotic patients who are mute and unresponsive.

"NERVOUS BREAKDOWN" This is a nonmedical term referring to all types of neurotic disorders in which emotional instability and conflict seriously incapacitate the person in normal life. The term has many unscientific implications which do not describe the situation accurately. Breakdown implies that the person has "gone to pieces" or otherwise "lost his mind," though this is actually not the case. (No one ever loses his mind in any true sense.) What is actually involved—as in all forms of nervous and mental disorder—is some loss or absence of normal self-control.

It is more exact to refer to "a period of emotional instability" or "a period of neurotic incapacitation." Modern psychiatry is now able to diagnose all kinds of personality disorders in more exact terms which are more hopeful because they imply that causes are known and can be treated with appropriate methods.

"NERVOUSNESS" Nervousness is a nonmedical term applied to many nervous and emotional symptoms occurring in neurotic conditions and personality disorders. More specifically, the symptoms of "nervousness" can be standard symptoms of neurotic anxiety tension states.

Symptoms. The underlying cause of

emotional instability is usually fear, which produces psychosomatic symptoms of restlessness, irritability, disturbing sensations from all parts of the body, nervous tremors or twitchings, feelings of generalized muscular tension, physical weakness, and vague fears of impending illness or doom. Most laymen are aware of the psychological origin of such symptoms. Frequently a vicious circle of increasing emotionalism and psychosomatic symptoms makes the person aware of an impending psychological crisis, as when the patient complains, "I feel I'm going to blow my top," or, "I feel something terrible is going to happen to me mentally." This rising crescendo of emotional instability associated with disturbing psychosomatic symptoms may lead to acute anxiety states associated with panicky feelings.

Treatment. Psychiatrists try to teach patients that nervous symptoms have a base in anxiety related to one's upbringing and perceptions. Individuals who feel unable to solve or cope with life's problems will of course experience anxiety. Persons with low self-esteem will be easily and markedly upset when criticized even mildly. Those who have not experienced durable and reliable relationships in early life may be inordinately upset over a mild marital spat. Unravelling the interconnectedness of past and current perceptions is an important task in psychotherapy and counseling. When counseling is successful, "nervousness" diminishes or disappears.

NEUROSIS Neurosis and psychoneurosis are almost synonymous psychiatric terms, describing a large number of functional disorders in which physical and mental symptoms are caused by emotional upsets. (The term functional refers to the fact that there is no permanent organic damage, but rather that the organism is simply functioning improperly.) The term neurosis is generally used to refer to minor functional disorders of emotional origin.

Everyone may be called neurotic to some degree, since every person has some emotional conflicts or instability which interfere with normal adjustment. Usually neurotic disorders do not involve the whole personality but are limited to some functions. In general they may be regarded as reactions to life-stresses, in which one or another psychological function breaks down under excessive pressure; for example, psychiatric studies in World War II showed that every soldier had his own characteristic threshold of neurotic breakdown when life-pressures became too great.

Symptoms. Each person tends to show his own characteristic pattern of neurotic reactions, depending partly on inherited weaknesses and partly on injurious emotional experiences in early childhood. The situation is comparable to a chain which gives way at its weakest link when excessive strain is placed upon it. The most disagreeable symptom in many neurotic states consists of emotional anguish, involving terrifying sensations and feelings that the person is about to go insane.

One of the most common patterns of neurotic disorder consists of psychosomatic symptoms developing in various organs in the body when a person becomes too emotionally conflictual. (The term psychosomatic refers to the fact that emotional upsets tend to disrupt the functioning of various organ-systems of the body, producing physical symptoms.) The most common psychosomatic symptoms occur in the gastrointestinal tract, where emotional conflicts produce a wide variety of symptoms including nausea, vomiting, gas, excess acidity, constipation, or diarrhea. The second most common type of psychosomatic disorder involves circulatory symptoms such as fast pulse, irregular heartbeat, high blood pressure, vascular flushing or paling in various parts of the body, fainting spells, and headaches.

Other types of (psycho)neurotic disorder include anxiety states, hysteria, obsession-compulsion neurosis, psychasthenia, neurasthenia, and psychoneurotic character disorders. In anxiety states, the basic pattern consists of symptoms of conscious and unconscious fear and anxiety. In obsession-compulsion neurosis, the characteristic symptoms involve obsessive ideas which the individual cannot get out of his head and irrational compulsions to commit acts which the person would not ordinarily perform. Hysteria is characterized by the conversion of emotional conflicts into a wide variety of physical symptoms such as hysterical blindness, deafness, and so forth. Psychasthenia is characterized by symptoms of extreme worry and guilt, reflecting an over-strict superego. Neurasthenia is a psychosomatic syndrome involving feelings of excessive fatigue, weakness, and lack of energy, usually accompanied by circulatory symptoms of low blood pressure and irregular heart action. Formerly, it was believed that these various kinds of psychoneurotic disorders represented essentially different conditions, but more recent psychoanalytic evidence indicates that they are only different manifestations of one basic process involving unconscious conflict.

Treatment. Most vital in getting the neurotic to accept treatment is to help him to accept the fact that his condition is completely psychological and that physical treatment can have no effect. This is often a problem, since neurotics are very sensitive and embarrassed about their symptoms and reluctant to admit that they do need psychological treatment.

Many neurotics would be greatly helped simply by accepting the fact that every person has some neurotic symptoms which he must learn to accept and live with. In certain instances treatment may teach the patient to be neurotic and like it; that is, to learn not to be panicked by neurotic symptoms. The patient should be reassured that he is not going to "lose his mind" and that the worst that can happen is that he will "feel bad" for a while.

Treatment of (psycho)neurotic conditions is a very complicated process which should be undertaken only by certified psychiatrists or clinical psychologists. It may require long and intensive specialized techniques to uncover the unconscious conflicts producing neurotic symptoms. Ultimately successful treatment usually involves some type of psychoanalysis in which the deep unconscious conflicts underlying neurotic symptoms are brought to light and dispelled after being consciously recognized.

NIGHTMARES AND NIGHT-TERRORS Insomnia, disturbed sleep, nightmares, night terrors and sleep walking occur in a variety of psychiatric disorders including anxiety states and depression. They may be symptoms of deep unconscious fears, emotional insecurities, or of underlying depression. States of emotional upset involving fear or anger may persist over long periods, causing anxiety symptoms during the day and sleep disturbances at night. On the other hand, sleep walking and night terrors in childhood are usually transient and may not be associated with emotional disturbance.

Symptoms. Nightmares and bad dreams usually involve horrible or tragic experiences, or fear of impending doom. They have the same psychiatric significance as daytime anxiety symptoms, and may reflect unexpressed anger and buried resentment. Occasional nightmares are common with preschool children, but children with recurrent nightmares are generally under emotional stress.

Treatment. As anxiety symptoms are due to fear and insecurity, anything which promotes feelings of greater security tends to counteract them. Children with occasional nightmares tend to respond to reassurance and emotional support. Treatment of recurrent nightmares and other anxiety symptoms usually involves psychotherapy directed at discovering and removing the sources of emotional conflict and stress. Use of sedative medication to treat transient insomnia may be helpful, but the use of barbiturates should be avoided.

OBSESSIONS Repetitious ideas which constantly return to consciousness in spite of a person's efforts to put them out of mind are one of the main symptoms of obsession-compulsion neuroses. Obsessive ideas may occur in all degrees of severity and extensity. Most normal people experience mild obsessions in the form of worries which they cannot put aside or musical tunes which run constantly through their heads. In more serious states the obsessive idea may be so intense that the person can think of nothing else. It is generally believed that obsessive-compulsive states are produced by intense unconscious conflicts involving forbidden impulses, which are striving to enter consciousness in a struggle with conscience (superego), which is striving to repress the socially undesirable impulses.

Treatment. As with all other psychoneurotic conditions, basic treatment consists of psychiatric evaluation and appropriate therapy. Symptoms often reflect deep unconscious conflicts which may be understood through psychotherapeutic treatment. The general principle of treatment is to teach the patient to pay less attention to the symptoms and to focus attention on underlying, unexpressed feelings or impulses. Sometimes behavioral therapy is useful in aiding the patient to cope with obsessive ideas. When the symptoms are severe, medication may be helpful in conjunction with other treatment methods.

OCCUPATIONAL THERAPY Psychiatrists long have recognized the importance of healthy work habits in mental health. Often one of the first symptoms of an incipient mental disorder is the breakdown of work habits; conversely, as mental patients begin to improve, one of the first symptoms of recovery is a return of an interest in working.

Occupational therapy consists of a comprehensive program of work projects in the arts and crafts to which mental patients are assigned as part of an overall plan to get them back into community living. During their waking hours mental patients should be assigned to an activity program which keeps them busy and gainfully employed. Occupational therapy has been found to be one of the most important elements in the rehabilitation of patients, retraining them in work habits suitable for their return to community life.

OEDIPUS COMPLEX The Oedipus complex refers to the strong emotional attachment and love relationship developed by male children toward their mothers. These positive feelings are often accompanied by other feelings of competitive rivalry, fear and resentment toward the father. This complex received its name from the ancient Greek legend which was the basis for Sophocles' tragedy, *Oedipus Rex*.

Freud early recognized the clinical significance of mother-son relationships, particularly in reference to the potential triangle of jealousy and conflict involving mother, son, and father. Love and longing toward mother, rivalry and resentment toward father, are commonly experienced by boys ages four to six; more intense emotional states (the Oedipus complex) typically reflect disturbed family dynamics. In some instances, the mother may be openly seductive toward her son or encourage excessive dependency. On other occasions, father may feel threatened by competitive and rivalrous impulses in his preschool son. In other instances, the child may feel emotionally deprived by both parents and become more demanding and dependent toward mother in an effort to obtain some love and caring.

Normally the male child resolves Oedipal feelings by forging a positive identification with his father and renouncing wishes to possess mother in favor of being protected and cared for by both parents. Emerging interest in activities outside the home, with peers or in school, facilitate the resolution of the Oedipal situation.

Given the importance of a healthy father-son relationship in resolving these developmental issues, the feelings linked to the Oedipal complex may be less successfully resolved when there is an absent or unavailable father—as sometimes occurs following divorce.

Treatment. Handling an unresolved Oedipus complex is sometimes a difficult psychiatric problem, requiring the cooperation of all concerned, including both parents and the child. Parents may need to correct maladaptive reactions to the boy's expression of normative Oedipal feelings, or they may need to examine unexpressed marital conflict which triangulates the child. Where the father is absent or relatively unavailable, as may occur following divorce, efforts should be made to promote increased contact between father and the child. As in other neurotic disorders, treatment is aimed at resolving disturbed patterns of family interaction and in helping the child to relinquish excessive dependence on mother and find alternative sources of gratification.

PARANOID STATES Paranoid thinking involves the psychological mechanism of projection, in which a person "projects" his own feelings and attitudes, mistakenly imputing motives to others which are actually his own. Paranoid thinking is always delusional in the sense that real events are misinterpreted by having the individual's own feelings and motivations projected onto them.

Symptoms. The most common type of

paranoid thinking involves the persecution complex, in which a person develops ideas that other people are "after him," saying untrue things about him, or otherwise persecuting him and causing him trouble. The paranoid may think that others are following him, watching him, trying to influence him over television, trying to poison him, or otherwise causing damage.

Paranoid thinking may be organized into complexes of all levels of severity and extensity, ranging from single paranoid ideas (such as that one's teacher is hostile) to the full-fledged psychosis known as paranoia, involving complex and systematized delusions. Paranoid thinking may be understood as involving defensive attempts to rationalize one's own personal inadequacies by blaming all failures on others. In extreme cases, paranoid states may be regarded as extensive reconstruction efforts, in which the patient tries to reorganize the world in line with his own motives.

A common symptom of paranoid states is auditory hallucinations, in which a person hears voices directing him to commit some act, such as killing another person, or setting fire to a building. The paranoid patient is always potentially dangerous because of his known tendency to take matters of law and order into his own hands in an attempt to correct fancied injustices or to punish or otherwise eliminate those he mistakenly perceives as enemies.

Treatment. Paranoid thinking is always unhealthy, and paranoid ideas should be corrected when first noted. One should always carefully examine any temptation to believe that others are the cause of failure or of systematic hostility, though in very occasional cases this may actually be true. Psychiatric experience indicates that paranoid states become increasingly difficult to treat and correct once paranoid ideas become incorporated into systematic and organized delusions that "the world is against me."

Paranoid conditions are among the most difficult to treat psychiatrically, and chronic paranoid states frequently never respond to treatment. Patients with well-established paranoid delusions of persecution are potentially socially dangerous and should be committed to mental hospitals for observation and treatment for as long as they remain delusional.

PERSONAL SOCIAL BEHAVIOR   Mental hygiene experience indicates that getting along with others is a vital factor in mental health; studies of the development of neurotic behavior in infants and very young children indicate that such problems often originate in early disturbed human relationships. Since every child is socially trained (conditioned) by his early contacts with parents and relatives, where parents or other important adults are neurotic or emotionally unhealthy, young children tend toward the same abnormal behavior patterns.

There is considerable evidence that many neurotic patterns are transmitted from older to younger generations by imitation and conditioning; for example, the neurotic mother who is fearful of many things in life such as darkness or water tends to communicate fears and anxieties by imitation in children who develop the same pattern.

It is now generally accepted that one of the major purposes of all social institutions—the family, schools, the church, law-and-order—is the conditioning of the child in healthy personal social behavior. Getting along with others is probably the most difficult psychological problem in life, and perhaps the most common cause for neurotic conflict when a person becomes socially maladjusted. To like other people, it is first necessary to like and respect one's self; those who are difficult to get along with frequently do not like themselves and are frustrated by their own behavior.

Treatment. A basic method in child guidance clinics (and psychotherapy in general) is the conditioning of the individual who is not getting along well in new kinds of personal social relationships. Frequently the therapist is able to establish a friendly, accepting, noncritical, and helpful relationship with the patient for the first time in the latter's life. Various forms of group play and therapy provide opportunities for the socially ill-adjusted to learn to relate in healthier ways than formerly.

PHOBIA   Phobias are intense, unreasoned fears, usually symptomatic of deep neurotic anxiety states. Contrasted with ordinary fears, in which there is usually a recognized conscious cause for the apprehension, phobias usually reflect deep anxieties of unconscious origin, so that the sufferer may not be consciously aware of the causes or sources of his irrational behavior.

Symptoms. Phobias may appear in early childhood in the form of unreasoning fear of darkness, mice, snakes, enclosed or high places, water, or disease. Frequently, all of a child's deep anxieties and insecurities are displaced onto one phobia. The form of any particular phobia is often a matter of chance, although conditioning and imitation of similar fears in adults may be predisposing causes.

Treatment. When phobias become disabling, some form of psychotherapy is indicated. The child should be referred to a child guidance clinic for psychiatric evaluation.

Specific phobias, such as fear of darkness, should not be reinforced in unhealthy ways as by taking the child into bed with the parents; this may only increase the child's neurotic dependency-needs. (It sometimes helps to leave the child's room dimly lighted, but otherwise the child should be calmly and firmly induced to stay in bed by himself.)

PSYCHIATRIST The psychiatrist is a physician specializing in the diagnosis and treatment of mental disorders. Under present qualifications, the psychiatrist must have had four years of medical education leading to a medical degree; an internship in general medicine of at least a year; one year of training in neurology; and at least three years of specialized psychiatric internship and residency involving mental-hospital and outpatient experience with children and adults. Certification in psychiatry by the American Board of Neurology and Psychiatry is achieved by passing examinations in all branches of the study of neurology and psychiatry.

PSYCHOANALYSIS; PSYCHOANALYST Psychoanalysis involves specialized theory and methods of treatment developed for the study of the unconscious and conditions caused by unconscious conflict. The specific term, psychoanalysis, usually refers to orthodox Freudian methods as further developed by students adhering to Freudian theories. How-

ever, the situation is complicated by the fact that many former pupils of Freud split away from his theories to form their own schools, so that today there are many types of psychoanalysis, labeled with confusingly similar titles.

All psychoanalytic methods involve "depth-analysis" of unconscious levels of personality integration. Psychoanalysts seek to discover the hidden (latent) unconscious meanings of overt manifest symptoms—which are regarded as only symbolic of the underlying unconscious processes.

Four of the special methods devised by Freud for psychoanalytic study of mental processes are described in the following paragraphs.

Free association. The patient lies down on a comfortable couch and is instructed by the analyst simply to say anything which comes to the mind. This process of undirected free association results in progressively deeper uncovering of forgotten memories, unpleasant experiences; personal conflicts, and a general reporting of all the contents of consciousness. The analyst usually assumes a more or less passive role, simply stimulating the patient to talk about himself on deeper and deeper levels and only occasionally interpreting the unconscious significance of the associations produced by the patient.

Dream interpretation. Freud early recognized that the obvious contents of dreams are heavily loaded with latent symbolic significance, reflecting unconscious conflicts. Through the interpretation of unconscious significance in dream symbolism the patient becomes aware of some of the underlying conflicts of his life.

Transference mechanisms. As a natural part of the psychoanalytic process, the patient tends to bring out and transfer to the analyst many of the key problems and conflicts which he has had with others. In the more healthy and healing atmosphere of personal relationship with his analyst, the patient learns more appropriate patterns of reaction.

Analysis of psychological abnormality (psychopathology) in everyday life. During the course of psychoanalysis the patient gradually develops deep understanding of the unconscious significance of such activities as symptom-formation, humor, wit, errors, slips of the tongue, and other forms of psychopathology in everyday life.

Although Freud did not require his own students to be physicians and argued that medical training might actually be a handicap in becoming a competent psychoanalyst, modern psychoanalysis has largely become a medical specialty in the field of psychiatry. The theories and methods of psychoanalysis largely remain scientifically unproven; the psychoanalytic movement has, however, achieved wide acceptance and recognition as a necessary foundation for modern psychiatry.

There are those who consider psychiatric training incomplete until the psychiatrist has become adept in psychoanalytic methods by being analyzed himself. There is increasing evidence, however, that although psychoanalysis has made invaluable contributions to modern psychopathology, it does not provide the complete answer to all psychiatric problems and must eventually take its place among a wide variety of other methods, all of which have specific application.

PSYCHOBIOLOGY; PSYCHOBIOLOGIST
Psychobiology is a school of psychiatry which was led by the late American psychiatrist Adolph Meyer. In contrast to psychoanalysis, which is concerned primarily with the study of the unconscious, psychobiology teaches that each person should be regarded as a biological organism in which physical and mental functions are integrated as a unit. The psychobiological method is based on the recognition that every person is a biologic organism which must be studied by all possible biological and psychological methods, in order to obtain a comprehensive understanding of all levels of behavior. Meyer emphasized a broad-spectrum approach, simultaneous study of all levels of behavior integration by suitable biochemical, physiological, neurological, psychological, psychiatric, and biosocial methods.

PSYCHODRAMA
Psychodrama is a form of group therapy in which mental patients are encouraged to take part in amateur plays or dramas related to their own problems. Psychiatric experience indicates that patients often derive great benefit from acting out their problems with other people who have lived through similar experiences. Often the psychiatrist supervising psychodrama assigns themes to be acted out which are close to the patients' own problems, so that each patient learns to express himself more openly and arrive at new solutions to his problem(s).

PSYCHOGENIC
Psychogenic is an adjective applied to symptoms or clusters of symptoms (syndromes) of psychological origin, as distinct from those produced by physical causes. Psychogenic disorders are usually caused by unconscious conflicts and complexes of emotional origin. Thus, psychogenic vomiting refers to vomiting caused by underlying emotional conflicts or unconscious complexes, while psychogenic headaches are psychological symptoms of anxiety tension states.

PSYCHOLOGICAL EXAMINATION AND TESTING
The use of scientific psychological tests by scientifically trained clinical psychologists for the purpose of testing higher mental functions has become increasingly common. Psychological testing usually involves the following special examination methods:
- life history studies, relating particularly to patterns and rates of development and maturation of the different processes and abilities;
- direct behavior observations, in which objective ratings made on all types of personal social behavior, are often later compared with ratings made by the subject himself;
- introspective reporting, in which the individual is encouraged to report in detail all the feelings, thoughts, and experiences of his life;
- objective tests and measurements, by means of which standardized tests are used to measure intellectual abilities and personality factors;
- projective tests—the use of ambiguous (unstructured) test-stimuli, such as the Rorschach ink-blot test, to draw forth purely subjective responses which reflect the deep psychic organization of the person.

Psychological tests may be employed in

many special situations, such as schools, hospitals, clinics, military service, courts, prisons, industry, and so forth. They are used to measure special abilities or disabilities which may have vital bearing on a person's functioning in the appropriate context. In all testing situations, psychological examinations should be administered by qualified psychologists with specialized scientific training.

PSYCHOLOGY; PSYCHOLOGIST Psychology is the science of behavior. It is basic to psychiatry and concerned with the innate and acquired factors which organize the normal personality. Modern psychology stresses the use of special experimental and statistical methods for the objective study of sensation, perception, learning, memory, thinking, feelings and emotions, judgment, and higher mental processes.

Training as a psychologist consists of at least four years of graduate study in normal, experimental, developmental, abnormal, clinical, applied, physical (physiological), educational, and animal psychology; the course of study leading to the A.M. and Ph.D. degrees. After completing formal academic study of basic psychology, many psychologists seek further training in special applications of their field—clinical, educational, industrial, business, advertising, personality-counseling, and so forth. Competence is attested by certification of a psychologist by the American Board of Examiners in Professional Psychology after demonstration of suitable qualifications and satisfactory completion of required examinations. In contrast to the psychiatrist, whose training is basically medical, the psychologist's training is basically academic and oriented within the specialized field of psychology.

PSYCHOSES Psychiatric classification of mental disorders involves two major groups: (psycho)neuroses and psychoses. The psychoneuroses include minor reactions, usually involving only part of the personality. They are generally considered as functional disorders, not involving organic disease or lesions, and caused by unresolved unconscious conflicts of emotional origin.

Symptoms. The psychoses, by contrast, involve deeper disintegration of the whole personality, to such an extent that mental functions are distorted in comparative entirety. The psychotic individual usually shows greater or lesser disintegration of normal personality functions and is recognized socially as not being responsible for what he does. Loss of control is a constant symptom.

In the so-called "functional" psychoses-schizophrenia, paranoid disorders, mood disorders (manic depressive psychoses), disruption of mental functioning by psychological conflicts and/or altered biochemistry is not attributable to any known physical disorders. With treatment, the outcome for the "functional" psychosis is variable. With the recent use of lithium carbonate and antidepressant medication, the outcome for manic depressive psychosis is generally quite favorable.

Treatment. The outlook in many psychotic conditions is much more hopeful than was previously believed. The prognosis for organic psychosis depends upon the treatability of the disease process which affects the brain. Organic psychoses associated with abuse of drugs generally remit when the patient is withdrawn from the offending substance. With the development of a variety of antipsychotic medications, many of the dramatic symptoms associated with organic brain disease may be sufficiently controlled, while attention is directed at the underlying physical disorder.

Functional psychoses, which are presumably caused by both genetic vulnerability and environmental stress, are best treated by medication and supportive psychotherapy. Often attention must be directed toward the reduction of stress factors in the patient's immediate environment.

PSYCHOSOMATIC Psychosomatic refers to the functional unity of physical and psychological components of the human organism. It is recognized that somatic conditions may determine psychological states and, conversely, psychological states may influence somatic conditions. Psychosomatic symptoms involve physical disorders reactive to psychological states. For example, gastric ulcers may be caused by chronic psychic tension states. Hypertension may develop in reaction to chronic anger and irritability. In other words, mind and body are inseparable; what affects one also influences the other. Mental content influences the condition of the body, and the condition of the body influences the state of the mind.

PSYCHOTHERAPY The term psychotherapy applies to special psychological methods for treating mental conditions by purely psychological techniques as contrasted with physical or chemical treatment. It is now generally accepted that functional psychological disorders respond only to distinctive psychological methods of treatment. Since most personality problems and psychoneurotic disorders are caused by disorders of learning or conditioning, and involve habits, ideational complexes, and emotional conflicts which exist on purely psychological levels, they can be treated only by psychotherapy.

All forms of psychotherapy ultimately depend on retraining methods whereby the patient learns how to solve life's problems in healthier ways. All psychotherapy involves some type of diagnostic process to discover the psychological causes of disorder, suitable conditions of rapport and understanding so that relearning can take place, and the use of suitable retraining methods by means of which the patient learns to cope more efficiently with his problems.

Among the more important established methods of psychotherapy are psychoanalysis, involving the "depth" study of unconscious complexes; personality counseling, involving specialized psychological tutoring in problem areas to help the client actualize himself in all areas of life; marriage counseling utilizing special methods for dealing with situational problems in marriage; vocational guidance, helping the client to discover what kinds of work he is suited for, and adjusting to work situations; group therapy where groups of patients with similar conditions meet with a psychiatrist to discuss mutual problems; psychodrama using plays and dramatic productions where mental patients can act out their problems; play therapy, usually with children, to provide an opportunity to act out deep emotional problems; and behavioral and emotional retraining to recondition behavior patterns in persons with conduct or personality disorders.

RATIONALIZATION Rationalization is a form of mental defense mechanism (originally described by Freud) in which a person seeks to excuse or defend his conduct by providing plausible, seemingly rational explanations. One may blame errors on others, depict one's self as the victim of circumstance, and attempt to invent reasons for explaining bad conduct.

Psychologists believe that the best defense is no defense at all, but rather a frank admission of error and the taking of steps to prevent its repetition in the future. The person who rationalizes is unconsciously seeking to avoid blame or responsibility for his own conduct; however, the only result is continuance or intensification of the original difficulty.

REGRESSION The term regression refers to a mental mechanism by which people retreat (regress) to more primitive stages of development on encountering frustration or failure in their attempts to adjust at higher levels of development. Thus a child experiencing severe emotional conflicts may show regression to infantile behavior such as bedwetting, baby talk, increased demand for protective care from the mother, and thumbsucking. Masturbation, after one has supposedly reached adult heterosexual levels of adjustment, may be regarded as regressive behavior in reaction to failures to adjust normally to the opposite sex. Since it is a constant struggle to maintain adult levels of adjustment, many types of regressive behavior are commonly seen in everyday life.

REPRESSION Repression is a mental mechanism described by Freud to explain the dynamics of unconscious mental conflict. According to Freudian theory, every child develops a conscience (superego) by internalizing moral codes imposed by society. The superego then operates by excluding (repressing) socially forbidden impulses from consciousness. To Freudians, the unconscious consists of unacceptable impulses, strivings, and painful memories which have been repressed from conscious expression and which can gain outlet only in disguised form, such as symptom formation, dreams, errors, or other types of everyday psychopathology. Repression mechanisms play an important role in the causation of the functional mental disorders, where unconscious conflict and complexes may be discovered and treated by insight-oriented psychotherapeutic methods.

RORSCHACH TEST The Rorschach test is a method for studying unconscious complexes and deep personality structure by eliciting spontaneous responses to ambiguous ink blots. The subject is presented with the ink blots, one at a time, and first simply asked to tell what they mean to him. Later the clinical psychologist administering the test questions the subject to discover which specific features of the ink blots elicited which responses. Clinical experience with the ink-blot responses of normal individuals and of clinical patients indicates that very important information is provided concerning deep personality-structure and unconscious conflicts, since these are projected into, and determine, the responses.

SCHIZOPHRENIA Formerly known as dementia praecox (mental disorder of the young), schizophrenia is one of the more serious and common psychoses, resulting in disabling mental symptoms. The term schizophrenia means splitting of the mind and is manifested by a splitting or dissociation of emotional and rational mental processes. Schizophrenia is regarded by many as a functional reaction, caused by personality inadequacies which result in inability to meet the demands of adult adjustment. The basic mechanism appears to be progressive withdrawal from contact with the real world, with regression to infantile or childish feelings and reactions.

Symptoms. No physical or organic cause has been demonstrated in schizophrenia. (Hereditary factors have, however, been suspected, since mental disorders and schizoid personality types are frequently observed among other members of the family.) Age of onset is most frequently adolescence or early adult life, but may occur as late as the middle years. Most psychiatrists now agree that schizophrenia is related to defects or weaknesses of basic personality structure caused by damaging childhood experiences, unconscious conflicts, and inability to express

instinctive—particularly sexual—drives. Several clinical types of schizophrenia have been classically described as follows:

Simple schizophrenia. This type is associated with gradual personality changes manifested by increasing withdrawal from contact with external reality and a lessened response to social demands in the form of a falling-off of emotional reactivity, interests, and ability to adjust to the community. In extreme form, the person may become completely apathetic, preoccupied with an inner mental life, and indifferent to group activity.

Hebephrenic schizophrenia. This form is characterized by silly, foolish, or inappropriate behavior; bizarre ideas reflecting an abnormal fantasy life; and frequent hallucinations, usually auditory. The patient shows a progressive disintegration of personality, becomes inaccessible to social contacts, and shows increasing immaturity and shallowness in emotional reactions, with regressive features such as failure to attend to matters of personal grooming and bowel or bladder control.

Catatonic schizophrenia. This is characterized by phases of truculence, silence, stupor, and excitement, frequently alternating suddenly. So-called "catatonic" symptoms include negativism, peculiar grimaces and gestures, and muscular immobility associated with inattention to bodily needs, refusal to eat, and neglect of toilet habits. In excited phases the patient is driven by purposeless overactivity motivated from within, which results in sleeplessness and rapid physical exhaustion. Catatonic patients have relatively hopeful prospects for cure, and the condition frequently clears up spontaneously.

Paranoid schizophrenia. This is characterized by bizarre delusional thinking combined with an otherwise relatively intact personality. The delusions, usually of persecution, apparently represent a defensive effort to "rebuild" the world in terms of the individual's own motivations, the symptoms representing a projection of inner conflict. Systematic paranoid delusions are highly resistant to treatment, and the long-term outcome is usually very poor. Paranoid schizophrenics are usually regarded as potentially dangerous because of their known tendency to take law and order into their own hands and to attempt to punish anyone they believe is persecuting them.

Treatment. Because of the difficulty in determining the exact cause of schizophrenia, treatment of the condition cannot guarantee absolute cure. A large percentage of schizophrenics have shown spontaneous improvement and may also have long periods of normality, although regression may take place. Drug therapies using tranquilizers such as chlorpromazine and trifluoperazine, and other substances, are an attempt to limit schizophrenic attacks, which can be aggressive, paranoic, or self-destructive in nature. Such drug treatment can increase the schizophrenic's contact with reality and help bring compulsive behavior under control. In combination with psychiatric therapy, which attempts to uncover the original causes of the disorder, treatment with drugs is phasing out other forms of treatment, such as electroshock therapy.

With proper treatment, usually involving both drugs and psychotherapy, and with the support of patient and understanding family and friends, many schizophrenics can improve their condition and function successfully in their community.

SELF-CONSCIOUSNESS Heightened awareness of the self is a common symptom in neurotic anxiety states. Normally, most bodily functions are "silent" in that they operate automatically on physical levels and the person is not aware of them. Most neurotic disorders, however, are associated with emotional disturbances producing symptoms on all physical and mental levels, of which the patient quickly becomes aware.

Symptoms. Classically related to self-consciousness are emotional conflict and insecurity manifested by lack of self-confidence, stage-fright, inability to perform well in public, and specific symptoms such as stuttering and stammering, inability to remember, and concentration difficulties in thinking.

Treatment. Symptoms tend to disappear spontaneously if the individual can gain some measure of success which will give him more self-confidence and emotional security. In general, success is nature's antidote for anxiety and can exercise a therapeutic influence under appropriate circumstances.

SEX INSTRUCTION AND SEX ORGAN CONCERN Concern on the part of children with sex matters and sex organs is today much more openly expressed and, by and large, given more serious thought by adults than was once the case. This holds true even with younger children. The age level of overt sex consciousness has dropped within recent times by at least two years; children now hear much more and think much more about matters of sex, hence the attention of parents must be attuned to these changes.

In almost all modern school curricula, even at grammar-school level, children are taught adequate anatomy and general physiology in relation to sex. At the same time, on the outside, they are exposed to a rather alarming amount of frank discussion among their companions—revelations which most parents completely fail to realize are going on.

There are, of course, countless books dealing with sex instruction, available to parents, unfortunately not all of them well written. The present author believes that detailed teaching regarding sex physiology, love, and related topics must be skillfully—and individually—handled, and should never be forced upon young children whose own curiosity has not yet been awakened. The child's wish to know should be the key to effective teaching. Given a little general reading, it should not be difficult for parents to determine the optimum method to use.

SHOCK TREATMENT Various methods have been used to produce artificial convulsions as a method of treating mental disorders.

In past, insulin shock therapy was used to treat many of the serious functional psychoses. The patient received a dose of insulin which lowered blood sugar and produced a subsequent convulsion. This method is, however, potentially dangerous and is no longer utilized. It was subsequently discovered that convulsions could be induced more safely and easily by administering a convulsive dose of electricity through paddles placed on one or both sides of the head. Shock treatment is generally administered to hospitalized patients but is occasionally administered on an outpatient basis to prevent recurrence of severe depressive episodes. Before the convulsion is induced, the patient is given a muscle relaxant to prevent bone fractures during the convulsive seizure, and an anesthesiologist is usually in attendance to monitor breathing and blood pressure. With proper administration, medical complications are unusual, even for patients with pre-existing physical disorders.

During early experimentation with shock treatment, beneficial effects were reported in treating all the functional psychoses. Currently, however, shock treatment is prescribed for patients with severe depressive psychosis, and occasionally to treat psychotic patients whose agitation and violence cannot be otherwise controlled. Shock treatment is generally utilized when depressive patients do not respond to antidepressant medication or when there is an imminent risk of suicide (shock treatment generally produces favorable treatment results faster than antidepressant drugs).

Although shock therapy has been criticized as a refined method of punishment or social control, many severely depressed patients have been unquestionably helped by this form of treatment. Though many patients fear electroshock treatment because of the progressive memory loss said to accompany treatment, amnesia is generally restricted to the immediate time period of the treatment itself. A typical course of electroshock treatment involves six to twelve induced seizures.

SIBLING RIVALRY   Sibling rivalry refers to competitive reactions, jealousies, and hostility developing between children in the same family. The first child in the family typically feels rejected and deprived when the birth of the second child diverts some of the attention he formerly received. Older children frequently become jealous of the youngest child who is treated as the baby in the family and gets the most attention. Middle children tend to get "lost in the shuffle" and to receive less recognition than either the oldest or the youngest child.

Sibling rivalry should be recognized as a normal phenomenon and can be minimized if the parents will attempt to prepare older children for the birth of younger ones and later attempt to divide attention equally among all children.

Intense sibling rivalry is a typical symptom of insecure children who feel deprived or rejected. Attention should be focused upon problems in the parent-child relationship or upon marital difficulties that impair parenting.

SLEEPING AND DREAMING   Studies over the past twenty years reveal that dreaming is a constant feature of normal sleep. It can be identified in the sleeping subject by picking up potentials generated by rapid eye-muscle movements (REM). REM sleep recurs approximately every 90 minutes throughout the night. Subjects awakened during the REM phase are generally able to give details of the dream. Further, if they are repeatedly awakened at the onset of REM, daytime irritability and concentration difficulties occur, and succeeding sleep is marked by greater than usual amounts of dreaming. These observations establish a role for dreaming as part of normal central nervous system functioning.

SLEEPWALKING (SOMNAMBULISM) Sleepwalking and other actions performed by a person while apparently asleep are evidence that certain brain areas become inhibited in sleep while others continue to function. This disorder typically occurs in middle to late childhood. During sleepwalking, the child arises from bed and walks about, appearing unresponsive during the episode, and experiencing amnesia for the episode upon awakening. In a related disorder Pavor Nocturnus or Sleep Terror Disorder, the child abruptly awakens after being asleep for a short period of time; there are signs of extreme anxiety present, and the child is usually unresponsive to efforts to calm him. Epileptic seizures arising during sleep may occasionally occur with a similar picture.

In any event, both sleepwalking and sleep terror disorders are generally innocuous and usually disappear in adolescence.

SOCIOPATHIC REACTIONS   These are personality states formerly referred to as moral imbecility or as psychopathic personality and characterized by a wide range of antisocial behavior combined with an otherwise relatively intact personality.

Symptoms. The sociopath tries to "take"

what people normally have to earn. Sociopaths show a lifetime history of lying, stealing, fraud, deceit, sexual promiscuity, alcoholism, and general personal irresponsibility—usually not corrected by punishment or experience.

Sociopathic reactions are not hereditary, since it is rare for more than one case to appear in a family. There is no evidence of underlying organic disease, except that a small percentage of cases shows abnormal brain waves, possibly indicating an underlying diffuse brain disease. Most sociopathic reactions appear to be learned, as various types of personal and social conditioning factors reinforce sociopathic tendencies. Thus, some particularly attractive children tend to be spoiled by parents, teachers, and other adults, all of whom allow the child to get his own way and escape normal punishment and corrective measures. Sociopaths in any community tend to flock together, teaching each other new methods of "getting away with murder" and encouraging each other in subtle ways to prey on the rest of the population.

Treatment. To date, only a few states have developed special resources for the treatment of sociopaths, who properly belong neither in prison, since their trouble is psychological, nor in mental hospitals, since they are not mentally ill in the ordinary sense of the term. Only a few psychiatrists have claimed much success in treating sociopathic reactions. Contrary to former opinion, which maintained that such cases did not show any normal anxiety or ability to learn from experience, the sociopath is highly adept at learning methods of swindling the public and of avoiding punishment.

Most sociopaths show improvement only when they can be led to recognize that their activities are too self-defeating and that the cost in mental anguish is not worth the gains obtained.

Many young people who are regarded as "black sheep" in early life tend to become more law-abiding as increasing age and experience result in a better understanding of themselves and of the costs of their anti-social behavior. One of the great psychiatric problems of the future is to develop special methods and resources in the community for diagnosing and treating young sociopaths before such patterns become too deeply ingrained.

SPLIT PERSONALITY   Cases of multiple personality disorder are typically described as following major childhood traumas, particularly sexual or physical abuse. Multiple personality may be explained psychologically as a dissociative reaction in which events triggering painful impulses or feelings linked to earlier traumas struggle for expression, and alternately gain outlet in the form of apparently incompatible personality reactions.

Symptoms. In states of multiple personality the same person may alternately act out two or more different personalities, enacting complex behavioral patterns while under different identities, calling himself by different names and behaving like different people. The patient may be amnesic for events enacted by one or more of the different personalities.

Treatment. The preferred treatment is long-term psychotherapy in an effort to establish a safe and protective setting which allows for the emergence of the different personality types. Sometimes hypnosis may be used in an effort to gain further understanding of the patient's childhood traumas.

STAMMERING AND STUTTERING
Stammering is hesitant, spasmodic speech with interruptions in which no sound is produced. It was once regarded as neurotic in origin, with strong emotional and environmental influences, but it is now recognized that an organic base in speech processing may be involved. Stuttering is a speech disorder whose chief feature is the repetition of certain consonant sounds in rapid succession. It is also known as "logoclonia." Stuttering is also used synonymously with stammering.

Treatment. Current therapy is twofold: speech correction and psychotherapy. In the former, the accent is on slowness. That is, the subject is encouraged to speak in an exaggerated and deliberate fashion at first, to the point of breaking words down to individual syllables; later, sentences are marked by prolonged spacing of words.

STRESS   In the course of athletic activity or work, the body may be subjected to physical forces that strain muscles, internal organs, bones, and joints. The body may also have its normal metabolic functioning and internal physiology disrupted by sickness, weather changes, injury, and emotional tension. All such influences can be considered forms of stress.

When stress is experienced for prolonged periods, or when the stress is sudden and overwhelming, disorders such as ulcer, asthma, migraine, colitis, constipation, cardiac dysfunction, and hypertension may result. Mental instability leading to schizophrenia may also be induced by physical or emotional stress.

The body possesses mechanisms that attempt to deal with stress. In preparation for stressful situations the adrenal glands produce the hormones epinephrine and norepinephrine, which act to increase cardiac activity, as well as to send an increased blood supply to muscle tissue and to promote the use of stored glucose. When stress occurs over an extended period of time, the body's energy reserves may be extended and the stress-triggered mechanisms may become less responsive. An individual's physical and mental health is then in jeopardy. Stress from various causes may also affect the fertility of both men and women.

Studies concerning "life events" that cause the most stress indicate that loss of a spouse or other family member, imprisonment, childbirth, personal injury, divorce, and unemployment are among the most stressful situations individuals can encounter. Urban life is also often associated with a lifestyle that is stressful—including physical stresses connected with air and noise pollution and the psychological stresses of career competition, traffic congestion, and anxiety about one's personal safety.

Maintaining regular exercise and sleep habits and taking vacations are known to alleviate the fatigue of some forms of stress. Important, too, is the discovery of the true cause of physical and emotional stress, with treatment of the cause, rather than merely focusing on the symptoms. Psychiatric counseling and a complete physical examination may uncover the true origin of undue stress.

TEMPER TANTRUMS   Tantrums are infantile uncontrolled rage reactions used to terrorize the environment and get one's own way. Every child learns early to control adults by crying or screaming in rage to get what it wants. Once it learns that temper tantrums are successful in controlling the environment, the child tends to organize these into a terroristic lifestyle in which the child constantly intimidates others to gain his own ends. Temper tantrums have become more common with the advent of progressive methods of education, the child being permitted and encouraged to express himself in all situations. The over-permissive parent tends to allow the young child early to escape from discipline, using temper tantrums and other undesirable behavior in unhealthy ways.

Treatment. Temper tantrums are more easily prevented than controlled once the pattern has been established. When the child first develops a tantrum, he should not be given his own way or allowed to acquire any secondary gains. Many parents make their first mistake in attempting to argue or reason with the child, who is out of emotional control; such methods are rarely effective. The child should be handled quietly but firmly, being isolated until he quiets down and is willing to listen to reason again. Above all, the parent should keep control of his own emotions and not allow himself to shout at the child or otherwise lose control of his or her own behavior.

TENSION SYMPTOMS   States of emotional excitability tend to be expressed in muscular contractions in all systems of the body and are experienced as unpleasant tension symptoms. In abnormal metabolic states such as hyperthyroidism, heightened metabolism in all body systems causes feelings of generalized tension.

Symptoms. Very similar symptoms occur in psychoneurotic anxiety states and anger reactions, in which an over-secretion of adrenalin causes generalized body tension. In situations of acute emotional reaction such as combat fatigue or war neurosis, the person may complain of a generalized unpleasant tension state in such words as, "I feel as if I'm going to explode, as if I'm going to blow my stack."

Localized tension states may reflect muscular contractions in any of the specific body systems. Tension headaches may be caused by spasm of the temporal or occipital muscles at the sides or back of the head. Tension in the facial musculature causes frowning or grimacing. Spasm of the throat and swallowing muscles causes the symptom of a lump in the throat (globus hystericus), with difficulties in swallowing. Spasm of the coronary arteries of the heart causes anginal chest pains and feelings of pressure in the chest; spasms of the diaphragm cause interference with breathing and sighing respirations; and spasms of the stomach or intestinal musculature cause quivering sensations ("butterflies in the stomach") or abdominal cramps. Tension in the arms, legs, and bodily musculature also frequently occurs in anxiety states as a symptom of nervousness.

Treatment. Since most tension symptoms are only symptomatic of underlying states of emotional excitement or conflict, basic treatment is to remove such causes of deep underlying conflict. However, much symptomatic relief can be achieved by learning methods of progressive muscular relaxation. This involves identifying specific muscular contractions and then inhibiting them voluntarily.

The tense person may discover that he is frowning, grinding his teeth, clenching his hands, and holding himself stiffly. By recognizing these tensions individually, it is possible for him to relax them one by one until a state of complete relaxation is attained.

Much tension can be prevented by learning to take a calm, tolerant attitude toward life, accepting what cannot be changed and attempting only what is possible. It is important to take life's problems and frustrations in stride, rather than overreacting emotionally in ways which progressively build up tension.

In severe anxiety, tension states in which upset emotions and bodily tensions have gotten completely out of control, it may be necessary to use tranquilizing drugs or sedatives to quiet the patient sufficiently so that psychotherapeutic methods can be used. In extreme cases it may be necessary to remove the person from a disturbing environment for a short period of hospitalization in order to re-achieve control.

Miscellaneous Health Conditions

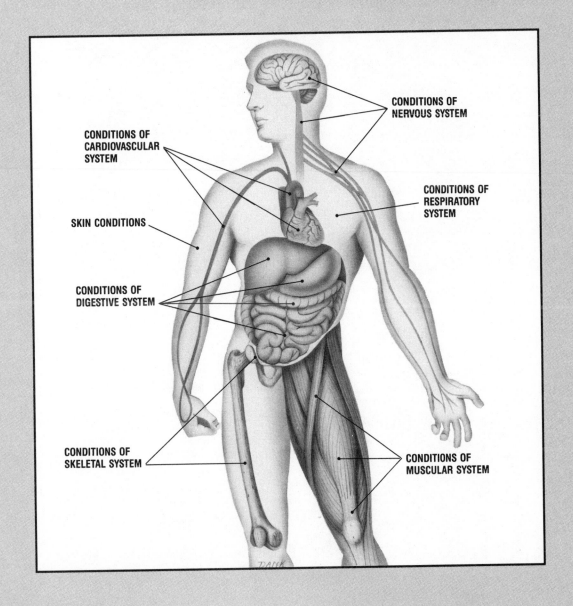

CONDITIONS OF
NERVOUS SYSTEM

CONDITIONS OF
CARDIOVASCULAR
SYSTEM

CONDITIONS OF
RESPIRATORY
SYSTEM

SKIN CONDITIONS

CONDITIONS OF
DIGESTIVE SYSTEM

CONDITIONS OF
SKELETAL SYSTEM

CONDITIONS OF
MUSCULAR SYSTEM

There are certain disorders, impairments, or departures from good health which do not fit into a neatly categorized system. Some are quite common; others occur rarely. Proper identification of symptoms is crucial in determining possible treatment.

This section concerns those topics which fall into a miscellaneous grouping. See also the questions on disagreeable breath (Q-5); lightheadedness (Q-32); difficulties in sleeping (Q-36) in the section QUESTIONS AND ANSWERS ABOUT COMMON SYMPTOMS.

The following is a list of terms identified in this section:

AUTOIMMUNE DISEASE
BENDS, THE (CAISSON DISEASE)
CYSTIC FIBROSIS
DIABETES, BRONZED
    (HEMOCHROMATOSIS)
DIABETES MELLITUS (SUGAR
    DIABETES)
DOWN SYNDROME
DUPUYTREN'S CONTRACTURE
ELEPHANTIASIS
FUNGI
GEOGRAPHIC TONGUE
GLOSSITIS
INGROWING TOENAIL
INSULIN
INSULIN SHOCK
JAUNDICE
LEPROSY (HANSEN'S DISEASE)
LITHIASES

LOW SALT SYNDROME
MEDICAL QUACKERY
MUSHROOM POISONING
OCCUPATIONAL DISEASE
PILONIDAL CYST
PINEAL GLAND
PROLAPSE
PYREXIA
ST. VITUS' DANCE (SYDENHAM'S
    CHOREA)
SCLERODERMA, DIFFUSE SYSTEMIC
SCLERODERMA, LOCALIZED (MORPHEA)
SMOKING
SPLEEN, DISORDERS OF THE
STONES (CALCULI)
SYNDROME
"TONGUE-TIE"
TRANSPLANTATION
WITHDRAWAL SYNDROME

AUTOIMMUNE DISEASE This is a general term for a wide variety of disorders that have in common the body's propensity to "attack" itself. The individual's immune system interprets incorrectly that a part of itself is foreign and attempts to destroy it. In the process, the individual becomes ill. Some of the diseases that are considered to be of autoimmune origin include diabetes mellitus, lupus erythematosus, multiple sclerosis, and some forms of Addison's disease. (*See* INDEX for these topics.)

BENDS, THE (CAISSON DISEASE) The bends occurs among divers and those who work under high air pressure in caissons (air-tight boxes for working on river bottoms). Unless the change from high to lower (normal) surface pressure is gradual, an individual may develop paralysis, also known as "diver's paralysis."

Symptoms. Indications of caisson disease do not manifest themselves until the subject has emerged into normal air pressure at which time he complains of joint pains; these are rapidly followed by paralysis, dizziness, headache, vomiting, confusion, and convulsions. In severe cases, breathing decreases and coma ensues. Patients frequently recover, but some of them may remain paralyzed for life.

Treatment. Prevention is the best treatment. Those who apply for work involving high air pressure environment must pass rigorous physical examinations. Emergence from high pressure areas should be through air locks in which the pressure is gradually reduced.

CYSTIC FIBROSIS This is a congenital, hereditary condition which is manifested by chronic bronchitis; persistent, large and very smelly stools; and growth failure—all with variable degrees of severity in different cases. In some the stool symptoms border on diarrhea and the lungs are affected only minimally. In others it may be just the reverse; the bronchitis is so bad that multiple abscesses and scar tissue form in the lungs, causing backpressure in the right side of the heart, heart-failure, and even death.

The condition is not too difficult to diagnose if suspected. A sample of the sweat is analyzed to determine the salt concentration; in cystic fibrosis this is usually high, and patients therefore do poorly in hot climates.

Treatment. Treatment can only be directed toward maintaining good nutrition (with digestive enzymes) and keeping the chronic bronchitis under control with antibiotics.

DIABETES, BRONZED (HEMOCHROMATOSIS) This is a rare disorder manifested by deposits of hemosiderin (an iron-protein compound found in all body tissues and possibly the result of decomposition of hemoglobin, the coloring element of blood). Hemochromatosis most often occurs in the liver and the pancreas. The cause is unknown; it is probably due to a deficiency in iron metabolism.

Symptoms. Hemochromatosis most often afflicts elderly males, three-quarters of whom show the classical signs of diabetes, bronzing of the skin, and cirrhosis of the liver. Other manifestations include atrophy (shrinkage) of the testicles, enlargement of the liver, and the formation of fibrous tissue in the heart muscle. Laboratory examination of the blood and/or microscopic study of a skin specimen determine the diagnosis.

Treatment. To prevent the building up of iron deposits in the tissues, weekly bleeding (usually a pint) of the patient is required until the iron in the blood serum is depleted.

DIABETES MELLITUS (SUGAR DIABETES) Diabetes mellitus occurs among all age groups, but most commonly makes its appearance between the ages of forty and sixty. Studies indicate that about 10 percent of those over age sixty have diabetes mellitus. Twice as many women as men have the condition. In the mid-1980's diabetes mellitus caused more than 26,000 deaths annually.

Equally significant is the mortality that diabetes produces as a contributory cause. For example diabetes aggravates atherosclerosis. It has been calculated that if diabetes could be eliminated a sixty-five year old diabetic would have 7.9 years added to his or her lifespan.

The diabetic person is not able to produce or regulate the hormone insulin, which is produced in the pancreas. Insulin is necessary to control the level of glucose (a type of sugar) in the blood. If glucose is not properly assimilated by the body, it will accumulate in the blood and tissues and be passed out of the body in the urine. This results in the loss of nutrients and energy the body needs in order to carry out basic activities.

There are two major categories of diabetes mellitus. Juvenile-onset diabetes appears in children or young adults and requires regular injections of insulin and strict dietary controls so that proper blood glucose levels are maintained. Juvenile diabetics have increased risk of developing degenerative changes and diseases of the eye and kidneys.

Adult-onset diabetes is generally less severe than juvenile diabetes. Sometimes the symptoms are so subtle the condition is overlooked. Usually adult-onset diabetes can be controlled with dietary restrictions alone or with added drug therapy. For adults, diabetes means a greater risk of eye disorders, such as cataracts, and greater susceptibility to infection, among other health problems.

Diagnosis of diabetes is made by the detection of sugar in the urine and abnormal amounts of it in the blood. It should be recognized that there is a normal level of sugar in the blood at all times, a level that varies somewhat, depending on the time of day and length of time after a meal. Usually, however, there should be no sugar in the urine. Diabetics may test for urine sugar by simple methods such as noting a color change when a piece of chemically impregnated paper is dipped into the urine. In some instances a sugar-tolerance test is performed in which the patient is given a measured amount of glucose solution, followed by analysis of blood and urine sugar concentrations at intervals of several hours. A number of other tests have been developed to detect diabetes in questionable cases.

Symptoms. The diabetic who is taking appropriate treatment should not normally feel ill. When treatment is inadequate, or when the initiation of the disease is sudden, acidosis and coma may result. This is a potentially serious condition and must be treated at once. It may be marked by a feeling of dullness and fatigue followed by nausea and vomiting. The senses become dulled and the patient becomes progressively more stuporous. Usually this condition is preceded by increased thirst together with increased urine output, which causes loss of large amounts of body fluids and minerals making the patient dehydrated. There is also a characteristic deep breathing described as "air hunger," as a result of the body's attempt to restore a normal balance of acids and bases.

Important late complications of diabetes are found chiefly in the eyes, kidneys, and blood vessels. The eyes may be afflicted by changes in the retina or by cataracts. If these problems are severe enough, blindness may result. Small blood vessels in the kidneys may also suffer damage, causing the kidneys to shrivel and decrease their ability to remove poisons from the circulation. Arteries may become narrower and calcium deposits may build up. This may lead to clotting in the arteries of the brain, thus producing strokes; and to the complete stoppage of arteries in the lower extremities, producing gangrene.

In children the onset of diabetes may occur suddenly with extreme thirst and increased output of urine. Itching in the genital region or elsewhere may also occur. One of the most common precursors of diabetes in adults is obesity. It is recommended that obese adults should have their urine checked for sugar at least yearly after the age of forty.

Treatment. Treatment of diabetes for the past fifty years has been primarily with insulin. During the past thirty years, however, substances have been developed that can be taken by mouth for patients with mild diabetes to lower the blood sugar and spare the pancreas. Attempts are also being made to manufacture synthetic insulin incorporating the techniques of genetic engineering. Currently insulin is processed from pork and beef pancreases. In any case, because the body is not able to manufacture insulin and vary its concentration, it is vital that the patient maintain a carefully regulated diet.

The balance of carbohydrates, proteins, and fats must be kept within close limits, and meals should be taken at regular intervals; each individual's dietary prescription should be worked out by the physician. The obese diabetic is put on a weight-reduction program. Exercise is carefully regulated and infections are carefully avoided. For older diabetics care of the feet is especially important. Corns and calluses should be cared for by someone acquainted with the diabetic's tendency to develop infections and gangrene. Proper footwear should be worn to prevent the development of corns, calluses, and ingrown nails.

An important contribution to treatment has been the invention of a small portable device with which a diabetic can monitor his or her blood sugar. A drop of blood from a finger is placed on a specially prepared tape and a color change proportional to the blood sugar can be read visually or by a reflectance meter which gives a readout. When close monitoring is necessary, the procedure can be performed several times daily and changes in insulin or medication made appropriately.

DOWN SYNDROME "Down syndrome" and "trisomy 21," is a congenital condition caused by faulty chromosome behavior in the fertilized human egg. The usual chromosome inventory for humans is 23 pairs. The Down syndrome individual, however, has an extra chromosome, creating a total of 47, instead of the normal 46. This abnormality produces an individual characterized by a broad face, stubby fingers, and upward-slanting eyes, plus various degrees of mental retardation and vulnerability to infection. Dwarfism, poor neuromuscular coordination, and congenital heart damage are also possible. Because of the genetic nature of the condition, there is no cure. Close to half of all Down syndrome children die before adulthood, often because of their susceptibility to lung and intestinal infections.

The incidence of Down syndrome is about one in every 600 births. However, as the age of the mother increases, the chances of a Down syndrome child also increase. For women over the age of forty-five the incidence rises to about one in every forty births.

Down syndrome children are usually pleasant and affectionate, as well as easily managed; but although they are docile, they can be a source of strain in the family because of their retardation. Even in adulthood, the average mental age is about eight years. However, cases have been documented showing that Down syndrome children are capable of developing vastly improved intellects when given increased parental attention, patience, and encouragement. In cases where retardation or other congenital defects are severe, or when financial requirements for medical care cannot be met, parents may decide to institutionalize their Down syndrome child.

For some parents who must deal with the birth of a Down syndrome child, guilt feelings and self-recrimination must be overcome. Consultation with one's physician and with other parents of mentally impaired children will help. If the decision is made to rear the child, then all family members should encourage the child to develop as much as he or she possibly can. Families should be aware that there is no treatment, contrary to the claims of unscrupulous hucksters, that transforms an afflicted child into a completely normal one. Parental patience, love, and encouragement are possibly the most appropriate therapy.

Because the risk of having an afflicted child greatly increases if the mother is over thirty-five, or if a family history of the condition exists, physicians may advise couples to obtain genetic counseling or, if the woman is pregnant, to undergo amniocentesis to determine the likelihood of producing a Down syndrome child.

DUPUYTREN'S CONTRACTURE This disorder, first described by the French surgeon, Dupuytren, occurs most often in aging Caucasian males. Benign tumors form in the palm of the hands. Under the microscope they appear as dense groups of a scar-like tissue and like a scar tend to pull on the adjacent tissues. This may lead to contraction of tendons going to fingers, most often the middle and ring fingers. It becomes impossible to straighten out the affected fingers and varying degrees of disability result. Various surgical procedures have been developed to restore freedom of motion. The condition is generally bilateral but may be much less noticeable in one hand than in the other. The condition is said to be more common in patients with such diseases as diabetes, epilepsy and alcoholism. Dupuytren's contracture may also be found in individuals free of any disorders. Its fundamental cause remains unknown.

ELEPHANTIASIS This is a condition most often seen in the legs, which are markedly enlarged due to excessive subcutaneous (beneath the skin) fluid and thickening of the tissues. There is obliteration of normal ankle and calf contours, giving the impression of elephant legs. The fundamental cause is blockage of the flow of lymph. In temperate and colder regions the disfigurement is usually due to a developmental defect present at birth (Milroy's disease). In other parts of the world the cause may be parasitic blockage of the lymphatics. However, elephantiasis may be seen after multiple attacks of erysipelas, a streptococcal infection of the skin and lymph vessels, and in other chronic infections involving the lymphatics.

FUNGI Of the thousands of varieties of fungi, a few are found on the cutaneous surface and cause no disease; even fewer produce infection of the skin (superficial mycosis) and of internal organs (deep mycosis). Fungi are the subject of many and diverse types of classification, according to their morphology, growth habits, and geographic distribution. In their ability to be provocative of disease, they can be divided into three groups: those capable of digesting skin keratin and using it for growth, and therefore capable of producing disease of destruction (ringworm of the hair and nails) or of allergic sensitization (ringworm of the groin and other skin sites); those incapable of digesting keratin and therefore unable to infect, except very superficially (tinea versicolor, erythrasma); and those capable of invading the skin and other organs and causing diseases the common feature of which is a fungating lesion or mass known as a granuloma (blastomycosis, sporotrichosis, histoplasmosis, coccidioidomycosis).

In addition to causing disease by invasion and growth, fungi are a common cause of allergic reactions of the respiratory tract, being responsible for a significant incidence of asthmatic attacks. The importance of fungi as a cause of disease depends to some degree on the geographic distribution of the organisms and their habits of growth, which are largely governed by climate, flora, geology, etc. However, the susceptibility (or resistance) of the individual host is undoubtedly the determining factor in the complexity of influences giving rise to disease. This has been strikingly demonstrated in this era of chemotherapy and of AIDS, both of which lead to an immunocompromised state. In both, severe systemic infections with fungi often occur.

GEOGRAPHIC TONGUE Frequently noted and thought to be of no importance is the changing appearance of the tongue due to temporary loss of papillae (tongue ridges) in areas of varying size and shape. The areas containing normal papillae seem to be enlarged and give the impression of being the mountain ridges of a bas-relief map. Changes in the sites of involvement result in new configurations of the "ridges" and "valleys." There are usually no associated symptoms, and there is no significance to either the change in appearance or the persistence of the condition. Geographic tongue exists as a medical oddity.

GLOSSITIS Inflammatory conditions of the tongue may result from bacterial infections, yeast-like infections (thrush), and from certain nutritional deficiencies. Because of the rich blood supply to the tongue, bacterial infections are uncommon in otherwise healthy individuals. Rarely, vitamin deficiencies can cause glossitis; specific replacement therapy will usually give dramatic results. Pernicious anemia may be accompanied by glossitis which is characterized by a disappearance of the papillae and results in a smooth shiny tongue. Such glossitis may be the first symptom of this serious condition.

INGROWING TOENAIL Ingrowing toenail occurs almost exclusively in the great toe. It is usually due to poorly fitting footwear. In the early stages, the form of the nail is unaltered, but the soft parts of the pulp are crowded over on its edge. Careless trimming of the nail on the edge predisposes to inflammation and to ulceration. Later, the edge of the nail becomes folded under, and by pressure on the pulp, aggravates the condition.

If treatment is continued for a sufficient time, a cure usually may be produced by keeping the parts free from pressure and by separating the overhanging skin from the nail either with a little cotton stuffed under the nail or by drawing the skin aside with adhesive tape, while the ulcer is treated with local antibiotic powder or ointment. The nail should be cut square across the top, and never trimmed down its sides. If a rapid cure is desired, the doctor can surgically remove the skin on the side of the nail affected (on both sides if necessary) by splitting the nail and grasping the portion to be removed by forceps.

INSULIN Insulin is a hormone necessary for the normal metabolism of sugar (carbohydrate). It is produced by "beta cells" present in a region of the pancreas known as the islets of Langerhans. Banting and Best, more than sixty years ago, first showed that the hormone (a protein) was necessary in metabolizing the blood sugar and tissue glucose. The disease diabetes mellitus is due to inadequate secretion of insulin, either in absolute amounts or relative to the body's needs. There is some evidence that many diabetics do indeed produce insulin, but that it is "bound," or in other ways ineffective.

Insulin consists of two long chains of amino acids linked together by sulfur-containing bridges, and the exact sequence of the constituent amino-acids has been determined. As a protein, insulin is digested and rendered ineffective if given by mouth and must therefore be injected. Insulin has been obtained from the pancreas commercially, from both beef and pork sources. More recently human insulin has been manufactured in the laboratory by recombinant DNA technology.

A number of modifications of the insulin molecule have been made so that its action may be prolonged, thus avoiding the need for multiple daily injections. The physician today has a choice of several insulins, permitting fine adjustments of dosage for the varying individual needs of the patient. Among the insulins now available are protamine zinc insulin, NPH (isophane), lente, semilente, ultralente, globin zinc, as well as unmodified "regular" insulin. Also mixtures of the different insulins can be made either by the patient or premixed often in combination of 30 percent regular insulin and 70 percent longer acting insulin. (See the table below.)

The dosage must be tailored for the individual patient and will vary from time to time, depending on the patient's health, weight, age, the presence of pregnancy or infections, the type of diet, and exercise. The dosage schedule must be regulated by the physician because an overdose of insulin leads to hypoglycemia (insulin shock) and inadequate dosage results in poor diabetic control. In rare cases, allergy or resistance (the latter necessitating ever higher and excessive doses) has been reported.

When insulin is given to a diabetic it enhances the entry of glucose into tissue cells, enhances the burning oxidation of glucose to carbon dioxide and water; increases the storage of glucose as glycogen in the liver; and promotes the formation of fatty acids from glucose. Insulin is essential for normal protein metabolism. A deficiency or lack of insulin therefore results in many widespread metabolic defects.

A number of oral drugs have been introduced which are useful for some diabetics. They probably act by stimulating the diabetic pancreas to produce more insulin. However, not every diabetic responds to these agents, and in times of stress (such as after injury or during illness or surgery) insulin is the preferred agent.

INSULIN SHOCK Insulin shock refers to an abnormally high concentration of insulin in the blood. It frequently occurs when too much insulin is administered to a diabetic, or if too little food is taken with a regular dose of insulin. The excess insulin then lowers the blood sugar level and the symptoms of a severe hypoglycemic attack may result. In psychiatry, insulin shock refers to a mode of treatment for certain psychoses, chiefly schizophrenia which has largely been replaced by electro-convulsive treatment (ECT).

Symptoms. Insulin shock may be signaled by sudden weakness, tremors, and sweating. Vomiting is rare, although there may be some drooling from the mouth. Respiration and blood pressure are usually normal, and the pulse is full and bounding. The hands may tremble, and in the late stages convulsive seizures and unconsciousness may occur. In a typical case of hypoglycemia there will be no sugar in the urine. (All of the features mentioned above differ from those seen in diabetic coma, caused by ketoacidosis, a condition produced by insufficient insulin.)

Treatment. In a mild case of insulin shock, a carbohydrate such as sugar or candy may be given. A rapid improvement should result. In more serious cases it is preferable to administer a glucose solution by injection. This may be required if the individual is unconscious. Another possible treatment consists of the administration of glucagon, a hormone from the pancreas that raises blood sugar. This can be

SOME INSULINS AND THEIR ACTIONS

	Onset	Peak Action	Duration of Action
Regular insulin	30 min.	2-4 hrs.	4-6 hrs.
NPH insulin	1-2 hrs.	6-12 hrs.	18-26 hrs.
Insulin-zinc suspensions			
Lente	1-3 hrs.	6-12 hrs.	18-26 hrs.
Semilente	1-2 hrs.	3-8 hrs.	10-16 hrs.
Ultralente	4-6 hrs.	12-24 hrs.	28-36 hrs.
Protamine zinc insulin	4-6 hrs.	12-24 hrs.	24-36 hrs.

injected under the skin, in the same way as insulin.

It is important that the diabetic be taught to recognize the symptoms of insulin shock. Sugar or glucose may be carried at all times and taken if blurred vision or sudden weakness or dizziness occurs.

An identification card, stating that the patient has diabetes and takes insulin, will be helpful in case of an accident or a severe hypoglycemic reaction. Young people and children who are diabetic should be encouraged to wear a medical alert bracelet as they often do not carry identification.

JAUNDICE   Jaundice results from the discoloration of tissues and body-fluids by bile pigment. There is a characteristic yellow color to the skin and mucous membranes. In dark-skinned individuals, the jaundice may not be readily apparent but is obvious in the white of the eyes. Occasionally, severe jaundice may cause a peculiar itching. This is usually seen in the obstructive type.

There are two major causes of jaundice: first is due to inability of the liver to dispose of the bile pigment which normally circulates in the blood—either because of increased formation of this pigment, or because of inability of the liver to secrete it into the bile (due to disease or liver-cell damage as seen in hepatitis); and the second results from a backing-up of the bile into the bloodstream due to obstruction on the bile-collecting system (obstructive jaundice). The obstruction may occur in the small canals of the liver itself, or in the bile ducts. An impacted gallstone in the bile ducts or acute inflammation of the gallbladder are the two most common causes of this type of jaundice. Tumors in the region may also cause obstructive jaundice.

Treatment. Deep painless jaundice demands thorough investigation, as tumors are common causes. The bile-staining does not in itself cause any particular harm, and after the cause has been relieved the jaundice will gradually fade.

LEPROSY   (HANSEN'S   DISEASE)
Known for over 2,000 years, leprosy is a disease of high incidence in the tropics, but is also present in many countries of the temperate zone. In the continental United States lep-rosy has been contracted occasionally in the southern-most states (Florida, Texas, Louisiana, and Southern California). Cases reported elsewhere in the United States have almost always been contracted in a tropical or sub-tropical area.

Commonly acquired in childhood and adolescence by natives of those areas of the world in which the disease is endemic, it is usually also acquired by adults whose childhood was spent in non-leprosy areas. Both sexes are affected, though males appear to be more susceptible to the acute (lepromatous) type.

The mode of transmission of the causative organism, *Mycobacterium leprae* (Hansen's bacillus), is probably through the skin or mucous membranes of the nose or throat. What determines the acceptance of the disease by an exposed person, or the type of disease acquired, is not known. Classification of the disease is often difficult, many cases belonging to an indeterminate or borderline group. More concise are the lepromatous (acute, infectious) and tuberculoid (usually non-infectious, less actively progressive) types.

Symptoms. These vary greatly, depending on the type and stage of the disease. Thickening of the skin, either in the form of small nodules or large plaques, or as a diffuse generalized condition, is common to all forms of the disease—as is involvement of the mucous membrane and septum of the nose. Ulceration, especially of the mucous membranes, produces great deformity and interferes with function. Nerve involvement results in loss of sensation and loss of sweating of the area, and finally in actual atrophy and absorption of tissue (especially of the fingers and toes).

Treatment. The heretofore universally used chaulmoogra oil has been replaced with several drugs often used in combination (sulfones, para-aminosalicylate, rifampin). The cortisone drugs are probably very effective in some types and stages of the disease, and are especially useful for at least temporary relief in the acute lesions of the eye and in the lesions based on an acute allergic response.

LITHIASES   Lithiasis is the formation of stones in an organ of the body. Specific types include gallbladder stones (cholelithiasis), and kidney stones (nephrolithiasis). Cholelithiasis is usually due to biochemical abnormality in the bile production. Kidney stones are caused by increases in calcium or urate or xanthine (a nitrogen compound). Stones, regardless of where they are located, can be quite painful.

Treatment. Depending on the severity, treatment includes medications, application of ultrasound waves to break up the stones or surgery. A recurrence of new stones is not unusual. (*See also* GALLSTONES in the section GASTROINTESTINAL CONDITIONS.)

LOW SALT SYNDROME   Also referred to as heat exhaustion, low salt syndrome is caused by the excessive loss of salt, usually during hot weather when a person is engaged in vigorous or prolonged exercise. Typically the person feels weak, has abdominal cramping, and is flushed.

Treatment. Treatment consists of replenishing both salt and water, moving to a cool location, and resting.

MEDICAL QUACKERY   Although everyone is presumably against quackery, it is by no means a dying business; its cost to the American people is estimated to be in excess of one billion dollars a year. This figure includes the purchase of some surprising items as well as some old "stand-bys." The American Medical Association believes, for instance, that most Americans buy vitamin pills not because they actually believe their diet requires this supplementation, but only in response to advertising which convinces them that the daily cost is so low that it is economical to be "on the safe side."

Of course, the "cures" for arthritis and muscular rheumatism—for which no true cures exist as yet—fall in a class of worthless medications second to none; nevertheless, they alone cost many hundreds of millions of dollars a year.

Surprisingly, the money spent on other false "cure-alls" is a comparatively small amount. In this category fall the more brazen quacks who appeal to those people who, for one reason or another, must surely have missed the point of all their high school biology and chemistry classes: such "cure-all quacks" peddle brass bracelets, magnets, boxes with colored lights, packages with bits of radio-active ores, and—more recently—concentrated sea-water plants.

In addition to this group there are, of course, the cancer-cure peddlers. The only cheery word in this otherwise dismal and dirty business is the A.M.A.'s opinion that most of the money is spent by people who do not really have cancer, but only imagine they do. Thus the source of testimonials—the quack's so-called "proof" of effectiveness—are claims of recovery from a non-existent ailment brought about by nonsense medicine. Persons with cancer not cured by surgery, radiation or chemotherapy will not be cured by carrot extracts, laetrile, macrobiotics, or exotic oriental plants. A moment's reflection should convince any adult that a true cancer cure would not need to be peddled—there is infinitely too much demand for it. The scramble for a cancer cure is now so universal that almost anything with even the faintest possibility of effectiveness is snapped up by industrial or government laboratories for evaluation.

But should the individual be so temporarily foolish as to seek the advice of a quack, let him immediately regain his senses if the quack offers testimonials as proof of effectiveness—especially if the quack laments the fact that "big-shot" doctors refuse to recognize him or his cancer cure. The quack really hasn't a leg to stand on; he depends upon his victims' ignorance of facts available to any reader of the daily newspaper.

The quack is dangerous because he may deprive his customers of proper medical care, especially in cases where time is of importance. Since he works on a personal basis, the quack's services are usually expensive. His operations are never advertised nationally, and as a result, he is actually difficult to track down, and even more difficult to convict. Unfortunately, conviction carries no heavy penalties and is not a real deterrent. More than any other single factor, it is probably the justified harassment by Federal agencies that has served to keep the quackery business down to its present level.

The American Medical Association has suggested that laws with stricter penalties for unlicensed practice of medicine be passed and enforced as a means of dealing with authentic quacks; the Food and Drug Administration

(FDA) has added to this a law requiring proof of the effectiveness of a drug before it can be released for public use and marketed. So it is that the burden of proof of effectiveness now rests with the individual who administers or sells a drug. In the absence of such proof, its sale becomes illegal, thus permitting the FDA to prosecute on this basis—a much easier and potentially more successful course of action, according to the FDA itself.

MUSHROOM POISONING Mushroom, or toadstool, poisoning is commonly due to consumption of the species of mushroom (toadstool) known as *Amanita muscaria.*

Symptoms. Symptoms begin within a few minutes to two hours after eating. There is formation of tears, salivation, sweating, vomiting, abdominal cramps, diarrhea, thirst, dizziness, confusion, collapse, and sometimes coma and convulsions.

In the form of mushroom poisoning produced by *Amanita phalloides* and related species, symptoms occur after six to fifteen hours and are announced by the sudden onset of abdominal pain, nausea, vomiting, and diarrhea. There is often blood in the stools and dehydration may be extreme. Jaundice due to liver damage follows in a few days. The liver itself is enlarged, the pulse is rapid, the blood pressure falls, and the temperature is below normal.

Treatment. In cases of poisoning from *A. muscaria,* atropine is a specific antagonist of nervous-system overstimulation. Where *A. phalloides* is the cause, a high carbohydrate intake—some via intravenous injection—is indicated to prevent severe liver damage.

OCCUPATIONAL DISEASE The term refers to an illness definitely traceable to exposure to work related materials. The risk of disease may be almost immediate or delayed many years after the employee has left the job. Lung disease in the form of a highly malignant cancer is seen in asbestos workers as long as 30 years after the prolonged exposure. A more benign and immediate illness is the eye strain and accompanying headache experienced after working many hours in front of a computer.

PILONIDAL CYST A pilonidal cyst is a result of congenital folding-under of tissues which are normally at the surface. As a result, skin-like structures—including hair and epithelial cells—are enclosed within a cyst located at the base of the spine. After repeated irritation, the area may become inflamed and cause a draining abscess.

Pilonidal cysts are most commonly seen in young males, particularly those who have more than average amounts of hair on the body.

Symptoms. The symptoms of this type of cyst are pain and tenderness at the base of the spine and repeated episodes of pus drainage.

Treatment. In chronic cases of pilonidal cyst the only treatment likely to give lasting results is surgical removal.

PINEAL GLAND The pineal gland is located deep in the brain, above and behind the pituitary gland. In animals such as lizards, the pineal is known to be an organ receptive to light. It has also been determined that numerous metabolic substances are manufactured in this gland. As improved techniques become available, it will be possible to study its function more adequately. Since tumors of the pineal gland which produce active metabolic substances have not been described, the chief importance of this structure, as seen in man at the present time, is as an indicator of the skull midline in X-rays, since it calcifies after adolescence.

PROLAPSE Prolapse, or collapse, may occur to certain organs. Sometimes due to complications in childbirth, or because of other disorders, the uterus may become displaced and drop into the vagina. This situation is known as a prolapsed uterus.

Prolapse of the rectum is also relatively common, especially among the elderly. This condition occurs when the rectum falls through the anus. It may be brought about by the muscle strain of chronic constipation, parasitic infections, or hemorrhoids.

Symptoms. A prolapse of the uterus will push the vagina down and out. Interference with urine excretion and trauma to the protruded vagina may occur. With a rectal prolapse the protruding rectal tissue is easily abraded, may bleed, or become infected.

Women are six times more likely to suffer some form of prolapse than are men.

Treatment. Most cases of prolapse can be corrected either by the implantation of a supportive appliance (a pessary), or by reconstructive surgery. As soon as a prolapse is discovered, a physician should be consulted. Rectal prolapse may require an abdominal operative approach to bring the rectum up inside. Uterine prolapse is also best managed by a surgical repair.

PYREXIA   *See* FEVER in the section INFANT AND CHILD CARE.

ST. VITUS' DANCE (SYDENHAM'S CHOREA) Sydenham's chorea, or St. Vitus' dance, is characterized by the sudden onset of spontaneous movements of the face, arms, and legs associated with poor coordination and muscular weakness. One-half of patients with chorea show evidence of rheumatic infection before, during, or after an attack of chorea. The disorder affects the basal ganglia in the center of the brain as well as other structures, and is probably related to hypersensitivity to streptococcus infection.

Symptoms. Most patients develop Sydenham's chorea between five and fifteen years of age. The child may be irritable and fatigue easily. While writing, eating, or playing games, he may notice difficulty in using one or both arms. He may complain of weakness; frequent involuntary grimaces of the face are noted; there may be difficulty in speaking and in swallowing; involuntary movements occur in the arms and legs.

Treatment. There is no specific treatment available for Sydenham's chorea although sedative drugs are effective in decreasing the involuntary movements. Complete recovery from the condition is the rule. However, if chorea is associated with rheumatic involvement of the heart, complications may then result from the cardiac disorder.

SCLERODERMA, DIFFUSE SYSTEMIC The cutaneous manifestation of this disease represents the visible evidence of a connective tissue disturbance of the entire body; this is usually the first symptom the patient is aware of. It is a disease of adult life, occurring earliest in adolescence and rarely in the elderly.

Symptoms. The replacement of normal pliable connective tissue by thick and brittle fibers causes a hardening of the skin which is usually noted by a restriction of muscular activity in the affected area. Thus the patient finds it increasingly difficult to smile, grin, or frown if the face is affected. Objectively, there may be an erasing of the lines and wrinkles of the face. Fine movements of the fingers are made impossible if those areas are involved. Swallowing or breathing can be labored from involvement of the skin of these areas or from lesions in the throat or the lungs.

The disease is irregular in its course; remission of many months and years are not uncommon. Although the hardness of the affected areas usually persists, extensive periods of remission of the disease may afford the patient continued "normal" activity.

Treatment. Relief of symptoms with massage, whirlpool baths, avoidance of cold (when the hands and feet are involved), and the application of emollient lotions may be helpful. The cortisone drugs are occasionally effective. Newer approaches utilize such chemotherapeutic agents as azothioprine and cyclophosphamide which in low dosage seem effective in some of the autoimmune disorders.

SCLERODERMA, LOCALIZED (MORPHEA)   *See* the section SKIN CONDITIONS.

SMOKING The American Cancer Society estimates that cigarette smoking is responsible for 83 percent of lung cancer cases among men and women.

Until the early 1950s, smoking was considered and discussed mainly in terms of its social and psychological implications. Since that time, increased emphasis has been placed on its potential harm to physical health, particularly as a contributing case of lung cancer, chronic bronchitis, and coronary heart disease. The cause against cigarette smoking has been overwhelmingly established in the statistical sense, but demonstration of a direct cause-and-effect relationship is still lacking. The best assembled summaries of presently available information on this subject can be found in the reports by the English Royal College of Physicians (Smoking and Health, 1962) and the U.S. Surgeon General's

Reports on Smoking and Health, published in 1963 and 1988.

About 300 different compounds have been identified in the tobacco leaf and about 260 in the tobacco smoke. Due to changes produced by combustion (cigarettes burn at about 1120° F.), only 98 compounds have been found in both leaves and smoke. This shows at a glance the enormous complexity of trying to extricate the one or more agents responsible for smoking damage. Of the isolated compounds, 16 substances have the potential capacity of producing cancer in some animals. Tobacco smoke contains gases, volatile compounds, and solid matter. No filter can completely remove all particulate matter. About 50 percent of inhaled smoke is retained in the respiratory system, mostly in the lung.

The physiological effects of smoking can be divided into local (upon the respiratory system) and general (upon the body), as a whole, after being absorbed. Local effects are mostly characterized by increase in the resistance to airflow in and out of the lung; stimulation of mucus-secretion; and delay of mucus-removal. The latter is the result of a slowing down in the beating of hair-like structures (cilia) located in the inner lining of the bronchial tubes, whose function is to remove normal mucus and to trap and expel foreign material entering with inspiration. The net result of these effects is to create a state of chronic irritation which perpetuates itself, particularly in heavy smokers. This irritation in turn is believed to initiate, by hitherto unknown mechanisms, the structural changes which may lead to chronic bronchitis or cancer.

The general effects of smoking are mainly due to the absorption of nicotine. The amount of nicotine which can be recovered from the mainstream smoke of an average cigarette is about 2 mg.; of this, the amount absorbed into the lung varies from 10 to 90 percent, depending on the smoker's habits (depth of inhaling, breathholding time, etc.). The main effects of the absorbed nicotine are transient increases in blood pressure and heart-rate, and decreases in skin temperature and urinary volume. The appetite is usually reduced.

There is very little exact information on the psychological effects of smoking. Smoking often relieves tension and anxiety and in some individuals provides pleasure. The pattern of smoking at different ages in the two sexes does not throw light on motivation. Studies of schoolchildren and young adults show a significant correlation between their smoking rates and the smoking habits of parents and siblings. The different ways of enjoying tobacco (cigars, cigarettes, water-pipe) bear a distinct relationship to prevalent cultural habits. Very little is known about the factors that lead people to discontinue smoking, but it seems evident that awareness and intelligent appraisal of the hazards involved are the most potent motivations for discontinuance of the habit.

There is no evidence that smoking promotes physical health. On the contrary, as stated previously, the statistically overwhelming evidence indicates that smoking is a causative factor in, or the most likely cause of, the worldwide increase in deaths from lung cancer; that it is an important predisposing factor in chronic bronchitis; that it increases the risk of dying from coronary heart disease, and accentuates the symptoms of vascular disease of the limbs; and that it has an adverse effect on healing of gastric or duodenal ulcers. Cigar and pipe smoking carry less risk than cigarette smoking, probably because the smoke is not inhaled; however, local lesions of the mouth and lips are more frequent. It is also important to point out that the mentioned risks of smoking are proportional to the amount of smoking. For all practical purposes, anything above twenty cigarettes daily is considered heavy smoking.

Although some smokers may never experience any serious ill effect as the result of smoking, there is no sure way to identify the minority who will not be affected. Full protection for all requires preventive measures of general application. Since at present we cannot yet identify the substance or substances in tobacco smoke which are deleterious to health, no claim of safety can be made on the basis of modified cigarette-tobacco or filters. Non-smokers who are exposed to smoke, for example, the non-smoking spouses of smoking partners, have been shown to experience a heightened risk of cancer. This has been referred to as "passive smoking" and is a major reason for the increasing bans on smoking in public areas.

SPLEEN, DISORDERS OF THE The spleen is an organ weighing, on the average, from three to five pounds, situated in the left upper abdomen, behind and below the stomach. It is made up of vascular components, reticuloendothelial and lymphoid elements, and connective (supportive) tissue. The reticuloendothelial system is that part of the blood's cellular elements concerned with "policing" and "cleaning" up the bloodstream and sites of invasion by foreign bodies such as germs; but it does not include the white blood cells.

The spleen destroys blood cells, an activity that is acclerated with splenic enlargement. It also stores up red blood cells. It has the capacity to "pick" deformed red blood cells out of the circulation. The spleen, it seems, plays some role in bodily defense against infection and has a function, as yet not determined, in protecting the whole blood-manufacturing process. The extent to which the spleen influences bone marrow function is not yet known.

The spleen is often involved in blood diseases, such as leukemia, anemia, and Hodgkin's disease. There are also splenic disorders due to pathology of the organ itself or localized pathology, such as cancer of the pancreas and high blood pressure in the liver's circulatory system (the portal system).

Two blood disorders in which the spleen is enlarged are Felty's syndrome and Banti's disease.

Banti's disease is a disease characterized by enlargement of the spleen, lowering of the white blood cell and platelet count, and cirrhosis of the liver. It is caused by increased congestion in the circulatory system in and about the liver, by clotting formation with the liver's circulatory system, or by cirrhosis of the liver.

Felty's syndrome is a disorder characterized by rheumatoid arthritis, enlarged spleen, and a lowered white blood cell count. Its cause is unknown.

Lowered white and/or red cell counts with enlargement of the spleen are observed in several other conditions for which surgical removal of the spleen is performed if the disease itself and the patient's condition do not make the operation unwise. On the other hand, splenectomy is rarely done in lymphomatous diseases such as Hodgkin's disease and leukemia.

STONES (CALCULI) Stone formation in body fluids is hastened by stagnation of heavily saturated solutions such as are found in the gallbladder, urinary system, pancreas, and salivary glands. Chronic infection may also hasten their formation. Because of their mechanical interference with normal flow of fluids they can cause severe symptoms; the pain associated with gallstones and kidney stones in particular can be very severe. If the stones become impacted they must be removed, but often they will pass spontaneously. (*See also* GALLSTONES in the section GASTROINTESTINAL CONDITIONS.)

SYNDROME A syndrome is a pattern of symptoms which together are indicative of a disease. Many diseases present characteristic syndromes (patterns) of signs and symptoms which are diagnostic.

"TONGUE-TIE" A web of tissue is found under the front and central part of the tongue and runs to the floor of the mouth, just behind the lower teeth; called the frenulum, it serves no purpose. It is worth mentioning only because there are some who feel that the membrane has some deleterious effect on the development of speech.

If the tongue is mobile enough to reach the lips, this membrane can have no effect on a child's speech. Many doctors, however, will snip it, because of pressure from parents and grandparents. This is probably a safe procedure, although an occasional baby will bleed alarmingly when cut here.

TRANSPLANTATION Successful transplantation of kidneys is now a routine procedure at many medical centers. Careful matching of donor and recipient and the use of immunosuppressive agents prevent organ rejection. Such kidney transplants may prevent death from uremia or abolish need for frequent dialysis on the artificial kidney. More dramatic and increasingly successful have been heart transplants. Between 80 and 90 percent of heart-transplant patients still do well a year after the surgery and in some instances patients have done well for as long as five years. Lung transplants have so far been uniformly unsuccessful. And only a minority of liver transplants have been successful. (*See also* HEART TRANSPLANTATION in the section CARDIOVASCULAR CONDITIONS; KIDNEY TRANSPLANT in the section URINARY CONDITIONS.) Variable results have been reported for pancreas transplants (for diabetes) and thymic and bone marrow transplants for immunologic and hematologic deficiencies.

WITHDRAWAL SYNDROME   This is the general term given to the symptoms experienced by an addicted individual who terminates the use of alcohol, tobacco, heroin, cocaine or other drugs.

Symptoms. Irritability, hallucinations and seizures are among the major symptoms. Restlessness, trouble in concentration, and insomnia are among the minor symptoms and may be noted in persons quitting use of tobacco.

Treatment. A switch to a less toxic drug, for instance methodone, may be a practical alternative, but then the patient may become addicted to methadone. In withdrawal from alcohol the benzodiazepine group of drugs may be of help. The drug clonidine has been shown to diminish some of the craving and discomfort when alcohol, tobacco, and even heroin are suddenly given up.

Nutrition and Health

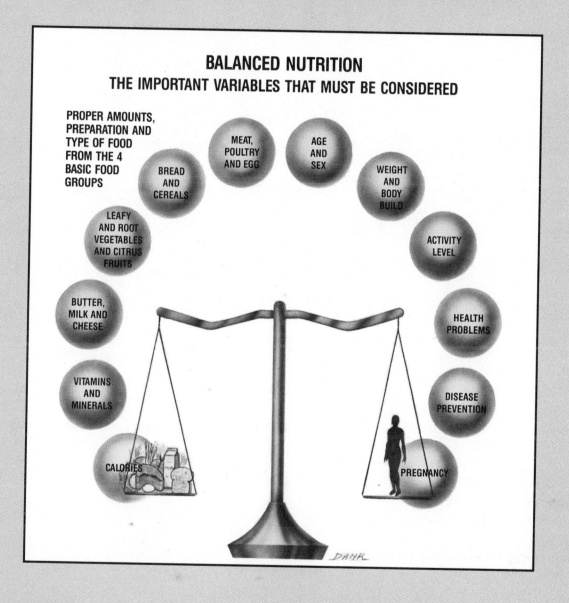

Despite the fact that the U.S. diet is the richest and most varied in the world, it is evident that the whole nutrition story has yet to be written. The Surgeon General's Report on Nutrition and Health issued in 1988 recommends that individuals

- Eat a variety of foods.
- Maintain desirable weight.
- Avoid too much fat, saturated fat, and cholesterol.
- Eat foods with adequate starch and fiber.
- Avoid too much sugar.
- Avoid too much sodium.
- If you drink alcoholic beverages, do so in moderation.

This section examines basic dietary concerns, vitamins and minerals, and disorders and conditions that arise from improper nutrition. *See also* the questions on why physicians object to overweight patients (Q-1); the role of fat in the diet (Q-2, Q-3); the validity of quick weight loss programs (Q-4); bland diet (Q-7) and vitamin supplements (Q-14) in the section QUESTIONS AND ANSWERS ABOUT COMMON SYMPTOMS.

The following is a list of terms identified in this section:

ABSORPTION

ALBUMIN

AMINO ACIDS

ANABOLISM (PROTEIN)

ANOREXIA NERVOSA

APPETITE AND HUNGER

"BASIC FOUR"

BIOTIN

BULIMIA

CALCIUM

CALORIE

CARBOHYDRATES

CHOLESTEROL

CHOLINE

DEXTROSE

DIET

ELEMENTS (MINERALS)

FATS

FOLIC ACID

INOSITOL

IODINE

IRON

LOW-CHOLESTEROL DIET

LOW-RESIDUE DIET

LOW-SALT (LOW-SODIUM) DIET

MINERALS

MONOSODIUM GLUTAMATE (MSG)

OBESITY

OVERWEIGHT

PELLAGRA

POTASSIUM

PROTEINS

RECOMMENDED DAILY ALLOWANCES

RICKETS

SCURVY

SODIUM

THIRST

UNDERWEIGHT

VITAMIN A

VITAMIN B_2 (RIBOFLAVIN)

VITAMIN B_6

VITAMIN B_{12}

VITAMIN B COMPLEX

VITAMIN C

VITAMIN D

VITAMIN E

VITAMIN K

VITAMINS

WATER

ABSORPTION Absorption, as used in a biologic sense, is the transport of materials across a barrier and incorporation into the tissue itself. Food and water, from one end of the alimentary canal to the other, may still be considered to be "outside" the body. Not until the substances cross the thin cellular lining of the stomach and intestines and are picked up by the circulating blood and lymph, do the products of digestion become part of the body, that is, become "absorbed."

Little except alcohol is absorbed in the stomach. The basic components of food (protein, fat, and carbohydrate) must be sufficiently digested, broken down into smaller basic molecular units, before they can be absorbed. Digestion is carried out through the action of enzymes, chiefly in the first foot or so of the small intestine (duodenum). Absorption of foodstuff, however, takes place largely in the latter part of the small intestine (jejunum and ileum).

Water is absorbed, excreted back into the digestive canal, and reabsorbed, in a continuous dynamic state of flux. Most of the water, including the liquid portion of the gastrointestinal juices, is finally absorbed in the large intestine. When motility is increased, there is insufficient time for water reabsorption; the bowel contents are then liquid (diarrhea). Prolonged activity of reabsorptive mechanisms leads to the dry stool of constipation.

Absorption involves complex physical factors, such as the size and concentration of the molecules; water-salt concentration; surface tension; and active transport by the cells, which do chemical work and use energy in the process of transferring molecules across cell membranes.

Proteins and carbohydrates are broken down into their component parts: amino acids and simple sugars, respectively. These are then absorbed directly in the blood capillaries in the intestinal walls and carried by the circulating blood to the liver where they undergo many chemical changes.

Fat is split into fatty acids and glycerol in the intestine. These, in a complex way, are absorbed by tiny lymphatic vessels (lacteals) which eventually collect into larger vessels that empty into the veins.

The absorption of drugs, vitamins, and minerals is also based on passive diffusion or active transport mechanisms.

ALBUMIN Albumin is an important protein found in all tissues. (Egg white is a form of this substance.) The albumin in blood serum is formed by the liver from amino acids resulting from protein metabolism. The normal serum concentration is from about four to five grams per one hundred milliliters of blood. When liver cells are damaged, formation of albumin is reduced and its serum level characteristically falls. The level also falls in severe malnutrition and in some forms of kidney disease in which there is a loss of albumin in the urine.

Albumin acts as a regulator of water and salt balance between the fluid in the blood and in the tissues, thus maintaining the total blood volume in equilibrium. It also acts as a transport mechanism for many natural compounds and drugs.

AMINO ACIDS Proteins, indispensable constituents of every living cell, are very large molecules composed of great numbers of building units: the amino acids. Although they vary in chemical structure, these units all have in common a nitrogen-containing (amino) group—NH_2—and an acidic (carboxyl) group—$COOH$. There are some twenty-two different amino acids found in nature. Hundreds and even thousands of amino acids are joined together in a chain-like arrangement to form the numerous proteins of the body. Proteins as varied as the hormone insulin and the critical ingredient of red blood cells, hemoglobin, differ only in the composition of their amino acids.

Food proteins are broken down into the component amino acids which are absorbed, enter the circulation, and reach the liver, where many new proteins are manufactured. The circulating amino acids then reach the rest of the body where cells extract what they need, replacing the tissue being lost by wear and tear. Some amino acids are converted into carbohydrate and fats; some may be burned for energy. The nitrogen part of the molecule is eventually split off and excreted by the kidneys as ammonia, urea, and other products.

The essential amino acids must be supplied

by food. These acids are phenylalanine, methionine, leucine, valine, lysine, isoleucine, threonine, and tryptophan. The nonessential amino acids are equally important but can be synthesized by the body. Among them are glycine, alanine, cystine, tyrosine, proline, histidine (which may be nonsynthesizable in children), and arginine.

Amino-acid solutions (made from milk or other proteins) are used in the treatment of certain nutritional disorders. The nutritional quality of a protein food is determined by its amino-acid composition; generally, animal proteins—meat, milk, eggs—supply more of the essential amino acids in a balanced ratio than do vegetable proteins.

ANABOLISM (PROTEIN)   Anabolism is a term meaning the build-up of tissue material. More specifically, the word is applied to the formation (synthesis) of protein. Recent investigation indicates that 30 to 50 percent of the body's protein is undergoing synthesis and breakdown (catabolism) simultaneously. Like a bank in which money is being deposited and withdrawn at the same time, the protoplasm of cells is undergoing anabolic and catabolic reactions.

During growth, late pregnancy, or convalescence, and during physical training when new muscle tissue is being formed, anabolism exceeds catabolism. When dietary protein is less than required, or when the caloric intake is significantly reduced, body protein is broken down faster than it is being built up; that is, catabolism exceeds anabolism. These processes are often measured by nitrogen-balance studies. Nitrogen is derived from protein (*see* AMINO ACIDS in this section), and the balance is measured by determining the intake and urinary output.

ANOREXIA NERVOSA   *See* the section MENTAL HEALTH: PSYCHIATRIC AND PSYCHOLOGICAL CONDITIONS.

APPETITE AND HUNGER   Appetite and hunger are not the same. Appetite is largely the conscious psychological aspect of the desire for food. It is conditioned by past experiences, cultural customs, and habit. Thus, the urge to eat a tempting dessert (appetite) may

exist long after the more physical sensation—hunger—has been appeased by an excellent meal. Hunger itself is not modified significantly by the past experience of the individual.

There are centers in the hypothalamus, a part of the base of the brain, which regulate feeding. One center regulates appetite, or the desire to eat; the other acts as a brake to prevent overeating and is called the satiety center. The nutritional roles of appetite, hunger, and the hypothalamic centers, despite extensive investigation, have still not resolved the growing incidence of obesity and of eating disorders.

"BASIC FOUR"   The term refers to the four categories of food considered essential for good health.

The value of the "basic four" concept is its emphasis on a varied diet. For a given individual, modifications may be in order. Thus milk-intolerant persons may need alternatives, perhaps yogurt, lactase treated milk, or calcium supplementation. For those with cholesterol problems, beef and pork may be limited with fish as the alternative, and eggs need to be limited because of their high cholesterol content. (*See* the entry DIET in this section for a selection from the "Basic Four" that will supply a daily balanced diet of about 1500 calories. For a diet containing 3000 calories merely double each selection by two.)

BIOTIN   Biotin is water soluble and is one of the B-complex vitamins. It is an essential nutrient and plays an important role in the metabolism of both fat and carbohydrate. It is widely present in food and is synthesized by the bacterial flora in the intestinal tract. Good food sources include liver, kidney, egg yolk, and some vegetables. Biotin deficiency is rare; however, raw egg white contains a substance—avidin—which combines with biotin, making the latter unavailable to the body. Experimental biotin deficiency can thus be produced by feeding large amounts of raw egg white. The symptoms are loss of appetite, muscle pains, and a dry, scaly skin condition (dermatitis). Retardations in mental and physical development, declines in the immune system, and hair loss have been reported in children with biotin deficiency.

BULIMIA   *See* the section MENTAL HEALTH: PSYCHIATRIC AND PSYCHOLOGICAL CONDITIONS.

CALCIUM   Calcium is an essential chemical element (a mineral) largely concerned with the structure of bones and teeth; a small portion is involved in bloodclotting and transmission of impulses from nerve to muscles. Absorption of calcium in the diet is enhanced by vitamin D. The element circulates in the blood where its concentration in the plasma is carefully maintained, in part by parathyroid hormone, at about 100 milligrams per 100 milliliters. Lack of calcium in the diet leads to a form of "leaching out" of bone mineral contents (osteoporosis), and when vitamin D is deficient, the condition known as rickets occurs.

Milk and cheese are essentially the only foods that supply large amounts of calcium. The dietary requirement for this mineral is between 800 and 1200 milligrams per day (one pint of milk supplies 300 milligrams). The woman who is pregnant or breast-feeding her baby may need additional calcium to protect her from the fetus's or baby's drain on her tissues.

Severe calcium deficiency (usually not dietary alone, but related to a deficient supply of vitamin D and deficient parathyroid hormone metabolism) results in tetany, a state of muscle spasm. Significant calcium excess (hypercalcemia and deposits in certain tissues) does not occur from dietary intake alone; it depends on excess vitamin D or excessive parathyroid secretion.

CALORIE   The calorie is defined as a unit of heat energy which raises the temperature of 1 kilogram (2.2 pounds) of water 1 degree centigrade ($1^{4}/_{5}°$ Fahrenheit). Because the source of our energy is food, and because energy can conveniently be expressed in terms of heat, it is in calories that we measure the energy supplied by our food.

Both by direct and by indirect means, we know that a gram of carbohydrate furnishes 4.1 calories; a gram of protein, 4.1 calories; and a gram of fat, 9.3 calories. For practical purposes we use the values 4, 4, and 9 calories, respectively.

To maintain body weight during health, the caloric intake must equal the caloric output. For growth or repair of tissue after injury or starvation, the caloric intake must be higher. Physical work or exercise performed has much to do with the caloric output; it is evident that obesity is frequently due to a caloric intake greater than such output. (Reducing food-consumption and increasing activity help reset the balance.)

CARBOHYDRATES   Carbohydrates are the main energy fuel of the body. Chemically, they are compounds containing carbon as well as hydrogen and oxygen, the latter two in the same proportion as in water. With but few exceptions, carbohydrates are of plant origin. They compose the group commonly known as sugars and starches.

Carbohydrates are synthesized by green plants from the carbon dioxide contained in the atmosphere and the hydrogen in water in the presence of sunlight in the process of photosynthesis. Life as we know it on earth depends on this process, for the carbohydrates of the plant kingdom are the major energy fuel on which the animal kingdom and man both exist.

These substances are classified according to their chemical structure as follows:

Monosaccharides.   These are the simple sugars composed of six carbon atoms in a ringlike structure. Glucose and dextrose are examples.

Disaccharides.   These more complex sugars are formed by condensation of two monosaccharides which can be split by the body. An example of this is sucrose, or common table sugar.

Polysaccharides.   These large complex molecules are the end product of the condensation of many monosaccharides. An example of this is starch, or glycogen in animal tissue.

When ingested, carbohydrates are split through the action of enzymes in the saliva, stomach, and intestine. The complex sugars are broken down into monosaccharides such as glucose, galactose, and fructose, which are then absorbed in the small intestine. From there these sugars are carried to the liver; some continue through the bloodstream to individual cells in the body where they are burned as a source of energy. Carbon dioxide, which we throw off in breathing, and water are the end result of this process. Other carbohydrates in the liver are stored in the form of aggregates (glycogen) to be reconverted into glucose when the need arises.

In this country, about 50 percent or more of our total energy requirements are met by carbohydrate. This varies depending on taste, economic factors, dietary habits, and so on. The foods largely concerned are rice, potatoes, cereals, flour products (bread, cake, etc.), legumes, and vegetables. Since these foods are generally considerably cheaper than meat, eggs, fish, and dairy products, which are the primary sources of proteins and fats, there is a tendency for the less economically favored as well as those living in underdeveloped areas to eat a high-carbohydrate diet. Insulin is necessary for the proper metabolism of carbohydrates, and when there is an impairment in this function, the clinical condition known as diabetes results.

CHOLESTEROL   Cholesterol is a dietary substance which is believed to play a role in atherosclerosis (hardening of the arteries, coronary heart disease, "heart attacks"). This complex molecule is a fatty substance, chemically a sterol alcohol.

Cholesterol is widely distributed in the animal body and is found in nervous tissue, blood, and in the bile. Bile salts and certain adrenal and sex hormones are derived from it. In the skin, cholesterol is the precursor of vitamin D, so that when it is irradiated by sunlight it is converted into the vitamin. Cholesterol is found only in foods of animal origin and is supplied by diets high in meats, glandular organs, and fat. However, the human body is not dependent on diet for its cholesterol supply, for it may be manufactured in the liver.

In the basic disease atherosclerosis, which causes so many deaths and so much disability in our country (through heart attacks, strokes, kidney disease, and so on), small deposits occur on the inner lining of the blood vessels. One of the substances in the deposits is cholesterol. In addition, patients with advanced atherosclerosis often exhibit elevated plasma cholesterol levels. It therefore seems logical to conclude that atherosclerosis can be retarded by the reduction of cholesterol in the diet.

Recent studies indicate that total cholesterol is composed of fractions which play different roles in the atherosclerosis process. High density cholesterol (HDL) represents cholesterol in transit from tissues such as the arteries back to the liver. The higher the HDL level the better, hence the term "good" cholesterol. In contrast is the low density lipid (LDL) or "bad" cholesterol; the higher its level the greater the degree of atherosclerosis. Total cholesterol of more than 200 milligrams per deciliter is considered a risk factor, and when it exceeds 240–260 milligrams per deciliter the condition requires medical attention. Treatment often consists of weight reduction, exercise, stopping smoking, reduction of cholesterol and total fats in the diet. Sometimes addition to the diet of vegetable oils and especially fish oils, and elements such as oat bran may prove helpful in lowering the cholesterol level. If these measures do not result in a

OUTER LAYER

MUSCULAR LAYER

INNER LAYER

BLOOD CHOLESTEROL

This is a cross section of a blood vessel showing the cholesterol (fat) particles invading the inner wall. A hard yellowish plaque forms which may eventually impede the blood flow.

satisfactory level, various cholesterol lowering medications, Gemfibrozil®, Lovostatin®, etc. and the vitamin nicotinic acid may be effective. It has been definitively established that the risk of cardiovascular disease is reduced as the blood cholesterol is lowered.

CHOLINE Choline is a nitrogen-containing compound. Little is known about its importance in human nutrition, except that it serves as coenzymes in metabolism. In animal experiments, administration of diets low in choline leads to a deficiency state characterized by an accumulation of fat in the liver. For this reason it has been used in the treatment of various forms of liver disease in man, but the results have not been clear-cut.

Choline is present in large amounts in the following foods: egg yolk, meat, fish, and cereals. The dietary requirements for choline are uncertain because the compound can be manufactured in the body. Human requirements are probably less than 500 milligrams daily; the average diet contains 250 to 600 milligrams of choline per day.

Choline is readily acetylated in the body to acetylcholine, an important neurotransmitter. Indeed a few hours after labelled choline is ingested, labelled acetylcholine can be detected between brain cells.

DEXTROSE Dextrose is the technical name of sugar, a white crystalline powder ($C_6H_{12}O_6$), also called d-glucose. This is derived from fruit sugar and from starch. Dextrose is the form in which sugar appears in the blood. A solution of dextrose may be dripped into the vein or administered through a tube passed into the stomach. Dextrose is a primary fuel in cellular metabolism. It is especially important in the brain cell where drops in this blood sugar level, rapidly lead to confusion and coma. It is equally important to the function of muscle where it is stored in an agglomerated form called glycogen.

DIET What a person eats has a profound effect on his well-being, but because individuals vary so much in age, height, weight, physical activity, inherited characteristics, and so on, there is no single "normal" diet plan. Current nutritional knowledge, however, indicates that a wide variety of foods helps to ensure a better diet for whatever the individual needs

DIETARY GUIDELINES TO REDUCE RISK OF CANCER

*Reduce amount of both saturated and unsaturated fats to 30 percent of total calories.

This can be accomplished by broiling, boiling, or baking foods instead of frying them. Excess fat should be trimmed off meat before cooking. Butter, cream, salad dressings, margarine, shortening and oil should be limited, and even reduced when cooking recipes call for such products. Labels of all packaged foods should be carefully checked for the amount of fat per serving before purchasing or consuming.

*Eat more fruits, vegetables, and whole grain cereals.

These foods have been found to help reduce cancer risk when eaten as part of a balanced diet. Certain vitamins and other nutrients—particularly vitamin A, C, and E, and dietary fiber—are felt to be of special importance. It should be noted, however, that the best way to consume these elements is through a balanced diet rather than through vitamin supplements.

*Limit consumption of salt-cured, smoked, and charcoal-broiled foods.

These foods, when consumed in excess, lead to cancer of the esophagus and stomach. This is generally not found to be as severe a problem in the U.S. where food processing and preparation methods are better than in other parts of the world.

*Alcoholic beverages should only be consumed in moderation.

These calories, which are empty of nutrients, may deprive the body of other elements of a balanced diet.

may be. One-sided and "crash" diets are apt to be deficient or harmful if consumed for more than a very short while. Furthermore, for many illnesses a physician's advice concerning diet is extremely important.

Caloric needs and food preferences vary widely, but there is a minimum of certain types of food (see BASIC FOUR in this section) which forms the basis of a normal dietary intake. Around this minimum a full diet can be planned with considerable freedom of choice of foods.

The basic daily diet plan for adults (which supplies about 1,500 calories) is briefly as follows:

Milk: 1 pint (low fat)
Meat, fish, or poultry: 1 average serving (about 3½ ounces)
Additional protein foods: 1 egg, ½ pint milk, or 1 ounce of fish or cheese
Vegetables: 2 servings of a leafy green or yellow vegetable and 1 serving of another vegetable
Fruits: 3 servings of citrus fruit or juice, or noncitrus fruit
Margarine: 3 teaspoons
Breads and cereal: 4 slices of enriched or whole-grain bread, or 2 slices of bread and ½ cup serving of enriched cereals and ½ cup of a starchy vegetable.

ELEMENTS (MINERALS)

Of the more than one hundred chemical elements now recognized, fourteen appear to be essential for human nutrition. These minerals (a preferred term) are widely distributed in foods, and under conditions of health there is little danger of a dietary deficiency developing. In certain disease states, however, abnormalities of mineral-nutrition do occur. Common examples might be the negative calcium balance with resulting osteoporosis in the menopausal state: deficient calcification of bone in the infant with rickets; kidneystones in disorders of the parathyroid glands; sodium and potassium may drop to a dangerous range in intensive diuretic therapy; potassium may rise to a dangerous level in kidney disease. Like vitamins, with which many are connected, minerals have important bodily functions.

The essential minerals are sodium, potassium, chlorine, calcium, phosphorus, sulfur, magnesium, iron, copper, iodine, manganese, cobalt, zinc, and molybdenum. Several are discussed in this section in separate entries under their own names. (See also MINERALS in this section.)

FATS

Fats are an important part of the everyday diet. They are more than twice as rich in potential energy as are carbohydrates or proteins, nine calories being released for each gram of the average type of fat processed by the body (metabolized). In other words, fats contain a large amount of energy in a small volume.

A meal high in fat tends to have a more prolonged effect on the sensation of "fullness"; fats also add to the palatability of food and serve as a vehicle for fat-soluble vitamins. Food energy not immediately utilized is stored in the form of fat within the body as a "reservoir" for future use. As tissue, fat serves as a protective cushion for certain organs and helps insulate the body against temperature changes.

On the basis of certain physical and chemical properties, the group of substances known as fats may be classified as follows:

- Neutral fats (triglycerides), which make up the greater part of the fats in the diet and are typical of fat in animal tissue such as meat. Triglycerides are composed of the simple chemical glycerol, attached to which are three fatty acids. The latter are simple, long chains of carbon atoms, perhaps eighteen to twenty-one atoms long, with an "acid" chemical configuration at one end.
- Waxes, which include the esters (fatty acids connected onto another substance) of cholesterol and vitamins A and D
- Phospholipids (containing phosphoric acid), present in all cells and particularly concentrated in certain portions of the central nervous system
- Glycolipids or cerebrosides, fatty material containing carbohydrate, found in the white matter of the brain
- Steroids, including cholesterol, certain hormones, vitamin D, and bile acids.

Fatty acids have been also classified on the basis of saturation. When the bonds between the carbon atoms, which are arranged in a long chain, are each covered with a hydrogen atom, the fatty acid is said to be a saturated fatty acid. Some of the more important fatty acids are partially unsaturated; that is, they have some bonds between the carbons which do not have hydrogen molecules attached. Three of the unsaturated fatty acids (linoleic, linolenic, and arachidonic) apparently cannot be synthesized by animals and man, and have been termed essential.

Foods of relatively high fat content include milk, cream, butter, egg yolks, fish liver, other meats (especially pork), and vegetable oils of various types. Margarine is manufactured from vegetable oils that have been saturated (hydrogenated) in order to make melting less likely at room temperature.

The average American daily diet contains about 100 grams of fat which supply about one-third of the total caloric intake. Perhaps two-thirds of the fats come from animal sources: meat, milk, eggs, dairy products, etc. The remainder come from vegetable materials. High fat, high cholesterol diets are strongly implicated in a high incidence of cardiovascular disease. They have also been associated with the higher incidence of cancer of the breast and colon found in the more advanced countries.

FOLIC ACID Folic acid (also known as pteroylglutamic acid or folacin) is a member of the vitamin B complex. It is best known for its effect on the bone marrow, and it plays an essential role in the normal development of the red blood cell.

In the absence of adequate amounts of folic acid, a certain type of anemia may occur, identified by the presence of large cells (macrocytosis) and characteristic changes in the bone marrow (megaloblastic anemia). This type of anemia may be present in pregnancy and in infancy. Folic acid deficiency may also occur at times in diseases of abnormal intestinal absorption found particularly in tropical countries.

Folic acid is closely related to vitamin B_{12} in that both play a role in the normal maturation and development of the red cells. Folic acid is present in foods in both free and combined (conjugated) forms. It appears that folic acid is converted in the body to folinic acid, also known as citrovorum factor, which may be the more active form. (There is some evidence that

ascorbic acid [vitamin C] assists in the conversion of folic acid to folinic acid.)

The best dietary sources for folic acid appear to be liver, green leafy vegetables, kidney, muscle meat, and whole-wheat cereals. The RDA is set at 200–180 mg. of total folacin activity in the diet. Folic acid is also synthesized by intestinal bacteria, and this may be an important source of supply in man.

Certain drugs have been used in the treatment of leukemia—a so-called "blood cancer"—by serving as antagonists of folic acid. By interfering with the use of folic acid, the leukemia cells are impaired in their growth and metabolic processes. When these folic acid antagonists are administered, symptoms of folic acid deficiency may be produced, including a red, inflamed tongue, diarrhea, and anemia.

INOSITOL Little is known of the role of inositol in the nutrition of animals or man. In chemical structure it is related to glucose. It is present in large amounts in the heart, brain, and musculature of man, and also in bacteria, plants, and grains. It has been administered, together with other agents, in the treatment of several conditions, including liver disease, but the results have not been conclusive. There is some evidence that inositol may be helpful in the therapy of disordered nerve function in diabetics and does function as coenzymes in metabolism.

IODINE The importance of the element iodine in human nutrition lies in the fact that it is necessary for the formation of thyroid hormone, which controls the rate of energy-production in the body. The human requirement for iodine is about 1 microgram per kilogram of body weight daily. The suggested daily amount, making allowance for physical activity, is 0.15 to 0.30 milligram; this amount can be supplied by the regular use of iodized salt.

Iodine is absorbed by the intestine and brought to the thyroid gland, which converts it into the active hormone. Various measurements of thyroid activity are based on iodine. Thus, one can measure the uptake of radioactive iodine by the thyroid gland. (This is increased in overactivity of the thyroid and decreased in underactivity.) In addition, the iodine in the blood, which is bound to protein and presumably represents circulating thyroid hormone, can be measured.

Iodine deficiency leads to the development of goiter, a swelling of the thyroid gland. Where the iodine content of the water and soil, and of foods grown therein, is low, the incidence of goiter is high. (However, it is important to note that goiter can be produced by factors other than iodine deficiency.) Where goiter is prevalent, cretinism, or congenital underactivity of the thyroid (hypothyroidism), is observed. Iodine is also essential for growth, normal fertility, and lactation.

Thyroid enlargement is also seen in normal situations during puberty and in pregnancy, during which time the need for iodine is increased.

Treatment. In the treatment of iodine deficiency, the mineral may be administered as an iodine solution (Lugol's solution), but the widespread use of iodized salt has greatly reduced prevalence of the typical iodine goiter seen in past generations.

IRON Iron, an essential element, is important chiefly because of its function in the blood. About two-thirds of the body's total amount of iron (four to five grams) is in heme, a compound which when linked to the protein globin forms hemoglobin, the red pigment in red blood cells. Hemoglobin is responsible for carrying oxygen to the tissue cells and for removing waste carbon dioxide. When the body is deficient in iron, the amount of circulating hemoglobin is reduced and anemia results.

Some iron is found in certain enzymes. About 15 percent of total iron is combined with a protein to form a storage compound known as ferritin.

The body tends to hold on to its store of iron; normal people excrete very little (about 1 milligram per day). Furthermore, most of the element released when red cells die is re-used. An important source of iron loss occurs in menstruating women; if the periods are heavy, the risk of iron deficiency anemia increases. World-wide iron deficiency anemia resulting from poor nutrition is still the most widespread chronic condition. Under normal circumstances, little dietary iron (perhaps 10 percent) is absorbed. However, when there is a need for iron, as in iron-deficiency anemia after a bleeding episode, the intestinal tract absorbs more iron from foods.

The recommended daily allowance for adults is 10 milligrams, with additional requirements during adolescence and pregnancy (15 mg/day). This amount is generally supplied by a well-balanced diet. In many states of (iron-deficiency) anemia, iron is administered by mouth as ferrous sulfate and other iron-containing compounds.

Iron in excessive amounts may be toxic. For this reason medications containing iron should be kept out of reach of children.

LOW-CHOLESTEROL DIET Recent research has found the common form of heart attack (actually coronary atherosclerosis) highly prevalent among people who (among other things) eat a diet high in saturated fatty acids. Such a diet, rich in animal fat, such as fatty meats, is often associated with a high level of cholesterol in the blood serum. Because cholesterol is present in the injured portions of the damaged heart, it seems logical to attempt to lower its serum-level. This is done by reducing the "animal" or saturated fatty acids and by increasing the so-called "vegetable"—a poor term—or polyunsaturated fatty acids. Other food items shown to be useful in lowering blood cholesterol include fish and fish oils, oatmeal, bran, and psyllium hydrocolloid. When diet is not sufficiently effective, chemical agents such as Lovostatin® may be useful.

Lean cuts of meat, with visible fat removed and cooked (medium or well-done) by methods which drain off fat, are recommended. When a source of fat is needed in preparation of food, an oil such as corn-oil or safflower-oil, high in linoleic acid (an essential unsaturated fatty acid), is to be used. These oils may also serve as a salad dressing but recent studies indicate that olive oil has the same effect. Frequent use should also be made of vegetables, nuts, and fruits.

A patient placed on a low-cholesterol diet will be told to avoid the following foods: butter, saturated margarine and shortening, lard, sweet cream, sour cream, and foods containing the above in large amounts.

Also to be avoided are bacon, ice cream, sausage, frankfurters, luncheon meats, brains, liver, kidney, sweetbreads, egg yolks

(3 per week allowed), and most cheeses except dry cottage.

Because fat, cheeses, and cream in any form should be omitted, macaroni, spaghetti, rice, or potatoes should be cooked without cheese, or fat-or-cream sauces.

FIBER AND THE DIET

What foods supply dietary fiber?

Choose foods such as beans, wheat and oat bran, fruits with skins intact and also bananas, whole grain cereals and breads, brown or wild rice, most vegetables, and popcorn.

How should I start adding fiber to my diet?

Fiber should be added gradually, since too much too quickly will cause cramps, diarrhea, and gas. Drink plenty of water. Use many different sources of fiber and try to add them at every meal. Be careful not to add unnecessary fats to high fiber items, such as rich cheese sauces to healthy vegetables.

LOW-RESIDUE DIET This is a diet used before and after surgery on the stomach and intestines in conditions of inflammation or irritation of the digestive (gastrointestinal) tract. The advantage of this diet is that it spares the digestive tract much work because it consists of small, frequent feedings that are easily digested and are low in residue.

Five meals a day are recommended—breakfast, midmorning snack, lunch, midafternoon snack, and supper. The patient should eat slowly and rest after each of the three main meals.

Foods to be avoided are: raw vegetables and raw fruits such as figs or raisins; whole wheat cereals and bread; spices, fried foods; excessively fat foods; rich desserts (pastries and pies); nuts; corn; beans, cabbage; onions; cucumbers; and rhubarb.

Among the foods that are allowed are weak coffee and tea, diluted orange juice without pulp and well-cooked cereals. Dairy products are limited to two cups. Among desserts, one can select tapioca, rice pudding, spongecake or angel food cake, jello, custard (and similar dishes), marmalades, jellies, and cooked or canned fruits. Most meats, fish, and poultry may be eaten; these should be baked, broiled, boiled, or roasted—*not* fried. Consommé and creamed soups are also permissible.

LOW-SALT (LOW-SODIUM) DIET Salt is often restricted in the diet of many patients with high blood pressure (hypertension), congestive cardiac failure, certain forms of kidney disease, fluid in the abdomen (ascites), and in certain disorders (toxemia) of pregnancy. This is done because salt—the sodium portion of it—retains fluid in the body. A low-salt diet is therefore helpful in ridding the body of excess fluids and in lowering blood pressure. Drugs and other therapeutic measures are usually also recommended.

The average American diet contains from 5 to 10 grams of sodium a day (not all in the form of salt); but this varies considerably, depending on the foods consumed. In mild restriction (total sodium intake kept in the range of 2.5 to 4.5 grams per day), no salt is allowed at the table and is used sparingly, or not at all, in cooking. In moderate restriction (about 1 to 2.5 grams) no more than one-fourth of a teaspoon of salt may be used in preparation or at the table. In a strict diet (under 1 gram), all foods are prepared and eaten without salt.

FIVE STEPS TO LOWER SODIUM LEVELS IN THE DIET

1. Don't add salt to prepared foods. Remove the salt shaker from the table.
2. Limit the obviously salty foods. Chips, pretzels, pickles, and salted nuts should be eaten in moderation only.
3. Learn to read package labels to discover hidden sodium. Since ingredients are listed in order of weight in the product, watch for salt or sodium listed near the top of any list. Compare brands; some manufacturers have lower sodium than other manufacturers' products.
4. Discover other spices and herbs to replace salt in food preparation.
5. Request that food ordered be prepared without salt or that dressings and sauces be served on the side.

Foods high in sodium include most processed and so-called convenience foods, cheeses, oil-packed tuna, bacon, ham, bologna, hotdogs, canned vegetables and soups, ketchup, prepared mustard, antacid medications, salad dressings, and fast food items.

The following dietetic recommendations are based on a strict low-salt ("salt-free" diet):

Basic list of low-sodium foods:
  Beverages:
    Coca Cola
    Cocoa powder
    Coffee
    Fruit juices (except tomato)
    Ginger ale
    Tea
  Seasoning Agents:
    Allspice
    Caraway
    Cinnamon
    Curry powder
    Garlic
    Mace
    Mint leaves
    Mustard powder
    Nutmeg
    Onions
    Paprika
    Pepper
    Peppermint extract
    Parsley
    Sage
    Thyme
    Tumeric
    Vanilla extract
    Vinegar
      Avoid onion salt, celery salt, and garlic salt. Also avoid all prepared sauces such as horse-radish, prepared mustard, Worcestershire sauce, and steak sauce.
  Fats and Oils:
    Margarine, unsalted
    Nuts, unsalted
    Olive oil
    Peanut butter, salt-free
    Salad oil
      Avoid bacon fats and other fats to which salt has been added.
  Miscellaneous: (These foods contain "empty" calories and should not be used if patient is overweight.)
    Coconut, dry
    Honey
    Jam
    Jelly
    Marmalade
    Sugar
    Pure sugar candy (Life Savers, lemon drops, rock candy, peppermints)

The above-listed foods are extremely low in sodium and may be used if desired to flavor and add variety to the diet without adding significantly to sodium intake. The use of herbs in cooking has always been advocated by the well-known good cooks; now when salt must be excluded from the diet, herb cookery becomes even more desirable. The addition of herbs and allowed condiments permits interesting flavors which compensate for the lack of salt. The use of a pressure cooker, too, enables the cook to preserve the natural flavors of the meats and vegetables and therefore make them more palatable.

Here follows a listing of, and commentary on, various foods in general—with particular regard to the problems posed by the necessity of holding sodium intake down to as low a level as possible.

Breads: Salt-free bread, 6 slices per day.
Cereals: Cooked cereals (do not use "quick-cook" brands) prepared without salt. Shredded Wheat, Puffed Wheat, or Puffed Rice may be used, but do not use any other prepared cereal.
Dairy Products: Milk—2 glasses daily, to be taken as a beverage or used in cooking; 1 serving of vanilla ice cream may be substituted for 1 glass of milk. One egg daily—cooked without salt. ¼ cup coffee cream daily. Salt-free margarine as desired. Salt-free cheddar cheese as meat substitute.
Fruits: Three servings daily. Any fruit—fresh, frozen, or canned—to be used unless a preservative agent has been added; read the labels to determine whether or not a preservative has been added. Serve a citrus fruit at least once daily.
Meats: 2½ ounces twice daily. Salt-free canned chicken, salmon, or tuna. Lamb, veal, beef, chicken (white meat only), or fresh fish.
    Bake, broil, or fry in vegetable oil. Do not use salt in preparation. Onions, garlic, herbs, paprika, and pepper may be used as seasoning. Do not use batters, bread crumbs, or other sauces that contain sodium.
Potato or Potato Substitutes: ½ cup serving twice daily. White potato, sweet potato, macaroni, rice, or spaghetti; dried

beans, prepared without salt, seasoned with fresh lean pork.

Cook without salt, and do not use cream sauce or cheese sauce. Fresh tomatoes, peppers, and onion may be added to give variety.

Other Vegetables: Two servings (½ cup) daily. Asparagus, beets (salt-free canned only), broccoli, Brussels sprouts, cabbage, cauliflower, corn, cucumbers, carrots, eggplant, green beans, lettuce, Lima beans, okra, onions, peas, peppers (red or green), parsnips, mushrooms, squash, tomatoes, and turnips.

Limit spinach, chard, fresh beets, or celery. Vegetables should be fresh, canned without salt, or frozen; limit the use of frozen peas or Lima beans. Cook without salt. Vegetables may be cooked or served as a salad. If served as salad, a vinegar dressing, lemon juice, or any oil-and-vinegar dressing without salt may be used. Do not use commercial dressings.

MINERALS Most of the minerals (*see also* VITAMINS in this section) are found in such profusion in all foods that, save for a few substances, it is impossible to have a deficiency. Sodium and chloride are of course present in common table salt. Calcium, important for the formation of teeth and bone, is found chiefly in dairy products. Since vitamin D is required for the absorption and utilization of calcium, it is today ordinarily added to commercially-distributed milk. Phosphorus, magnesium, manganese, potassium, zinc, sulfur are all essential to the diet but are readily available in the child's average diet of meat, fruit, vegetables, grains, and dairy products.

Certain minerals, though normally present in sufficient quantities, may be brought to the doctor's attention by a condition caused by their deficiency. Thus, an insufficiency of iron will result in anemia. Furthermore, trace elements of copper and cobalt are apparently necessary for optimum utilization of the iron itself. A deficiency of iodine will lead to a goiter condition; but today this is almost unheard of, because of the universal use of iodized salt. Lack of fluoride in the diet will result in increased incidence of dental cavities (caries);

many communities add this substance to their watersupply, with universal improvement in the soundness of teeth.

Many parents have been deluded by food faddists into believing that giving their children this or that element will increase pep, provide strength, and even forestall arthritis, hypertension, and the like; there are those who will go so far as to drink sea water or diluted mud if bottled attractively! The salesmen for these elixirs-of-life reap huge profits and the victims only lose money—as most of these remedies are at best no more effective than the soup one may have had for lunch.

MONOSODIUM GLUTAMATE (MSG)
Known under the brand names of Accent, Vetsin and Ajinomeoto, MSG is a food additive with a meat-like taste. It is said to enhance other flavors. Used in some oriental cooking it may produce chest pain, headache, facial pressure, a burning sensation and excessive sweating. These symptoms, usually temporary, experienced following a meal containing MSG are now referred to as Chinese restaurant syndrome. The continued use of this product as a food additive especially in baby foods has been questioned. If requested by the patron most restaurants will omit the MSG during the preparation of the ordered food.

OBESITY Obesity, or the state of being overfat, is not the same as overweight. This subject is one of the most important, common, and controversial in all medicine. It is important because it is well recognized that excessive weight is a detriment to good health. Obesity aggravates heart disease and arthritis and increases the possibility of high blood pressure, atherosclerosis, hernia, and gallbladder disease. It may bring out latent diabetes, it makes surgery and pregnancy more hazardous, and increases the mortality rate. In spite of this, perhaps 20 percent of adults in the United States are significantly overweight, that is, more than 15 percent above average weight for their height and age.

It is important to accept the fact that obesity is not entirely due to overeating. In spite of what is being written in various publications, people who are already overweight may actually be eating no more than those whose weight is normal. It was during the period when they were in the process of gaining weight that their food consumption was more than they could use, and they must now cut down in order to get rid of the surplus.

Obesity seems to run in families, but this may be so because of the establishment of familial eating patterns. It has been well established that the total number of fat cells in the body is the same despite weight fluctuations. After strenuous reduction, the fat cells are smaller but still capable of being repleted. Overfeeding in childhood may spur the body's production of fat cells and leave the adult with an increased base for his obesity. Increasingly, nutritionists believe that plumpness in children should be actively discouraged as a long-term prophylaxis against the problem of obesity.

Emotional and psychological factors are extremely important in the overall picture of obesity. There is gratification and pleasure in eating. Eating also offers relief from unsettling experiences such as home sickness, death of a dear one, and so on. Metabolically speaking, there is the fact that some patients may be converting more of their total caloric intake into fat deposits than others do. The fact remains that one cannot lose weight unless one reduces his caloric intake.

Treatment. The treatment of obesity is generally unsatisfactory. A long-range project, it will invariably be unsuccessful unless the patient is adequately motivated—that is, if he really and sincerely wants to lose weight and is willing to undergo a long period of discomfort in the process.

Although dietary manipulation is the simplest and easiest part of the therapy, it is not the most important one. A low-calorie diet, that is, a diet lower in calories than the body needs, is considered essential. (The usual recommendation is a 1,200 to 1,500-calorie diet, high in carbohydrates and moderately restricted in fats and proteins.) Equally essential, however, is some form of increased physical activity, be it merely an hour's walking a day or participation in some mildly active sport. It is more important to maintain physical movement frequently and regularly during the day, every day, than to perform strenuous exercises intermittently.

As essential as the reduction in diet and the increase in exercise is some attempt, generally made with the aid of the physician, toward psychological retraining.

The use of bulk-producing substances or of drugs such as those said to be appetite suppressors has not been successful. Thyroid extract is no longer prescribed in obesity therapy. Responsibility for the ultimate solution of the problem remains with the patient.

Prevention is always the most desirable approach in the treatment of this stubborn condition. Therefore, any weight gain in children and young people should be carefully watched by parents in order to forestall obesity in the first place. (*See also* the section QUESTIONS AND ANSWERS ABOUT COMMON SYMPTOMS.)

OVERWEIGHT Overweight is not the same as obesity (overfatness). It merely means that a person weighs more than the average range of the so-called "normal" for the same age and height. The excess weight may be due to heavy musculature.

The average body consists of about 20 percent fat; 38 percent muscle; 42 percent bone, blood, organs, and other tissues. If the body-fat content is normal, but the bony frame heavy with much muscle development, a person may be overweight as determined by the usual height-weight-age tables. In contrast, another individual may be "overfat" (obese) with poor muscle development and more fat, yet his total weight may be "normal" according to the standard tables. By and large, however, the person who is overweight is also overfat.

The problem of normal or ideal weight is very complex. The young man of today is somewhat taller and heavier than a man of the same age one or two generations ago. Is this good? We do not know, since we do not know what weight is most conducive to good health. Many people gain weight as they grow older. This may be the average situation, but probably represents an accumulation of fat and a decrease in muscle-mass.

The tables on pages 488–489 give average (not necessarily ideal) weights in "ordinary clothing." Each merely represents what a large number of Americans weigh. A deviation of 10 percent above this may be overweight. A deviation of 25 percent represents obesity.

What a person should weigh at age twenty-

1983 METROPOLITAN HEIGHT-WEIGHT TABLES
DESIRABLE WEIGHTS FOR WOMEN*†

Height	Small Frame	Medium Frame	Large Frame
		-----lb-----	
4'10"	102–111	109–121	118–131
4'11"	103–113	111–123	120–134
5'0"	104–115	113–126	122–137
5'1"	106–118	115–129	125–140
5'2"	108–121	118–132	128–143
5'3"	111–124	121–135	131–147
5'4"	114–127	124–138	134–151
5'5"	117–130	127–141	137–155
5'6"	120–133	130–144	140–159
5'7"	123–136	133–147	143–163
5'8"	126–139	136–150	146–167
5'9"	129–142	139–153	149–170
5'10"	132–145	142–156	152–173
5'11"	135–148	145–159	155–176
6'0"	138–151	148–162	158–179

FRAME SIZE FOR WOMEN††

Height in 1 Inch Heels	Elbow Breadth for Medium Frame
4'10" to 4'11"	2¼" to 2½"
5'0" to 5'3"	2¼" to 2½"
5'4" to 5'7"	2⅜" to 2⅝"
5'8" to 5'11"	2⅜" to 2⅝"
6'0"	2½" to 2¾"

†Weights at 25 to 59 based on lowest mortality. Weight in pounds according to frame (in indoor clothing weighing 3 lb., shoes with 1" heels).

††Elbow breadth is measured with the forearm upward at a 90 degree angle. The distance between the outer aspects of the two prominent bones on either side of the elbow is considered to be the elbow breadth. Elbow breadth less than that listed for medium frame indicates a small frame. Elbow breadth greater than that listed for medium frame indicates a large frame.

*Courtesy of Metropolitan Life Insurance Company. Reprinted with permission.

five to thirty is probably the ideal weight no matter what the age. It should be noted, however, that these averages are collected from a mixed population. In some racial groups the average weight for a certain age and height may be considerably different than for other groups.

PELLAGRA Pellagra is a serious disease characterized by mental, nervous-system, and skin symptoms produced by the deficiency of niacin (nicotinic acid) or its related substances, niacinamide and nicotinamide. Such deficiencies are usually associated with a diet overly rich in corn, and pellagra may be endemic in areas where this food plays a large part in daily nutrition. Secondary deficiency may result from prolonged diarrhea and certain forms of liver disease. (Protein containing the amino-acid tryptophan protects against low niacinamide intake because tryptophan is a raw material from which niacinamide is formed.)

Symptoms. In advanced pellagra the tongue is red, swollen, and tender, and the whole mouth appears inflamed. There is a characteristic skin lesion which forms at similar sites on both sides of the body at exposed

1983 METROPOLITAN HEIGHT-WEIGHT TABLES
DESIRABLE WEIGHTS FOR MEN*†

Height	Small Frame	Medium Frame	Large Frame
		----lb----	
5'2"	128–134	131–141	138–150
5'3"	130–136	133–143	140–153
5'4"	132–138	135–145	142–156
5'5"	134–140	137–148	144–160
5'6"	136–142	139–151	146–164
5'7"	138–145	142–154	149–168
5'8"	140–148	145–157	152–172
5'9"	142–151	148–160	155–176
5'10"	144–154	151–163	158–180
5'11"	146–157	154–166	161–184
6'0"	149–160	157–170	164–188
6'1"	152–164	160–174	168–192
6'2"	155–168	164–178	172–197
6'3"	158–172	167–182	176–202
6'4"	162–176	171–187	181–207

FRAME SIZE FOR MEN††

Height in 1 Inch Heels	Elbow Breadth for Medium Frame
5'2" to 5'3"	2½" to 2⅞"
5'4" to 5'7"	2⅝" to 2⅞"
5'8" to 5'11"	2¾" to 3"
6'0" to 6'3"	2¾" to 3⅛"
6'4"	2⅞" to 3¼"

†Weights at ages 25 to 59 based on lowest mortality. Weight in pounds according to frame (in indoor clothing weighing 5 lb., shoes with 1" heels).

††Elbow breadth is measured with the forearm upward at a 90 degree angle. The distance between the outer aspects of the two prominent bones on either side of the elbow is considered to be the elbow breadth. Elbow breadth less than that listed for medium frame indicates a small frame. Elbow breadth greater than that listed for medium frame indicates a large frame.

*Courtesy of Metropolitan Life Insurance Company. Reprinted with permission.

areas such as the hands and face. The bright scarlet color of the tongue and mucous membranes of the mouth, together with soreness of the mouth and increased salivation, are characteristic findings. Diarrhea is also a serious sign.

Among the nervous-system disorders that may be found in pellagra are non-specific weakness or apathy, and later, psychoses characterized by impairment of memory, disorientation, and confusion (sometimes with excitement, mania, and delirium). The extremities may be rigid, and there may be uncontrollable sucking and grasping reflexes in more advanced cases. In pellagra, the "three d's" are diarrhea, dementia, and dermatitis—although many cases do not show these features.

Treatment. Specific therapy includes niacinamide in large doses, both by mouth and by injection. However, the total nutritional state must be corrected because the patient who develops pellagra has generally been on an inadequate diet for a long time. Pellagra-preventive foods include liver, lean meat, peanuts, potatoes, legumes, milk, and eggs. The last two furnish little niacin but are excellent sources of tryptophan, an amino acid which is the precursor of niacin. The minimum niacin requirement of the adult is 6.6 niacin equivalents per 1000kcal. and not less than 13 niacin equivalents per 2000kcal. The requirement of an infant up to six months of age is 8 niacin equivalents per 1000kcal.

Fortunately pellagra is no longer common in this country, a fact which points out the advantages of widespread preventive measures and dietary supplementation.

POTASSIUM Potassium is an important electrolyte in the body which is intimately associated with sodium metabolism. The normal intake of potassium is about one to four grams and is related largely to the meat and fruit content of the diet. Unlike sodium, which is extracellular (in the external body fluids rather than in the cell), potassium is to a great extent intracellular.

Potassium deficiency develops through excessive loss from the kidneys or bowels. It occurs in certain types of complex kidney disease and in various types of overactivity of the adrenal gland. Patients with diarrhea or those who chronically use cathartics may lose potassium in excessive amounts in the stool.

But the most common cause is the group of diuretic drugs which promote excretion of fluid, sodium and potassium.

In severe potassium deficiency, muscle weakness and paralysis may develop, leading to difficulties in breathing and changes in the heart.

In certain diseases, both potassium and sodium concentration need to be adjusted. For this the physician uses certain drugs (diuretics) or hormones to stabilize the electrolyte pattern of the body. He often replaces deficiencies in these substances by administration of intravenous fluids in the hospital. For mild disorders, potassium pills and foods high in potassium are widely used.

PROTEINS Proteins are an essential constitutent of all living things, from bacteria to man. Every cell contains some members of this large family of complex molecules. For growth; for maintenance and replacement of loss by "wear and tear"; for the creation of enzymes which initiate chemical reactions; and for hormones (such as insulin) which direct how, when, and where these reactions proceed, proteins are essential. About 17 percent

LOW SODIUM-HIGH POTASSIUM FOOD LIST

Fruits	Serving	K(mg.)	Na(mg.)
Apple, fresh	1 medium	152	
Apricots, canned in heavy syrup	½ cup	302	
Avocado, cubed	½ cup	453	
Banana	½ cup	440	
Cantaloupe, fresh cubed	½ cup	201	
Dates, chopped	½ cup	577	
Figs, fresh	2 medium	194	
Fruit cocktail, canned in syrup	½ cup	206	
Honeydew, fresh cubed	½ cup	214	
Orange, fresh	1 medium	263	
Peaches, fresh, sliced	½ cup	172	
Plums, fresh, Damson type	½ cup	254	
Prunes, cooked with sugar	½ cup	312	
Raisins, sun-ripened	½ cup	553	
Fruit Juices			
Apricot Nectar	½ cup	190	
Grapefruit Juice, canned, sweetened	½ cup	203	
Orange Juice, frozen (dilute 1 to 3)	½ cup	252	
Pineapple Juice, canned, unsweetened	½ cup	187	
Prune Juice, canned	½ cup	301	

LOW SODIUM-HIGH POTASSIUM FOOD LIST—continued

Fruits	Serving	K(mg.)	Na(mg.)
Tomato Juice, low sodium	½ cup	275	
Vegetable Juice Cocktail	½ cup	268	
Vegetables			
Beets, sliced, cooked	½ cup	177	
Broccoli, frozen, cooked	½ cup	196	
Brussels Sprouts, frozen, cooked	½ cup	229	
Carrots, sliced, cooked	½ cup	172	
Potatoes, diced, boiled	½ cup	221	
Potatoes, French Fried, 4″	10 pieces	509	
Potatoes, instant mashed, seasoned	½ cup	300	243
Potatoes, Sweet, fresh, mashed	½ cup	310	
Pumpkin, canned	½ cup	294	
Spinach, fresh or frozen, cooked	½ cup	342	54
Squash, Winter, boiled, all varieties	½ cup	330	
Tomatoes, fresh	1 medium	366	
Tomatoes, canned	½ cup	262	157
Legumes			
Blackeyed Peas, canned	½ cup	449	301
Great Northern Beans, low sodium, cooked	½ cup	375	
Kidney Beans, cooked	½ cup	315	
Lentils, mature, cooked	½ cup	249	
Lima Beans, frozen, cooked	½ cup	362	
Peanut Butter	2 Tbsp.	200	
Pinto Beans, dried, cooked	½ cup	468	194
Soybeans, cooked	½ cup	486	
Milk and Dairy Products			
Buttermilk, commercial, skim	1 cup	204	319
Chocolate Milk, commercial, whole	1 cup	365	118
Ice Milk, soft serve	1 cup	350	119
Milk, skim	1 cup	355	127
Milk, whole	1 cup	351	122
Yogurt, skim	1 cup	350	125
Yogurt, whole	1 cup	323	115
Meats			
Beef, lean	3 oz.	204	45
Chicken	3 oz.	351	54
Fish, (Cod, Haddock, or Halibut) broiled	3 oz.	447	114
Lamb, lean	3 oz.	246	60
Liver, beef	3 oz.	324	156
Pork, fresh, lean	3 oz.	333	57
Tuna, low sodium	3 oz.	237	36
Turkey	3 oz.	282	75
Veal, lean	3 oz.	426	69
Miscellaneous			
Bouillon, Beef, low sodium	1 cube	570	
Bouillon, Chicken, low sodium	1 cube	641	
Molasses, Light	1 Tbsp.	183	
Molasses, Blackstrap	1 Tbsp.	585	
Salt Substitute	1 pkt (900 mg.)	430	

of an adult body is protein tissue, chiefly muscle tissue.

Chemically, proteins consist of hundreds or thousands of small units, (its "building blocks"), known as amino acids, all of which contain nitrogen as well as the usual elements, carbon, hydrogen, and oxygen.

Tissue proteins such as albumin cannot be formed unless all the essential amino acids are present in the diet and sufficient calories are supplied from fats and carbohydrates to provide the energy needs. If there is a deficiency in intake of either proteins or calories, the body tissues waste away. One ill effect of protein deficiency is that the formation of protective antibodies against infection is lessened and the malnourished patient may become more susceptible to infectious conditions.

Protein requirements vary in health and in disease; they also vary at different ages. They are proportionately highest in infancy, when the body is rapidly creating new cells and tissue (that is, during growth). Under certain circumstances such as pregnancy and breast-feeding, infections, burns, serious injuries, and hyperthyroidism, the protein requirements also rise.

The recommended daily average protein requirement is 0.6 gram per kilogram of body weight. Thus a man weighing about 70 kg needs about 56 grams of protein a day.

The daily intake in our country varies from about 50 to 100 grams; occasionally wider variations are seen. However, these requirements apply to "good" protein—that is, protein high in essential amino acids. Animal sources, chiefly meat, fish, and poultry, supply these in well-balanced amounts. The protein of vegetables is less satisfactory. Because starches, rice, roots, fruits, and vegetables form the basic diet in many Oriental and African regions, millions over the world today suffer from inadequate protein intake. The precise needs for protein in terms of quality and amino-acid balance are still uncertain.)

Unlike fat, protein cannot be stored in appreciable quantities. Excess dietary amino acids are metabolized, and it is therefore not economical to feed the relatively expensive high-protein foods in very large quantities.

Because protein is so basic to the living processes, deficiency symptoms are widespread and varied. They include weight loss, stunted growth, fatigue, lack of energy, slow wound healing, and prolonged convalescence. The liver does not function normally. The serum albumin falls and edema develops. Infections are another common symptom. The resulting anemia is a reflection of inadequate formation of the critical blood protein, hemoglobin. In certain tropical areas a serious disorder of protein malnutrition, known as kwashiorkor, occurs in young children; there is wasting, liver damage, accumulation of fluids (edema), growth-failure, and changes in skin and hair. Unless vigorously treated, this may prove fatal.

A well-balanced diet will protect against protein deficiency. High-protein diets, often used in convalescence, consist of larger proportions of meats, fish, poultry, milk, cheese, and eggs. (Egg white is pure protein.) Products made of wheat, rice, and potatoes contain some protein, but not in large amounts. Because high-protein foods are also usually more expensive than foods rich in starches or fat, many people, even in this country, do not eat enough protein.

RECOMMENDED DAILY ALLOWANCES In 1941 the Food and Nutrition Board of the National Research Council established a guide for nutritional recommendations. These have been called Recommended Dietary Allowances, and have been revised periodically since that time. It is important to note that the specific recommendations are designed for the maintenance of good nutrition of practically all healthy persons in the United States; but because of individual variations and requirements, these figures do not cover every person. Furthermore, it is not true, as is sometimes stated, that amounts below the RDA are inadequate.

The recommended allowances can be attained with a variety of common foods. Other nutrients, vitamins, and minerals for which human requirements are uncertain at this time are not included. When used as suggested (see RECOMMENDED DIETARY ALLOWANCES chart in this section), the recommended dietary allowances offer the best available estimate of dietary recommendations for the average healthy American. The needs in illness or under unusual circumstances may be different.

Food and Nutrition Board, National Academy of Sciences—National Research Council

RECOMMENDED DIETARY ALLOWANCES,[a] Revised 1989*

Designed for the maintenance of good nutrition of practically all healthy people in the United States

Category	Age (years) or Condition	Weight[b] (kg)	Weight[b] (lb)	Height[b] (cm)	Height[b] (in)	Protein (g)	Fat-Soluble Vitamins — Vitamin A (µg RE)	Vitamin D (µg)	Vitamin E (mg α-TE)	Vitamin K (µg)	Water-Soluble Vitamins — Vitamin C (mg)	Thiamin (mg)	Riboflavin (mg)	Niacin (mg NE)	Vitamin B6 (mg)	Folate (µg)	Vitamin B12 (µg)	Minerals — Calcium (mg)	Phosphorus (mg)	Magnesium (mg)	Iron (mg)	Zinc (mg)	Iodine (µg)	Selenium (µg)
INFANTS	0.0–0.5	6	13	60	24	13	375	7.5	3	5	30	0.3	0.4	5	0.3	25	0.3	400	300	40	6	5	40	10
	0.5–1.0	9	20	71	28	14	375	10	4	10	35	0.4	0.5	6	0.6	35	0.5	600	500	60	10	5	50	15
CHILDREN	1–3	13	29	90	35	16	400	10	6	15	40	0.7	0.8	9	1.0	50	0.7	800	800	80	10	10	70	20
	4–6	20	44	112	44	24	500	10	7	20	45	0.9	1.1	12	1.1	75	1.0	800	800	120	10	10	90	20
	7–10	28	62	132	52	28	700	10	7	30	45	1.0	1.2	13	1.4	100	1.4	800	800	170	10	10	120	30
MALES	11–14	45	99	157	62	45	1,000	10	10	45	50	1.3	1.5	17	1.7	150	2.0	1,200	1,200	270	12	15	150	40
	15–18	66	145	176	69	59	1,000	10	10	65	60	1.5	1.8	20	2.0	200	2.0	1,200	1,200	400	12	15	150	50
	19–24	72	160	177	70	58	1,000	10	10	70	60	1.5	1.7	19	2.0	200	2.0	1,200	1,200	350	10	15	150	70
	25–50	79	174	176	70	63	1,000	5	10	80	60	1.5	1.7	19	2.0	200	2.0	800	800	350	10	15	150	70
	51+	77	170	173	68	63	1,000	5	10	80	60	1.2	1.4	15	2.0	200	2.0	800	800	350	10	15	150	70
FEMALES	11–14	46	101	157	62	46	800	10	8	45	50	1.1	1.3	15	1.4	150	2.0	1,200	1,200	280	15	12	150	45
	15–18	55	120	163	64	44	800	10	8	55	60	1.1	1.3	15	1.5	180	2.0	1,200	1,200	300	15	12	150	50
	19–24	58	128	164	65	46	800	10	8	60	60	1.1	1.3	15	1.6	180	2.0	1,200	1,200	280	15	12	150	55
	25–50	63	138	163	64	50	800	5	8	65	60	1.1	1.3	15	1.6	180	2.0	800	800	280	15	12	150	55
	51+	65	143	160	63	50	800	5	8	65	60	1.0	1.2	13	1.6	180	2.0	800	800	280	10	12	150	55
Pregnant						60	800	10	10	65	70	1.5	1.6	17	2.2	400	2.2	1,200	1,200	320	30	15	175	65
Lactating	1st 6 months					65	1,300	10	12	65	95	1.6	1.8	20	2.1	280	2.6	1,200	1,200	355	15	19	200	75
(Nursing)	2nd 6 months					62	1,200	10	11	65	90	1.6	1.7	20	2.1	260	2.6	1,200	1,200	340	15	16	200	75

[a] The allowances, expressed as average daily intakes over time, are intended to provide for individual variations among most normal persons as they live in the United States under usual environmental stresses. Diets should be based on a variety of common foods in order to provide other nutrients for which human requirements have been less well defined. See text for detailed discussion of allowances and of nutrients not tabulated.

[b] Weights and heights of Reference Adults are actual medians for the U.S. population of the designated age, as reported by NHANES II. The median weights and heights of those under 19 years of age were taken from Hamill et al. (1979) (see pages 16–17). The use of these figures does not imply that the height-to-weight ratios are ideal.

*Reprinted by permission.

RICKETS   Rickets is a disease of childhood and is due to vitamin D deficiency. It is usually found in areas where the intake of vitamin D is low and where there is insufficient exposure to ultraviolet rays. (*See* VITAMIN D in this section.) At times it may be caused by failure to absorb the vitamin, as in patients with chronic intestinal disorders.

The basic disturbance is inadequate calcification of growing bones; that is, the basic bone structure is formed normally but does not become calcified or hard. There is also enlargement of the structures at the ends of the bones.

Infants with early rickets are restless and sleep poorly. They continually move their heads on the pillow, which denudes the head of hair. Such infants do not sit, crawl, or walk at an early date. Later there may be enlargement of the frontal bones (the bones in the forehead), enlargement of the cartilage at the ribs (known as the rachitic rosary), and disturbances in the leg and hand bones. Bowlegs, knock-knees, and pigeon breast may develop. X-ray examination shows these signs early.

If vitamin D deficiency is severe but develops later in adult life, a condition known as osteomalacia occurs. This is a demineralization of the spine, pelvis, and legs, producing bowing of the legs and abnormalities in the spine and pelvis.

In rickets, the serum calcium level may fall abnormally low, and the patient may develop tetany, or muscle spasm.

This once common disease can easily be prevented by giving infants vitamin D, beginning in the third or fourth week of life. The child who already has rickets responds slowly to doses of vitamin D, and these doses have to be larger.

It is important to remember that there is danger in giving excessive amounts of vitamin D. Therefore, no parent should feel that if a little vitamin D is good protection against rickets, much more can be safely given. One should always follow the recommendations of the physician or the manufacturer of the product used.

SCURVY   Scurvy indicates vitamin C deficiency. A typical case is suggested when a baby between six and twelve months old (who has not been getting enough vitamin C as fruit juice or as vitamin supplement) fails to gain weight, becomes irritable, cries when it is moved, and seems to have pain and tenderness in its legs. There may be swelling around the knees or other joints. Deformities at the junction of ribs and cartilage are seen. The gums are swollen and bleed easily; there is fever, increased pulse and respiration. Severe, untreated scurvy is fatal.

X-ray examination of the limb bones shows a distinctive pattern. Anemia is common, and tests for fragility of the capillaries are positive. In adults, weakness, irritability, weight loss, anemia, and muscle and joint pains come on gradually. Bleeding gums and loosening of teeth follow. The patient bruises easily. The level of ascorbic acid in the blood (white cell layer) is very low.

Treatment.   Both young and old with scurvy usually respond rapidly to large doses of vitamin C. Because this serious illness is so easily prevented, it is the obligation of all parents, physicians, dietitians, and others involved with dietary planning to ensure an adequate intake of this nontoxic substance for all.

SODIUM   Sodium is an essential mineral that plays a critical role in normal electrolyte metabolism. The average intake of sodium in the diet varies widely: from two to perhaps 15 grams of sodium chloride (common salt) per day. Intake depends to a large extent upon the amount of table salt added to the food and is a matter of taste. Some salt is present in foods. Salt is excreted mainly in the urine, and although its content in the body depends largely on the intake by mouth and output in the urine, its concentration in the blood is regulated in part by hormones. The adrenal glands, for example, produce a salt-retaining hormone.

Because the kidneys normally are efficient sodium conservers, sodium deficiency practically never develops due to low sodium intake. If the kidneys are diseased or if there is excessive loss from the bowels in diarrhea or through the skin in sweating, there may be excessive loss of salt and sodium deficiency may develop. Adrenal disease (with accompanying loss of salt-regulating hormone) allows wastage of sodium. Such a deficit is accompanied by dehydration or acidosis. Excessive fatigue, muscle cramps, and mental confusion are characteristic of sodium deficiency. Sodium excess is accompanied by overhydration and edema.

THIRST   The sensation of thirst is regulated by a highly specialized group of nerve endings that respond to changes in the volume and composition of the various body-fluids. This is part of an intricate system that regulates urine excretion, sweating, blood volume, and the amount of fluid in tissue cells. While an individual is aware of being thirsty when his mouth and throat are dry, the degree of thirst is not dependent on these sensations, since dryness is relieved after the first swallow. Nevertheless, the total intake of fluid is generally regulated precisely so as to provide the amount necessary for maintenance of proper fluid composition. Excessive thirst may be due to a hot environment, increased perspiration, intake of alcohol or spicy or salty

---

The Surgeon General's Report on NUTRITION AND HEALTH (1988)[1]
RECOMMENDATIONS
Issues for Most People:

- *Fats and cholesterol:* Reduce consumption of fat (especially saturated fat) and cholesterol. Choose foods relatively low in these substances, such as vegetables, fruits, whole grain foods, fish, poultry, lean meats, and low-fat dairy products. Use food preparation methods that add little or no fat.

- *Energy and weight control:* Achieve and maintain a desirable body weight. To do so, choose a dietary pattern in which energy (caloric) intake is consistent with energy expenditure. To reduce energy intake, limit consumption of foods relatively high in calories, fats, and sugars, and minimize alcohol consumption. Increase energy expenditure through regular and sustained physical activity.

- *Complex carbohydrates and fiber:* Increase consumption of whole grain foods and cereal products, vegetables (including dried beans and peas), and fruits.

- *Sodium:* Reduce intake of sodium by choosing foods relatively low in sodium and limiting the amount of salt added in food preparation and at the table.

- *Alcohol:* To reduce the risk for chronic disease, take alcohol only in moderation (no more than two drinks a day), if at all. Avoid drinking any alcohol before or while driving, operating machinery, taking medications, or engaging in any other activity requiring judgment. Avoid drinking alcohol while pregnant.

- *Fluoride:* Community water systems should contain fluoride at optimal levels for prevention of tooth decay. If such water is not available, use other appropriate sources of fluoride.

- *Sugars:* Those who are particularly vulnerable to dental caries (cavities), especially children, should limit their consumption and frequency of use of foods high in sugars.

- *Calcium:* Adolescent girls and adult women should increase consumption of foods high in calcium, including low-fat dairy products.

- *Iron:* Children, adolescents, and women of childbearing age should be sure to consume foods that are good sources of iron, such as lean red meats, fish, certain beans, and iron-enriched cereals and whole grain products. This issue is of special concern for low-income families.

[1]DHHS (PHS) Publication No. 88-50211. Reprinted by permission.

foods, or may herald such conditions as diabetes. Internal bleeding can sometimes be suspected in a patient with sudden excessive thirst, because of the reduction in circulating blood. Shock due to extensive burns or bleeding from any source is usually accompanied by thirst in the conscious patient.

UNDERWEIGHT Below average weight may be normal for an individual, in the absence of pathology, and must be differentiated from "loss of weight." In the healthy person, underweight is actually desirable. In 1962, an investigation involving a million men revealed that a person who was not merely at normal weight but below normal weight had a 79 percent greater chance of never suffering heart disease of any kind. Numerous studies since then have affirmed that the lean have less diabetes, less hypertension and even somewhat less cancer. The mechanisms that lessen the incidence of these diseases in the underweight are probably different from one person to another. A classic study of caloric restriction in the rat showed that when the restriction was moderate to severe, the life span was greatly prolonged. (*See also* ANOREXIA NERVOSA and BULIMIA in the section MENTAL HEALTH: PSYCHIATRIC AND PSYCHOLOGICAL CONDITIONS.)

Loss of weight may result from starvation, under- or malnutrition, protein deficiency, vitamin deficiency, mineral deficiency, disease processes, and emotional disorders. Once the physician has ascertained the cause of underweight, then he may prescribe the proper treatment. This may include diet—even surgery if tumors, etc, are the cause of the loss of weight.

VITAMIN A Vitamin A is an essential fat-soluble vitamin or "accessory food substance." It is involved in vision since it is a part of the purple visual pigment, rhodopsin. It is also needed for the proper maintenance of a very thin layer of cells (the epithelium) which lines or coats certain bodily structures. In deficiencies of vitamin A, the tissues involved are the eyelid and eyeball linings (conjunctiva), the windpipe (trachea), the hair follicles, and the kidneys. Bone growth is also affected by vitamin A levels.

The vitamin is present in such animal food as liver, egg yolk, butter, and cream. It is also derived from many green and yellow vegetables, which contain a plant pigment—carotene—that is converted into the vitamin in the intestinal lining.

Vitamin A deficiency results from a poor diet and inadequate intake. It also follows from failure to absorb the vitamin, as in chronic diarrhea, sprue, certain forms of childhood indigestion (celiac disease) and premature birth, as well as from failure to convert carotene to vitamin A. This last is seen occasionally in diabetes mellitus and advanced liver disease.

Children deficient in vitamin A show retarded growth and, like deficient adults, are susceptible to infections. Night-blindness (nyctalopia), or inability to adjust the eyes to darkened conditions, is the result of inadequate retinal pigment, rhodopsin. A dry, thick roughening of the skin (follicular hyperkeratosis) appears on the arms and legs. In advanced cases, the conjunctiva of the eye is dry and wrinkled, and infections are frequent.

Treatment. The recommended daily allowance for a healthy adult on a mixed diet (receiving two-thirds of the vitamin as carotene) is 5,000 International Units. In treatment, doses of 10,000 to 50,000 Units a day are used for children and 50,000 to 100,000 Units for adults.

Whereas vitamin A is easily stored and slowly excreted, it follows that repeated large doses may lead to excessive accumulation and "poisoning." A number of instances of abnormal excess of the vitamin in the body have been reported, especially in children. Symptoms of this condition are weight loss, headache, low-grade fever, changes in the bones and hair, anemia, and an enlarged liver. These symptoms usually disappear within one to four weeks after stopping the vitamin.

VITAMIN B$_2$ (RIBOFLAVIN) Riboflavin is a member of the water-soluble vitamin B complex. It is essential for proper growth and tissue function. Deficiency of this vitamin (ariboflavinosis) results in characteristic oral, skin, and eye lesions. The deficiency may be present when there is an inadequate consumption of milk and other proteins. More often it is found in patients with chronic diarrhea; liver disease; chronic alcoholism; or when, after an operation, infusions are given into the vein for some days without preventive vitamin therapy. Pure riboflavin deficiency rarely occurs. It is more likely to be present with other deficiencies of the vitamin B complex.

In vitamin B_2 deficiency, the corners of the mouth may be the site of the first signs of riboflavin deficiency. They may become reddened, and there may be cracks or maceration of the mucosal lining in the angles. These cracks often leave scars in healing. A series of disturbances in the oil-secreting (sebaceous) glands of the skin may also occur, with the following sequence of symptoms: increased oiliness; appearance of yellow, flaky scales—often in the folds between the nose and the mouth, sometimes behind the ears; and later, plugging-up of sebaceous-gland pores and roughening of the skin. In some cases, the cornea of the eye may develop a prominent network of tiny blood vessels. This may be accompanied by burning, tearing, and itching sensations.

Treatment. General nutritional therapy is essential, and riboflavin may be given by mouth in large doses. In rare instances, it may have to be given by injection. The recommended daily intake for the adult is between 1 and 2 mg. a day. The minimum requirement is less. Riboflavin is widely distributed in foods, but it is destroyed on exposure to light, and considerable loss can occur in such foods as milk.

VITAMIN B₆   Actually a group of closely related compounds, vitamin B_6 is often designated as pyridoxine. This member of the B complex has a function in the processing (metabolization) of amino acids, the basic components of protein. It also plays other less well-understood roles. Vitamin B_6 can relieve a form of neuritis sometimes observed by patients taking isoniazid (a drug for tuberculosis). Another preliminary report suggests that it contributes to the protection against dental caries (cavities) in children. A few cases of anemia in adults respond to large doses if the normal dietary intake is inadequate and a specific high requirement exists. Recent evidence suggests that vitamin B_6 may be required in heightened amounts during pregnancy.

The minimum daily requirement has not been firmly established, but the best estimates are that 2.0 mg. per day is an adequate amount for adult males and 1.6 mg. for adult females.

Vitamin B_6 is abundant in foods, and a spontaneous dietary deficiency is not likely to occur. However, infants, and perhaps some adults, subsisting on an artificial processed diet not supplemented with vitamins could become deficient. In a few instances of proven vitamin B_6 deficiency, the patients (infants) developed anemia, impaired growth, and convulsions. In experimental deficiency in adults, a type of skin condition (seborrheic dermatitis) developed on the face. In addition, weakness, loss of appetite, a burning tongue, and inflammation around the eyes were noted.

Treatment. For treatment of vitamin B_6 deficiency, large doses of pyridoxine are given by mouth or injection. Ideally, the possibility of vitamin B_6 deficiency can be avoided by giving the vitamin precautionarily in multivitamin preparations—especially to infants, pregnant women, and others who may be eating poorly or whose requirements are higher.

VITAMIN B₁₂   This member of the vitamin B complex family is one of the most biologically active substances known. The average daily requirement is only about 2.0 micrograms. It is found in liver, beef, pork, organmeats, and eggs and milk products, among other sources. Chemically, it is a cobalamin, meaning it contains the element cobalt—the only nutritionally significant compound that does contain it. The usual form used as medication is cyanocobalamin and is derived from microbiologic material—that is, it is produced by certain bacteria when grown under special conditions.

Vitamin B_{12} is necessary for the normal development of red blood cells. If there is a deficiency of this vitamin, the cells do not grow to maturity and the patient becomes anemic. True B_{12} dietary deficiency is extremely rare; certain people, however, lack a substance in their gastric juice called "intrinsic factor" which binds and carries vitamin B_{12} across the intestinal membrane. They therefore cannot absorb the vitamin B_{12} in food. Such patients develop a serious disease known as pernicious anemia, characterized by severe anemia and a progressive deterioration of nerve tracts in the spinal cord, the outcome of which used to be fatal.

Treatment. Some years ago liver (raw or cooked, and later as an injectable extract) was the standard treatment for pernicious anemia. With the discovery of vitamin B_{12}, it became possible to treat the disease with monthly injections of this nontoxic vitamin. The disease is also treated by daily oral administration of vitamin B_{12} plus intrinsic factor obtained from animals. More recently, large oral doses of the vitamin alone have also proved to be effective. So it is that pernicious anemia, a disease of vitamin B_{12} deficiency, is no longer the fatal condition it was a mere generation ago.

VITAMIN B COMPLEX   Vitamin B complex is the name given to a number of nutritional factors differing widely in chemical structure, but having in common an essential role in human nutrition. Many of the vitamins in this complex are components of one or more agents which play an important part in the activity of other bodily substances. Included in the group are thiamine (vitamin B_1), riboflavin (vitamin B_2), niacin, pyridoxine (vitamin B_6), and panthothenic acid, together with the "anti-anemia" vitamins, folic acid and vitamin B_{12}. (Choline is also usually included in the B complex.)

Deficiency of B-complex vitamins is a form of malnutrition frequently encountered in medical practice. Many of these vitamins occur in the same foods, and multiple deficiency is therefore observed more often than deficiency of a single substance. Some of the vitamins in this group are closely interrelated, and the clinical signs of deficiency may be similar, whatever the particular vitamin present in adequate amounts.

Deficiency of vitamin B complex does not necessarily result from inadequate diet alone. Numerous abnormal conditions may bring on, and contribute to, the deficiency. When the metabolic rate is above normal, as in hyperthyroidism, fever, or leukemia, there is an increase in the requirements for thiamine, riboflavin, and niacin. These vitamins also function in the metabolism of carbohydrate, and the requirement is increased following high carbohydrate consumption.

Vitamin B complex may be poorly absorbed or lost from the body in diarrheal diseases, inflammation of the digestive tract, and certain circulatory disorders. Furthermore, the body may use the vitamins in an abnormal manner in such diseases as diabetes mellitus and cirrhosis of the liver.

The administration of antibiotics by mouth may have an effect on vitamin B complex; in some instances, production of a B vitamin by intestinal bacteria may be impaired by the antibacterial effects of the drug. In other instances the antibiotic may actually reduce vitamin requirements by destroying the bacteria that utilize them.

VITAMIN C   Vitamin C, also known as ascorbic acid, is an essential water-soluble vitamin unrelated to the B complex. Its primary function is to maintain healthy connective tissue such as is found in bone and teeth. Ascorbic acid also has a role in the body's handling of iron and in the functioning of the adrenal gland whose hormones are essential in man's response to stress. For this reason, it is often administered in prolonged stressful situations, as after burns or extensive injury.

Vitamin C deficiency (scurvy) usually occurs in children from failure to supplement the diet with this essential item. All infants need vitamin C during the early months of life; for without it serious illness develops. In adults, a deficiency may develop from a poorly balanced diet. It may occur in elderly people who live alone, cook their own food without much concern about nutrition, and rarely if ever drink fruit juices.

The chief dietary source is citrus fruit, orange juice being the most likely source in this country. Other sources are tomato juice, tomatoes, cabbage, and potatoes. The vitamin is rather easily destroyed by cooking (oxidation with exposure to heat and light).

The average daily requirement for normal children is from 30 mg. (infants) to 60 mg. (boys, 13 to 15 years). Adults need about 60 mg. a day (80 mg. a day in pregnancy). Most well-balanced diets supply this amount. The vitamin is essentially nontoxic, and larger amounts may be given safely if there is reason to think the requirements are high or the diet poor in citrus fruits (grapefruit, lemons, and limes, as well as oranges and tomatoes).

VITAMIN D   Vitamin D is an essential fat-soluble food substance which has its primary effect on the calcium and phosphorus content of body fluids. It is actually a group of closely related substances, chemically resembling cholesterol and certain hormones. A unique feature of vitamin D is its formation in the skin on exposure to sunlight or ultraviolet rays (hence the name sunshine vitamin). The body is therefore only partially dependent on the dietary supply. Deficiency is rarely seen in adults and is becoming uncommon in infants due to the widespread use of dietary supplements and fortified milk(s) in early life. (Milk irradiated with ultraviolet light has an increased vitamin D content.)

Vitamin D increases the absorption of calcium, and possibly phosphorus, from the intestine and helps to maintain the levels of these minerals. A deficiency of the vitamin results in the condition known as rickets. Normal bone and tooth formation requires, however, dissolved in the body-fluids, an adequate supply of calcium and phosphorus as well.

The vitamin is particularly abundant in fish and fish livers. Cod liver oil was for years the main medicinal source. Nowadays vitamin-enriched, irradiated milks and milk products, margarines, etc., permit a reasonable intake which (with exposure to sunlight) meets the vitamin D requirement of many, but not all, children and adults. Many popular vitamin preparations also contain vitamin D.

Treatment. The recommended daily allowance in medical treatment is approximately 400 International Units a day, or about 10 micrograms of crystalline vitamin D_2, known as calciferol. In the darker-skinned races the requirements are about 50 percent higher because skin pigment interferes with vitamin D production. Premature infants require much larger amounts, often in a water-mixed preparation, because of immature fat absorption.

Massive doses given over long periods of time may lead to toxic reactions such as elevation of serum calcium levels, deposit of calcium in abnormal and unwanted sites, vomiting, and diarrhea. Death may occur from kidney failure. *Note:* The fat-soluble vitamins A and D are the only ones in which the danger of overdosage is a realistic possibility.

VITAMIN E   Vitamin E (also known as alpha-tocopherol) is a fat-soluble vitamin which has an essential but still poorly understood role in metabolism. It is widely distributed in foods (especially high in wheat-germ oil and eggs), so that dietary inadequacy is rare. An uncommon form of anemia in infants has been shown to be specific to vitamin E deficiency.

Vitamin E may also prevent some of the retinal damage that may occur in premature infants receiving oxygen therapy. Vitamin E deficiency in the adult has been shown to produce muscle and neurologic damage as well as breakdown of red blood cells in some animal experiments. Vitamin E deficiency leads to failure of normal progression of pregnancy, hence the occasional reference to vitamin E as "the fertility vitamin." Its relevance to human pregnancy is debatable. Hence the older idea that vitamin E was without a role has been abandoned. Still in actual practice vitamin E deficiency is extremely rare, and many of the claims advanced for its use, as in heart disease and osteoarthritis, have not been substantiated.

VITAMIN K   Vitamin K is essential for the formation of prothrombin, a substance necessary for blood coagulation. In vitamin K deficiency, hemorrhage in any tissue or in mucous membranes occurs. Such deficiency, however, is rare unless there is some underlying disturbance. Vitamin K is present in a large variety of foods and is synthesized by bacteria in the intestinal tract. The adult human requirement is easily supplied by the ordinary diet, in addition to the amount produced in the intestines. Natural forms of vitamin K are fat-soluble; deficiencies are therefore observed in conditions in which fat absorption is impaired (jaundice or malabsorption).

In infants whose mothers have not received vitamin K before birth, there is the danger of an inadequate intake in the first ten days of life. Cerebral hemorrhage may be present in such a case. Vitamin K deficiency may be diagnosed by estimating the prothrombin activity of blood.

VITAMINS   Some vitamins cannot be manufactured in the body, hence must be included in the diet. There is, in fact, a tendency to dose children with them too liberally, on the theory that whatever the organism does not need will simply be thrown off, and that an oversupply is safer than an undersupply. This is not accurate: doctors and nutritionists have positive knowledge that here "too much of a good thing" can be harmful. Nevertheless, vitamins may indeed be needed in increasing amounts during periods of rapid growth, during stress, and while convalescing.

Babies especially need to be given vitamins—but only according to the doctor's recommendation—because of their very rapid growth and because they are seldom exposed to the rays of the sun. What is usually prescribed for them is a multivitamin mixture, to be continued through their first year of life; but as soon as the diet becomes reasonably balanced and some meats, fruits or vegetables, as well as grain and dairy products, are consumed almost daily, the vitamin supplement becomes a needless expense and may even be dangerous. In this case, as in so many others, the wise parent will be content to be guided by the advice of the family doctor or pediatrician rather than rely on well-meaning friends or on advertisers.

WATER   Like air (oxygen), water is absolutely essential for life. Indeed, one can live for weeks without food but only a few days without water. Water is lost from the body through the kidneys as urine, by which means certain waste products are removed; through the bowel in stools, by which means solid wastes are removed; through the lungs in maintaining the air moist in the respiratory passages; and through the skin (both with and without sweating). Even without sweating, as much as a liter (approximately a little over a quart) is lost every day; with sweating, of course, the amount is considerably higher.

This water must be and is replaced by drinking it in beverages, by whatever water exists in solid foods, and by the small amounts of water produced by the metabolism of foodstuffs. (The words dehydration and overhydration refer to the balance between the amounts of water and of solids in the body.)

About 60 percent of the total weight of an adult is fluid. Of this total body water, about half is contained within the cells. The remainder is distributed in the blood plasma, in lymph (which circulates between cells), and in other tissues. Dissolved in the body fluids are the electrolytes, such as sodium, potassium, calcium, and magnesium, all of which are essential for normal bodily functions. These electrolytes are very carefully balanced by nature so that precise amounts are present both in and outside the cells. Many serious disturbances associated with disease occur because of abnormalities in the electrolytes.

When water deficiency exists, whether through inadequate intake or excessive loss, the results, in addition to thirst, are concentrated urine and a rise in body temperature; the patient becomes irritable, weak, and tired, his muscles may twitch, and eventually death may result. On the other hand, when there is an excessive amount of fluid, urine volume increases maximally; there may be headache, confusion, nausea, vomiting and muscle cramps.

SPORTS-RELATED HEALTH CONDITIONS

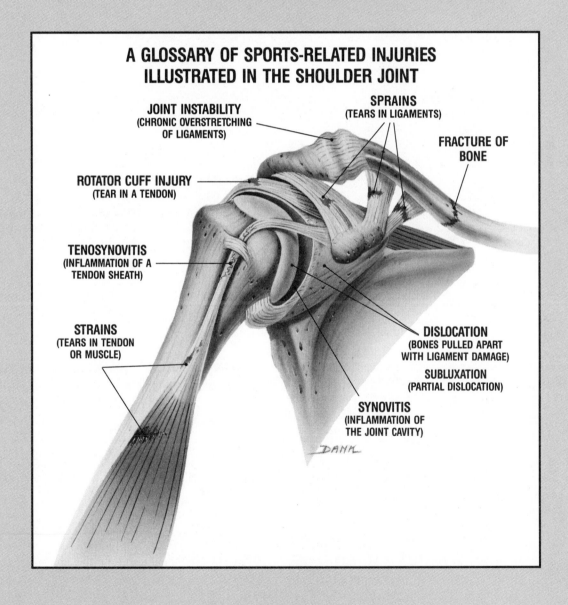

A GLOSSARY OF SPORTS-RELATED INJURIES ILLUSTRATED IN THE SHOULDER JOINT

JOINT INSTABILITY
(CHRONIC OVERSTRETCHING
OF LIGAMENTS)

SPRAINS
(TEARS IN LIGAMENTS)

FRACTURE OF BONE

ROTATOR CUFF INJURY
(TEAR IN A TENDON)

TENOSYNOVITIS
(INFLAMMATION OF A
TENDON SHEATH)

STRAINS
(TEARS IN TENDON
OR MUSCLE)

DISLOCATION
(BONES PULLED APART
WITH LIGAMENT DAMAGE)

SUBLUXATION
(PARTIAL DISLOCATION)

SYNOVITIS
(INFLAMMATION OF
THE JOINT CAVITY)

DANK

In the last decade more people have seen the importance of fitness in maintaining good health. Recreational sports participation has increased among all segments of the population. With increased usage of muscles and tendons without the proper preparation for exercise, injuries may result. Most disorders arise from repeated use of the injured tendon; treatment is directed at eliminating the activity which caused the problem until the problem corrects itself.

The physician who is concerned with the sports health field will counsel the patient about substituting less strenuous forms of exercise while maintaining the level of fitness achieved. This section examines the tendons most commonly affected in this type of injury, symptoms and treatments, and method of preventing recurrence of the injury.

The following is a list of topics identified in this section:

ACHILLES TENDINITIS
  (ANKLE AND FOOT)
ANTERIOR CRUCIATE LIGAMENT (ACL)
HALLUX RIGIDUS (BIG TOE PAIN)
IMPINGEMENT SYNDROME (SHOULDER)
LIGAMENTOUS INJURY
MEDIAL COLLATERAL LIGAMENT (MCL)

MENISCAL INJURY
OLECRANON BURSITIS
PATELLA (KNEE) PAIN
PLANTAR FASCIITIS (HEEL SPUR)
POSTERIOR TIBIAL TENDINITIS
TENNIS ELBOW
ULNAR NEURITIS

ACHILLES TENDINITIS (ANKLE AND FOOT) The term Achilles tendinitis describes combinations of posterior calf and heel pain with associated stiffness that usually occurs after sports requiring running, and particularly those that require bursts of acceleration. Examples are jogging on hills, tennis, squash, and basketball. The most common cause of Achilles tendinitis is simple overuse without adequate warm-up or sufficient rest between exercise sessions. Overuse causes failure first at a microscopic level in the fibers of the tendon. Without adequate rest, the disorder leads to progressive degeneration within the tendon with greater pain and weakness.

Abnormalities of the posterior heel can, at times, be responsible for Achilles tendinitis. Known commonly as "pump bumps" or spurs, these bony prominences can cause abnormal pressure on the Achilles tendon and degenerative changes within the tendon.

Symptoms. The typical patient with Achilles tendinitis complains of chronic heel pain initially occurring after he stops exercising. Later, the pain is present during exercise and finally occurs during even simple movements.

Examination reveals tenderness of the tendon to touch. If the disorder is chronic (particularly in patients over 40 years of age), there may be swelling in the tendon.

If a patient has spurs, the site of tenderness will be in the lowermost aspect of the tendon, but in the majority maximal tenderness is at a somewhat higher level. Range of motion of the affected foot should be compared with the opposite extremity; most cases will demonstrate some loss in the ability to flex the foot.

Treatment. Most patients see a physician at the earliest stage of tendon disorder, that of reversible inflammation. With rest from stressful activity, plus a supervised program of Achilles stretching and strengthening, and a short course of non-steroidal anti-inflammatory agents (for example, ibuprofen) complete resolution should be expected in one to three months. For patients with chronic tendinitis particularly those with extensive swelling of the tendon, initial treatment is the same. But, expected recovery time is considerably longer, being approximately three to six months. The worst prognosis is in long distance runners, in whom full return to activities with established Achilles tendinitis is unlikely.

Surgical treatment is rarely indicated, but the cleaning away of devitalized tissue (debridement) will predictably provide relief of symptoms present during simple movement but rarely allows return to full sporting activities. The best candidates for surgical treatment are patients with a demonstrable spur seen on the X-ray. After removal of this bony prominence the tendon is relieved of abnormal pressure. However, ultimate healing of the damaged tendon is slow, because of the relatively poor vascular supply of the tendon.

ANTERIOR CRUCIATE LIGAMENT (ACL)

The anterior cruciate ligament is an intraarticular structure that originates from the lateral femoral condyle to insert on the anterior portion of the tibia. It is the primary restraint to anterior movement of the tibia on the femur. Unlike the medial collateral ligament complete disruption of the ACL is more common than partial disruption.

Symptoms. As with MCL injury, the patient may recognize the moment of injury, as a pop will be felt and often heard by the patient. Almost immediately the knee will swell. Unlike the MCL injury the isolated ACL injury is not significantly painful. Meniscal injury occurs frequently with ACL injury and should be considered if significant pain is present. If the patient attempts immediate return to activity he often experiences instability of the knee.

Physical examination reveals marked diffuse swelling of the knee. If aspiration is performed a bloody effusion will be noted. Stability testing is best performed with the knee at 20° of flexion supported by a pillow. With the patient relaxed the examiner stabilizes the femur with one hand and pulls the tibia forward with the opposite hand. This should be compared to the contralateral knee.

Treatment. ACL insufficiency in the aggressive athlete in sports requiring lateral knee motion is usually poorly tolerated. Immediate ligament repair is recommended for them. In all other individuals conservative treatment is initiated with crutches and a hinged brace until swelling diminishes. Therapy is concentrated on hamstring strengthening to restrain anterior tibial translation. Return to sports with a brace is allowed in six to eight weeks.

HALLUX RIGIDUS (BIG TOE PAIN)

Hallux rigidus describes a form of osteoarthritis involving the first metatarsal phalangeal joint at the base of the big toe. Because of repeated high load stress (such as that occurring in running in tennis) the joint develops bone spurs. The osteophytes cause pain on joint motion and ultimately severely restrict its motion.

Symptoms. The typical patient is a manual laborer, jogger, exercise walker, or tennis player over 35 years of age. The patient has pain localized to the metatarsal phalangeal joint of the great toe. The pain is present initially only with exercise and later occurs with simple movement. With advanced disease one may note bone spurs especially on the upper surface (the dorsum) of the toe. Rarely, if ever, is a significant bunion deformity present. The most striking feature is the marked reduction in passive motion of the metatarsal phalangeal joint usually with pain at the extremes of motion.

A radiograph of the great toe will reveal bone spur formation on both sides of the joint although there will be preservation of central joint space.

Treatment. Initial treatment is conservative with shoe modification—placing a rocker bottom beneath the ball of the foot to minimize motion at the joint. If full return to vigorous activity is desired, conservative treatment generally is inadequate and surgery is indicated. Surgery consists of removal of the bone spurs to eliminate blockage of motion and the associated discomfort. Post operative return to full activity without significant discomfort can be expected within four to six months.

IMPINGEMENT SYNDROME (SHOULDER)

Impingement syndrome is a term used to describe degenerative disorders to the rotator cuff and biceps tendon occurring after repetitive overuse of the shoulder. This is commonly known as bursitis of the shoulder.

An important component of the shoulder socket is the long head of the biceps tendon.

This runs from the biceps muscle through a groove on the upper arm to insert on the superior portion of the shoulder socket. As the biceps tendon travels from the humerus, it lies in intimate contact with the rotator cuff tendon.

At risk are individuals who repetitively use the arm in an overhead fashion, in activities such as tennis, throwing, swimming, or golf. The cuff tendon and biceps tendon can undergo repetitive microtrauma setting up a progressive inflammatory and degenerative process within the rotator cuff tendon.

Symptoms. Patients complain of anterior shoulder pain. The pain worsens during and after activities requiring overhead use of the arm. As the disorder progresses, significant night pain will develop as the patient sleeps on the inflamed shoulder. If left untreated, and with continuation of activity, the rotator cuff will undergo degeneration and the patient will notice a definite loss of power.

As the disorder progresses the patient exhibits difficulty in achieving maximal overhead elevation of the arm. Often marked shrugging of the affected shoulder is noted on this maneuver. Rotator cuff strength is best assessed by testing ability of the patient to externally rotate the arm against resistance and abduct with the humerus internally rotated against resistance. The acromial clavicular joint can be independently assessed by (1) directly palpating the joint to see if tenderness can be elicited; (2) by the examiner maximally adducting the patient's arm across his chest. If this elicits pain it is a sign of acromial clavicular joint inflammation. The biceps tendon is tested by asking the patient to forward flex and supinate the forearm against resistance. If bicipital tendinitis is present, these maneuvers will elicit pain in the anterior portion of the shoulder. In case of advanced tendinitis rupture of the long head of the biceps can occur. This will be evident on physical examination; when the patient is asked to contract his biceps the muscle will appear shortened, and curled into a ball.

Initial radiographs of the shoulder may be normal. As the disorder advances bony thickening, spurring, or calcifications within the rotator cuff tendon can be seen.

Treatment. The majority of patients with impingement syndrome respond favorably to conservative therapy. If gross weakness is not present on the initial examination the patient is advised to refrain from activity, given oral anti-inflammatory agents, and placed on an exercise program for rotator cuff muscles. If no response is obtained within one month, soluble cortisone is injected into the subacromial space and another course of anti-inflammatory medication is given. Return to activity is allowed gradually once the pain is substantially abated.

If profound weakness is present initially or the patient fails to respond to conservative measures over a three to six month period, an arthrogram (X-ray after a dye injection) of the shoulder is obtained. This will document the presence of a full thickness rotator cuff tear. If no tear is present but pain continues, surgery is recommended to prevent further trauma to the rotator cuff. If a tear is present in a symptomatic active healthy individual, surgical repair is recommended.

LIGAMENTOUS INJURY The knee is a complex joint allowing for flexion and extension as well as rotation. Stability is provided by the four primary ligaments: the anterior and posterior cruciates and the medial and lateral collaterals.

The most commonly injured ligaments in the athlete are the anterior cruciate and the medial collateral ligament. Analogous to meniscal injury, damage to these ligaments occurs when the knee is subjected to abnormal motion. In fact, meniscal damage occurs frequently in conjunction with ligament rupture. The forces required to cause ligament damage are much greater than those producing meniscal damage alone. The most commonly associated sports are football and skiing. The mechanism of injury is different in the two sports; in football the foot is planted in the turf and as the athlete tries to change directions quickly or is hit, the femur rotates externally on the fixed tibia. In skiing, the leg is unweighted during a fall and the tibia externally rotates as the knee hyperextends.

MEDIAL COLLATERAL LIGAMENT (MCL) The medial collateral ligament arises from the medial aspect of the femur to insert on the medial tibia, and is a primary restraint to stress. The medial collateral ligament is made up of two portions, a deep short portion and long superficial portion. It is the longer superficial portion that is primarily responsible for medial stability of the knee. Isolated medial collateral ligament injuries are rarely complete ruptures.

Symptoms. The patient will localize the injury to the knee and occasionally hear a pop or feel a tearing sensation on the medial aspect of the knee. Immediate swelling generally occurs.

Physical examination usually reveals mild swelling. Tenderness is localized to the medial aspect of the knee.

Treatment. Conservative treatment of the isolated MCL injury is always successful. The patient is immobilized in a hinged brace and kept on crutches until the initial pain abates. Full weight bearing is then initiated. The range of motion as well as quadriceps exercises are begun after four weeks. A return to sports is permitted with use of the brace.

MENISCAL INJURY Meniscal injury specifically refers to tearing of the structure of the medial or lateral meniscus. This common athletic injury occurs when the knee is twisted in an unusual fashion during rapid directional changes, especially in football, soccer and basketball.

The menisci are C-shaped cartilage pads lying on each of the two tibial plateaus. At their periphery they are attached to the capsule of the knee while the inner edge lies free in the joint. They distribute compressive loads applied to the knee and aid the ligamentous structures in stabilizing the joint. During excessive stress of the joint the meniscus is susceptible to being torn. Tearing occurs more frequently in the medial than the lateral meniscus.

Symptoms. The patient with a meniscal tear will often describe a definite injury usually a sudden twist of the knee, and pain associated with a sensation of a pop. Gradual swelling will develop during the first day after injury. The patient will note knee pain specifically localized to the inside (medial meniscus) or outside (lateral meniscus) at the level of the joint line. Activity increases the pain, often precluding continued participation in sports. If the tear allows displacement

of the meniscus the joint may lock so that the patient is unable to extend the knee.

Physical examination may reveal quadriceps atrophy of the affected side if the individual has been favoring the knee. The joint will often be swollen due to secondary inflammation. Tenderness will be present at the joint line as the examiner applies pressure. Internal rotation of the tibia on the femur will reproduce the medial pain and external rotation reproduces the lateral pain. An ordinary X-ray of the knee will not demonstrate any abnormalities, but arthrography or magnetic resonance imaging (MRI) can provide further confirmation of the diagnosis.

Treatment. It is rare for a meniscal tear to heal spontaneously. If symptoms do not abate, surgery is recommended. Repair of the meniscus is indicated if a large part of the meniscus is involved. Smaller tears may also require excision of the damaged portion. Surgery performed arthroscopically minimizes operative trauma to the joint and allows faster recovery. The results of repair/excision for isolated meniscal injury are excellent for full functional return.

OLECRANON BURSITIS Olecranon bursitis is a common disorder which produces swelling and discomfort over the back of the elbow. It occurs more commonly in active individuals over forty.

In any area of the body where a bony prominence must glide under the skin during joint motion, a bursa is interposed. A bursa, in its normal state, is a thin walled sac lined with cells that provide the lubrication needed for proper gliding. When irritated by direct trauma, or overuse, the bursa walls thicken and fluid accumulates. Bony changes may also occur with the formation of a spur at the point of the elbow (the olecranon).

Symptoms. The common complaint is of elbow swelling. The pain is usually mild. In the initial stages the swelling will be present only after activity. As the disorder progresses the swelling will become more constant.

Physical examination reveals a cystic mass localized to the olecranon process of the elbow. Palpation causes only mild pain. X-rays of long standing cases will reveal a small olecranon spur.

Treatment. Initial treatment is reduction

of activity, or anti-inflammatory agents and a compressive elastic elbow sleeve with a relief over the olecranon process. If swelling does not diminish within one month aspiration of the cyst is performed followed by an injection of soluble cortisone. After aspiration and injection, the patient resumes use of the elastic elbow sleeve, as directed by the physician. Only in rare cases (usually those with a large bone spur) is surgery indicated. In severe cases bursa and bone spur are excised.

PATELLA (KNEE) PAIN Patella pain is the most common cause of knee pain. It occurs with greater frequency in athletic individuals particularly in adolescence when generalized ligamentous laxity is present.

The patella is a bone within the tendon of the quadriceps muscle; when viewed in cross section it is diamond shaped. The patella articulates with the lowermost part of the femur which has a V groove which conforms to the patella shape. In a normal individual the patella moves symmetrically within the femoral groove during flexion and extension of the knee. Abnormal tracking of the patella has been associated with several anatomic factors, such as a long patella tendon, and a shallow femoral groove. Abnormal tracking causes abnormally high pressures on the articular cartilage of the patella, causing inflammation and pain.

Symptoms. The patient typically complains of insidious onset of knee pain. The pain is poorly localized occurring both in the front and the back of the knee and is often bilateral. The pain is present on sporting activities or daily activities involving knee flexion such as walking stairs, squatting or arising from a seated position. Occasionally, straight ahead buckling of the knee will occur. On physical examination these patients will often demonstrate "squinting" knee caps. When viewed during normal standing the patella will appear to be pointed inward. Examination, with the patient supine, demonstrates hypermobility of the patella and tenderness when the undersurface (articular surface) is palpated. Direct compression of the patella onto the femur will also cause pain.

Treatment. Treatment is initially directed at reducing inflammation with rest and oral anti-inflammatory agents. To improve tracking, quadriceps exercises are initiated. However, only straight leg raising is allowed initially. Leg extension exercises from a flexed position can worsen cartilage inflammation, because it involves increased patella-femoral contact pressure. In addition, an elastic brace with a cut-out over the patella is used which will splint the patella to help improve patella tracking. Conservative care is successful in the majority of cases. Only in refractory cases is surgery indicated to realign the extensor mechanism. Shaving down the articular cartilage of the patella alone is uniformly unsuccessful.

PLANTAR FASCIITIS Deep within the sole of the foot lies a band of tough tissue called the plantar fascia. Since it originates from the base of the heel, it forms a ligament for the arch of the foot traversing to the base of the metatarsal heads. Plantar fasciitis is an inflammation of the fascial layer that occurs uniquely at its origin at the base of the heel. Causes include a tight Achilles tendon since lack of an adequate range of motion of the foot during use transmits abnormal stresses to the heel insertion site of the plantar fascia, resulting in inflammation; and acquired flat foot, which is usually due to weakening of the tendon supporting the foot. Abnormal stresses are thus placed on the plantar fascia with resulting inflammation.

Symptoms. Typical patients are those participating in repetitive activity on a hard surface, such as exercise walking, jogging or tennis. Patients complain of pain, often severe, occurring during activity and when walking barefoot. The pain is characteristically in the sole of the foot at the heel.

Treatment. Initial treatment involves rest from repetitive activity, non steroidal anti-inflammatory agents, and Achilles stretching exercises. If flat feet do not exist, a simple heel cup, scooped out to relieve pressure over the affected area, is placed in the shoe. If flat feet are present, full-length custom shoe inserts with a molded arch support and heel relief are ordered. Relief can be expected in four to six weeks with a return to full activity in two months in a majority of cases. Surgery is rarely indicated. Simple debridement of the heel spur has met with uniformly poor results. Relief can be provided by release of the heel attachment of the plantar fascia. Although pain relief is good for the procedure, return to sporting activity is poor, because of resultant weakness in the push-off stage of gait.

POSTERIOR TIBIAL TENDINITIS

This muscle originates from the medial aspect of the tibia, becomes tendinous above the ankle and traverses the medial side of the foot. The posterior tibial tendon provides dynamic support for the arch of the foot. Loss of this support results in acquired flat foot deformity.

This condition begins as an inflammatory process within the tendon sheath. It occurs in the older athlete, usually over fifty years of age and is a sequel to abnormalities of gait, most often hyperpronation (flat foot). The excessive inward rotation of the foot places great stress on the tendon and leads to inflammation. If it progresses, it can lead to a chronic degenerative process within the tendon and possible subsequent rupture. Posterior tibial tendinitis in the younger age group (under thirty) is usually associated with an anatomic abnormality of the tendon at its origin.

Symptoms. The patient will complain of pain along the medial border of the foot often radiating to the area above the ankle. In severe cases the patient will note progressive flat foot deformity and uneven wear of the shoes. Physical examination will usually reveal swelling and tenderness along the course of the posterior tibial tendon.

Treatment. In the early stages of the disorder conservative treatment is successful in the majority of cases. Patients are advised to refrain from vigorous activities and are given a course of nonsteroidal anti-inflammatory agents as well as molded shoe inserts with a firm medial arch support.

If advanced degeneration or rupture of the tendon is present with flat foot deformity, surgical treatment is needed to reconstruct the posterior tibial tendon by use of one of the toe flexor tendons. Results for return to painless motion have been good but full return to vigorous activity is uncertain.

TENNIS ELBOW The term tennis elbow implies an inflammation at the muscle ten-

dons responsible for motion of the wrist and hand. Tennis elbow occurs most commonly at the outer aspect of the elbow which is the bone of the upper arm (lateral epicondyle of the humerus). It can occur at the inner side also (medial epicondyle).

Lateral Tennis Elbow

This refers to an inflammation of the muscles responsible for extension of the wrist and fingers. Anatomic studies have shown the site of inflammation may be mostly in a single tendon.

Although known as tennis elbow, this disorder develops frequently in the non-athletic population as well. Due to repetitive overload of the wrist extensor mechanism, it may occur in any activity requiring use of a firmly held wrist against a resistive force. Typical examples besides tennis are carpentry and gardening.

Symptoms. In the early stages of the disorder the patient complains of pain, occurring after activities. With progression the pain occurs during the activity. As the tennis ball is struck, the patient will experience immediate pain in the lateral part of the elbow often radiating to the lateral forearm. In its most severe stages pain will occur during simple activities of daily living such as handshaking and writing.

Treatment. The foremost principle of the initial treatment is rest from the activity causing pain. This period of rest varies with the severity of the disease. Usually a minimum of three weeks is required. Unless contra-indicated in a particular patient a three week course of nonsteroidal anti-inflammatory agents is also given. To minimize further trauma to the tendon occurring during activities of daily living, a removable wrist splint which positions the wrist in a slight dorsi flexion is prescribed. Progress is monitored by the physician at three-week intervals. Once the pain has diminished considerably a gradual program of strengthening and gently stretching exercises is initiated. Beginning with an object such as a soup can, the patient performs wrist dorsi flexion exercises and the weight is slowly increased to a 5 lb. maximum. The patient maximally flexes the wrist with the elbow flexed at a right angle. While keeping the wrist flexed, the elbow is gradually extended to the point where discomfort occurs. With progress the patient will be able to comfortably achieve maximum wrist flexion with full elbow extension. Once the patient can successfully carry out the initial phase of exercise without discomfort a gradual return to activities is allowed. A tennis player's stroke should be analyzed by a registered professional. Any tendency toward late contact with the ball or lack of proper body rotation should be corrected as these factors are clearly related to lateral tennis elbow. Bracing (elbow strap) is usually indicated only in those individuals greater than 50 years of age who are at the beginning or low intermediate level of the skill.

If pain persists despite this course of treatment, cortisone injections can be attempted. Due to possible detrimental effects on tendon structure, no more than two injections should be given, spaced one month apart. Only in rare instances is surgery indicated. At present the patient usually requires a minimum of six months of conservative therapy before considering surgery.

Medial Tennis Elbow

Much less common than its lateral counterpart, medial tennis elbow is not an affliction of the weekend tennis player or homemaker. It occurs almost exclusively in the elite level tennis players and baseball pitchers who place extraordinary force on the elbow during the serving and pitching motion.

During the cock-up portion of the tennis serve and baseball pitch, the arm is placed above and behind the body, the elbow is maximally flexed and the hand maximally supinated. From this position the athlete accelerates the hand forward with tremendous force. Much of this acceleration force is developed by the muscle tendon group originating on the medial epicondyle, those muscles responsible for forearm pronation and finger flexion. This repetitive microtrauma can cause overload and subsequent inflammation of the common flexor/pronator tendinous origin.

Treatment. Treatment is carried out using the same principles as with lateral tennis elbow. Initial rest including administration of anti-inflammatory medication is followed by a careful stretching/strengthening program with a gradual return to activity.

ULNAR NEURITIS   Occurring almost exclusively in a throwing athlete, ulnar neuritis is an inflammatory process involving the ulnar nerve as it traverses the elbow. Analogous to medial tennis elbow it occurs due to repetitive stress placed on the elbow during the throwing motion.

The ulnar nerve originates in the armpit area and travels through the upper arm in the anterior muscular compartment. Above the elbow it becomes posterior in position, then traverses the elbow joint lying in a bony tunnel, the cubital fossa (the "funny bone"). It next travels anteriorly in the forearm splitting the two heads of a flexor muscle. Thus the ulnar nerve is constrained at either end of the forearm. In a small percentage of individuals hypermobility of the nerve at the elbow exists. When these individuals participate in throwing sports they are at particular risk for inflammation of the ulnar nerve.

Symptoms. The athlete will complain primarily of numbness and tingling in the little and ring fingers whose sensation is supplied by the ulnar nerve. In neglected cases, atrophy of the hand will be noted as well as weakness of the fine muscles of the hand that allows spreading of the fingers.

Treatment. Initial treatment is conservative with anti-inflammatory drugs and avoidance of activity. If this fails surgery may be required to allow the patient to return to competitive sports. The surgery moves the ulnar nerve permanently out of the cubital fossa, and stabilizes it behind the muscle fascia layer.

FIRST AID AND EMERGENCIES

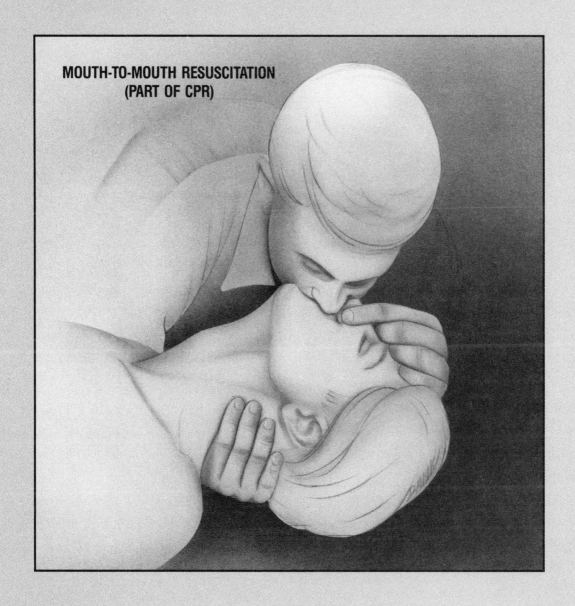

MOUTH-TO-MOUTH RESUSCITATION
(PART OF CPR)

First aid and emergency care should be included as a fundamental part of preparation for living. An educated person might reasonably be expected to know how to give mouth-to-mouth resuscitation; he should have some general ideas about the treatment of severe bleeding; and he should know that in moving an accident victim a simple fracture might be made into a compound fracture. Unfortunately, emergencies strike unexpectedly. Prompt, intelligent action may convert a dangerous, even life-threatening situation into a controllable one.

First aid measures are based on the use of common sense. It is important to understand the why and wherefore of each procedure and the reason or principle governing each action that is taken. This section examines the first principles which will enable a person to act correctly in most situations.

The following is a list of topics identified in this section:

ACCIDENT PREVENTION
ARTIFICIAL RESPIRATION
BEE STINGS
BITES
BITES AND STINGS (INSECT)
BITES (SCORPION) (TICKS)
BITES (SNAKE)
BITES, SPIDER (BLACK WIDOW)
BITES, SPIDER (BROWN RECLUSE)
BLEEDING
BRUISES
BURNS
**CARDIOPULMONARY RESUSCITATION
  (CPR)**
CHOKING

CONVULSIONS
CROUP
CUTS
ELECTRICAL SHOCK
FAINTING
FALLS AND FRACTURES
FOREIGN BODIES, INSERTION OF
FRACTURES
FROSTBITE
HEART (CARDIAC) EMERGENCIES
HEAT EXHAUSTION
HEAT STROKE
NOSEBLEED
POISONING
TABLE OF COMMON POISONS

ACCIDENT PREVENTION Not all accidents can be prevented, but analysis of thousands of them indicates that with care and forethought, many can be avoided. For example, it is generally agreed that most of the serious cases of childhood poisoning can be prevented if certain precautions are taken. Not all falls are avoidable, but those that occur in a bathtub—because of no rubber mat—most certainly are avoidable. Slippery scatter rugs are a special threat to elderly or feeble individuals and to children, and could well be firmly anchored or removed. The evidence that safety belts can drastically reduce our enormous automobile casualty rate cannot be disputed. We are naturally concerned about the food our children eat and the education

they get. But are we equally concerned and equally alert when it comes to protecting them against accidents? Accidents are, in fact, the number one threat to the young child's life.

In first aid, major emphasis should be on prevention, and the first and last points stressed in first-aid courses should be the preventability of accidents. Dr. Harry Raybin, of New York City's famous Poison Control Center, has said: "A knowledge of antidotes will not satisfactorily substitute for prudent housekeeping." Here are some safety tips, derived from the sad experiences of others, which you should carefully consider and profit from:

• When there are small children in the

home, be sure to keep medicines where they cannot be reached by creeping, climbing toddlers. Some of the newer medicine chests have safety locks which cannot be opened by the small child. If yours can be opened too easily, you should keep it free of all medicines. This applies especially to aspirin, which is the most common single cause of childhood poisoning. Find a location for medicines which you are sure is inaccessible to the children. A sliding latch placed high on the bathroom door is one solution you might consider.

• Other common causes of childhood poisoning include bleaches, disinfectants, and cleaning agents which are often kept virtually at floor level in the kitchen. Most detergents are not likely to produce serious poisoning, but bleaches and lyes are major threats. They are best kept under lock and key, or in some inaccessible place.

• Never leave small children unattended. A minute's negligence can result in tragedy.

• Many falls in the home can be prevented by using rugs with nonskid backing, by not waxing floors too highly, and by avoiding rickety step-ladders, or chairs balanced together, for doing repairs. Night lights are also an aid in avoiding falls.

• Children's falls out of windows can be completely prevented by having adequate window-guards.

• Falls out of bed are always a possibility with the young and the elderly, especially when certain drugs are being taken or when there is fever, confusion, or serious debility. These falls can be prevented by placing chairs against the bed, by side rails, or by similar methods.

• A small fire extinguisher in the kitchen may be more useful than any other gadget there. It may prevent a grease fire from spreading to wooden cupboards and to curtains.

• Kerosene, gasoline, benzine, turpentine, and other cleaning fluids are potential poisoning agents as well as fire hazards. Keep them in a safe place or, unless the need for them is frequent, do not keep them at all.

• Never take a medicine without reading and rereading the label.

• Do not store cleaning fluids, lye solutions, or any other hazardous substances in soda bottles, wine bottles, or milk containers. Do not trust to your memory to identify chemicals you may have stored away for some vague future use—a moment taken to label them is a worthwhile safety provision.

By their very nature, accidents can occur even to the most careful among us. One should therefore be prepared to cope with many kinds of accidents and emergencies. They can occur in someone else's home, as well as in your own, or on the highway, at the beach, in the woods, or the countryside, at some distance from a medical center or a doctor's office.

ARTIFICIAL RESPIRATION *See* color insert First Aid and Life Saving, plates F4-F5. *See also* Emergency Survival Guide on the endpapers.

BEE STINGS More deaths occur each year in the United States from bee stings than from the bite of any other insect or animal. This is because certain individuals have allergic or hypersensitive reactions to the sting of bees. Such persons can suffer sudden collapse or respiratory obstruction. Usually, they have shown sensitivity to a bee sting on one or more previous occasions, with reactions such as unusual local swelling, marked weakness, asthmatic breathing, or severe drop in blood pressure. Once an individual has shown some unusual reaction of this kind, special precautions are thereafter necessary. Desensitization, much as one desensitizes for the pollens or against horse serum, should be seriously considered; while this has been shown to have marked protective value, it is still not widely enough employed. In the absence of desensitization, the hypersensitive person should take special precautions to avoid bees and to wear protective clothing and netting if exposure is unavoidable. If such exposure is unavoidable, certain emergency drugs for use after a bee sting may easily be carried on the person. One of these is a tablet (Isuprel®), which can be placed under the tongue; as it is absorbed, it has an adrenalin-like effect. Another remedy is one of the several different types of pocket inhalers used by asthmatics. A few inhalations of this will prevent bronchial spasm. Some highly allergic persons carry emergency injectible epinephrine with them when they expect to be in contact with bees.

BITES Animal and insect bites may be daily events in the lives of some people, and only a small percentage constitute a threat. Obviously, a minor bite from a household pet need hardly cause concern. On the other hand, a child bitten by a stray dog may not only sustain a severe laceration requiring stitches, but the question of rabies inevitably comes up. This is even more true of skunk and bat bites. Every effort must be made to locate the stray animal and have it placed under observation until the question is resolved. Recently, only one or two cases of human rabies per year occurred in the United States (none in 1988), but it remains a serious disease with a virtually 100% mortality rate. In general, an animal bite may be allowed to bleed at first, for this washes out bacteria, bits of clothing, or other contaminants. The wound may then be washed with soap and water; if bleeding continues, it may be treated as described under BLEEDING in this section.

Most cat bites, like cat scratches, are not likely to be of any consequence. Fever and swelling of nearby lymph glands can occur, often well after the original injury has healed. This is a viral disease known as cat-scratch fever. It is quite rare, however. Bruising without cutting of the skin may occur after some animal bites, such as a horse bite. This is best treated initially by cold water or ice applications which slow down both bleeding or swelling.

BITES AND STINGS (INSECT) Most insect bites fall into the nuisance category. Thus, while mosquito bites in certain parts of the world do transmit such diseases as yellow fever and malaria, the transmission of any disease from mosquito bites in the United States is rare. In recent years, the public health authorities have been concerned over a few cases of encephalitis which have been traced to viruses carried by the mosquito. Generally, however, all one needs to do is apply some household remedy, such as calamine lotion; and one can dismiss the idea of coming down with an illness from mosquito bites. The bites of certain other insects fall into an entirely separate category, and with these, appropriate medical measures as described under the proper heading should be taken.

BITES (SCORPION) (TICKS) Scorpion bites are not life-threatening, as is widely believed, but the venom of the bite can produce considerable local pain and symptoms of illness. First aid may consist of ice applications. Wood ticks often attach themselves to people passing through certain wooded areas of the United States. They may transmit the disease known as Rocky Mountain spotted fever. In such areas, immunization against the disease is advisable. A more recent tick-borne disease which may become chronic and simulate arthritis, meningitis, and skin disorders is Lyme disease. Ticks that have attached themselves to the skin may be removed by covering them with mineral oil, vaseline, or kerosene. The injured or dead tick is then readily removed. (*See* Lyme Disease in the section Infectious Diseases).

BITES (SNAKE) Most snakes are harmless; they are useful scavengers, and they flee from human beings. If by chance they do bite, the bite produces two curved lines or serrations resulting from the indentations of their small, blunt teeth. Poisonous snakes, however, possess fangs, which are specialized hollow, long teeth through which the snake can expel his venom. When a poisonous snake strikes, sharp puncture wounds are produced which appear as two needle-like wounds fairly close together. The injected venom produces severe inflammation with marked swelling, discoloration, and burning pain. The aim of first aid is to limit the absorption of venom, and to draw it out of the wound site.

The following steps should be taken:

• Place a tourniquet above the puncture wounds and tie tightly enough to make the veins stand out prominently. The tourniquet can be a handkerchief, a belt, twine, or anything else that can adequately encircle the limb, for most snake bites are on the extremities. Too tight a tourniquet will shut off the circulation entirely; this can be recognized by failure of the veins to fill up.

• With a sharp razor blade, a pocketknife, or other sharp object, make a short longitudinal cut into each fang mark. Avoid cutting into a vein or any of the cordlike structures under the skin, which are the tendons, and make the cuts approximately one-quarter inch long and one-quarter inch deep.

• Due to the tourniquet, fairly free oozing of blood should occur. The former advice to suck the wound is no longer recommended, but if a suction device is available, as with a snake bite kit, it can be used repeatedly.

• Snake bite kits are available for those who go camping and hiking in areas known to be inhabited by such poisonous snakes as the rattlesnake or the cottonmouth moccasin, the copperhead, and the coral snake. These kits enable you to give first-aid attention promptly. They should be carried along as a routine part of outdoor equipment in such areas.

• Once the tourniquet is on properly, with veins bulging, do not disturb it, for the venom spreads more quickly when the pressure of the tourniquet is loosened. *Do not* give whiskey or other spirits—these are valueless and, in fact, tend to accelerate the spread of venom.

• If available, place ice around the bite. It slows the spread of the venom.

BITES, SPIDER (BLACK WIDOW)

The black widow spider (*Latrodectus mactans*), resident in all the Americas, is encountered most frequently in dark, dry places (under rocks, in trash piles, basements, tree roots), is jet black with orange-red markings, and has an hourglass pattern on the abdomen.

Symptoms. The site of the bite becomes painful, swollen, and occasionally blue-black from hemorrhage. Generalized symptoms develop rapidly and are those of shock and toxic poisoning (vomiting, sweating, aching of muscles, abdominal cramps, faint generalized rash). Not all of these symptoms may be present in each case. Suspicion that the bite is by a spider, and appearance of any of the symptoms of shock or toxicity, make treatment imperative.

Treatment. The patient should be transported to the nearest hospital emergency room as quickly as possible. Treatment for shock and administration of the specific antiserum are highly effective. Though the symptoms are formidable, reports of fatalities are rare.

BITES, SPIDER (BROWN RECLUSE)

A type of spider bite being reported with increasing frequency is that of the brown recluse spider. Like the black widow spider, it is found mostly in the southern part of the United States, most of the cases being reported from Texas, Arkansas, and Louisiana. The brown recluse spider gets its name from its pattern of living in dark, secluded locations of man-made dwellings, cellars being a favorite haunt. This spider has to be molested before it bites, and children could be well advised of this fact. It can be identified by its brown color and the violin-shaped figure on its abdomen. Its bite produces a breakdown in the skin, which is sometimes extensive, and it may produce general symptoms such as chills, fever, and anemia.

One can apply ice to the bite itself as a temporary measure. Medical attention is mandatory and hospitalization may be required. Local injection of cortisone-type drugs have been found useful in the treatment of recluse-spider bites. These bites ulcerate and require wound treatment.

BLEEDING

The most widely applicable method for the control of bleeding is direct pressure, using a compress. By this is meant the exertion of sufficient pressure on a bleeding area to compress bleeding vessels. For most bleeding, even from fairly large veins, such direct pressure should bring the hemorrhage under control. In most emergency situations, one can use any clean cloth for the compress: a handkerchief, towel, shirt, sheet, or pillowcase folded on itself to make a multilayered wad. Using either the fingers or the palm of the hand, apply the emergency compress over the bleeding area and exert firm pressure against it. Maintain pressure for ten minutes or so. One may then diminish the pressure, occasionally lifting up part of the compress to judge whether the bleeding has come under control. Pressure can be maintained more or less indefinitely, if necessary. However, if brisk bleeding continues despite firm pressure, particularly if the bleeding comes in good-sized spurts (as may happen when an artery is involved) one should turn to other first-aid measures. The two other are the pressure point and the tourniquet methods.

Pressure Point Method. This method can be used for bleeding from a limb and for hemorrhage where a tourniquet is not applicable. (When a tourniquet is to be used, finger pressure should be applied to stem the loss of blood while the tourniquet is being prepared and applied.) The pressure point method is based on the principle that some of the major arteries can be directly compressed to a point where bleeding from one of their branches is either considerably cut down or abolished altogether. The application of pressure should always be between the cut and the heart. There are standard pressure points at which major arteries going to the head and extremities can be readily compressed. You can identify these locations on yourself by feeling for your pulse. In fact, it is a good idea to gain some familiarity with their location in this manner. Some of these locations are the following:

• *Brachial.* The brachial artery is the major vessel going to the arm. It emerges from the region of the armpit and runs down the inner side of the upper arm. Direct pressure on the inner part of the arm presses the artery against the bone; with sufficient pressure, its pulse can be abolished. This maneuver will control bleeding from any injury of the arm, forearm, or hand below the level at which pressure is being exerted.

• *Carotid.* The carotid arteries are the major vessels supplying the head, including the face and the brain. Ordinarily they can be readily felt on either side of the windpipe, and are compressible against the spinal column below. Pressure on the carotids should be applied only as a last resort, since it may lead to complications attendant on cutting down brain circulation. Prolonged pressure could, in fact, produce paralysis. One may consider intermittent or partial carotid artery pressure (for brief intervals of a minute or so) as a temporary first-aid method, to be followed by direct pressure. In no case should both carotids be compressed simultaneously. For an extensive bleeding wound of the head region where facial and temporal pressures (see below) are not applicable, cautious use of carotid pressure can be of value.

• *Facial.* The facial artery, a branch of the carotid, winds over the jawbone, about halfway between the angle of the jaw and chin. Pressure at this point may successfully control bleeding from the face and jaw.

• *Temporal.* The temporal artery winds over the bone just in front of the midportion of the attachment of the ear. This is an artery whose pulsations are often visible in older individuals. Pressure on it will control bleeding from the upper part of the head on that side.

• *Femoral.* The femoral is a large artery which emerges from the pelvis to nourish the lower extremity. It produces an obvious pulse which can be easily felt in the crease between the thigh and abdomen at about its middle. Pressure here will control bleeding from the thigh, leg, and foot.

Several further pointers to remember about bleeding are these:

• There is no reason why combinations of the above methods cannot be used. Thus, one might combine a compress on the actual wound site with pressure on one of the standard pressure points. Actually, because arterial circulation may form a network (this is known as the collateral circulation), some bleeding can occur from a wound even if the pressure point method is correctly utilized. The bleeding that escapes the pressure point is usually modest, however, and controllable by a local compress to the wound.

• Another tip to be remembered is that elevation of a limb tends to decrease bleeding and should be routinely employed when possible. Thus, with a bleeding wound of the hand, the first approach might well be to apply a compress with firm pressure to the wound and to elevate the arm as high as possible.

• Where bleeding is extensive, there is always the possibility of shock. The preferred position for incipient or actual shock is for the victim to lie stretched out flat on his back.

Tourniquet. A tourniquet is a tightly applied device which encircles a limb and controls the circulation through it. When the pressure exerted by the tourniquet is of sufficient degree, no more blood can flow through the arteries, and the limb is deprived of its circulation. It is this complete cutting off of the blood supply that makes the tourniquet a method to be used only as a last resort, and then only with extreme caution. The overzealous use of a tourniquet for a period of several hours may endanger the entire limb.

A tourniquet is made easily enough by using a handkerchief, strap, belt, suspenders, a strip of cloth, necktie, towel, rubber tubing, or similar material to be tied about the limb. Do not use wire, cord, or anything that will cut the flesh. Place a hard pad or object over the artery so that when the tourniquet is tightened, it will press the pad or object against the artery. Next, a stick or any substitute such as a pencil is placed between the tourniquet and the skin. Twisting the tourniquet one or more times produces an increase in pressure. At first the veins may bulge up, but as the pressure of the tourniquet is increased and the circulation through the artery is cut off, the limb turns white and all visible blood vessels collapse. At this point, bleeding should stop. Continued bleeding indicates that more pressure needs to be applied. Occasionally a stouter tourniquet may be needed to accomplish this.

A tourniquet should never be left in a concealed position where its presence escapes notice. Opinions vary as to how long a tourniquet may be safely allowed to stay on. United States Armed Forces experience indicates that a tourniquet can remain on for several hours without causing damage. However, the wise course is to release it before one hour has passed. One may check after twenty minutes or even less to determine whether bleeding has been controlled. Sometimes, one can use the tourniquet to gain rapid control of bleeding, then switch to the direct pressure method (described above) with considerable success. This also circumvents the drawback of continued use of the tourniquet.

BRUISES   *See* FALLS AND FRACTURES in this section.

BURNS   Burns are generally described in terms of their extent and their depth. Extent refers to the area of skin involved, and is sometimes stated in percentage. Thus, an extensive burn involving the skin of the arm would be an 8 percent burn, whereas one involving most of the back would be a 16 percent burn. A first-degree burn is one that produces reddening of the skin; a second-degree burn produces blister formation; a third degree burn produces injury of tissue at deeper-than-skin level. Extensive third-degree burns may produce shock, and often may require skin grafts to cover the denuded surfaces. Shock may also result from extensive second-degree burns with blistering. Shock results from the rapid loss of fluid, as well as from toxic chemicals produced by the burn. The initial first aid

for shock is to stretch the patient out and keep him warm.

Minor Burns. Minor burns involve a limited surface and present no threat of shock or similar reaction. A good first-aid measure for the usual minor burn of the fingers or hand is immediately to dip the hand into ice-cold water. This stops pain almost at once, and tends to cut down the degree of tissue injury. For such burns, a vaseline dressing, which has a protective effect, may be all that is necessary. Annoying blisters of the fingertips may be pricked with a sterile needle and allowed to collapse. The possibility of this leading to infection is quite remote, but one should observe the usual precautions of washing with soap and water and applying a surface disinfectant.

Major Burns. Extensive second- or-third-degree burns are major burns. These generally require hospitalization. It is best not to attempt treatment such as cutting away burnt clothing, since this may further aggravate the injury. Also *do not* apply burn ointments or other ointments. An exposed burned area may be covered with the inside portion of a clean pillowcase or sheet which is likely to be relatively free of bacterial contamination. Clothing that adheres to the burned area should not be pulled at, nor should any attempt be made to undress the victim. The patient should be kept covered. If medical aid or removal to a hospital is not possible for some time, and if there is no vomiting, the patient may be given fluids by mouth, since thirst is a common complaint. The fluid might consist of fruit juice to which a sprinkle of salt has been added. "Shock solution" is another fluid that has been advocated. This consists of one teaspoon of salt plus one-half teaspoon of baking soda dissolved in one quart of water.

A chemical burn is produced by the corrosive effect of such agents as lye (caustic soda [Drano®] and similar products), hydrochloric acid (muriatic acid), sulphuric acid, and carbolic acid (phenol). Burns of the skin resulting from phenol, creosote, or carbolic acid should be dabbed or rinsed with alcohol followed up with water. (Alcohol, of course, cannot be used when these substances enter the eye or have been swallowed.) Other chemical burns should be promptly washed with water. Burns due to an acid may then be covered with a paste made of bicarbonate of soda, or with vaseline. Chemical burns are usually quite destructive to tissue and hence heal slowly.

CARDIOPULMONARY RESUSCITATION (CPR). This emergency technique can save the life of someone who has suffered a heart attack, electric shock, or some other condition that has caused the heart to stop beating and interrupted the flow of oxygen-rich blood to the brain. The technique consists of clearing the airway, breathing into the mouth of the victim, and providing artificial circulation by manually compressing the chest. CPR must be initiated immediately and continued until the individual revives, a rescue team equipped with life-saving equipment arrives, or until the individual can be transported to a hospital emergency room. The Red Cross and American Heart Association offer six- to twelve-hour classes in the technique, often at hospitals, schools, and at places of employment. Once trained, anyone who weighs 90 pounds or more can effectively administer CPR.

CHOKING An error in the complicated swallowing mechanism may result in a lump of food covering the entrance to the air passage or even entering the passage itself. This will produce a breathing obstruction and severe coughing. The coughing itself may dislodge the foreign body. Otherwise, gasping or difficult respiration, together with the classic purplish appearance of the victim, can produce a terrifying sight. Heimlich Maneuver is the preferred method of relieving the obstruction. This is based on the principle that suddenly applied pressure to the upper abdomen will push the diaphragm up. This raises the pressure in the lungs and bronchial tubes and acts to expel the obstructing object. (*See* color plates F8B-F8C.) If this fails and the victim is a child, he should be turned upside down and vigorously slapped between the shoulder blades several times. An adult may be positioned over a chair or bed in a head-down position, and similarly slapped between the shoulder blades.

If these simple measures fail and the victim is still in great distress, call the doctor. In some cases, where the obstruction is partial and the victim continues to have a purplish color, artificial respiration (*See* ARTIFICIAL RESPIRATION in this section.) should be maintained while rushing the patient to the hospital.

CONVULSIONS The most common form of convulsion is seen in epilepsy. It is sometimes referred to as a fit or a seizure. Often there is a brief warning which the patient may recognize, known as the aura. This is usually followed by his falling to the ground and undergoing a generalized stiffening. Following this, a series of severe and involuntary muscular contractions occur, generally accompanied by grinding movements of the jaws and the appearance of a foamy saliva on the lips. Involuntary emptying of bowels and bladder is usual. The attack lasts for a minute or more, stops abruptly, and is followed by a period of sleep. The victim will have no recollection of what happened.

The aim of first aid is to prevent self-inflicted injury as a result of the powerful, involuntary muscular movements. Biting of the tongue may be severe. In any case, proceed as follows:

• Insert any handy object between the teeth, such as a wadded handkerchief, the victim's own tie, even a pencil. This will prevent the tongue from being bitten and chewed.

• Loosen the collar and necktie, and move the patient away from any object that he may strike during the seizure.

• As soon as the convulsive movements have stopped, turn him on his stomach so his tongue will not fall back into his throat.

In infants and young children, a high fever may produce a seizure. It is important to reduce the body temperature as quickly as possible by an alcohol rub or by wrapping the child in a cool wet sheet. A doctor should be promptly notified. These febrile seizures in children have no relationship to the possible development of epilepsy later in life.

CROUP Croup is produced by an infection involving the larynx and vocal cords, in which a spasm occurs. The spasm may be brought on by a bout of coughing, and most often occurs at night. Croup is generally limited to children with respiratory infections, and is also seen in whooping cough. The usual pattern is for the child to wake at night with a violent attack of coughing followed by obvious difficulty in catching his breath. The attempt to breathe in produces a noisy whooping or crowing sound, and the child turns a dusky red, but normal color is restored as the spasm subsides. This sequence of events may take place night after night. In addition to treating the infection with antibiotics, these measures will be of aid:

1. The child's room should be kept warm and free of drafts.

2. High humidity should be maintained, with one or more vaporizers going all the time. As a routine precautionary measure against possible burns, vaporizers should be placed at a safe distance, with the steam projected toward the head of the bed.

3. Partially covering the crib or the bed with a sheet, as was done in the old-fashioned croup tent, will make a semi-enclosed area which has a high moisture content. Another possibility is to take the patient into the bathroom and run the hot water which will quickly steam up the room. Hot liquids may be of help. (*See also* the section RESPIRATORY CONDITIONS.)

CUTS   In contrast to a laceration, which is an irregular tear of the skin, a cut is inflicted by a sharp edge. It often produces a linear opening into the skin. Most cuts are accompanied by bleeding, and if one of the larger vessels is involved, the bleeding may be quite brisk. (Control of this is discussed in the entry BLEEDING in this section.) Minor cuts generally require no special measures. Cuts received out of doors, as for example when walking barefoot on the ground, may require tetanus antitoxin, a decision which has to be made by the doctor. Sometimes the question arises as to whether or not a cut needs to be stitched. The purpose of stitching is to bring the gaping edges of skin together to facilitate healing. Unless this is done, healing is slower and leads to a broad and perhaps unsightly scar. Obviously, then, if the cut is of some length and the skin edges become separated by perhaps one-eighth to one-quarter of an inch or more, then sutures (stitches) will lead to more rapid healing and better cosmetic results as well. Cuts about the face are generally sutured with very fine material, with the stitches closely spaced to secure the least noticeable scar.

ELECTRICAL SHOCK   The usual contact with a 110-volt AC household outlet is not dangerous unless one happens to be wet—in a bathtub or otherwise in an electrical contact that completes the circuit. Most serious injuries are a result of contact with main power lines carrying high currents. Such contact may produce weakness or paralysis, unconsciousness, and a local burn. Under no circumstances should you touch the victim directly, for the current can be conducted to you. Be sure to proceed quickly but calmly. If a switch controlling the line is the fastest thing that can be shut off, do that first. Otherwise push the victim away from the line, or the line away from the victim, always being sure to use a nonconductor such as a long piece of dry wood or cardboard, a dry broom handle, or dry rubber hosing. Dry ropes or dry cloth can also be used. Make sure your hands are dry and you are standing on a dry surface. Pushing the victim off the wire will break the electrical circuit involving the victim. In severe cases, respiration will have usually stopped and artificial respiration may be necessary. (*See* ARTIFICIAL RESPIRATION in this section.) In addition, if the pulse is feeble or absent, try pounding the area over the heart several times fairly hard with a clenched fist. Maintain artificial respiration until medical help arrives.

FAINTING   A sudden, rapid drop in blood pressure with a resulting decrease in circulation to the brain will produce fainting. There may be warning symptoms such as dizziness, lightheadedness, spots before the eyes, sweating, pallor, and a sinking feeling. A simple faint seldom lasts more than a minute. If caught during the stage of early symptoms, fainting may be prevented simply by stretching the victim out on his back. No other measures are usually necessary, although inhaling spirits of ammonia and wiping the face and hands with cold water may be useful. Fainting may be brought on by bad news, or by a disagreeable sight. It occasionally occurs in a physician's office following a needle puncture.

Feeling faint, and fainting, may be secondary to such serious disorders as internal hemorrhage or unusual drop in the blood sugar. A single fainting spell in someone not ordinarily subject to them, should be accounted for, and a doctor consulted. In a known diabetic patient, a faint spell due to low blood sugar is sometimes referred to as a reaction. It may be prevented or counteracted by taking sugar or fruit juice, and it generally indicates that the routine medications being taken by the patient need adjustment.

FALLS AND FRACTURES The extent of damage sustained when somebody falls can vary from a mild bruise to a major fracture. Sometimes the injury seems disproportionate to the accident; thus, when elderly persons trip inadvertently, the result may be so serious a fracture as a major break involving the thighbone. It is wise to be alert to the possibility of fracture, and it is a basic rule that if such a possibility exists, the victim should be treated as though he had one. It is safer to put on an unnecessary splint than to ignore the possibility of fracture and allow further serious damage to occur. The truth is that even an expert may not always be able to distinguish between a bad sprain and a fracture until an appropriate X-ray film has been taken. However, there are some leads that should alert one in this connection:

• Obviously, an accident in which the individual has undergone considerable impact, such as falling down a flight of stairs or being knocked down by an auto, makes the probability of fracture high.

• A fracture will generally produce a deformity, such as an abnormal bulge or a peculiar contour to the surface of an extremity, or a similar obvious change from the usual appearance. One important exception to this rule is skull fracture, which cannot be detected without medical examination.

• False motion may be produced by attempted movement. What happens is that a muscular contraction acting on the broken bone will produce a type of motion that is obviously abnormal, such as a movement in the middle of the thigh or forearm.

• A peculiar grating sound may be produced as one lightly runs his hands over the region of the fracture. This is due to the crackling produced by the fragments of bone as they move. It is known as crepitus.

• Sometimes an obvious shortening of the limb occurs, due to the overriding of the broken bone ends. For example, after a thighbone fracture the entire leg on the affected side may be one or more inches shorter than the other leg.

If any of these findings are present, the victim should be treated for fracture, and special care should be taken not to aggravate the injury while trying to help. A natural impulse when seeing somebody stumble and fall to the ground is to rush over and help him up. It would be wiser first to check for the possibility of fracture. Otherwise, helping the person to his feet may transform a simple fracture into a compound—that is, one where the bone penetrates the skin and is exposed—or such help may aggravate the injury in other ways, since the broken ends of the bone may produce damage to neighboring structures. Also, one may have to deal with the possibility that the injured person will be unable to bear weight, and may collapse again. Hence, the old first-aid maxim of "splint them where they lie."

One should be particularly careful where the possibility of an injury to the spinal column exists, as for example, after a fall on the back or an accident in which considerable force has been directed against the neck. Here it is always possible that the underlying spinal cord may be damaged, and any aggravation of such injury could produce paralysis.

Once it is clear that no fracture exists and that one is dealing with a bruising injury or contusion, the best first-aid treatment is promptly to chill the affected area. Probably the easiest way to do this is with ice cubes, but if no ice is available, cold compresses may be applied instead. Immediate application of ice serves two purposes: It cuts down bleeding from any vessels that may have been torn, and it diminishes both the local pain and the extent of inflammation and swelling set up by the injury. An ice bag suitably replenished from time to time is a good expedient. For exactly how long this can be continued has never been accurately determined. For severe sprains with evidence indicating a torn vein, the ice bag can be kept on for hours.

At one large Eastern university, the practice in treating athletic injuries, such as a twisted knee, is to strap an ice bag around the injured part by means of an elastic bandage. Fresh ice cubes are added as needed, and this does not interfere with the athlete's attending classes. The ice bag may be kept on not only throughout the day of the injury, but on the following day as well. Bleeding, soreness, and pain have been considerably lessened by this procedure. For smaller injuries, probably a few hours of off-and-on ice applications will do, particularly if it becomes apparent that one is not dealing with extensive bleeding or with torn tissues and ligaments. Sometimes cold or ice applications are recommended for the first day, and thereafter heat—as from a heating pad or hot compresses—may be substituted. The idea here is that the cold will cut down the initial bleeding and swelling, while heat on the following day may aid in resorption of swelling and in increasing local circulation.

Following some falls with torn blood vessels, a large local accumulation of blood with an obvious swelling may occur. This is known as a hematoma. Usually, in addition to the swelling of the hematoma, there is obvious discoloration for some distance beneath the skin as the blood diffuses through the tissues. This process may go on for a period of days so that what initially seemed to be a small black-and-blue spot becomes larger and larger. It also undergoes color changes, turning from the black-and-blue stage to yellowish-brown or a lighter tone. What is happening is that blood in the tissue is acting as a foreign body and may produce local reactions. It can even undergo calcification. The doctor may therefore decide to aspirate a large hematoma in order to evacuate the blood from it. (*See also* FRACTURES in this section.)

FOREIGN BODIES, INSERTION OF If children find a hole, they love to put something into it. All the openings of the body have been subjected to this maltreatment with various effects.

The nose is probably the most accessible site and many objects have been inserted into it. If a child insists on repeating this activity, it may mean that he has a nasal allergy and is trying to scratch the lining. Most of the objects put into the nose are harmless and will soon ride out on the extra mucus secreted and/or be ejected by a healthy sneeze.

The nose is not the only body orifice into which the child may insert foreign bodies, however. Stopped-up ears will usually have to be washed out with a syringe and lukewarm water by the physician. An object left in the vagina will, after only a few days, begin to produce a very disagreeable odor; special lights and instruments, and occasionally an anesthetic, will sometimes be necessary for surgical removal of the object inserted here.

When an object is successfully swallowed, it will usually pass through the entire tract, for the most narrow segment is from the throat to the stomach. Sometimes it will not pass the exit from the stomach (pylorus) but if it reaches the stomach it is assumed the object will continue on through. Occasionally, however, an oblong or irregular-shaped object must be "teased" through the anal opening by the physician using direct visualization.

FRACTURES A fracture is a break in the structure of a bone. The two general types are simple (or closed) and compound (or open) fractures. A closed fracture is one in which the bone is broken but the overlying skin remains intact. An open fracture, on the other hand, is an injury severe enough not only to break the bone but also damage the overlying soft tissues and lacerate the skin. An open fracture is far more serious both because it is the result of a more violent injury and because of the danger of contamination of the bone-ends through the skin laceration. Every attempt should be made to minimize further damage and contamination of the injured limb while in transit to the hospital. It should be supported by a splint or a roll of newspaper or magazines, and if there are any lacerations, dry sterile dressings should be applied.

Fractures heal slowly in comparison with soft-tissue injuries. While a skin laceration will be well healed in about ten days, a finger fracture may require one month to heal, and a large bone such as a shin-bone (tibia) four to six months. Bones require not only ample time for healing, but also proper adjustment (reduction) to restore correct position and sufficient immobilization to maintain it through the long healing period.

Closed (non-operative) reduction is chosen whenever possible. Traction is employed to "unwedge" (disimpact) the fracture and regain length; the fractured limb is then manipulated so as to correct any deformation that may have developed. After clinical and X-ray examination have revealed satisfactory position, a plaster of paris cast is applied to retain the reduced fracture until bony healing occurs. In some situations closed reduction is unsatisfactory and open reduction is required. Under general or spinal anesthesia, with the fracture site directly visible, the orthopedic surgeon may employ various nails, plates, and screws to aid in the retention of the fracture after reduction has been achieved.

It is very important that the patient be as active as possible while the fracture is healing. Joint stiffness from disuse is one of the most troublesome fracture complications, and is to a large degree avoidable. With a fractured wrist, for example, the fingers and shoulders are free and should be vigorously exercised even while the forearm and wrist are immobilized. The shoulder should be put through a full range of active motion by swinging it freely like a pendulum, and the fingers exercised by squeezing a bar of soap or a mass of clay.

The correct first-aid treatment for a fracture is immobilization, for example, splinting. The basic principle is to run a relatively rigid support, customarily extending down to the adjacent joint, alongside the region of the break. Strapping or tying the support to the limb will help prevent motion of the fracture. Most first-aid stations have padded splints of various sizes available.

In a great many circumstances, however, one has to rely on makeshifts. Such makeshifts may simply be reasonably rigid objects, such as a branch broken off from a tree, a stick, a broom handle, a piece of piping, or even such an odd object as an umbrella. The object can be tied in place with a necktie, strings or rope, torn pieces from a shirt, a man's belt—in short, anything that is handy. Some of the possibilities for dealing with different fractures are to be seen in the illustrations, First Aid and Life Saving, Plates F1-F8. Here is what one can do for specific kinds of common fractures:

Wrist. Fractures of the wrist occur most commonly as a result of a fall on the outstretched hand. The impact may snap the bone of the arm just above the wrist. The deformity that results is sometimes referred to as the silver-fork deformity, since the break results in the hand and wrist presenting a curved elevation somewhat like the curved part of a fork. Technically it is known as a Colles' fracture. The splint should be laid over the upper and lower parts of the wrist. Appropriate ties attaching it to the hand and forearm are made to hold the splint in place. In addition, a sling—or pinning the sleeve to the shirt or coat—will give useful support.

Sometimes, instead of a typical Colles' fracture, a fracture occurs involving one of the small bones of the wrist. It may be hard to distinguish this from a sprain, except by X-ray. Needless to say, this and any other suspected fracture should be routinely X-rayed.

Finger. Crushing injuries in falls may produce a fracture of one of the three little bones that make up the finger. They may be difficult to distinguish from a bruising injury with swelling. A short narrow piece of wood, even a pencil or a portion of a tongue depressor, can be applied with gauze or adhesive strapping as a first-aid measure. Not uncommonly, instead of a fracture there may be a subluxation. In this, the supporting tissues present at each of the individual joints of the finger bones are torn, so that there is a displacement at the joint. It becomes obvious from observation that a portion of the finger is out of alignment. First-aid treatment for this is the same as for a fracture. Ice may be of help in relieving pain.

Forearm and Arm. Fractures of these bones are treated with splints in the usual manner. In addition, a sling or pinning of the sleeve to another part of the clothing will help support the limb. If no splints are available, one should consider any arrangement that will keep the arm or forearm immobilized against the trunk—for example, strapping of the upper arm to the trunk with strips of adhesive tape.

Thigh. Fractures of the thigh are most likely to occur in elderly persons, more often in women than in men, and generally as the result of a fall. Because of the brittleness of the thighbone in the elderly, it may fracture as a result of the impact of falling, most often high up in the region of the hip. A fracture is generally recognized by its pain, shortening of the extremity, and the fact that the leg tends to turn outward, in what is known as external rotation. Splints should be applied to the entire length of the thigh and extend down over the knee.

Knee. Fracture at the knee can occur in the

thighbone, just above the knee joint, or may involve one or both of the two bones of the lower leg, below the level of the joint. The latter is sometimes referred to as a bumper fracture, the name deriving from the fact that it is often sustained as a result of the direct impact of an automobile bumper. Fractures in this area will be recognized by the abnormality of contour, and are often compound, meaning that the bone ends protrude through the skin. As with all fractures or suspected fractures, no attempt should be made to help the patient up; he should be splinted where he lies.

Ankle. It is sometimes difficult to distinguish between a bad sprain and an outright fracture of the ankle joint. In both cases there may be a considerable amount of swelling, usually on the outer aspect, just above the ankle joint. If in doubt, treat as a fracture, and do not allow weight-bearing.

Neck and Back. In cases of fracture or suspected fracture of the neck and back, first aid should be directed toward avoiding potential spinal-cord injury. The best procedure may well be to allow the patient to lie where he has fallen, with no attempt to move him until proper medical aid has arrived. If circumstances are such that he must be moved, the basic principle is to avoid any manipulation or motion of the spinal column. Avoid any movement of the back and any rotation of the head. The victim must not be allowed to turn from one side to the other on his own. It takes at least three people properly to move someone with a suspected back injury. One should support the head and neck, a second the trunk, and the third the lower extremities. All the motions should be synchronized in such a way that twisting of the head, the trunk, or the hips is avoided. The basic principle is to keep the patient stiff and immobile. If he has to be transported, it should be on a flat, hard surface such as a door, on which he rests flat on his back. If a litter is used, the patient should be transported in the face-down position.

Skull. Some head injury is an inevitable accompaniment of skull fracture. If the person is knocked out and then recovers consciousness, this is spoken of as a concussion. If someone who has been knocked out comes to, and after a period of consciousness becomes unconscious again, there is a strong suspicion that bleeding within the skull has occurred. There is no specific treatment for a skull fracture, except to transport the patient to a medical institution and not to permit walking.

Rib. Blows and crushing injuries to the chest will often fracture one or more ribs. This will produce severe pain in the affected ribs, made worse with breathing or movement. Sometimes the pain produced by attempting to breathe is so marked that involuntary splinting occurs and the breathing is noticeably shallow. Rarely, a broken fragment of rib may penetrate the lung surface. The pain of a rib fracture is often relieved if the patient lies on the affected side. This will diminish the respiratory motion on that side. If medical aid is not readily available, one may attempt to splint the side with the fractured rib by means of adhesive taping. To do this, the victim is told to breathe out as much as possible. Wide (two to three inch) adhesive tape is run from back to front over the region of the presumed rib fracture. The tape should extend beyond the midline both in back and in front. Two or three such tape strips placed above and below the part of the rib cage involved, will cut down the motion imparted by breathing and will diminish the pain. (*See also* FALLS AND FRACTURES in this section.)

FROSTBITE   Injury to tissues (generally to fingers, toes, nose, or ears) produced by exposure to severe cold is referred to as frostbite. Initially, the affected area looks very white, and is obviously quite cold and stiff to touch. Later, variable amounts of reddening, often accompanied by an increase in pain, may be noted. Severe frostbite lasting many hours may lead to death of the involved tissues, a condition known as gangrene. Such extensive frostbite is seldom seen except in mountain climbers, in persons who are lost in the bitter cold, or in someone who has been injured and remained unconscious out-of-doors during a severe freeze. First-aid treatment of frostbite is to immerse the area in warm water at approximately 105° to 110° F.—in short, to warm up the area as rapidly as possible. In addition, a physician may give anticoagulant drugs or other medications which have been shown to cut down on the extent of cold injury. Rubbing the part with snow is an old procedure which has been completely discarded. It may in fact increase the extent of cold damage.

HEART (CARDIAC) EMERGENCIES

Patients with acute cardiac conditions are urged as soon as practicable to enter a hospital where constant observation and care may prevent a sudden unnecessary complication, or even death. With efficient drugs and special equipment, adverse changes in blood pressure, heart output, lung blockage, heart-rate and -rhythm, and cyanosis can in many instances be effectively met and overcome.

It is not always possible to distinguish between a longer-than-usual bout of angina and a new heart attack. Hence many patients have to be admitted to a coronary care unit (CCU) for observations. This common cause for admission is often abbreviated to ROMI (rule out myocardial infarction). All this illustrates the difficulty in identifying a possible new heart attack or similar emergency and is the reason for haste in bringing the person to the nearest medical facility. This expeditious action should be borne in mind especially if the doctor can't be reached or his or her office is further away than the nearest emergency facility.

Taking the pulse may furnish useful information, the more so if the attack is short-lived. A very slow pulse, 40 or under, may point to conduction difficulties in the heart, the Stokes-Adams attack, as a cause of angina or fainting. Conversely, a rapid irregular rate points to a paroxysmal arrhythmia as a cause for the patient's complaint. If no pulse is palpable, some authorities advise giving a few short thumps to the chest wall above the heart and instituting cardiopulmonary resuscitation.

It is not always possible to distinguish some cardiac emergencies from some lung emergencies. People who wake up at night with wheezing and shortness of breath may fall into either category but previous history may be useful in identifying the category. In allergic persons with previous seasonal attacks the cause is likely to be bronchial asthma. In persons with poorly controlled high-blood pressure the attack may be cardiac asthma. In either of the two forms of asthma victims breathe better when sitting bolt upright in a chair, perhaps next to an open window. Natu-rally, oxygen if available is very helpful, and some chronic cardiac or bronchial asthma patients learn the value of keeping an oxygen tank at home for emergency purposes.

HEAT EXHAUSTION Heat exhaustion is most common during spells of hot, moist, damp weather. It is sometimes seen among persons gathered into tight crowds who have to stand for prolonged periods. The victim generally complains of faintness, weakness, and dizziness. This is often due to a drop in blood pressure. The skin is moist, but not hot, and the pulse may become weak and rapid. If there has been a good deal of perspiration, there may be further complaints of muscular or abdominal cramps, sometimes associated with nausea and even vomiting. The following steps are useful:

1. Stretch the victim out in a cleared area so that he may benefit from whatever air in motion is available.

2. Give small amounts of cold drinks, such as fruit juices to which a pinch of salt has been added. If there has been excessive perspiration, one might give salt tablets, or a diluted salt solution made by adding a teaspoon of salt to a quart of water.

3. Mild stimulants such as coffee or tea may also be useful.

4. A cold, brisk sponging of the head, face, and arms, and inhaling of spirits of ammonia, stimulate the heart and circulation.

HEAT STROKE During heat stroke the body's temperature-regulating mechanism goes astray. Such a stroke generally comes on after overexposure to the sun, on very hot days, in places such as open fields or beaches. The victim is obviously hot to the touch, and very high temperatures ranging up to 104° or 106° F. are not uncommon. The skin is hot and dry, the pulse full and bounding. The chief complaint is complete weakness.

First aid consists of getting the victim out of the sun and into as cool and as shady a spot as possible. Vigorous measures to lower the body temperature should be taken immediately. These may include pouring cold water over the victim's head and shoulders, or applying ice bags to these areas. Immersion in cool water or rub-downs with alcohol may also be helpful in lowering body temperature. For further evaluation the patient can be wrapped in a cold moist sheet and transported to a hospital for further treatment.

NOSEBLEED More than 90 percent of all nosebleeds come from the lower half of the nose and from the nasal septum, the midline structure which divides the nasal pathway into two separate halves. The nasal septum has a very extensive blood supply and is easily damaged when picked at. Its delicacy of structure explains why nosebleeds occur as often as they do. Injury, various kinds of infection, and overstrenuous blowing are the usual causes; very rarely do they result from high blood pressure. This statement also applies to individuals known to have elevated blood pressure but who nevertheless can have nosebleeds for the same reasons as people with normal blood pressure.

Most of the suggested treatments for nosebleed, as, for example, the one that calls for applying ice to the back of the neck, are of little value. The most satisfactory method of controlling it is by direct compression of both nostrils. The nostrils should be firmly grasped with the fingers, exerting an even pressure on the entire fleshy portion of the nose. Maintain the pressure for approximately ten minutes, then cautiously release to see whether the bleeding has stopped. The clot that forms is easily dislodged, so do not blow the nose or poke about in it for some time after a nosebleed.

When nosebleeds are frequent, cauterization of the septum or similar procedures may occasionally be resorted to by a physician. Nosebleeds that occur behind the fleshy part of the nose may sometimes be severe, and not controllable by the form of compression described here. A possible first-aid measure would be to take a large wad of cotton, sprinkle it with a few drops of nasal decongestant such as neosynephrine nose drops, insert, and then compress the nasal tissue. Severe nosebleeds may require packing by a physician.

POISONING Many cases of poisoning occur only because suitable precautions are not taken. Remember that there is nothing a toddler may not sample in his travels around the household, including objects of unpleasant taste and odor. Warning notices, or skull and crossbones identification, will certainly not

hold him back. Eternal vigilance is the price not only of liberty, but also of child rearing. The fact that bathrooms come equipped with medicine chests is not necessarily a valid reason for keeping medicines there. With a young child around the house, medicines should be placed under lock and key. See that detergents, bleaches, lye, and acid solutions are completely inaccessible to him. Poisoning precautions should extend to the basement, the attic, the garage, the barn, and the woodshed and kept in mind on visits to relatives' homes. Children have been known to swallow insecticides, rodenticides, herbicides, algicides, and fungicides (the so-called "economic poisons") many of which are potentially serious threats.

Treatment. Call your doctor *immediately* or if the situation is obviously urgent go to the nearest emergency facility. If it is known what the child took, antidotes for temporary relief are given in the TABLE OF COMMON POISONS on the following pages. Advice on first aid and/or temporary measures may often be obtained by calling the Poison Control centers, which exist in many large cities. A phone call to a hospital or city health department is another quick means to obtain instant advice or help.

Here are a few basic facts to keep in mind in relation to chemical poisoning:

1. Milk is a good everyday antidote usually available in every household. It will neutralize various acids and alkalis, fluorides, and other poisons. Therefore, even if you do not know the exact nature of the poison, or its antidote, you will do well to give milk.

2. With few exceptions, the basic aim of first aid in chemical poisoning is to produce vomiting. Vomiting can be induced by scraping the back of the throat with a spoon or a finger, or by giving an emetic (an agent that produces vomiting), such as ipecac. Other easily made up emetics are a tablespoon of salt or of mustard in a glass of warm water. These can be repeated.

3. The exceptions to the above rule are the corrosives and the carbon tetrachloride, kerosene, and benzine group. The corrosives—agents which produce tissue burns—such as acids and alkalies (lye, Drano®, battery acid) produce whitish changes of the lips and mouth. If any of these has been swallowed, *do not* induce vomiting.

4. Some of the substances swallowed by children are not necessarily poisonous. However, when in doubt, produce vomiting anyway. In all cases make sure that a doctor or a Poison Control Center is called, and if a doctor cannot get there readily, plan on bringing the victim rapidly to a hospital where the stomach can be washed out if necessary.

5. A universal antidote, active against many different types of poisons, may be purchased at most drug stores. It consists of activated charcoal, tannic acid, and magnesium hydroxide. This will neutralize and absorb various poisons. If available, give a tablespoon of the universal antidote with water or milk. With most poisons, one can induce vomiting after one to two minutes. The alleged household "substitute" for the universal antidote, consisting of burnt toast and tea, is completely worthless. Milk is much better.

6. Always save the container that held the ingested substance. Its label will often specify the exact ingredients and may also give directions for treatment of accidental poisoning. If the victim is brought to a hospital, take the container along.

TABLE OF COMMON POISONS

Poison	Treatment
Acetone. This is found in some nail polish removers and some paint solvents. Small amounts are not dangerous.	Induce vomiting, then give one to two teaspoons of bicarbonate of soda in water.
Acids. Battery acid, sulfuric acid, etc., are corrosive, give off irritating fumes and produce burns about the mouth and lips.	Avoid vomiting. Give milk, repeated doses of milk of magnesia, baking soda, Tums®, or other household remedies for hyperacidity.
Alkalies. Chiefly lye (Drano® and similar products), ammonia, quicklime, produce chemical burns.	Avoid vomiting. Give large amounts of milk, vinegar diluted with water, fruit juices.
Arsenic. Found in some mouse seeds, some ant and rat poisons.	Induce vomiting. Give milk, milk of magnesia, egg white.
Aspirin. (Also found in Anacin®, Empirin®, APC, etc.) Taken in overdoses produces sleepiness, flushing, deep breathing, burning in upper abdomen.	Induce vomiting. Give one to two teaspoons of baking soda in water.
Barbiturates. Phenobarbital, and sleeping pills such as seconal, amytal, nembutal, are poison if taken in overdoses.	Induce vomiting unless the patient is in a coma. Give large amounts of coffee or tea. If comatose, give artificial respiration.
Bleach.	See CHLORINE.
Carbolic Acid (creosote). A corrosive which produces burns on the lips and mouth.	Avoid vomiting. Give large amounts of olive oil, cottonseed oil, or egg whites. Follow with one ounce of Epsom salts in a pint of water.
Chlorine. Found in bleaches.	Give an emetic and produce vomiting. Follow with diluted ammonia water (one teaspoon household ammonia to a glass of water).

TABLE OF COMMON POISONS—continued

Poison	Treatment
Cleaning Fluids: Benzine, kerosene, gasoline, carbon tetrachloride, etc., are poisonous both in liquid form and if inhaled as fumes.	Avoid inducing vomiting unless the cleaning fluid is known to be carbon tetrachloride. Give strong coffee or tea. Artificial respiration as necessary.
Copper. Bordeau mixture, blue vitriol, found in garden sprays.	Produce vomiting. Give milk or egg whites and repeat vomiting.
DDT. Contained in insect poisons and sprays.	Give one ounce Epsom salts in water and repeat vomiting.
Detergents. Not likely to be dangerous, except those few containing phosphates.	Give milk and induce vomiting.
Digitalis. A common heart medicine, and its derivatives (digoxin, gitalin, digitoxin). Produces weakness, slow pulse, collapse, and delirium.	Within first half-hour, produce vomiting. Otherwise do not do so. Give strong tea.
Fluorides. Found in many ant and mouse poisons. The amount found in children's antidental decay preparations is not likely to be dangerous, even if a whole bottle is taken.	Induce vomiting. Give milk repeatedly.
Iodine. Found usually as tincture of iodine or Lugol's solution.	Give enough of corn starch or flour to induce vomiting; repeat.
Lead. Found in some paints and in white and red lead, may be inhaled in dangerous amounts.	Induce vomiting. Give large amounts of milk.
Narcotics. Demerol, morphine, codeine, paregoric, tincture of opium, all narcotics. Produce drowsiness and coma, markedly constricted eye pupils, depressed breathing.	Give strong tea, or universal antidote consisting of activated charcoal, tannic acid and magnesium hydroxide. It may be purchased in any drugstore. Induce vomiting. Give artificial respiration.
Oil of Wintergreen. Produces symptoms similar to aspirin poisoning.	Give one to two teaspoons of baking soda in water. Induce vomiting and repeat.
Phosphorus. An ingredient of some roach and rodent poisons. May fume and has a pungent, garlicky odor.	Avoid vomiting. Give one half to one glass of hydrogen peroxide.
Strychnine. Found in some rodent poisons.	Induce vomiting. Give universal antidote (*see* above), strong tea, or coffee.
Turpentine. Produces burning of mouth and stomach, weakness and shock.	Induce vomiting. Give one to two ounces of Epsom salts in a pint of water.

HOME NURSING CARE

Every individual will experience some form of illness at some point in life. For most disorders, proper rest and home medical care is a vital part of the recuperation process. The kind of care depends upon the illness. It may be brief or prolonged. Giving sponge baths, taking temperatures, and administering medication can make a profound difference in the rate of recovery of a home-bound patient.

This section examines the basic skills required in home nursing care and outlines the procedures that should be familiar to every adult member of the household. The following is a list of topics identified in this section:

ALCOHOL RUB An alcohol sponging may be necessary for high fever. Performed correctly, it may bring the temperature down by two degrees or more within minutes. In addition, it has a soothing, cleansing effect, and leaves the patient feeling refreshed. Alcohol is a sterilizing agent; in addition to killing off bacteria, it cleanses the skin of accumulated oils and perspiration. Several precautions should be kept in mind, however:

• Keep alcohol away from the eyes, the genital and anal areas, and from any open cuts or surfaces.

• Avoid chilling the patient. Make sure that the room is warm and that there are no drafts. If the patient complains of being chilly, interrupt the sponging.

• Frequent alcohol sponges may be excessively drying to the skin. When frequent sponging is necessary, follow it up with the application of a body lotion or cream.

• Be sure to protect nearby furniture, since splashing with alcohol may harm the finish.

The actual sponging can be done with straight 70 percent rubbing alcohol, particularly if one wants to bring the temperature down rapidly, or with a mixture of equal parts of alcohol and tepid water. In addition to the basin of alcohol, provide yourself with two washcloths and two bath towels. The doctor may also request that an ice bag be placed on the patient's head. Proceed as follows:

1. Wring out one washcloth in the alcohol (or alcohol-water mixture) and place on the abdomen. The cloth can be dipped into the alcohol from time to time as it dries.

2. Dip the second washcloth in alcohol, and rub each part of the body slowly. The direction of the rubbing may be in rotation from the arms, to the trunk, then to the legs, and finally to the back. Place the bath towel under each part of the body as you go along. Keep rubbing for approximately five minutes. Dry each part as you proceed.

3. Help the patient back into night clothes. Take the temperature approximately thirty minutes after the alcohol sponging. If a high fever persists, and the doctor so orders, repeat the sponging.

BED BATH Giving a bath in bed is not as difficult as it sounds. It is a refreshing procedure gratefully received by most patients. A full or partial bed bath may be given daily, and even more often in hot weather, when the patient is perspiring freely, or in the presence of continued fever. Be careful not to chill the patient. The room should be warm, and drafts should be avoided. In cold weather windows should be closed. For extra warmth, use a small electric heater, or turn up the heat as the circumstances indicate. Newspapers placed under the basin of water and on the floor may be a useful precaution. In addition to the basin of water, bring soap, two washcloths, and two large bath towels to the bedside. You may pull the covers all the way back and place a bath blanket, if one is available, over the patient. Proceed as follows:

1. Place a bath towel under each part of the body as it is washed in rotation, from the arm to the trunk and down to the legs.

2. Apply soap with one washcloth and remove it with the other, rinsing out the cloth as you proceed. Dry each part with a towel. After washing the upper part of the body, turn the patient over and do the back.

3. The patient may be allowed to wash the anal and genital areas himself, if he prefers.

4. The bath may be followed by a short alcohol rub of the back. Next apply a body lotion or cream, and finally powder. Powder may also be applied to the crotch area and between the toes.

5. When bathing a patient, use the opportunity to observe the patient's skin for any sign of breakdown.

BED MAKING Not all beds in every household are suitably transformed into sick beds. For example, a patient who must occupy a too-soft or sagging bed continuously for a long period of time may develop backaches to add to his other miseries. For this reason, most hospital beds are fairly firm. A sag in the middle of a mattress may be partially compensated for by placing bed boards under the middle of the mattress. Sometimes, newspapers piled underneath the mattress may also compensate for sagging.

On the other hand, a too-firm mattress with no "give" may make it more difficult for the patient to rest; the unyielding surface may predispose to bed sores if the illness is of any duration. A polyurethane foam "topper" may be useful for correcting this. Hospital-type beds which have adjustable tops and bottoms may be worth the cost for cardiac and other patients, when the illness is expected to be long-lasting.

Foot drop is one of the complications of prolonged bed rest. The continued weight of the sheet and blankets pressing down on the toes and the top of the foot can, over a long period, leave the patient with a foot weakness or complete inability to raise the feet toward himself at the ankles, hence the term foot drop. One solution to the foot-drop problem is to place a board lengthwise at the foot of the bed. This may be a wooden plank wrapped in a bed sheet, or anything at all like it. Such a board enables the feet to rest against it in a right-angle position, which is the preferred position for avoiding foot drop. Another solution is to place a rolled-up blanket at the foot of the bed so that the feet can rest against it, thereby lifting the weight of the sheet and blankets off the feet. Still another solution—which has been employed in some children's hospitals—is to allow patients to wear their shoes in bed. Unorthodox as this appears, it is an excellent way of preventing foot drop.

Occasionally the bed must be changed while the patient remains in it, but this is not as difficult as it sounds. The basic idea is to make up one longitudinal half of the bed at a time. Proceed as follows:

1. Remove the top bedding. If the room is cool, cover the patient with a spare blanket. Stand on one side of the bed and move the patient and his pillow to the far side.

2. Loosen the bottom sheet on the near side and push it toward the center as far as you can.

3. Now lay the clean sheet down, lengthwise. Tuck it in at the sides and at the head and the foot securely. The part of the sheet that will go onto the occupied side of the bed can be fan-folded and placed next to the patient.

4. Now proceed to the other side of the bed. Help the patient move over to the half of the bed containing the fresh sheet. You can now strip the used sheet off the bed, and make up the remaining half of the bed.

5. A new top sheet and the original covers can then be placed over the patient.

BED SORE   A bed sore is an area of skin breakdown which generally occurs over a bony prominence in the bedfast patient. It results from long-continued pressure on the skin, which is compressed between the mattress below and the bone above. Perspiration or wetting of the skin due to incontinence aids and abets the process of skin breakdown. Common locations for bed sores are over the sacral area, the bony prominences of the hips and shoulders, and on the heels. In the absence of good nursing care, almost anyone who is bedridden more than a week or two may develop a bed sore. It is most likely to occur in thin and debilitated individuals who have difficulty turning by themselves, and who are therefore likely to lie in one position too long.

In the beginning, a bed sore usually appears as a reddened area over a bony contour. The skin may then turn darker, perhaps even black, become more moist, and finally break down, thus forming an ulcer which can become quite deep. Sometimes bacteria invade the area of skin breakdown, and because bodily resistance at that point is low, serious infection can result.

It is a good deal easier—and far better—to prevent bed sores than to treat them. Preventive measures include frequent turning of the patient in bed to avoid unduly prolonged pressure on any area. The patient who insists on lying on his back should be gently turned to the left side for a time, and then to the right side. With pillows propped up behind his back, he can also be placed with comfort in various intermediate positions. Unless there is some reason why this should not be done, the patient should also be encouraged to sit up part of the time, with appropriate support for his back. Placing the patient in a chair, if medically permissible, should also be considered. Attention to skin hygiene is important. This includes bathing, the frequency of which may be determined by such factors as hot weather and excessive perspiration. Following the bath, one can gently rub cocoa butter or body lotion into the skin, especially in areas of pressure. If the patient is incontinent, he should have his bedding changed promptly and not be allowed to lie wet for any period of time.

If, despite this care, reddening or other signs of trouble appear, measures directed to relieve pressure on the reddened area should be initiated. Thus, if the areas involved are the heels, pillows may be placed under the calves in such a manner as to elevate the heels off the mattress. If a pressure area appears over the sacrum, the patient should be encouraged to lie on either side; a rubber ring or pillows can be arranged under the lower back and hips to relieve pressure. Occasionally, patients may be turned onto their abdomens and kept there most of the time, if necessary, to relieve pressure on some part of the back. Still other approaches may have to be considered: One is to have the patient lie on a sheepskin, a specially prepared pure white skin which is placed on top of the sheet. The woolly side is allowed to come into direct contact with the bed sore. It may be wise to have two sheepskins available so that one can be used while the other is being laundered. The sheepskin seems to work by providing a soft but resilient surface for the bed sore, and its absorbent quality tends to keep the sore area dry. Another, more elaborate device is known as an alternating pressure pad. This is a special mattress pad that is kept in gentle undulating constant motion by a motor. This type of device is used for very stubborn cases, such as patients with paralysis, where bed sores are especially prone to develop. Finally, a widely-used device is the "egg-crate" mattress, actually a polyurethane pad whose surface resembles an egg container. It too, relieves some of the direct pressure.

CONSTIPATION   Constipation, which is likely to be a problem in the bedridden patient, may be due to such factors as inactivity, bland sickroom diets, or fever. There are a great many drugs and treatments for constipation, and many individual preferences. A medicine, food or procedure known to be effective for a particular patient should be tried first. This may be prunes, prune juice, or figs, or perhaps a glycerine or other type of suppository. Milk of magnesia and cascara sagrada, sometimes in combination, are well known, as are derivatives of senna. Many proprietary laxatives are also available. Stool softeners, such as Colace®, are sometimes given daily to keep the stool from hardening and drying out. Stimulating agents such as bran or the extract of psyllium known as Metamucil®, are preferred by some. Any of these may be suitable for temporary use if cleared with the attending physician.

One of the end results of prolonged constipation in a bedridden individual is the accumulation in the rectum of a large amount of hard, dried-out stool. This is known as an impaction, and it may be impossible for the patient to pass it. Sometimes the accumulated stool produces local irritation, which may result in an almost continuous dribbling fecal discharge. Impaction in the bedridden can be avoided by keeping track of bowel behavior. One should be sure that there is no prolonged period without a movement. When an impaction occurs, multiple cleansing enemas (*see* ENEMA in this section), rectal instillation of oil, and sometimes even manual removal may be necessary.

DIARRHEA   Causes of diarrhea vary from the trivial to the serious. Spoiled foods, certain viral infections, overindulgence in alcohol, acute anxiety, and mucous colitis are among the less serious or temporary causes for overactivity of the large intestine. Dysentery generally refers to infection of the colon by various bacteria and occasionally by amoebae, with resultant diarrhea. Some of the bacillary dysenteries are mild and self-limited; others produce great toxicity and are quite serious. In addition, various kinds of tumors and polyps as well as a condition known as diverticulitis may lead to diarrhea. In some instances, it may take all of a doctor's diagnostic ability plus X-rays and similar studies to determine the cause. In other instances, the cause may be clear and the chief problem one of tiding the victim over a bad day or two. Bland and low-residue foods are generally prescribed. These are foods that are nonirritating, readily digested, and leave little or no residue after the digestive process is over; hence they are not stimulating to the intestine. Such foods include cereals, such as cream of wheat, oatmeal, rice, and tapioca, also bread or toast, eggs, milk, jelly, sugar, jello, and custards.

Laxative and high-residue foods are to be avoided in the presence of diarrhea. The foods include such stimulating items as raw fruits and vegetables, prunes, figs and dates, and bran. Even eating moderate amounts of bland foods may act as a stimulus to the large intestine, due to what is called the gastro-colic reflex, which is the tendency of the bowels to contract reflexly when food is placed within the stomach. A further difficulty sometimes experienced is dehydration due to the loss of large amounts of fluid from the body. This can be corrected by the giving of fluids. Important elements such as potassium chloride, and bicarbonate are also lost in diarrhea, a loss which may produce weakness and collapse. In severe cases, intravenous feeding, in which some of these elements are replaced, is sometimes resorted to. In milder instances, such loss of salts will be made up over the course of a few days of ordinary eating and need not be specifically treated as such.

Two of the traditional drugs used in the treatment of diarrhea are paregoric and kaopectate. In most states, paregoric and other derivatives of opium require a doctor's prescription. One of the modes of action of paregoric is to slow down the transit time in the large bowel. By thus allowing more time for absorption of fluid, paregoric will cut down on the intensity and severity of the diarrhea. Other drugs are available for cutting down the motility of the large intestine; these are called antispasmodics and have a direct inhibiting effect on the overactive bowel. Kaopectate and similar medications are presumed to have an absorbent action, and thus tend to form a more solid stool. Whether they are as useful as tradition indicates is open to some question. Over recent years the drugs loperamide (Imodium®) and diphenoxylate (Lomotil®) have largely replaced paregoric.

When there is evidence of a bacterial infection, a physician may prescribe an antibiotic or related drug. Some of these are standard antibiotics, others are special drugs which are poorly absorbed from the bowel but are highly effective against the bacteria within the intestine. Before the advent of these drugs, no specific measures of value existed to attack and clear away the invading bacteria. With the drugs, it may be possible to bring relatively serious dysenteries under control, sometimes quite promptly. Antibiotics have some drawbacks, and their administration presents some complexities. Obviously, they should be taken only under the direction of a physician.

Occasionally, for diarrhea accompanied by cramps, a hot water bottle, heating pad, or other source of heat applied to the abdomen may have a soothing effect. Heat thus applied has value in relaxing the irritable intestinal musculature.

ENEMA An enema is the instillation of a fluid directly into the rectum. The fluid may be nothing more than tap water, which acts by mechanically distending the bowel. This results in contractions (sometimes felt as cramps), and in emptying the retained stool. Sometimes a small amount of lather is worked up in the water with a mild white soap; this is known as a soapsuds enema and is somewhat more stimulating to the bowel. In addition, several commercially prepackaged enemas are available in squeeze bottles with lubricated nozzles. These enemas contain various kinds of salts, so that a relatively small amount of fluid is effective. Their chief advantages are their convenience and disposability.

There are several points to keep in mind when giving an ordinary enema:

• Use one and a half pints for an adult; half a pint is generally enough for a small child.

• The temperature of the fluid should be approximately body temperature. Cold water is likely to be debilitating and harder to retain. A temperature of approximately 101° to 104° F. is desirable.

• Use a well-lubricated nozzle (vaseline is a good lubricant) and insert it into the rectum by exerting gentle pressure with a slight rotating motion.

• The water should be introduced gradually, not abruptly. For an adult, hold the enema can approximately one and a half feet above the level of the rectum, for a child no more than a foot. If the water runs out too rapidly or if the patient complains of cramps, cut down or interrupt the flow briefly.

• The patient can lie on his left side while receiving the enema. Perhaps even better is the knee-chest position, in which the patient supports his weight on his knees and elbows. The enema can be retained for five or more minutes before being expelled. If a very thorough cleansing is required, such as before an X-ray examination of the large intestine, the enema may be repeated until the returns are clear.

If the enema and its evacuation are to be performed in bed, the liberal use of newspapers, and perhaps a plastic sheet is a wise precaution. Use of the bedpan in bed is difficult, as well as objectionable to some patients. An alternative is to set the bedpan on a chair next to the bed, or to use a bedside commode. The patient may prefer to be alone when evacuating the enema. If no risk is involved, it may be wise to leave him alone. Make sure that there is toilet paper at the bedside.

In addition to the prepackaged fluid enemas mentioned above, units containing mineral oil are also available, as are suppositories of various sorts. When effective, these are a good deal simpler then enemas, and can be a satisfactory answer for temporary constipation.

EXERCISES IN BED If bed rest is to be prolonged—and if the doctor gives permission—mild, repeated exercises, particularly of the lower extremities, may be desirable. One of the risks in prolonged bed rest is the occasional occurrence of clotting in the veins of the legs. Thrombosis of a leg vein (phlebothrombosis in medical terminology) may produce some pain and tenderness in the calf, possibly with swelling of the involved leg. However, phlebothrombosis may occur with little or no external signs. When clotting in the vein is extensive, the return circulation from the leg may be interfered with. A permanent swelling of the leg can be one of the consequences. This used to occur frequently in the days when women who had given birth were kept in bed for a week or longer following a delivery. Clotting in a major leg vein was then so frequent that it was referred to as "milk leg."

A potentially serious consequence of clotting in leg veins is that a portion of the clot may break loose and travel on through the system of veins. The veins increase in size and are easily traversed; the clot passes through the heart and finally winds up in the lungs, a condition called a pulmonary embolus. A small embolus may go unnoticed, but larger ones produce a variety of symptoms, including hard, difficult breathing, chest pain, and sometimes serious circulatory and cardiac complications. Indeed, some authorities feel that the major reason for putting victims of heart attacks on anticoagulants (drugs that diminish the clotting time of the blood) is to prevent such a complication as thrombosis in veins. The possibility of thrombosis is increased in elderly individuals, in those who have had a history of a previous thrombosis, or when bed rest is prolonged.

No specific rules for exercises can be given to prevent thrombosis. It is known that even mild wiggling motions of the feet will stimulate the circulation in them and prevent slowing of circulation in the veins, which is a prelude to clotting. Probably more important than the *kind* of exercises is their *frequency*. It is preferable to do the exercises frequently, perhaps every hour or even more often, throughout the day. The patient can wiggle both feet fifteen or twenty minutes every hour on the hour, and bend each leg at the knee an equal number of times in addition. Check with the physician on this, however; in some illnesses there may be good reasons for not engaging in even such mild exercise. A procedure sometimes used, as after an operation, is the application of elastic hosiery to the legs. Because it accelerates flow through the deep veins, this is of value in preventing clots. A nurse or physician can prescribe the kind of hosiery and the method of putting it on.

Another reason for exercising is to prevent weakness and diminished walking ability once the patient is finally allowed up. As soon as anyone takes to bed, loss of muscle strength, and shortly thereafter, muscular wasting become apparent. If you look at the thighs and legs of anyone who has been in bed for a week or more, you are likely to see evidence of shrinkage. This shrinkage is referred to as atrophy. Atrophy can be reversed through use, but is, of course, preferably prevented. Atrophy is less likely to be seen in the upper than in the lower extremities, simply because the bedridden patient is likely to use his arms for a variety of movements such as reaching, eating, hair combing, and so on. Even in the upper extremities, however, the effect of immobilization can sometimes be seen, as in fracture of the arm when a cast is necessary. This often leads to considerable atrophy of the muscles of both the arm and the hand. Sometimes a doctor will order the patient to wiggle the fingers or perform what-

ever other motions are possible in the cast, in an effort to maintain some manual strength and dexterity. Again it must be stressed that the time to begin exercises, and their kind and frequency, should first be discussed with the doctor.

HAIR, CARE OF Care of the hair may present little or no problem during a short illness. If the patient has a large amount of long hair and will be bedridden for a considerable period, a short haircut may be indicated. But often, shampooing the hair is a desirable cleansing and refreshing procedure, and is also good for the morale of a patient long confined to bed. A specially designed plastic trough is now available for use in shampooing the hair in bed. The patient's head and hair are placed within the trough, and are soaped and rinsed in it. The rinse water runs out into a basin through the open side of the trough. A similar device can be improvised at home in the following manner:

• Roll up two bath towels tightly lengthwise. The shape of the roll can be maintained by pinning at suitable intervals. Arrange the towels to form a horseshoe-shaped trough. This is placed sideways on the bed with the open end over the side.

• Shape a shower curtain or plastic sheet over the towels to make a waterproof area into which the patient's hair goes. The free end of the curtain or sheeting extends over the side of the bed and into a pail or similar receptacle.

• The patient's head and hair can now be positioned so that the water used in washing will make its way down the trough and into the pail. A second piece of plastic sheeting and, in addition, a towel for covering the patient's neck and chest will be useful.

After washing, dry the hair with towels. A plastic sheet beneath a towel may be placed on the pillow to protect it from being further dampened. A hand hair dryer or similar device will make the drying easier. Also, an ordinary lamp placed close to the hair will hasten drying. Avoid placing it too close, however. Nor should the patient be allowed to become chilled. Close windows and doors to prevent drafts; when necessary, turn up the heat.

A "dry shampoo" may be quicker and easier. A suitable preparation in powder form may be secured at many druggists. The powder is worked into the hair, then combed or brushed out. Or one may take pledgets of cotton dipped in bay rum or cologne and wipe strands of hair from the scalp outward. Clean pledgets should be used at frequent intervals as one proceeds from one lock of hair to the next. It is sometimes possible to get a barber or beautician to come into the home to do the hair. This can be a most welcome visit.

HEAT TREATMENT AND COMPRESSES

Heat in one form or other is commonly used for a variety of disorders. Heat may relieve pain of many kinds—for example, the pain of an abscessed tooth, a spastic stomach or colon, or the cramps of menstruation. Dry heat is probably the easiest form to administer. The source of heat can be an infrared bulb or even an ordinary electric bulb, a hot-water bottle suitably wrapped in one or more layers of toweling, or a heating pad adjusted to an appropriate level. Moist heat may be more efficacious for certain conditions, as when trying to bring a boil to a "head." When applying moist heat, it is customary to cover the skin of the area with vaseline or cold cream. Usually, a towel or washcloth is wrung out in hot water (approximately 116° F.), folded, and applied to the skin. As the hot towel cools, it can be dipped and wrung out again, and reapplied. Ordinarily, however, it is more efficient to cover the hot wet compress with a dry towel, or if possible, to wrap some plastic sheeting around it. A hot-water bottle may be applied over it to maintain the heat, as may also an electric heating pad. Ordinarily one should guard against water getting into a heating pad (by interposing plastic sheeting), though some heating pads are now wetproof. An electric light may also be used to maintain the heat of the compress. Heat treatments of this kind can be given for periods of half an hour or more, as directed by the doctor, and can be repeated at intervals throughout the day.

Several precautions should be kept in mind when applying any form of heat treatment:

• Beware of burns. These are more likely to occur when the patient is semi-conscious or unconscious, either due to the illness itself or to various tranquilizing or pain-killing drugs.

Do not leave such a patient unattended when heat treatment is in use. Also check the skin at intervals to be sure that it is not turning too red.

• Never apply heat to a part where circulation is impaired. This is particularly true in elderly or diabetic individuals with impaired circulation to the feet. In such patients, heat treatments may produce a breakdown of tissue.

ICE, APPLICATIONS OF

It is a curious fact that ice applications are sometimes used instead of heat applications for very similar conditions. For example, the pain of a sore throat is sometimes helped more by cold than by the more commonly employed heat treatments. Ice has a numbing, pain-killing effect and also acts quite promptly. For immediate control of pain, therefore, it may be more efficient than taking pills by mouth. The pain-relieving properties of ice are sometimes used for superficial burns of the fingers or hand, where prompt application of ice compresses may give relief of an otherwise severe and distressing pain. In acute bursitis, severe pain is produced by the pressure of accumulated fluid in the enclosed area of the bursa, a pocket between tendon and bone. Not infrequently, heat will increase the swelling and make this pain worse, but cold will relieve the pain.

It is sometimes impossible to predict which treatment will be better. One can first try heat and, in the absence of significant relief, shift to cold. It is generally agreed, however, that with injuries such as sprains, or after falls or bruising injuries to the extremities, the prompt application of ice-cold compresses can be very helpful. Bleeding into the tissues, swelling, and pain will be diminished. There are various ways of doing this:

• An ice bag may be convenient. After cracking some ice in a bowl, cover for a minute with tepid water, which will round any sharp edges, then fill the bag with ice, wrap it in a towel or similar covering, and apply to the affected part. If the sensation of cold becomes distressing, the bag can be removed for a time, then reapplied. If the skin turns quite red, and stays that color with the ice removed, this may be a sign of over-long application; one should then cut down on the duration of the application. Generally, the cloth covering the ice bag tends to get damp and should be replaced.

• Another method is to wring out a cloth in a basin of ice-cold water and repeatedly apply the cloth to the skin. One can keep rotating such cold applications by using two or three cloths. Determine the duration of cold treatments with the physician. After an interval of twelve to twenty-four hours following an injury, a shift to local heat may be prescribed.

MEDICINES, GIVING OF Some people take medicines too freely and too light-heartedly; others are overly cautious. One should steer a middle course and always check with the doctor. Sometimes even a simple, everyday drug may present problems. For example, many people regard aspirin as a harmless household remedy. It is a fact, however, that aspirin is irritating to some people's stomachs and should be taken cautiously, or not at all, and preferably not without specifically discussing its use with a physician, by anyone who has a history of an ulcer or who is taking anticoagulant drugs. Remember, too, that aspirin is the most common cause of childhood poisoning; like all drugs, it should be kept entirely out of the reach of children.

Errors in taking medicine are far more common than is supposed; the degree of error is sometimes a surprise to the physician, and can be unpleasant or threatening to the patient. Make sure that you know exactly what the dose of a medicine is; make equally sure that drugs which look or act alike are not confused and taken by mistake. For example, digitalis, a drug often used in heart disease, comes in many dissimilar-appearing pills. Cardiac patients sometimes overdose themselves by unwittingly taking more than one digitalis preparation at a time, although they are in all innocence following the directions on the labels.

It is no longer possible to tell medicines by their appearance, and no one should rely on his memory to identify medicines in the sickroom or the medicine chest. Some doctors give the name of a drug or indicate its effect on the label. This is a good idea. Thus, such identifying marks as "pain pill," "water pill," "penicillin," or "sleeping pill" on the label will cut down the possibility of medication errors.

In giving a medicine to a patient, follow the "three times rule"—the rule used in hospitals. Look at the label and the medicine when you pick up the container, look again before taking the medicine out, and again when replacing the container.

Medicines should sometimes be taken on an empty stomach; sometimes they are tolerated better after a meal. In general, they act more rapidly when taken on an empty stomach, and have a slower and longer-lasting effect taken on a full stomach. Almost all medicines can be taken together, a fact that surprises some patients who feel that one medicine may not "go" with another. Thus, one can take a digitalis pill, a diuretic (urine producing) pill, and a potassium tablet—these three are often prescribed for certain cardiac disorders—at one time, without hesitation. Along with these, one can take an antibiotic, two aspirins, and a cup of coffee, plus some orange juice, without even a second thought. However, in some situations timing is important, and unless one knows definitely whether or not different medications can be taken in combination, and whether before or after meals, one should check the prescription label or check with the doctor.

Some medicines have expiration dates, others undergo virtually no change even after months have elapsed. When in doubt, never take an aged medicine. Always check with a doctor or pharmacist as to whether a medicine that has been on hand for some time can still be used. Some medicines retain their effectiveness longer when kept chilled, as in the refrigerator, and they age more rapidly in hot weather or in hot climates. Biological products especially, such as liver extract, insulin, and certain vitamin preparations, preferably may need to be refrigerated.

MOUTH CARE Like anyone else, the bedridden patient awakens in the morning with a less-than-pleasant taste in his mouth. Cleansing of the teeth and mouth is desirable and refreshing, as well as hygienic. If the patient can brush his own teeth, provide him with his toothbrush, paste, a glass of water, and a suitable receptacle which he can use to rinse out his mouth. A small towel "placed" about the neck may be a good precaution. If the patient is feeble, the teeth can be brushed for him, starting, of course, at the gum line and brushing toward the free surface of the tooth. Or one can cleanse the teeth by using pledgets of cotton dipped in a mouthwash.

Patients with dentures should remove them at night, placing them in a suitable container at the bedside. The dentures can be brushed clean from time to time. The patient may be given any standard mouth rinse, or warm salt water solution, to rinse his mouth in the morning prior to inserting the dentures. In some bedridden patients who undergo weight loss, the dentures may become loose or ill-fitting. This can often be corrected, or at least improved, by a dentist. In some illnesses, an increased furriness of the tongue may be noted. The fur may be white, yellowish, even brown or some other colors. It is generally harmless, but there is no objection to brushing the tongue lightly with brush and toothpaste, or wiping it with a moist washcloth.

NAUSEA AND VOMITING Nausea and vomiting are symptoms frequently encountered as a result of food poisoning, viral illnesses, reactions to drugs or alcohol, or in association with pregnancy, migraine headaches, and numerous other causes. In addition to nonthreatening and essentially temporary conditions, nausea and vomiting may be a sign of more serious illness. Hence, the evaluation and diagnosis of these symptoms is properly a physician's task. If it is clear that they are not the result of a serious condition, the following pointers will prove helpful in guiding treatment:

• There is no point in forcing solid foods or liquids in the presence of definite nausea, if the condition can be expected to improve spontaneously. Twelve to twenty-four hours with little food or fluid intake can be tolerated under normal circumstances.

• After the nausea has partially subsided, only small amounts of food should be taken at a time. One can sneak in a few tablespoons of a substance from time to time without producing a reaction; in contrast, to give a larger amount when the stomach is still in an irritable state may produce another bout of nausea and vomiting.

• To give chilled or ice-cold liquids is sometimes the most successful approach. One may give the patient small chips of ice to suck on; this is also refreshing. Sips of cold carbonated

drinks, such as ginger ale, may also be successful. These should be given cautiously at first, perhaps at intervals of several minutes.

• A remedy favored in some parts of the country is to give an undiluted cola syrup in teaspoonful doses at intervals of every ten to fifteen minutes. This seems to be tolerated even when nausea is very trying. The caffeine in the syrup may have a desirable and mildly stimulating effect.

After these measures have succeeded, one can cautiously and slowly go on to foods, preferably bland at first and offered in small amounts. Farina, oatmeal, or similar cereals, toast with jelly, and tea are among the more commonly used food items following severe bouts of nausea and vomiting. From these, one can go on progressively to such other bland items as eggs, chicken, and soups. The rate at which one approaches the usual diet should be gauged by how the patient feels as well as by how he responds to the increasing food allowances.

In recent years, some drugs useful in allaying nausea have appeared. They can be given by mouth, by injection, or by suppository. Some of these are tranquilizers. All of them are prescription items and should be taken only as directed by a physician.

The nausea of pregnancy has not been satisfactorily accounted for but is thought to be due to hormonal action on the digestive tract. It is generally worse in the morning, and often improves spontaneously later in the day. Various drugs can be employed for this. Sometimes, eating just dry toast or a few salty crackers, first thing in the morning, is helpful. It may be desirable, particularly in the morning, to cut down on the amount of fluids, and to make the intake of food at any particular time relatively small. To control nausea and vomiting in pregnancy may occasionally require energetic measures, and a woman who is losing weight or showing severe symptoms should be under medical management early in the pregnancy.

PULSE, TAKING OF A knowledge of how to take the pulse rate is often useful and can provide valuable information to the physician. It may make a great deal of difference in the doctor's diagnostic thinking if someone who complains of palpitations can also state with accuracy that his pulse at the time was 90 and not 140. In some heart conditions in which digitalis is prescribed, the pulse rate may govern the dose. Here, especially, observation of the pulse may be all-important. It is also a fact that the pulse rate goes up about ten beats for every one degree of fever. Thus, a rough estimate of the height of a fever can be made by taking the pulse.

The pulse can be taken in any of a number of locations. This is because the pulse represents the thrust given to the bloodstream by the heartbeat, and can be felt in many places. In thin individuals or where the heart is enlarged or the beat especially forceful, the heart rate can be taken by placing the hand over the heart itself. An easy location to feel the pulse is in the neck just below the jaw, but only palpate one side at a time. Most often the pulse at the wrist—the radial pulse—is checked. The easiest way to learn about the pulse is to take one's own. Turn the arm so that the hand faces you. Place the middle three fingers of the other hand on the wrist at the base of the thumb, in a line extending toward the forearm, and about a half inch in from the outer border. With a little exploration you should be able to feel the pulse in this location.

The pulse is generally regular, that is, the interval between the beats is the same. The impact one feels is also usually the same from beat to beat. When it is markedly diminished, we speak of a feeble pulse; if unusually vigorous, it is a bounding pulse. Occasionally, the interval between beats is prolonged in an irregular way, or there may be other departures from the normal; this is referred to as an arrhythmia. With some practice, major abnormalities of the pulse rate can be easily detected.

Generally speaking, healthy people should avoid taking their own pulse, for what is often thought to be a worrisome abnormality far more often has no medical significance. In fact, the pulse of healthy individuals can be quite variable. It may go up with exertion, excitement, anxiety, or after too much coffee or other stimulants. It may be fuller after several cocktails, and less vigorous when one is resting. A resting pulse of 70 is normal for one person, while one of 96 may be normal for another. In short, just as with blood pressure and weight, considerable range is entirely normal.

SICKROOM EQUIPMENT   The extent to which one invests in sickroom equipment will be determined by the needs of the patient, the duration of the illness, the financial circumstances, and the like. Obviously, the situation will vary widely between a child sick at home with the chicken-pox and an elderly individual suffering from the after effects of a stroke. If an illness is of some duration, the purchase of suitable sickroom equipment may be a worthwhile investment in terms of the return in comfort, efficiency, and safety for both the patient and those about him.

Thus, with a cardiac patient whose breathing is eased by sleeping in a nearly upright position, a hospital bed, the head of which can be raised, is a great comfort. Such a bed and similar equipment need not always be bought outright; it can often be rented from appropriate local agencies or businesses. In the absence of the hospital bed, one can use several alternatives: the most common is to pile three or four pillows one on top of another. Another way is to place pillows, or preferably firmer objects, between the box spring and the mattress at the head of the bed, to elevate it. One or two chairs can be upended and placed between box spring and mattress in such a way that their backs elevate the mattress. The type of backrest commonly used at beaches may also prove useful.

Some of the more recent models of hospital-type beds are adjustable to two heights and are called "hi-lo" beds. The adjustable heights make it easier for attendants to change the bed and to care for the patient; they also facilitate the patient's getting in and out of bed by himself. If the bed in the home is too low, suitable blocks can be either made or purchased for elevating all four corners. In addition, there are now commercially available beds that can be adjusted by the patient himself.

Reference has been made to mattresses under the entry BED MAKING in this section. In most modern hospitals, mattresses are made of a foam rubber and are of moderate firmness. The rubber mattress adjusts to the various positions of the patient's frame better than does an ordinary spring mattress, and it can be cleaned and sterilized more readily. Polyurethane foam, a synthetic rubber-like material, is showing up more and more frequently in mattresses; it possesses many of the advantages of rubber, but is generally cheaper. It is extremely light, and therefore much easier to handle. It can be bought in various thicknesses. (Most mattresses are either four or six inches thick.) A one- to two-inch thickness of this material makes an excellent topper for an ordinary mattress. But be sure to get one of some density; otherwise it may collapse too readily under pressure.

Both polyurethane foam and foam rubber are somewhat warmer than standard mattresses. This may be an advantage in cold weather and a disadvantage in very hot weather. Plastic and rubber sheeting are useful items. They will protect the mattress against soilage from draining wounds, or from an incontinent patient. They can also be used to protect the surface of bedside furniture, and are relatively easy to keep clean and to sterilize.

A bed table (so constructed that it fits over the bed) is desirable and useful for someone who is bedridden. On this flat surface the patient can eat or write, or keep a few small objects. In hospitals, it is a standard bedside item. It comes on wheels so that it can be moved about, and has a lever for vertical adjustment to the best height for the patient. Many models have a concealed mirror, to be used when shaving or putting on makeup. For temporary purposes, the following substitutes for a bed table may be useful:

• A plank or ironing board resting on the backs of two chairs placed on either side of the bed

• A wooden crate or heavy cardboard box with its center section partially cut away to fit over the legs of the bedfast patient

• A bed tray—essentially a tray with folding legs. When the legs of the tray are unfolded, it forms a table which is elevated and placed over the patient's thighs.

The bedside commode is a toileting device that can be kept in the sickroom. Some bedside commodes are fairly elaborate and costly. Others are basically simple chairs, with an opening in the seat and room for a bedpan directly underneath. A simple homemade device consists of a chair with a seat suitably cut out and a pail underneath. Lining the pail with the heavy plastic liners, the kind available for garbage disposal, may facilitate cleaning. Ordinarily, the patient may have to be helped or even lifted out of bed to get to the bedside commode. If the restriction is such that the patient must be toileted in bed, then a bedpan must be obtained. This is essentially a shallow basin made of metal or plastic, which can be worked under the patient's hips. For a patient who is flat in bed and cannot sit up, special bedpans with a low sloping contour, known as fracture pans, are available.

For the urination needs of males, a urinal may be purchased. These are made of glass, plastic, or metal. Any wide-mouthed, good-sized bottle can obviously serve as a substitute. Other aides and comforts to be considered for the sickroom are the following:

• A little bell or bedside buzzer attachment for securing attention

• A telephone extension or telephone jack placed at the bedside. This is especially desirable if the patient is unattended during part of the day. For those unable to use dial telephones, the telephone company will supply an old-fashioned phone which has no dial and communicates directly with the operator.

• A large, sturdy brown paper bag pinned to the bedside mattress is a suitable receptacle for the disposal of minor items such as soiled tissues

• A television set with a remote-control device may be extremely valuable to a shut-in.

• If the patient is unable to walk, a wheelchair may be the means to enable him to go from one room to another, or to get out of the house. In its simplest form, this may be an ordinary kitchen chair to which wheels are attached. The most complex is a battery-driven, motorized wheelchair which will enable even a person with considerable disability in the upper extremities to get about. In between are a variety of chairs, generally collapsible, an advantage for storage or when going on automobile trips. Wheelchairs come in various widths. Before buying or renting a wheelchair, be sure to measure the width of the doorways. It sometimes happens that only a wheelchair of the narrowest width can pass through the doorways of a particular building.

A walker is a device that enables someone who is weak or convalescent, and whose walking ability is uncertain, to practice walking more or less safely. The more complex and expensive walkers are contrivances on wheels possessing a heavy frame and a retractible seat. This enables the patient to walk supported by the frame, or, if he tires, he may sit in it. The walkerette is a lighter and cheaper device which may answer the same purpose. It has a relatively simple, tubular framework approximately waist high. Some walkerettes have two front wheels which the patient can push in front of him while he holds on to the framework for steadiness and support. A wheelchair can also be used for this purpose. The patient pushes the wheelchair before him much as an attendant would, the heavy chair acting to steady him. Still another possibility is to take an ordinary kitchen chair and place metal domes (the so-called "domes of silence") on the leg bottoms. The chair can be pushed much more readily with these domes than without them.

Finally, it is important to think of safety features in the sickroom. Elderly patients not infrequently fall out of bed. This common accident may occur to anyone, particularly if he is dazed by illness or drugs. Side-rails can be applied even to an ordinary bed. Several chairs lined up on either side of the bed may also prevent a fall. As a rule, the chairs need to be placed only along the upper half of the bed. Unless scatter rugs have nonskid bottoms, they may pose a special hazard to the patient. Such rugs are best removed. Very often the furniture in the sickroom can be used by the patient to support himself if he is weak or totters. However, a piece of furniture may be hazardous if it is too light, or if it has sharp edges, protruding knobs or legs. A night light in the sickroom may be a useful safety feature, and may also serve to orient a confused older person to his surroundings. Similar lights may be desirable in the bathroom and in hallways.

SITZ BATH   A sitz bath is often prescribed for cleansing or healing purposes in the rectal and genital regions. It is commonly prescribed for the pain of hemorrhoids (piles) and after rectal operations. It is literally a "sit bath" and can be performed in several ways. One may draw a basin partially full of warm to hot water. (The temperature will be prescribed by the doctor, and is commonly about 115° F.) The basin is placed in a convenient location, for example on a chair, or on top of a toilet or commode. As an alternative, one may draw four or five inches of water into a tub.

The patient then sits in the basin or the tub.

This brings the hot water into contact with the affected area. A sitz bath generally lasts fifteen to twenty minutes, or even longer, and may be repeated several times a day. Small amounts of warm water may be added to maintain the temperature, if desired. Most often, plain water is used for the sitz bath. An ordinary tub bath, though it too may be cleansing, will not provide the local heating effect for which a sitz bath is usually prescribed.

TEMPERATURE, TAKING OF   It is often necessary to follow the course of an illness by keeping track of the degree of fever. Sometimes a complication of an illness is indicated by a rise in temperature; conversely, improvement or response to drugs may be indicated by a drop in temperature toward normal. In recent years, flat thermometers (as against the older rounded ones) have been made available, and are easier to read. The trick in reading a thermometer is to rotate it slowly so that the light catches the mercury column at just the correct angle. When this occurs, the line of mercury becomes evident and the height which it has reached can easily be read off. Here are some further hints about thermometers:

• Never wash a thermometer under hot water. Wash with soap and water under the cold tap. This is ordinarily sufficient to get rid of bacteria, but one may be doubly certain by keeping the thermometer in alcohol for a few minutes, or by wiping it down with a pledget of cotton soaked in alcohol.

• Always check the reading prior to usage. It may still be elevated from previous use. If so, shake the mercury column down. This is done by holding that end of the thermometer which is away from the bulb *firmly* between thumb and forefinger, and then with several snapping motions of the wrist the mercury column can be forced downwards into the bulb. In doing this, make sure not to strike the thermometer against a nearby object.

• For mouth temperatures, the thermometer is placed under the tongue for five minutes. The patient should have had neither hot nor cold drinks for at least ten minutes prior to taking a reading. Do not use the oral method in out-of-control or confused persons; they may bite and break the thermometer. For rectal temperature, the lubricated thermometer tip should be inserted with a gentle motion to one-third of its length. It should be left in for approximately three minutes. With children and with unconscious or confused adults, one should stand by during the temperature-taking to make sure the patient does not roll over while the rectal thermometer is in place. Remove the rectal thermometer, wipe the lubrication off, read, and then proceed to wash as described above.

• The normal mouth temperature is 98.6°F., but in some individuals it may be as much as a degree lower. The normal rectal temperature is 99.6°F., hence mention should be made of whether the temperature was taken orally or rectally. It may be noted that while rectal thermometers have a shorter, stubbier bulb than oral ones, their calibration is the same. An unused rectal thermometer will give a perfectly correct mouth temperature.

A specially calibrated thermometer in which the calibrations are widely spaced is sometimes used for women to study their reproductive cycles. Small fluctuations are more readily read with this kind of thermometer. At about the middle of the menstrual cycle, it is sometimes possible to detect a rise of a few tenths of a degree, which is believed to be due to the release of an egg from the ovary.

VAPORIZERS Vaporizers are convenient ways of adding moisture to the air of a room. To increase the humidity is soothing to the nose, throat, and bronchial passages in various respiratory illnesses. It may help allay cough and make the bringing up of phlegm easier. In some viral illnesses in which there is severe cough with little production of sputum, humidification may also be desirable. This is especially so for children with an irritative, frequent cough. Croup generally refers to a cough in children, and is associated with spasm of the muscles of the larnyx, which may produce difficulty in breathing in. A vaporizer or steam-producing device directed toward the child may be the most important measure employed for croup. Keep in mind precautions against burns.

Many vaporizers of various sizes are available. To avoid frequent refillings, it is wise to get a vaporizer of at least one-gallon capacity. Most have an automatic shut-off device when the water level drops too low. Large sizes will easily run twelve hours without refilling. Vaporizers may be employed routinely for someone with a respiratory illness whenever the room is heated by steam or by hot air. Indeed, even in the absence of any infection of the respiratory tract, adding moisture to the air of the usual heated winter apartment has much to be said for it. "Cold steam" vaporizers are more expensive but are superior to the regular type of vaporizers. However they may produce a certain kind of clamminess to the air and also can require a good cleansing or sterilization from time to time.

Humidifiers are devices that disperse water vapor into a room without the preliminary heating that occurs in vaporizers. No steam is produced, which may be an advantage when a heating effect is not desired—for example, in warm weather. From a practical point of view, the vaporizer and the humidifier may be interchangeable in a sickroom for purposes of adding moisture to the air.

A simple method for increasing air moisture is to set pans of water on or under radiators. An even more efficient way is to place wet towels or sheets on the radiator, their ends dipping into pans of water. A large amount of water will continually evaporate into the air, but frequent refilling of the pans may be necessary.

QUESTIONS AND ANSWERS ABOUT COMMON SYMPTOMS

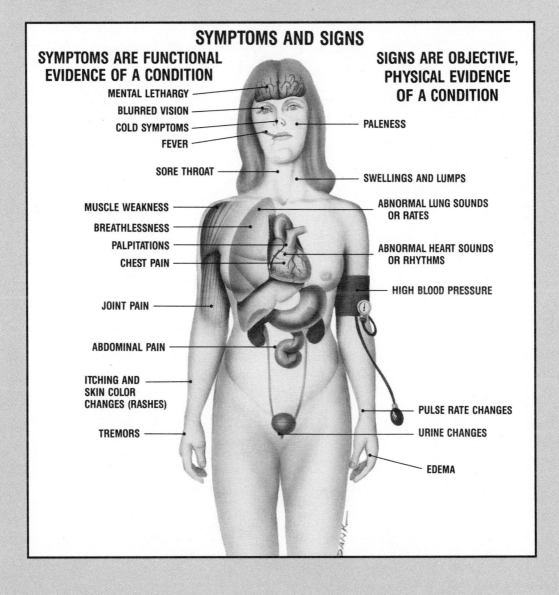

SYMPTOMS AND SIGNS

SYMPTOMS ARE FUNCTIONAL EVIDENCE OF A CONDITION

- MENTAL LETHARGY
- BLURRED VISION
- COLD SYMPTOMS
- FEVER
- SORE THROAT
- MUSCLE WEAKNESS
- BREATHLESSNESS
- PALPITATIONS
- CHEST PAIN
- JOINT PAIN
- ABDOMINAL PAIN
- ITCHING AND SKIN COLOR CHANGES (RASHES)
- TREMORS

SIGNS ARE OBJECTIVE, PHYSICAL EVIDENCE OF A CONDITION

- PALENESS
- SWELLINGS AND LUMPS
- ABNORMAL LUNG SOUNDS OR RATES
- ABNORMAL HEART SOUNDS OR RHYTHMS
- HIGH BLOOD PRESSURE
- PULSE RATE CHANGES
- URINE CHANGES
- EDEMA

Some of the most frequent questions heard daily in any doctor's office are discussed in this section. It is hoped that this material will serve to illustrate and clarify the many interesting aspects of medical practice. It should be emphasized, however, that the field of diagnosis is a complicated one, and that no layperson should attempt to match any symptoms against those in a particular paragraph and conclude that he or she is necessarily suffering from the specific condition described. Doctors themselves often have difficulty determining which of a great many possible disorders the patient being examined may have. This difficulty belongs under the heading differential diagnosis. To do a differential diagnosis properly may require specialized procedures such as blood counts, X-ray studies, examinations of stones, and the like. Sometimes batteries of tests of this sort may be necessary to evaluate a chest pain or an abdominal pain. Hence, in reading the material which follows, the reader is urged not to attempt self-diagnosis. Rather, one should consider this section only as a run-down of some of the various disorders that may afflict one of the most complicated of all machines—the human body.

Q-1. *For years I have been plump around the hips and abdomen. Why do physicians often object so strongly to overweight?*

A. Medical objections to obesity have steadily increased in recent years. The average person may look upon his excess weight as something that gives him a bulge around the midriff, necessitates larger clothing sizes, and makes him puff a bit when climbing stairs. A physician regards obesity as a disease which predisposes to many other diseases. Many ailments or conditions which shorten life are associated with excess weight.

Exactly why an overweight person is so much more susceptible to a variety of other illnesses has not been entirely clarified. Sometimes the association is understandable. Thus overweight people are prone to pain and discomfort in their knees and hips, generally in the form of osteoarthritis, because of the abnormal load borne by these joints year after year. The correlation between obesity and certain other diseases is less easy to explain but nonetheless real. For example, there is a significantly higher incidence of diabetes among the obese. Reducing the weight of patients with mild diabetes may clear up the diabetic condition. Even if it does not, the weight loss may permit them to escape taking special drugs for the diabetes.

High blood pressure is likewise more frequent in people who are overweight, and also tends to drop with a curbing of calories and consequent loss in weight. High blood pressure in the obese in turn contributes to the high incidence of such circulatory ailments as heart attacks and strokes. Obese individuals with normal blood pressure are subject to greater degrees of hardening of the arteries than those of normal weight.

It is no secret that treatment of strokes, diabetes, heart attacks, and similar disorders has considerable limitations, and that prevention is preferable to treatment in these disease categories. Hence the emphasis on keeping weight down as a form of prophylaxis against a variety of serious disorders. The influence of weight is dramatically underlined by the fact that, while individuals of normal weight live longer and have fewer illnesses than those who are overweight, the underweight do even better than those of normal weight. All human statistics and even animal experiments indicate that mild undernutrition tends to maintain good health. In short, the thinner the better. (*See* OVERWEIGHT in the section NUTRITION AND HEALTH.)

Q-2. *I avoid cream, butter, ice cream, and fat cuts of meat. Is this advisable?*

A. In recent years a considerable body of data has been accumulated proving some relationship between the kinds and amounts of fats in the diet and hardening of the arteries.

One important aspect of hardening of the arteries is the deposit of fats in the lining of the blood vessels. As this process goes on the arteries narrow, and eventually the blood may clot in a constricted passage. This is known as thrombosis.

A coronary thrombosis, a clot occurring in one of the arteries of the heart, results in a heart attack. A similar process in one of the blood vessels of the brain may produce a stroke.

More than seventy years ago it was demonstrated that a considerable portion of the fat deposited in the arteries consists of a waxy substance, cholesterol. When large amounts of cholesterol are fed to experimental animals, deposits are found in their arteries too. Because of these findings, the first diets brought forward in relation to hardening of the arteries were low in fats, especially cholesterol.

Cholesterol is found in large amounts in eggs, cream, whole milk, and milk products such as cheese and ice cream. At one time advocates of the dietary approach recommended a reduction of all fats as well as low cholesterol content. This called for such measures as avoiding all fatty foods and trimming all visible meat fat. It was found that the amount of cholesterol in the blood dropped in many subjects when they were shifted from their usual diet to a diet low in cholesterol and in saturated fats.

More recently it has been discovered that reduction of saturated fats (the fats of animal origin, such as those found in meats, butter, and milk) and addition of unsaturated fats (corn oil, safflower oil, and various vegetable oils, coconut oil being the sole exception) produces a further drop in the level of blood cholesterol. In the most recent formulations of the dietary approach to hardening of the arteries, diets have been worked out which are low in saturated fat and contain moderate amounts of unsaturated fats in the form of oils added in cooking and in salads.

There is already evidence that persons who have had heart attacks or other vascular diseases do better if they switch to such diets. The American Heart Association now recommends these diets for everyone, not only for heart-attack victims. Other dietary authorities feel that diseases of the heart and blood vessels are so common that everyone could well go on a diet of this kind or at least modify the customary intake of fats to conform to the general guidelines proposed for heart-attack patients.

Given below are some examples of diets which are high in polyunsaturated and low in saturated fats. In general, these diets can be approximated by the approach, recommended by the Bureau of Nutrition of the New York City Department of Health, termed the "prudent diet."

The prudent diet emphasizes fish, lean cuts of meat, and liquid vegetable oils.

The following further suggestions are made:

Fish, Meat, Eggs. Fish and shellfish at least four to five times a week, for any meal. The fat in fish is an excellent source of polyunsaturated fatty acids. Poultry may be taken often; it is low in fat. Veal may be taken frequently; it is a lean meat. Beef, pork, and lamb—not more than three to four times a week, with the serving not to exceed four ounces of cooked meat. Eggs, because of their very high cholesterol content (230 mgm per egg) are perhaps best avoided by adults and certainly they should not consume more than four a week.

Avoid very fat meats, bacon, sausage, corned beef, pastrami. Select lean cuts of all meats. Trim off all visible fat. Keep portions moderate—four to six ounces before cooking (four ounces after cooking).

Milk and Milk Products. The fat in whole milk is predominantly saturated and is not recommended. Two cups of skim milk daily for adults; two to four cups of milk daily for children—two cups of this milk allowance may be whole milk. More than four cups of milk is not recommended for children, even for adolescents. Use cottage, pot, or farmer cheese often. Avoid butter, cream, ice cream, cream cheese, hard cheeses, and other milk cheeses.

Fats. Vegetable oils should be used for their polyunsaturated fatty acids. To have more of these than saturated fatty acids, use vegetable oils daily. Olive oil, a monounsaturated oil, has recently been found equal to the polyunsaturates in these dietary programs. Use 1½ ounce (3 tablespoons) daily in cooking and at the table. Make salad dressings with oil. Substitute oil for other fats in cooking and baking. Butter, ordinary margarine, and other hydrogenated fats must be kept at a minimum. (*See* CHOLESTEROL in the section NUTRITION AND HEALTH.)

Q-3. *Everything I eat seems to turn into fat. Why is this so?*

A. Undoubtedly you are consuming more calories than you need for your bodily functions and activities. The only way the body can deal with excess calories is to convert them to fat. A switch from high-caloric to low-caloric items might make the difference. Some foods in ordinary portions pack a good deal more in the way of calories than others. When a normal portion of a food is very high in calories, it is referred to as a high-caloric item; when the opposite is true, as a low-caloric item. The difference may easily be illustrated when the choice of desserts facing a dieter is between half a cantaloupe (40 calories) and a three-inch wedge of lemon meringue pie (300 calories). Although a person may become too calorie conscious, a general knowledge of the caloric content of foods can be useful.

For example, the following are desserts fairly high in calories: a brownie, 2 x 2¾ inches, contains 140 calories; a typical chocolate almond bar, 200; a chocolate sundae, 335; an iced cupcake, 250; an ordinary doughnut, 140. In contrast, an apple or an orange has 75 to 100 calories; an average portion of melon, such as honeydew or cantaloupe, perhaps 50 calories; a banana, 75 calories. Not to be disregarded in this connection are the alcoholic beverages, for an 8 ounce glass of beer contains 120 calories, while the usual cocktails, such as martinis or Manhattans, 150 to 175 calories.

Icebox raiders should know that a hamburger on a bun usually represents well over 300 calories; a frankfurter on a roll, 250; a half cup of potato salad with mayonnaise, 200; and 8 to 10 large potato chips, 100. Nuts are high in calories, too, 4 to 5 cashews running to 100, as do 6 pecans. Certain bulky vegetable items, on the other hand, are quite low in calories, including salads with lettuce, tomatoes, and cucumbers, and many of the so-called "5 percent" vegetables. The 5 percent vegetables include string beans, wax beans, asparagus, broccoli, Brussels sprouts, and carrots. Ordinary portions will have about 20 to 30 calories. Sometimes with a little effort the number of calories in a food item can be readily decreased. Thus, eating a hamburger made from lean ground round steak, or drinking skim milk instead of whole milk, will cut the calories by half. Dieters are often advised to eat broiled meats and to cut away the visible fat, two methods of getting rid of the highly caloric fat portion.

Similarly, cottage cheese made from skim milk contains fewer calories than pot cheese made from whole milk. The common rather oily cheeses are almost as high in calories as straight butter. Cheeses can be either high- or low-caloric items and have to be identified before they can be classified. (*See* the section NUTRITION AND HEALTH.)

Q-4. *Are there special programs which will slim me down fast?*

A. These are the programs usually referred to as crash diets or formula diets. Crash diets and special-formula diets are usually too restricted in their range and in their caloric content. They are designed to achieve extremely rapid weight reduction and are sometimes used to start off a long-term reducing program by producing a large initial weight loss. The drastic reduction that can be brought about by a crash program seems to firm up a person's desire to continue reducing, and so, on psychological grounds, the crash diet may be defended. Physicians also feel that the problem of excess weight fundamentally demands a long-term solution of the disproportion between intake of food and actual need, so that short, painful bursts of dieting are not really the answer.

Formula diets generally consist of flavored skim milk-oil preparations to which vitamins have been added. A representative specimen runs 225 calories per serving so that when taken four times a day, it is a 900-calorie diet, which will certainly induce a loss of weight.

There is very little oral satisfaction in downing a drink of this kind, and a sense of deprivation that users may experience is the absence of chewing satisfaction. Some people cannot tolerate the liquid preparations and have digestive disturbances as a result. One of the secrets of the success of the formula diets is that they permit no leeway. Apart from coffee or tea and sometimes a raw vegetable such as celery or carrot, the dieter has no alternative. He can hardly cheat. From a nutritional point of view, however, a low-calorie diet has the virtue of including the four basic food groups, of not being monotonous, and of affording some eating satisfaction.

Over the last few years special physician-supervised low calorie dietary programs have emerged. Some run from 400 to 600 calories per day and dispense specially concocted packets on a weekly basis. They are drastic but do work predictably.

In general, crash diets and starvation programs are last-ditch maneuvers or programs for the desperate. There is no reason why a well-balanced, reasonable diet program which will provide satisfactory weight loss week after week cannot be maintained by the average overweight person. Because the overweight problem is chronic and long-term, crash programs which provide only short-term results are bound to fall short of the solution desired. (*See* OVERWEIGHT in the section NUTRITION AND HEALTH.)

Q-5. *Several people have told me my breath is sometimes unpleasant. How can I handle this problem?*
A. A number of different factors may contribute significantly to disagreeable breath. Perhaps the most common is the eating or drinking of certain kinds of foods or liquors. Among some of the items that may cause bad breath are garlic, onions, and various alcoholic beverages. Certain constituents of these substances are excreted through the lung into the air we expire and contribute their odor to the breath. (This is one of the principles behind the breathalyzer test for concentration of alcohol in the blood.) Some of these odorous constituents may also be excreted in the saliva and the sweat.

Decaying food particles impacted between the teeth may contribute an odor to the breath. A particle of meat caught between the teeth undergoes a chemical change by bacterial action in the mouth, and as a result can become somewhat odorous. The use of dental floss—a good hygienic idea—often reveals that meat fragments undergo softening and chemical changes which alter their initial odor. The extent to which particles lodge in the teeth

varies in different people and depends upon the structure of their teeth. In a normal set of teeth, there are narrow spaces between the teeth at the gum margin. Thus, the dental arrangement which collects food is a normal one.

Various disorders of the nose, throat, and oral cavity, particularly certain kinds of inflammation, may contribute to breath odor. They include various infections of the gums (gingivitis), abscesses, tonsillitis, and others. A condition of the nose and throat known as ozena, which is associated with dryness and crusting, will produce an odor. It may be helped by snuffing up water into the nasal cavity and washing away the crusts.

Various digestive disorders may create an unpleasant breath. Although normally the muscular activity of the digestive tract tends to propel in only one direction—onward from the stomach—there are various conditions in which this movement may be interrupted or reversed to produce regurgitation, burning sensations, unpleasant tastes, and odors. Constipation produces a furry tongue and unpleasant breath. Bad breath may be present in certain fevers and also in some women when they are menstruating.

The treatment of bad breath is, of course, indicated by the cause. He who insists on eating garlic, onions, salami, dill pickles, frankfurters, and similar food may find that his breath produces some social problems. The same may be said for certain kinds of liquors and wines, but reputedly straight gin and vodka do not create breath odor. Good mouth hygiene, including frequent brushing of the teeth and the use of dental floss, may relieve many common forms of bad breath. However, even with due care for all of these factors, there are occasional individuals whose breath will still have a distinct odor. In the absence of any specific cause, the only solution left may be camouflage by the use of mints and special sprays. (*See* HALITOSIS in the section DENTAL HEALTH.)

Q-6. *I often have a burning feeling high up in my stomach. What can I do for it?*
A. This is probably simple heartburn. Heartburn is a commonly experienced symptom of disordered digestion which is usually described as a burning sensation high in the up-

per central abdomen. It is sometimes located in the lowest portion of the chest cavity at the tip end of the sternum or breast bone. Heartburn is generally attributed to irritation of the lining of the gullet (lower esophagus) and stomach wall. In some individuals it regularly follows the eating of certain offending foods for which they have low tolerance. These may include onions, cucumbers, radishes, spicy, smoked, or heavily salted foods; too much coffee or very strong coffee, alcohol, mustard, garlic, chocolate, and certain fried or greasy foods.

It is probable that stomach acids play an important part in this complaint. For example, neutralizing the stomach acids with an alkalinizing agent such as ordinary bicarbonate of soda may give prompt relief of the burning sensation; the common over-the-counter medicinal alkalinizers are also usually helpful. In this respect, heartburn may be compared to the symptoms experienced by peptic ulcer victims, in whom pain is produced by exposure of the ulcerated area to acid stomach fluids. Here, too, neutralization of the stomach acids will relieve the pain. However, heartburn occasionally occurs in individuals who have no acids in their stomach juices, and it may well be that not all heartburn is due to the same cause.

Although heartburn is most often a mild disorder and ordinarily does not signify any grave disease, it may be the chief symptom of an ulcer. Also, in the condition known as hiatus hernia in which a portion of the stomach is above the level of the diaphragm, irritative and even ulcerative states of the pouch or stomach above the diaphragm are often described as heartburn. Some forms of heartburn which are experienced chiefly at night seem to be due to a reflux of acid gastric juices from the stomach up into the lower esophagus. Since the esophagus does not tolerate such exposure to stomach acids, the usual reaction consists of a sort of burning pain. This condition is sometimes referred to as peptic esophagitis. Certainly, if heartburn is not specifically related to a particular food item, and becomes more than just an occasional event, it may require a doctor's checkup to ascertain the cause. (*See* HEARTBURN; ULCER AND ULCERS in the section GASTROINTESTINAL CONDITIONS.)

Q-7. *I've been told that I have a "delicate stomach." What sort of foods should I eat?*
A. Probably a bland diet may be of value, once it has been ascertained that a special need exists. A bland diet is a specially selected dietary program consisting of foods that are relatively easy to digest and that are not likely to be stimulating or irritating to the digestive tract. Spicy, highly seasoned, fried, smoked, marinated, and pickled food items are prohibited. Also eliminated from the bland diet are some so-called "gassy" vegetables, nuts, and fatty cuts of meat. Many people almost automatically put themselves on a bland diet when they have a digestive upset. They may have cooked cereals, toast, jam, and tea for breakfast instead of their usual fried eggs, pork sausages, and two cups of strong coffee. Bland diets are recommended after digestive upsets that have included nausea, vomiting, and diarrhea. They are also recommended for certain stages of active ulcer, for functional colitis, for various illnesses in which there is fever and malaise (feeling poorly), and for gallbladder disease.

The following are guidelines for a strict bland diet. The omission of caffeine-containing beverages, such as coffee and tea, is due to their acid-producing characteristics. However, many bland diets permit weak tea or coffee.

General Rules:

• Meat should be well cooked and tender; it may be baked, boiled, broiled, or roasted.

• Skins, seeds, nuts, spices, or coconut should be avoided.

• Fruits or juice should be taken after some food has been eaten or at the end of a meal.

• Small frequent feedings are better tolerated than large meals.

• The food should be not only bland, but of moderate temperature.

DAILY FOOD ALLOWANCE:

Milk	3 cups or more
Vegetables	2 portions or more
Fruits	2 portions or more
Cereals, bread, cakes, or starches	6 portions or more
Eggs	1 or more
Meat, fish, or cheese	6 ounces or more
Fats	2 tablespoons or more

(*See also* the section NUTRITION AND HEALTH.)

Q-8. *Sometimes my stomach swells up, and I have to burp or pass gas. What causes this and how can I take care of it?*
A. This appears to be a common form of digestive disturbance often described as bloating and "gaseousness." By bloating most persons mean a distention of the abdomen, often accompanied by sensations of fullness. By gaseousness what is usually meant is either eructations, "burping," or flatulence, the passage of gas rectally. Sometimes all these conditions may occur together, in which case a patient will complain of abdominal swelling, burping, and annoyingly frequent passage of wind. They may also be dissociated from each other and can occur singly. They are all common complaints, and very few individuals have not experienced them at one time or another. However, in some people they occur with far greater frequency and may be a daily event.

When symptoms of this sort appear for the first time in middle or late life, a physician may suspect some organic disease or inflammation in the digestive tract. In fact, he may be impelled to order X-rays or other appropriate studies in order to get at the cause of the underlying difficulty. If, however, the complaints have occurred again and again over the years, it is apparently clear that no new or very threatening disorder can underlie them.

Certainly these complaints are encountered in persons who otherwise are in excellent health. For a long time it was thought that they were more common in individuals with gallbladder disease, but a recent study indicates that people without any gallbladder difficulties whatever may have these complaints as often as those with chronic disease of the gallbladder. The causes of bloating and gaseousness vary and include the following:

• Certain mild chronic disorders of the digestive tract may produce these symptoms. Among them are gastritis, a mild inflammation of the stomach lining; hiatus hernia, a protrusion of part of the stomach above the level of the diaphragm; and pylorospasm, a spasm of the muscle between the stomach and the intestine. Any of these disorders can lead to upper abdominal fullness, belching, or related conditions.

• Anxiety and tension may produce symptoms of this sort. The digestive tract frequently faithfully reflects emotional upsets and changes. Many people know that when they are upset they seem to "fill up" very rapidly, or they become "gassy." When they are nervous, some individuals, with or without being aware of it, make repeated swallowing movements which send air down into the stomach. The swallowed air may produce upper abdominal distention and burpiness.

• Conditions of this kind are sometimes associated with the hormonal changes in the female cycle. Bloating often occurs at the time of menstruation, and not infrequently heartburn and gaseousness are among the complaints of pregnancy. It is known that the hormonal changes which accompany menstruation and pregnancy can affect the behavior of the digestive tract.

• Reactions to certain foods, sometimes termed idiosyncrasies, produce these symptoms in many people. Among the common offenders are onions, cucumbers, radishes, cabbage, and smoked or spicy foods. Certain rich or fat foods, including pork, some cuts of beef, large amounts of buttery and creamy substances, chocolate, and fried and greasy foods commonly are also offending items.

• Constipation, though often without other symptoms, may produce bloating, distention, and gaseousness.

Obviously the treatment of these complaints should be directed to the cause when it is ascertainable. It may mean a process of learning from experience and thereupon avoiding offending foods. The "cast iron stomach" is more of a myth than a reality, and there are few individuals who are not aware that certain foods will give them indigestion accompanied by fullness, bloating, and gas.

In such cases an ounce of prevention is worth a pound of cure. Eating bland and very light foods, particularly when one is nervous or upset, may also be effective. Cutting down on the amount of fats in the diet or, in some cases, on fermentable starchy items may also be useful. When symptoms are frequent, one should go over one's diet and perhaps one's manner of living. This should be done in consultation with a doctor.

For mild or infrequent cases, a physician may prescribe certain drugs. Among them may be an alkalinizer containing familiar neutralizers such as bicarbonate of soda. Per-

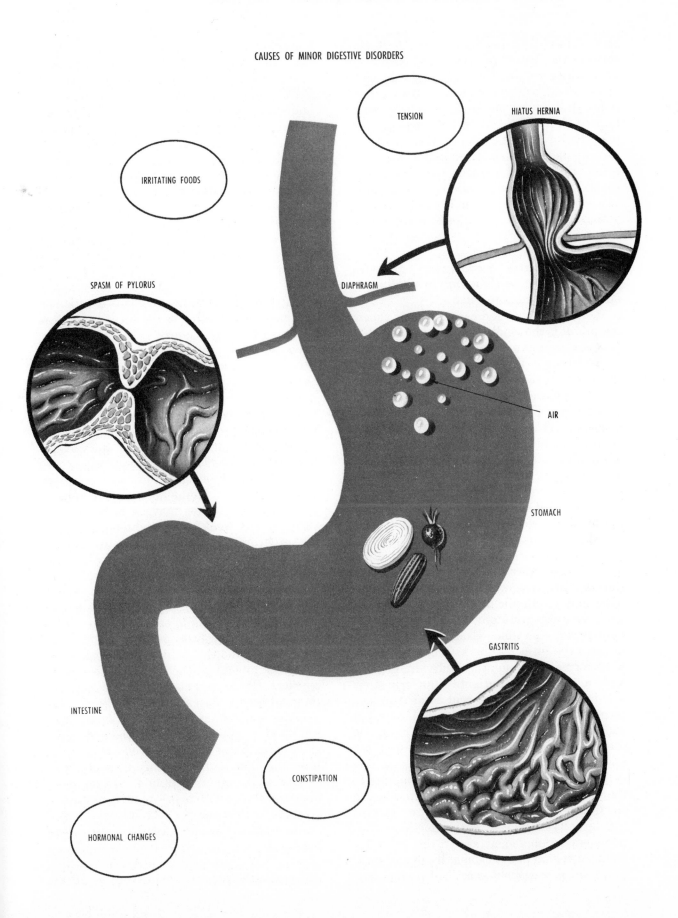

CAUSES OF MINOR DIGESTIVE DISORDERS

TENSION

HIATUS HERNIA

IRRITATING FOODS

SPASM OF PYLORUS

DIAPHRAGM

AIR

STOMACH

GASTRITIS

INTESTINE

CONSTIPATION

HORMONAL CHANGES

haps this will "bring up the gas," relieving some of the distention. An antispasmodic—a drug which relaxes the digestive tract—may be of value, as may a sedative or tranquilizer. Some individuals seem to be helped by activated charcoal tablets or by a few drops of peppermint in water. A hot-water bottle or heating pad on the abdomen may give prompt relief. Finally, for persons with chronic or spastic forms of constipation, regularization of bowel habits will possibly alleviate many of these symptoms. (*See* INDEX for specific entries.)

Q-9. *I regularly experience gnawing pains between meals which are helped by eating. What causes this?*
A. One of the common causes of this type of complaint is the condition termed peptic ulcer. A peptic ulcer is an opening or a small defect in the lining of the digestive tract caused by the action of the digestive juices of the stomach. The peptic ulcer is most commonly found in the upper part of the small intestine, the duodenum. This is ascribed to the fact that during the digestive process this area is sprayed with acid stomach juices. Such ulcers are known as duodenal ulcers. However, ulcers can form within the stomach itself (gastric ulcer) and occasionally in the lowermost portion of the esophagus (esophageal ulcer).

Peptic ulcer is a very common disease. An estimated 10 percent of the population will, at some time or other, develop an ulcer. For reasons that are unknown, the tendency to peptic ulcer may be chronic in some people who suffer from ulcer symptoms off and on for very long periods of time. Exactly what distinguishes the unlucky few with chronic peptic ulcer formation from other individuals is not known. Peptic ulcer patients often form stomach juice with a higher acid content and in larger amounts than normal individuals, but such excessive acidity is not in itself a cause of ulcer. It is believed that some process in the stomach lining weakens it so that a portion becomes susceptible to acid digestion, and so the ulcer is formed. But what this process in the lining is, remains unknown.

Characteristically, ulcers produce pain that is generally felt somewhere in the upper abdominal region and occasionally in the back. The pain is variously described as burning, gnawing, and like a hunger sensation. Typically, the pain is relieved by eating, drinking milk, or taking an alkalinizing medication. Peptic ulcer pain ordinarily occurs some hours after a meal, is relieved by eating, then recurs several hours later. The characteristic cycle of the ulcer, therefore, is pain . . . eating . . . relief . . . pain . . . eating . . . relief, and so on. Night pain, which arises for the same reason, namely, the accumulation of acid secretion in an empty stomach, occurs frequently. Pain may awaken the patient night after night at approximately the same time. It, too, is relieved by eating or by alkalinizers.

These basic facts about peptic ulcer imply the method of its treatment. Neutralization of acid promotes healing of the ulcer, and alkalinizers (Maalox®, Gelusil®, Tums® etc.) are used for this purpose. The newer agents ranitidine, cimetidine and others known as the H_2 antagonists, act by inhibiting acid formation by stomach cells. They have strikingly improved the peptic ulcer problem and virtually abolished the need for surgery.

Some physicians forbid alcohol, spicy foods, mustard, and fried or greasy foods, but otherwise allow a diet as close to a normal one as possible. Since caffeine seems to stimulate acid formation, coffee may be forbidden entirely or only weak coffee and tea permitted. One program calls for taking something every hour—either food, milk, or an alkalinizing tablet or liquid. If night pain is a problem, the patient may be asked to set the alarm so that he wakes up prior to the expected onset of pain and takes something to eat. Cigarette smoking seems to aggravate peptic ulcer in some individuals, and the incidence of peptic ulcer is higher among smokers than among nonsmokers. Hence patients with peptic ulcer are often advised to stop smoking.

For an unfortunate group of patients, clearing up of a peptic ulcer is not the end of the story. Months or possibly even some years later they may suffer another bout of peptic ulcer. A still more unfortunate few find themselves suffering with peptic ulcer symptoms a good deal of the time. For such intractable and chronic cases of peptic ulcer, and also where bleeding has occurred from an ulcer—especially if it has occurred more than once. A full anti-ulcer program including the H_2 antagonists may have to be maintained almost indefinitely. There are various surgical procedures in the treatment of ulcer. With one or another of these, it is often possible to promise the victim of a chronic peptic ulcer relief from his longstanding distress. (*See* PEPTIC ULCER in the section GASTROINTESTINAL CONDITIONS.)

Q-10. *I have had severe abdominal pains and have been told my X-ray shows stones. What is going on?*
A. The pains produced by the movement of stones is referred to as colic and occurs in either the bile-fluid system or in the urinary tract. There may be biliary colic or renal colic. These share the reputation of being among the most severe pains produced by any disorders of the human body.

In biliary colic, the pain is generally due to the movement of a stone either down the duct of the gallbladder or down the major bile duct, which runs to the intestine. The patient usually experiences severe pain in the upper abdomen, either in the line of the right nipple or in the central area of the abdomen above the navel, the epigastric region. The pain may double the patient up, and is generally completely incapacitating. It is sometimes felt in the back or in the region of the right shoulder.

Occasionally, there is an onset of steady pain in the region of the gallbladder which mounts in intensity. Waves of intensified pain may then be superimposed on this. The pain may be caused by movement of a stone within the gallbladder, with the communicating channel between it and the bile duct closed off. Or it may be due to the passage of a stone from the gallbladder into the bile duct where it may either lodge, perhaps producing jaundice, or pass on, with relief of the obstruction.

Renal colic refers to the pain produced by the passage of a stone anywhere in the urinary tract, but generally between the pelvis of the kidney and the bladder. The pain has a severe and knife-like quality. It too may come and go in waves, and when the movement of the stone stops or the stone is passed, the pain may end. The character and location of the pain depend on the location of the stone and its movement. When the stone is high up, perhaps moving from the pelvis of the kidney into the first part of the ureter—the channel which runs from kidney to bladder—pain may be experienced in the flank or in the back, adjacent to the lowest ribs and the spine. As the stone moves outwards and downwards, the pain may be experienced in the side, and radiating down toward the bladder and the genital region. As it moves further along the ureter, it is felt at lower levels, and in males may extend into the scrotum.

Both biliary and renal colic are variable in duration, sometimes lasting only a minute or two, but more often one or more hours unless they are relieved by a potent pain-killing drug. Second and third doses of drugs must often be given before complete relief is possible. The intensity, character, and location of the pain will generally indicate its probable cause to the doctor. In both biliary and renal colic, it is possible to confirm the diagnosis by X-ray studies. Any patient undergoing an attack of renal colic might be well advised to save a urine specimen from the time of the attack. The urine often contains red blood cells, a common accompaniment of the movement of a stone in the urinary tract. A doctor may request a patient to urinate through cheesecloth in the hope that the stone may be preserved; it can then be analyzed chemically and used as a guide for dietary or other treatment. (*See* BILIARY COLIC in the section GASTROINTESTINAL CONDITIONS; URINARY STONE FORMATION in the section URINARY CONDITIONS.)

Q-11. *Off and on for years I have had loose bowel movements and sometimes pass mucus. What causes this?*
A. If no organic disease is present, this is the condition called colitis. Functional colitis is a disorder of the large bowel that generally results in frequency of bowel movements and irregularity of bowel pattern. Sometimes increased amounts of mucus are passed; occasionally, when there is an impulse to move the bowel, nothing much more than some stained thick mucus may be passed. There may be departures from normal patterns of bowel behavior. Constipation may alternate with mild diarrhea; thus, after two or three days without a movement, there may come a day in which there are three or four fairly active ones. Another pattern is for two or three loose stools to be limited sometimes only to the

morning, sometimes scattered throughout the day. This pattern is often related to nervous stress or other tension. (*See* COLITIS; DIARRHEA in the section GASTROINTESTINAL CONDITIONS; DIARRHEA in the section HOME NURSING CARE.)

Q-12. *I often skip a day or two without having a bowel movement. Why?*
A. This is generally referred to as constipation. Constipation is a common problem, yet it is not so common as many people think. To skip a bowel movement for a day is not necessarily a sign of constipation, and there are perfectly normal individuals who have a bowel movement every other day and seem to be in excellent health. On the other hand, one can have a daily bowel movement and still be constipated if by constipation one means the passage of an overly hard, pellety, somewhat smaller than normal stool.

Constipation appearing for the first time in middle age can be serious, especially if it is progressive. Unfortunately, so much functional constipation appears in middle age that X-ray examination of the large intestine and other special procedures may be necessary to determine whether or not it is caused by an organic condition such as a tumor.

In the absence of a disease process in the large intestine, one can make a diagnosis of functional constipation. There are various approaches to the problem:

• Sometimes constipation is due to inadequate roughage and stimulating foods in the diet. This frequently occurs in individuals who are reducing, and may simply be due to a reduction of food bulk intake. Diminished bulk, or the absence of stimulation produced by such foods as salads, vegetables, and fruits, may result in sluggish action of the colon. One way to correct this, of course, is to add bulk and stimulating foods to the diet.

• Inadequate intake of water may play a part in some cases of constipation. When fluid intake is inadequate, the colon may abstract more than the usual amount of water from the stool, resulting in a dried-out stool and constipation. This is easily corrected by increasing fluid intake.

• Other essentially minor dietary manipulations may successfully alleviate mild degrees of constipation. Taking prunes or prune juice, figs, or dates may be of value. Some individuals seem to be helped by drinking a cup of hot water the first thing in the morning.

• Some cases of constipation result from the pressures of early-morning rush. Often, regularity of bowel habit can be restored by establishing a special time to go to the bathroom every morning and adhering to it whether or not a strong urge to move the bowels is present.

• Laxatives may be indicated when constipation persists despite restoration of a balanced diet and routine habits. Laxatives fall into various classes:

1. Bulk stimulants are substances that mix with the stool and take up water. The increased bulk acts as a mechanical stimulant to evacuation. Extracts of psyllium seed, one commercial preparation of which is known as Metamucil®, are an example of this.

2. Saline cathartics (a dose of "salts") act by pulling fluid into the bowel and result in an increased watery type of movement.

3. Direct stimulants are agents that act on the smooth muscle of the intestine, stimulating it to increased activity. Many of them are found in proprietary drugs sold over-the-counter. They include phenolphthalein, cascara, anthraquinone derivatives, and that old standby, castor oil.

4. In recent years stool softeners, which tend to keep the stool from losing its moisture and thereby its bulk, have been used increasingly. One such agent is known as dioctyl sodium sulfoccinate, found in Colace®.

On the whole, it is preferable to start with the milder agents, such as the bulk-formers and stool-softeners, rather than those that are essentially laxative, such as the salts. It may not be necessary to take them daily. Sometimes a dose every other day will work. One should use the smallest dose compatible with getting results. For occasional constipation, fast-acting suppositories and prepackaged enemas are available. These can bring relief within minutes. (*See* CONSTIPATION in the sections HOME NURSING CARE and GASTROINTESTINAL CONDITIONS.)

Q-13. *I can feel several small round growths protruding from the opening after a bowel movement. What are they?*
A. Most probably this is the condition termed

piles. Piles—known medically as hemorrhoids —are small, dilated veins just within or protruding from the rectal opening. They may be compared to the varicose veins seen on the lower extremities, but they are, of course, much smaller. Internal hemorrhoids are covered by the anal lining and are situated within the canal. External hemorrhoids are covered by skin and can be present individually or as a cluster around the opening. Why some people have difficulty with hemorrhoids and others escape them altogether is not known. Pregnancy, chronic constipation, and several other medical conditions may predispose to their formation. (*See* HEMORRHOIDS in the section GASTROINTESTINAL CONDITIONS.)

Q-14. *Some days I feel a lack of energy. Can I take vitamin supplements?*

A. The widespread promotion and consequent widespread consumption of vitamins has no real relationship to the dietary deficiencies or vitamin needs of most consumers. Many people take vitamins because they believe that this will increase their general health, enable them better to fight off colds and other viral illnesses, or give them more of that vague quality known as "pep." Carefully controlled scientific observations do not support these beliefs.

Divide a large number of individuals, all of them on an adequate diet, into two groups, give one group vitamin supplements and the other sugar pills, and approximately one-third of the persons in each group will claim that they feel better. In other words, the sugar pill works as well as the vitamin pill. The positive effect results from the individual's belief.

It is true that the ill health of individuals suffering from vitamin deficiencies is *corrected* by taking vitamins. But it is not true that the health of individuals not suffering from vitamin deficiencies is *improved* by taking vitamin pills. Neither is it true that large amounts of vitamin C taken at the start of a cold are of any special help. Furthermore, most inflammation of the gums seen in doctors' and dentists' offices is not due to vitamin C deficiency, nor does it respond to increased consumption of vitamin C. Claims that vitamin B improves the circulation to the heart have repeatedly been demonstrated to be untrue.

After a thorough examination of the various claims for various vitamins, the American Medical Association's Council on Nutrition concluded that the average American on the usual balanced diet does not benefit from taking vitamin supplements. The Council recommended that such supplements be taken by women during pregnancy, by individuals on bizarre or restricted diets who persistently refuse to include some important group of foodstuffs, and by certain geriatric patients on poor intakes. Vitamins A and D are recommended for the infant and the growing child. It should be noted, however, that children can be overdosed with these vitamins, and that an overdose of vitamins A or D can produce striking examples of poor health.

It is probable that individuals who dislike vegetables and will eat none of them, as well as strict vegetarians who shun anything resembling meat, may profit from taking a vitamin supplement. But those who think that the consumption of larger and larger amounts of vitamins does more and more good should be warned that there is such a thing as overdosage, that some vitamins produce fermentation and gassiness, and that water-soluble vitamins (such as those of the B complex) cannot be stored in the body—any excess taken in is promptly excreted in the urine.

Another point to remember is that there are still some unknown vitamins and necessary food factors which the manufacturers have been unable to isolate and put into their capsules. Those genuinely interested in securing a balanced vitamin intake must recognize, therefore, that nature puts its vitamins into food and not into pharmacies. (*See* RECOMMENDED DAILY ALLOWANCES; VITAMINS in the section NUTRITION AND HEALTH.)

Q-15. *Since taking birth control pills I've noticed some bloating and swelling of the breasts. What is the pill doing?*

A. The birth control pills work by interfering with the action of the gland regulating the ovary, the pituitary gland. This gland, situated at the base of the brain, controls all the processes going on in the ovary. Pituitary secretions are responsible for the growth of the egg (ovum) and for its release. Taking the birth control pill, which contains hormones similar to those usually produced by the ovary, in effect signals the pituitary gland that enough of these are present in the woman's body. As a result, the pituitary does not produce the hormones that stimulate ovarian activity. The final result is that the ovary does not go through the usual cyclic changes, no egg comes to maturity or is released, and hence the woman remains infertile. However, changes resembling those of the normal cycle do take place in the uterus and the breasts because of the hormones contained in the pills.

If, after taking the pills for three weeks and experiencing these transformations, the pills are stopped, menstruation will ensue. Menstruation occurs whenever the hormone level in the body drops to a significant extent. Whether the hormonal drop occurs normally, or is produced by stopping medication, a menstrual flow will occur.

As a birth control measure, the hormone pill is just about 100 percent effective, and indeed is considered by most authorities to be the most effective method of contraception presently available. In order to work reliably, however, the pill should be taken daily, as skipping even one day may permit the pituitary to start ovarian stimulation. However, little is known with certainty about all the side-effects of some of these pills, and as recently as 1989 they were accused of raising the expected incidence of breast cancer. (*See* CONTRACEPTION in the section FEMALE HEALTH CARE.)

Q-16. *Why do I have pain and bloating between periods?*
A. The release of an egg from the ovary (ovulation) is sometimes accompanied by lower abdominal pain, tenderness, and/or bloating. Sometimes the abdominal pain is severe enough to make it difficult for a doctor to decide whether a young woman complaining of pain in the lower right abdomen is suffering from appendicitis or is having ovulatory pain. Ovulatory pain or discomfort do not necessarily occur in every menstrual cycle, and many women never experience it.

In others, however, they may occur so regularly that they can be used as a fairly reliable indication of the time of ovulation. Discomfort most often appears between the twelfth and sixteenth days of the usual menstrual cycle, but it can also vary from cycle to cycle.

The discomfort seldom lasts for more than twelve hours, then tends to subside. It is sometimes referred to as *Mittelschmerz*, German for middle pain. Very occasionally it is accompanied by an increased discharge of mucus and occasionally a trace of blood appears with the discharge. Such a pink-stained discharge in midcycle is sometimes referred to as ovulatory bleeding. Again, this may be found in only an occasional cycle. A physician must of course rule out other possibilities that may produce similar symptoms, such as cervical erosions, polyps, and tumors. Women who undergo *Mittelschmerz* may find it of interest (and it may be of use to their physicians) to chart their menstrual cycles on a calendar, and to note the days on which this type of discomfort is experienced. Such information may be of considerable value in family planning. (*See* MENSTRUAL CYCLE in the section FEMALE HEALTH CARE.)

Q-17. *What can I do about discomfort during menstruation?*
A. Various degrees of discomfort are often noted, particularly on the first and second days of the menstrual flow. They may consist of backache, a feeling of heaviness in the pelvis due to congestion, a tendency to urinate frequently, and an overall subpar feeling. It is known that a mildly toxic substance may originate in the lining of the uterus during menstruation, some of which is absorbed into the body. This is referred to as menotoxin and undoubtedly contributes to the feeling experienced. Certainly many women do not look their best at this time. They may appear paler than usual, have puffiness under the eyes, and feel headachy. However, the complaints most likely to be disabling are those relating to the rhythmic cramps originating in the menstruating uterus, medically termed dysmenorrhea. Dysmenorrhea is most common on the first and second days.

Painful uterine cramps are more likely to occur during the early reproductive years. With the passage of time, and especially after a pregnancy, dysmenorrhea is greatly diminished or ceases altogether. There seems little reason to doubt that dysmenorrhea arises in the thick muscular wall of the uterus, which is capable of severe contraction. Among the helpful procedures for uterine cramps are the following:

• A hot-water bottle or heating pad applied to the lower abdomen.

• Antispasmodic drugs, similar to those used for pains arising in the digestive tract, may also relax the muscle of the uterus and thus cut down the intensity of painful cramps.

• Many of the drugs used for arthritis, known as steroidal anti-inflammatory drugs (NSAIDS) have proved useful for dysmenorrhea. A further advantage is that they do not promote bleeding as does aspirin. Examples of the drugs are Ibuprofen®, Motrin®, Advil®, and Nuprine®.

• Occasionally a doctor may find some organic cause contributing to painful uterine cramps. The reason can be an underdeveloped uterus (juvenile uterus) or an abnormally narrow opening of the womb. Hormone injections may be given to build the uterus to mature size, and slight dilatation of the opening is easily done. (*See* MENSTRUATION in the section FEMALE HEALTH CARE.)

Q-18. *Before my period I feel nervous and snap at everyone. What causes this?*

A. Premenstrual irritability is a common phenomenon which is experienced by some women during every one of their menstrual cycles. It is sometimes of minor degree and passes unnoticed, but it can also be quite marked and produce intense subjective feelings of tension and nervousness. Depression, the "blues," and a tendency to tearfulness may also occur. Not infrequently there are also physical symptoms such as headache, bloating, swelling of the extremities, and tenderness or painful engorgement of the breasts. Usually, with the onset of the menstrual period or by the second day of the flow, symptoms are markedly alleviated. It is generally conceded that most, if not all, of these changes are due to the action of the hormones of the ovary. An important factor is the water retention these hormones produce. The swollen, bloated feeling is due to fluid retention. It is also believed that water retention in the cells of the nervous system may be responsible for premenstrual tension states.

Minor degrees of premenstrual tension are often tolerated without treatment, with the help of the knowledge that the symptoms will pass with the period. For jumpiness and nervousness, mild sedatives or tranquilizers may be prescribed. Where the chief complaint is of feelings of depression, drugs of the dexedrine-benzedrine group may be ordered by the physician. Where water retention seems to be significant (some women gain four to five pounds of fluid in the last week or so of the menstrual cycle), diuretic drugs may be administered. These are drugs which promote the excretion of fluid from the body by way of increased urination.

The diuretics seem to be equally successful in reducing bloat, the swelling of the extremities, and some of the psychic and emotional changes that accompany fluid retention. There are various schedules of administration of the diuretic drugs. They may be given every day or every other day for the last week or ten days of the menstrual cycle, during the phase of increasing fluid retention. (*See* PREMENSTRUAL SYNDOME in the section FEMALE HEALTH CARE.)

Q-19. *Some of my menstrual cycles are longer than others. Can I use the rhythm method of birth control?*

A. A knowledge of the "safe period" is the essential approach to the rhythm method of birth control. It is used by many couples who wish to diminish the possibility of pregnancy without using pills or other mechanical techniques.

Calculation of the safe period is based on the following basic considerations:

• The egg or ovum is released from the ovary only once during a menstrual cycle and remains fertile for only about twenty-four hours after release from the ovary. If a day or so passes, the egg is no longer capable of being fertilized by the sperm.

• Ovulation does not necessarily occur on the same day in each cycle, and the exact cycle-length varies also. Many women who are sure that they menstruate at twenty-eight day intervals find on charting that the interval may vary from twenty-six to thirty days, or even more widely.

• Because of fluctuation in cycle length and the day of ovulation, it is necessary to record the dates of menstruation for at least a year in order to calculate the safe period accurately. A cycle always begins with the onset of menstruation, and can conveniently be charted by marking off the dates of menstruation on a calendar.

• Once the length of the menstrual cycle is

known, there are various formulas for calculating the safe period. The following one offers less chance of error than some others: Subtract fifteen days from the shortest recorded cycle and subtract four more—this gives the first day of the fertile period. Subtract fifteen days from the longest cycle and add four more—this gives the final day of the fertile part of the cycle. For example, suppose that during the preceding year the cycles have varied from twenty-five to thirty days. Subtracting 15 from 25 gives us 10, subtracting 4 more gives us Day 6. Subtracting 15 from 30 gives us 15 and adding 4 more gives us Day 19. Hence Day 6 to Day 19 represents the range of the fertile period. Sexual relations before and after these days would be most unlikely to result in pregnancy.

• The smaller the variation in the menstrual cycle, the more precisely can the fertile period be calculated and the shorter it is. Thus, if all menstrual cycles during the preceding year have fallen between twenty-seven and twenty-nine days, the calculations give a fertile period from Day 8 to Day 18. On the other hand, if cycles are very irregular, safe period calculations and the rhythm method cannot be used accurately. (*See* CONTRACEPTION; MENSTRUAL CYCLE in the section FEMALE HEALTH CARE.)

Q-20. *I feel waves of heat and perspiration many times a day in recent months. What can I do for this?*

A. They are probably menopausal flushes. Flushes, or as they are also sometimes called, "flashes," are transient sensations of warmth experienced by women during the menopause or "change of life." The warm sensation characteristically travels from one part of the body to another—for example, starting in the head and face and moving down to the trunk.

Flushes are often associated with perspiration. Sometimes the waves of perspiration are frequent and annoying, and may be a predominant symptom. The sensation of warmth may be so marked and realistic that the person experiencing it may be impelled to open a window or insist that the furnace is sending up too much heat. Not infrequently the flushes and sweats come on during the night.

It is generally agreed that the flushes are manifestations of a drop in the amount of fe-

male hormone in the system. They usually appear at about the time that the menstrual periods become scanty, irregular, or are skipped altogether. They are likely to vary considerably from day to day, and are aggravated by nervous tension, fatigue, or fluctuations in the weather. Waves of warmth and similar sensations, experienced by a woman who is still menstruating regularly, need not necessarily be regarded as a sign of oncoming menopause.

The flushes may come and go in erratic manner for months and even years. Following an initial period during which they are mild and occasional, they may increase in intensity. Then, after a period of months or even years, they slowly begin to decrease, both in number and intensity. Occasional flushes may be experienced even years after the menopause.

Where the flushes are marked, and considerable discomfort and annoyance are repeatedly experienced, a physician may prescribe moderate amounts of female hormone. These are usually taken in decreasing amounts over a period of time. Their purpose is to give enough female hormone to tide a woman over the acute period of hormone withdrawal. By gradually decreasing the amounts taken, the period of withdrawal is less abrupt, and there are fewer symptoms. The hormone can be given orally or by injection, both methods being of equal efficacy. (*See* MENOPAUSE in the section FEMALE HEALTH CARE.)

Q-21. *I have noticed some red tingeing to the semen. What causes this?*

A. This is generally due to the presence of some blood in the semen. Men are occasionally disturbed to notice a pink or bloody tinge to the ejaculated semen. There is a great deal of circulatory congestion in the genital region during sexual stimulation, and this is the usual background for some slight bleeding that may occur in the male reproductive system at the time. Most commonly, it is an isolated event which happens once or twice and may not be seen again for a long time.

Very rarely, it occurs frequently. A doctor will check for various possible contributory causes, including considerable prostatic enlargement, possible chronic inflammatory disease in the prostate or seminal vesicles, or other potentially aggravating or causative factors. Very often no specific cause can be determined in the more usual types of investigation. The man who sees some blood in the semen should not be unduly alarmed, although he should of course take the precaution of reporting to a doctor. (*See also* the section MALE HEALTH CARE.)

Q-22. *I have a slight irritation around the vaginal area. Sometimes moist secretions go with it. What is this?*

A. This is probably due to mild inflammation of the vagina, called vaginitis. There is usually vaginal discharge with this. However, not all vaginal discharges are signs of disease. In some women, there is sufficient hormonal stimulus to secretion at certain times in the menstrual cycle to produce a slight mucous discharge. This may occur around the middle of the cycle, and is not infrequent just prior to the onset of menstrual flow. In such cases, there may be enough secretion to stain the underclothing, but there will be little or no accompanying itching or other irritation. Perhaps the most common cause of vaginal discharge is a very common organism known as the trichomonas. This produces a slightly greenish, frothy discharge accompanied, when marked, by some redness of the external genital parts. (*See* VAGINITIS in the section FEMALE HEALTH CARE.)

Q-23. *I have had chills, fever, and aching in both flanks. What can be the cause of this?*

A. This is most probably a urinary tract infection, known as pyelitis, which involves the kidneys. Pyelitis refers to an infection in the central collecting portion of the kidney, into which the urine flows. This central collecting portion has a distinctive white irregular lining, and narrows into the ureter, the duct that runs from the kidney to the bladder. Although pyelitis is an old and well entrenched term, it is doubtful that a pure form of pyelitis ever exists. In all instances there is associated inflammation of the kidney itself, so that a more descriptive term is pyelonephritis, indicating a mixed infection both of the pelvis of the kidney and of the kidney substance itself.

Acute pyelonephritis is generally easy to recognize. There are chills and fever, pain in the flank, turbid urine, and such general symptoms as weakness, headache, and malaise. There are also chronic forms of pyelonephritis, in which careful search reveals the continuous existence of excessive bacteria in the urine, perhaps with such other evidence of infection as casts and white blood cells in excess. Occasionally there is also bleeding, which quite often accompanies infection of the urinary tract.

However, only in recent years has the existence of very stealthy and quiet forms of chronic pyelonephritis been recognized. Careful studies have shown that very low-grade persistent infections may be present in the kidneys for months or years without producing significant symptoms. They may lead to such eventual difficulties as impaired renal function and high blood pressure.

It is not always clear how the kidney becomes infected. Bacteria in the blood stream undoubtedly may be filtered out through the kidney and set up an infection in that organ. It is also likely that in many instances the infection reaches the kidney from the bladder below. It is common for a woman who first has symptoms of bladder inflammation, such as frequent urination and a sense of inability to empty the bladder completely, subsequently to suffer chills and fever and other symptoms indicating that the infection has spread up into the kidney. In young children, particularly girls, it has been demonstrated that there may be a reflux of urine from the bladder up the ureter and into the kidney because of inadequacy of the valve-like arrangement between bladder and ureter. Whenever there is obstruction of the free flow of urine from the bladder, infection appears in the bladder urine first, then often ascends into the kidney. This is true whether it occurs in a child with a congenital obstruction of the bladder opening, or in an elderly male with obstruction due to an enlarged prostate.

Prevention of chronic pyelonephritis can be accomplished only by recognition and full treatment of cases of acute pyelitis or pyelonephritis. It is very easy to bring an acute urinary-tract infection under apparent control within a few days. Appropriate antibiotics or other medication quickly bring the fever down to normal, and many of the symptoms disappear. However, in order to eradicate the lingering traces of infection within the kidney itself, experience has shown that the drugs should be continued for a longer period—perhaps even weeks—after the original symptoms have subsided. Otherwise the door may be opened to a chronic kidney infection.

It may also be necessary to investigate the reasons for recurrent attacks of acute pyelitis. Repeated attacks may be due to a complication of some kind, such as a stone or some structural change producing partial obstruction; this may vary from a stricture or narrowing of a portion of the urinary channel to pressure on it externally from an enlarged prostate. Recurrent pyelitis can be avoided only if such a predisposing condition is corrected. If, as occasionally happens, it cannot be corrected, a doctor may decide to place a patient on medication designed to prevent infection on an almost indefinite basis.

A great many medications are available for the treatment of both acute and chronic pyelonephritis. They include various antibiotics and various sulfa drugs. In practice, the problem is not starting treatment with the appropriate drug; rather the question is how long to continue treatment before there can be assurance that the infection in the kidney is completely eradicated. (*See* PYELITIS in the section URINARY CONDITIONS.)

Q-24. *I have to urinate frequently. What causes this?*

A. In women, the most common cause of frequent urination is cystitis, an inflammation involving the bladder. The channel between the bladder and the exterior of the urethra is very short in women—less than one inch long—and it is not difficult for an infection to work its way up the urethral passage into the bladder. Inflammation of the bladder produces a group of symptoms, often including the following: a frequent desire to void, pain or burning on urination, and a sensation of fullness in the bladder even after voiding. The desire to urinate may be felt at intervals of only a few minutes, and only a few drops may be passed with each voiding. With severe cystitis, there may even be some bleeding with urination, more frequently at the end of urination. Cystitis is generally treated by giving an antibiotic or other medication to clear the bacterial infection.

In men, the most common cause of frequent urination is enlargement of the prostate gland, an accessory sex gland located just at the base of the bladder. Enlargement of the prostate occurs in a considerable number of men as they grow older. The enlarged prostate may impede the passage of urine from the bladder, producing such symptoms as weakness of the stream, difficulty in starting (hesitancy), dribbling, difficulty in ending the stream, and the feeling that complete emptying is impossible. The bladder does not in fact normally empty entirely with the act of urination. A certain amount of urine is left behind; this is called residual urine. The residual urine normally does not exceed one ounce, but in some men with enlarged prostates from four to twelve ounces may remain. A doctor can determine the amount by passing a catheter, a hollow tube, into the bladder after urination and draining it.

Not infrequently, bladder infection occurs in the presence of retention of urine, and the symptoms of cystitis that the male then experiences are much like those noted above for the female. Mild enlargement of the prostate requires no treatment. It simply results in higher urinative frequency with perhaps a need for getting up one or more times at night. More advanced enlargement, producing severe symptoms, may require surgery.

Other causes of frequent urination are numerous. Nervousness often gives rise to repeated desire to void. Sometimes exposure to cold, or wading in cold water, produces a contraction of the bladder and a need for voiding. Certain substances in the diet may stimulate or irritate the bladder and produce a desire to void. There are also substances called diuretics which promote the passage of urine. They result in passing larger amounts of urine more frequently than usual. Among common substances that may have diuretic effect are coffee, tea, alcohol, and a variety of drugs used in the treatment of certain conditions of the heart and of blood pressure. In diabetes, the spillover of sugar into the urine is associated with an increased amount of fluid passing through the kidneys and bladder; consequently, one of the early symptoms of diabetes is frequent urination.

Other causes may be noted. Tumors and stones in the bladder may lead to a desire to urinate often. In some women, swelling of the uterus or womb at the time of menstruation may lead to pressure on the bladder and result in frequent urination. Other structures pressing on the bladder may do likewise. Finally, various kinds of inflammation and scarring in the bladder may produce contraction with a need for frequent urination because of the loss of normal bladder capacity. (*See* INDEX for specific entries.)

Q-25. *Over recent years, I have had frequency of urination, difficulty in starting urination, and dribbling. What causes this?*

A. In a man past fifty the most likely cause of this is enlargement of the prostate gland. There are all degrees of enlargement of the prostate occurring in aging men. Even in the complete absence of symptoms, routine examination may reveal a considerable enlargement of the prostate. This is so because considerable enlargement can occur without obstruction of the bladder. On the other hand, a prostate which is not much larger than normal may result in considerable obstruction. In general, however, there is a proportionate relationship between the amount of prostate enlargement and the degree of obstruction associated with it. Obviously, if extensive enlargement produces no particular symptoms, no problem exists and the man can consider himself lucky.

The early symptoms due to obstructive enlargement of the prostate usually consist of frequency of urination and weakness of the stream. Frequency of urination may increase from three or four times daily to six or eight times. Instead of urinating once at night, a man may find himself getting up two or three times. This state of affairs may level off and persist unchanged for months and years. However, if obstruction progresses, the frequency usually increases until the need for voiding may be felt as often as hourly throughout the day, with a further increase in nocturia, the passing of urine during the night. Difficulty in starting the stream, weakness of the stream, and a prolonged dribbling conclusion rather than a sharply cut off end to urination are characteristic.

Infection and complete obstruction often follow. Whenever there is obstruction of the urinary tract, a condition favorable to infection exists. It is therefore not uncommon for a urinary tract infection to occur at some point in the development of prostatic enlargement with obstruction. This generally takes the form of cystitis, with the usual symptoms of a need for voiding, painful urination, frequency of urination, and a constant sense of incomplete evacuation. These may be followed by the symptoms of an ascending urinary tract infection, which include chills, fever, and other signs. An equally threatening and more dramatic event is the sudden onset of complete obstruction. After months or years during which difficulty in voiding and other signs of enlargement have been experienced, there may be a fairly abrupt onset of total obstruction. The patient finds himself unable to urinate despite an increasing accumulation of bladder urine and consequently pain.

Certain measures may be salutary in these circumstances. The application of a warm, moist towel to the genitals, a warm bath to induce relaxation, or the application of an ice-cold compress to the pubic region may stimulate the desire and the capacity to void. If none of these maneuvers works, catheterization may have to be resorted to. This consists of the passage of a flexible hollow tube into the bladder to permit the urine to drain. The catheter may be kept in for a considerable period of time—catheter drainage—since it is likely that it will be necessary to drain the urine again within a few hours.

Although a man may successfully "live with" moderate symptoms due to enlargement of the prostate, repeated episodes of infection, or complete obstruction, indicate the need for surgical intervention. Individual urologists favor various surgical approaches to the enlarged prostate. In addition to removal of portions of the obstructing prostate by an instrument passed into the urinary channel itself (transurethral resection), several direct operative approaches to the prostate gland are used. One involves an abdominal operation and a one- or two-stage removal of the prostate gland. Another (the perineal prostatectomy) avoids the abdominal approach by operating in the region between the anus and scrotum, the perineum.

Each of the various surgical approaches has its merits and drawbacks and involves the pros and cons of many technical considerations. Suffice it to say that relief of obstruction can be definitely promised. (*See* PROS-TATITIS in the section MALE HEALTH CARE.)

Q-26. *I have been passing a reddish urine. What is the cause of this symptom?*

A. This is most likely due to the presence of blood in the urine, a condition referred to as hematuria. There are many causes but a few are far more common than all the others combined. Congestion, infection, stones, and tumors are among the leading causes. Among the most common conditions in which hematuria occurs are the following:

Bladder infection (cystitis). Perhaps the most common cause of hematuria is that associated with infections of the bladder, most often seen in women. In addition to such "bladder symptoms" as frequent desire to void, and pain in the bladder region with feelings of fullness not relieved by urinating, some bleeding may occur. The bleeding sometimes takes the form of a terminal hematuria, the passage of a small amount of blood after passing the urine. In men, similar bleeding associated with a bladder infection can occur. With the clearing of the infection, the bleeding promptly ceases.

Congestion, especially prostatic. Congestion, especially when there is prostate enlargement, may lead to some bleeding. It is likely to be made worse by alcohol, sexual stimulation, and intercourse.

Stones. Stones at various levels of the urinary tract may produce bleeding. Stones can occur at any level, from the pelvis of the kidney to the ureter, the bladder, and even the urethra, the channel between the bladder and the outside. The movement of a stone often produces severe pain, known as renal colic, and there is frequently associated bleeding into the urine. When the possibility that there is a stone in the urinary tract is being considered, it is important that the patient save the urine to be examined for blood cells.

Tumors. Various kinds of tumors of the bladder and of the kidney may produce enough bleeding to color the urine.

Other disease. A variety of other conditions may produce bleeding into the urine. Among them are acute nephritis, blood disorders, even including infectious mononucleosis, circulatory disorders involving the kidney blood supply, overdosage of anticoagulant drugs,

damage to the kidney due to direct blows or other causes.

Finding the specific cause for hematuria may be easy—for example, when cystitis is present—or very complicated, when one of the less common causes is operating. Then the investigation may require various technical procedures for visualizing the kidney and its passages, procedures which are generally performed by a specialist known as a urologist. (*See* INDEX for specific entries.)

Q-27. *I have recently noticed a yellow tinge to my skin and eyeballs. What is this?*

A. This is probably the condition known as jaundice. It is due to the accumulation of bile pigments in the blood and tissues, and the degree of yellow staining roughly parallels the degree of accumulation of bile substances. One of the chief constituents of bile, bilirubin, is formed by the breaking down of red blood cells, a process that goes on continuously in the body. Massive sudden destruction of red blood cells (as in hemolytic anemia) may produce so much bilirubin that the capacity of the liver to handle it is temporarily overwhelmed. Transient jaundice will result. In ordinary circumstances the bilirubin is passed into the bloodstream, brought to the liver, and excreted by it into the bile. Two common mechanisms which may interfere with the process, and therefore produce jaundice, are injury to the liver resulting in impairment of its function, and obstruction of the bile ducts, reducing the volume of fluid they can carry.

Damage to the liver may be caused by a variety of agents, including drugs and heavy and prolonged alcoholism; but perhaps most commonly occurs as a result of the inflammation produced by the virus of hepatitis. Hepatitis can exist without jaundice, in which case it may then go undetected. Jaundice, however, is such a striking finding that it always demands a diagnostic explanation. In viral hepatitis, liver cells may be so greatly damaged that they are unable to function adequately, and usually enough bilirubin accumulates in the bloodstream to produce obvious jaundice. The urine turns dark because of the overflow of bile into it. In many cases of hepatitis, the jaundice intensifies for one or more weeks, and severe degrees of it may be encountered.

In the average case, the recovery process sets in after some weeks; the liver cells begin to return to normal functioning and the jaundice slowly subsides.

In healthy persons, there is a continuous secretion of bile by the liver cells into a system of fine canals which increase in size until finally they empty into a pencil-size canal known as the common bile duct. Obstruction of the flow of bile through this duct leads to a backing up of the bile, and a reversal of the normal process occurs: The accumulation produces a dilation of all the ducts, and there is a reverse flow of bile into the bloodstream. Because of the continued production of bilirubin and the continued inability of the liver to excrete it, increasing bilirubin accumulation and jaundice occur as a result of obstruction of the bile duct. Among the common causes of such obstruction are a stone or a tumor pressing on the duct. Obstruction can result from inflammation and swelling, leading to a narrowing of the duct.

It is not always easy to tell which of the various possible causes are producing the jaundice. Certain tests tend to draw a line between hepatitis and obstructive jaundice. Sometimes a needle biopsy of the liver is indicated. Examination of tissue under the microscope may lead to a diagnosis. It may sometimes seem quite probable that a stone is the cause—for example when there is a history of gallstones—and although an exact diagnosis cannot be reached by testing, it may be considered wise to operate in order to relieve the jaundice produced by the presumed stone.

Although X-raying the upper digestive tract may occasionally suggest the possibility of a tumor, operation may again be necessary to arrive at a final conclusion. In recent years, with new and potent drugs coming into use, some of which occasionally lead to jaundice, the problem of distinguishing among the various causes of jaundice has become somewhat complicated. Serial tests and prolonged observations may be necessary before a sound opinion can be reached. (*See* JAUNDICE in the section MISCELLANEOUS HEALTH CONDITIONS.)

Q-28. *I have been told several times now that I have anemia. Why do I get it?*
A. Anemia is a deficiency of red blood cells. The red cells are formed in the bone marrow, and the process can be retarded in any of a number of ways, with anemia as a result. By far the most common form of anemia is iron-deficiency anemia. This results from a lack of iron, which is an essential building block in the formation of hemoglobin, the basic constituent of the red blood cell. Iron deficiency can cause a reduction in the number of red blood cells. Individual cells may be smaller and more irregular than normal and contain less than their normal amount of hemoglobin. Insufficient iron in the diet may be an important factor. Even in infancy, iron-deficiency anemia can occur when the child is maintained on milk alone for a year or more. Similarly, at puberty, the combination of an inadequate diet and a rapidly growing organism may result in a form of anemia, which once was known as the green sickness—chlorosis.

Occasionally, women in whom menstrual blood loss is excessive suffer from iron-deficiency anemia. In other forms of bleeding in which iron is lost, such as bleeding from an ulcer, prolonged nosebleeds, or bleeding from hemorrhoids, iron-deficiency anemia may result. The treatment of iron-deficiency anemia is relatively simple and consists of the administration of iron in a number of ways. The body will quickly utilize any iron furnished under these circumstances, and the correction of anemia takes place quite promptly.

Other forms of anemia not involving the iron mechanism may also occur, although they are less common. Absence of certain essential elements in the diet or in the body may interfere with the proper maturation of blood cells in the bone marrow. One well-known form of this condition is known as pernicious anemia. In this disease, the system fails properly to assimilate vitamin B_{12} from the diet, and severe anemia may result. The condition is rapidly correctable by direct administration of vitamin B_{12}. A somewhat similar form of anemia due to metabolic difficulties with another substance, folic acid, is occasionally seen in pregnant women and in persons suffering from certain nutritional disorders, or in association with disorders of assimilation in the intestinal tract.

Various disorders of the bone marrow may lead to anemia, sometimes quite severe. The activity of the bone marrow may be inhibited by a number of known factors, and also probably by some unknown ones, so that its cells are reduced in number—a condition known as aplastic anemia. In leukemia and similar disorders, there seems to be an overproduction of white blood cells together with a severe reduction in the number of red blood cells, so that anemia may be the most prominent feature. There are some disorders in which there is a rapid destruction of red blood cells, or hemolytic anemia. Inhibition of bone marrow activity accompanied by anemia is found in uremia. All of these causes of anemia are relatively uncommon, but of course require consideration for accurate diagnosis and treatment. This may mean referral to a hematologist, a physician who specializes in blood disorders. (*See* ANEMIA in the section CARDIO-VASCULAR CONDITIONS.)

Q-29. *I seem to lack pep. Could this be a glandular trouble?*
A. The chief gland regulating the rate at which the body functions is the thyroid gland. The thyroid gland is held responsible for many of the difficulties about which people commonly complain. Thyroid underactivity is blamed for the tendency to put on weight easily, for proneness to fatigue, for lack of "pep," for sluggishness and inertia, and for subpar feelings. The truth is that these complaints are seldom due to underactivity of the thyroid. Most overweight, whatever its real basis, is not specifically related to inadequate amounts of thyroid secretion. Overweight is generally due to a combination of sedentary living and an overhealthy desire for foods, particularly for carbohydrates. Tiredness, fatigue, and inertia—the common complaints of many people—are seldom due to a single cause; they are seldom traceable to the thyroid.

True underfunctioning of the thyroid is referred to as hypothyroidism. Most commonly seen in middle-aged women, it usually comes on very gradually. Surprisingly, many hypothyroid persons are not overweight; rather, they appear puffy. This puffiness may be noted in the skin generally, but is most marked around the eyes. The condition is referred to as myxedema.

One of the characteristic findings of hypothyroidism is excessive dryness of the skin. The skin looks and feels dry. There is a strik-ing absence of both oils and sweat. In severe cases the skin may have a leathery appearance. The best body site to observe this is not on the hands and forearms—which in many housewives are often dry due to excessive exposure to soaps and detergents—but on the skin of the trunk. The scalp and hair also tend to dryness. Hair loss and thinning of the eyebrows are other common complaints. The pitch of the voice commonly drops to the point of marked huskiness.

There are various degrees of hypothyroidism, but in the advanced stages everything appears to be slowed down—thinking and speaking appear slowed, the appetite seems less than normal, the bowels are sluggish, and there is a lack of drive and energy. Menstrual periods often go awry, the periods being prolonged and the menstrual cycle itself being shortened. Chronic headache is sometimes a major problem, and so are occasional nervousness, irritability, and depression. Considerable derangement of brain functioning may occur in advanced stages, and there is little doubt that some people who are considered mentally ill may be unrecognized hypothyroids.

Diagnosis of hypothyroidism includes special blood tests, basal metabolism tests, or uptake of radioactive iodine by the gland. In borderline cases, a "therapeutic test" with thyroid may be undertaken. This is simply administration of thyroid in gradually increasing doses while the patient's reaction is being observed. Hypothyroid persons are very sensitive to even small doses of thyroid, and will generally show a prompt response: there will be clearing of the puffiness, while the skin becomes more moist and more supple, the pulse rate speeds up, and general stimulation is discernible. On the other hand, individuals whose thyroids are reasonably normal—whatever their other symptoms of fatigue or weight gain may be—do not possess the same unique sensitivity to administered thyroid. Hence, little improvement of consequence will occur if they take thyroid. (*See* HYPOTHYROIDISM in the section GLANDULAR CONDITIONS.)

Q-30. *I am high-strung and thin. Can this be a glandular problem?*
A. The only gland that could contribute to this is the thyroid when it becomes overactive,

a condition called hyperthyroidism. In hyperthyroidism, an excessive amount of thyroid hormone is secreted. The condition is a good deal more common in women than in men. It is frequently precipitated by psychic stress such as death, a separation, or an accident in the family. It may come on during or after pregnancy, and it has been known to occur in several members of a family, as for example, a mother and a daughter. In young women the condition is sometimes referred to as Graves' disease. There may be an obvious swelling in the thyroid region (the thyroid is located in the lower part of the neck to either side of the windpipe) along with a rapid heartbeat, a forceful pulse, excessive perspiration, and, not infrequently, a bulging appearance of the eyes.

Hyperthyroid women usually complain of heat sensations, nervousness, and crying spells. They may manifest restlessness, jitteriness, sleeplessness, and similar signs of overstimulation. There may be various abnormalities of the menstrual cycle, including scanty periods or disappearance of the periods. Marked weight losses can occur as well as a variable amount of overactivity of the bowels, including frank diarrhea. Milder cases may go unrecognized and may even seem to abate for a while, but then a recurrence of symptoms is likely.

In the older age group, hyperthyroidism may be milder and harder to recognize. All degrees of an overstimulated state between the normal and the obviously hyperthyroid may be found. Hence mild degrees of hyperthyroidism may exist for years, manifested only by a rapid pulse, palpitations of the heart, a tendency to excessive perspiration, feelings of warmth, or various symptoms likely to be attributed to "nervousness."

There is now a choice of treatment for hyperthyroidism. In addition to surgery, in which a large portion of the thyroid gland is removed, drugs are available that will cut down thyroid hyperactivity. In certain individuals, partial destruction of the thyroid by radioactive iodine may be employed. Some of the complaints of rapid heart rate are improved by the class of drugs known as beta-blockers which slow the heart-rate and may lower blood pressure. Of course, most nervous states are not due to excessive thyroid activity. On the other hand, no person should be characterized as being "just plain nervous" unless the possibility of thyroid overactivity has been investigated. (See OVERACTIVE THYROID [HYPERTHYROIDISM] in the section GLANDULAR CONDITIONS.)

Q-31. *What can be done for swelling of the legs?*

A. Swelling of the legs is known medically as edema. When advanced it is often referred to as dropsy by the layman. The condition generally results from an accumulation of fluid in the skin, and is due to various factors. Probably the most common of them has to do with simple mechanics and is brought on by gravity. When a person has settled down in a chair, with legs hanging down, or has stood for a long time, a noticeable degree of swelling may develop in his feet or ankles. This happens to many perfectly normal individuals, particularly on a hot day.

Another factor related to edema is any difficulty, new or old, a person may have with the veins and the circulation through them. An aftereffect of a clot in one of the larger leg veins may be a tendency to troublesome swelling of that extremity. The usual factors that aggravate this condition are a dependent position of the legs, inactivity, hot moist weather, and increased amounts of salt in the diet. Swelling often occurs in association with varicose veins, since in a varicose vein the return blood flow from the legs is impaired. Other factors that augment pressure within the veins may also predispose to swelling. Thus, clots of the large veins of the pelvis into which the leg veins drain, or pressure upon these veins from nearby organs, may sometimes result in leg swelling.

The condition known as congestive heart-failure is followed by a rise in pressure in the veins, and congestion can occur in various parts of the body. Frequently this results in leg swelling. Sometimes the puffiness may be marked.

In addition to cardiac causes, certain diseases of the kidney may underlie leg swelling, particularly conditions in which albumin is lost in the urine. When loss of albumin in the urine occurs for any length of time, body tissues puff up, and this may be most marked in the legs. It should be kept in mind, however, that such relatively trivial things as altered circulation in the veins are responsible for swelling of the legs most of the time, and that the heart and kidneys are most usually in no way involved.

There are various ways of dealing with troublesome leg swelling. Obviously, if disorders of the heart and kidney are involved, a physician will direct treatment specifically toward these organs. If the swelling is due to local circulatory disorders, as mentioned above, the patient will be advised to keep the affected leg in an elevated position as much as possible to diminish the force of gravity. The use of elastic stockings may also be advised, and the patient will be told to curtail the salt content of his diet. Finally, diuretic drugs may be prescribed. By pulling salt and water out of the kidneys, these drugs may rapidly diminish the degree of swelling of the legs. (*See* EDEMA in the section CARDIOVASCULAR CONDITIONS.)

Q-32. *I sometimes have a lightheaded feeling and things seem to swim about. What is responsible for this condition?*
A. This is generally referred to as dizziness, and dizziness is very variable. It can vary from a mild sensation of lightheadedness or giddiness (which is not truly dizziness) to what is medically known as true vertigo, in which objects around the patient seem to be in motion; this sensation is often accompanied by nausea. At the risk of a slightly inaccurate stretching of the term to include all of these sensations, the following may be considered as important causes:

• Mild sensations of lightheadedness or giddiness may be due to insufficient sleep, to a hangover from alcohol or drugs, and sometimes to a psychosomatic disturbance resulting from depression or emotional stress.

• Some viral illnesses attack the labyrinth —the semicircular canals of the internal ear which regulate equilibrium. This disturbance is called labyrinthitis and may produce severe symptoms of dizziness, nausea, and vomiting. The slightest attempt to get up or even a movement of the head may produce a marked increase in all these disagreeable sensations.

• Ménière's disease affects the labyrinth, and comes and goes in irregular fashion. It is usually found in individuals past middle age, most often men, and is frequently associated with a diminished sense of hearing on the affected side. The attacks often come without warning and produce intense dizziness and vomiting. These attacks may last from minutes to hours, during which time the patient is quite prostrated. Ménière's disease is considered to be a primary disturbance of the semicircular canals. The symptoms may be precipitated by an excessive distention with accumulated fluid. Occasionally, they may be brought about by stressful situations. Other neurological disturbances can lead to such symptoms as head noises and dizziness.

• Finally, dizziness may be secondary to disturbances such as very low blood pressure, hemorrhage, or severe anemia. This is sometimes observed when patients who are taking drugs for high blood pressure experience a sudden drop in blood pressure, as may occasionally happen when the person remains standing for any length of time. The reverse of this is also seen: high blood pressure by itself may produce moderately severe sensations of dizziness. Bouts of dizziness are also seen in elderly persons and may be associated with circulatory changes to the brain.

The treatment of dizziness will depend upon the particular cause. If due to anemia, the anemia will have to be corrected; if due to high blood pressure, judicious lowering of the blood pressure may be helpful; and if due to the effect of drugs, changes in the drug program may be necessary. Acute attacks of dizziness such as seen in Ménière's disease do not usually last long, and it is often difficult to tell whether any drug has been of help or whether the attack has not in fact passed spontaneously. Where the disturbance seems to be in the semicircular canals, as with some viral illnesses, the drugs that have been developed for the treatment of motion sickness (seasickness) are often quite useful. Among these are Dramamine®, Bonamine®, and Marezine®. These drugs seem to break up the "seasick" feeling and may markedly diminish nausea and the tendency to vomit.

The physician will prescribe the appropriate dosage of the drug. If it cannot be taken by mouth, injectable and suppository forms are available. In the case of some individuals who have frequent attacks of labyrinthitis, moderate doses may be taken for fairly long periods of time. Various forms of vitamin therapy are employed in the treatment of Ménière's disease, and may produce a diminution in the frequency and severity of the attacks. (*See* INDEX for specific entries.)

Q-33. *I have headaches and sometimes dizziness. Several members of my family have had elevated blood pressure. What can I do?*
A. High blood pressure frequently exists without producing any symptoms. The diagnosis can only be made by having the blood pressure measured in the doctor's office. If your symptom is due to elevated blood pressure, here are some facts you should know.

High blood pressure is a common disease. It affects about 20 percent of the population; it seems to run in families; and it is found to an increasing degree in the older age groups. The old definition of normal systolic blood pressure as consisting of 100 plus the age implied a recognition of the aging factor. Actually, there are many exceptions to this, and the saying has relatively little significance. It seems quite clear that elevated blood pressure contributes materially to the aging of the heart and the blood vessels. Thus hardening of the arteries, heart attacks, and strokes have an increased incidence among people with elevated blood pressure, as compared to those with normal blood pressure.

Treatment for high blood pressure was unsatisfactory for many years. It consisted of difficult programs such as rigid salt restriction, or special dietary programs such as the rice diet. The problem of treatment has been greatly eased over the years by a variety of new drugs. Indeed, the physician may now choose from a range of medications, some of which are for mild cases, others for the more severe ones. Depending upon the patient's reaction to the drugs and to the degree of elevation of blood pressure, a combination can be worked out for controlling the pressure, usually with gratifying results. First, however, it must be established that none of the less common causes of high blood pressure are present. Among these are certain tumors of the adrenal gland and various kidney disorders. On the other hand, most cases of high blood pressure are known as essential hypertension; that is, no specific disease of an organism seems to underlie the elevated pressure. (*See* HIGH BLOOD PRESSURE in the section CARDIOVASCULAR CONDITIONS.)

Q-34. *I often have dull aching in the forehead, which is sometimes throbbing. What could be responsible for this?*
A. These sensations in the head are classified as headaches. There are literally dozens of factors that may produce headache, some uncommon, others so common as to be almost everyday occurrences. A very incomplete list of some common causes of headache includes the following: tension, inadequate sleep, oversleeping, colds and other respiratory illnesses such as flu, menstruation, elevated blood pressure, sinus infections, eye strain, constipation, missing of meals, overindulgence in tobacco or in alcohol, and a variety of illnesses in which fever is also a symptom. Other far less common causes of headache include brain tumors, infections within the brain or its coverings, marked anemia, lead and certain other forms of poisoning, hemorrhages and clots within the arteries of the brain (strokes), uremia, severe hemorrhage, and sunstroke.

Some headaches have a throbbing quality, with the throbs synchronous with the pulse, and are sometimes referred to as vascular headaches. One well-known type of vascular headache is migraine, which has a hereditary component, since it seems to run in some families. Typically, it produces a throbbing headache on one side of the head, generally followed, before it runs its course, by nausea and often by vomiting. In some allergic persons eating certain kinds of foods may precipitate a headache.

Many apparently healthy persons have an occasional headache which cannot readily be accounted for. However, many people learn to identify the various likely causes of their own headaches. An alcoholic hangover on Sunday following a Saturday night drinking bout, or an emotional upset, or staying up very late looking at television all regularly lead to headaches in some people. However, the cause-and-effect relationship may not operate all of the time. Thus it is well known that some patients with elevated blood pressure have headaches when their pressure is high; but since the levels of the blood pressure vary, sometimes headache may be experienced even when the blood pressure is in the lower range. (*See* HEADACHE; HEADACHE, MIGRAINE in the section NERVOUS SYSTEM CONDITIONS.)

Q-35. *What can I do for pains in the head?*
A. It is commonly desirable to determine the cause of the headache as the first step in treatment. If the ache is due to some organic disease, the doctor will attempt to define the disease and institute appropriate treatment. This may mean taking medication to reduce the blood pressure, perhaps giving up smoking, or perhaps changing dietary habits so that the blood sugar does not drop too low. One may suspect that a definite disease process is producing headache if the headaches are frequent or chronic and if this is a new occurrence; if their location is different from previous headaches; if they do not follow the pattern of headaches in the past; or if they are resistant to the usual simple measures.

In order to determine the cause of headaches, a physician may have to make extensive examinations. In addition to determining the level of the blood pressure and studying the chemistry of the blood, a skull X-ray, a study of brain-wave patterns (electroencephalogram) and, perhaps, careful examination of the eyes and of the nervous system may all be necessary. A migraine headache may be spotted by the existence of a family history of it, a tendency to recurrence under certain circumstances such as undue stress, excessively hard work, or perhaps menstruation, and also because the headache pursues a progressive course involving throbbing, visual disturbances, nausea, and vomiting. Certain drugs are now available for the treatment of migraine, and even for its prevention.

It must be conceded that in more than 80 percent of the cases an organic cause for headache may not be found. Sometimes talking things over with a doctor or psychiatrist may relieve some of the stresses that form a background to migraine and other tension headaches.

However, most headaches are simple headaches and not a sign of an underlying threatening or severe disease process. Most people take a couple of aspirins for them and try to do the best they can. Occasionally, stronger medications, such as combinations of aspirin with codeine or other pain killers, may be required. Some patients find that an ice bag applied to the head may give considerable relief. For some of the headaches that arise in the back of the neck and are due to stiffening of muscles or to an arthritic involvement of the upper portion of the spine, heat is useful. They may be further helped by following up with some massage.

Sometimes tension-producing experiences may lead to repeated headaches, and the best answer may be a change in environment, as for example, a switch to another job if a person cannot develop a less intense attitude toward the stresses and strains of his life. Sedatives or tranquilizers, sometimes combined with muscle relaxants, may be useful drugs in the treatment of headache due to nervous tension. Finally, when eyestrain or sun glare are the causes, appropriate glasses or smoked lenses may clear up the headaches. (*See* HEADACHE in the section NERVOUS SYSTEM CONDITIONS.)

Q-36. *I have such trouble falling asleep at night. I also wake up frequently during the night and find it difficult to get back to sleep. What can I do?*
A. Difficulties in falling asleep or in staying asleep are common symptoms of nervous tension. Insecurity and anxiety frequently contribute to insomnia. The student worried about a major final exam, the executive harried over a difficult decision he must make, the mother worried over her child's illness, or the husband and father about losing his job—all of whom may have sleep difficulties. The difficulty may take various forms. It may consist of an inability to fall asleep reasonably quickly, or of a light and uneasy slumber with many awakenings during the night. Sometimes it may take the form of early-morning insomnia in which the person falls asleep much as usual, but wakens several hours ahead of schedule.

Whatever form it takes, a sleep difficulty can be very trying and can lead to intense feelings of wretchedness and tiredness. Its widespread existence no doubt accounts for the many popular remedies against it. In addition to counting sheep—which apparently no one ever does—recommendations have included: a warm tub bath, a glass of warm milk prior to retiring, a nightcap such as beer or some other alcoholic beverage, strict avoidance of coffee and similar stimulants, reading or looking at television until the eyes get tired and the lids droop, and taking a walk before retiring. Another suggestion is to disregard the problem of sleeplessness altogether, that is, to stay up and just hope that sooner or later normal sleepiness and the sleep pattern will be restored. But this seldom works.

There is no doubt that insomnia may be due to sedentary patterns of living. Many sedentary people living in cities have no physical activity, and when bedtime arrives, the lack of normal physical fatigue may contribute to difficulty in sleeping. Also, many persons are exposed to various kinds of nervous stimulation throughout the day and find themselves in an overstimulated state at bedtime, unable to relax and fall asleep. Thus, many businessmen find that they are unable to stop thinking of their business problems when they go to bed.

Sometimes an appropriate change in one's pattern of life may be necessary before relief from bouts of insomnia can be achieved. A program of increased physical activity may be of value to some. A shift to a less tension-producing job may be helpful. Certainly, when insomnia is frequent, reexamination of one's pattern of life and stresses, perhaps in consultation with a physician or psychotherapist, may be worthwhile.

Ours has been described as a sleeping-pill age. Widespread use of pills to induce sleep is perhaps more of a reflection on the kind of world in which we live than on the many sleepless persons in it. Sleeping pills are not recommended as an initial solution to sleeplessness, but it may also be a mistake stubbornly to refuse any kind of medication when insomnia is producing great fatigue and difficulty in concentration and in work. A great many medications are available, other than the typical sleeping pill, which may be of help in solving the problem. Mild sedatives and tranquilizers and some of the antihistamines (these are not sleeping pills but are drugs used for allergies, and often produce mild drowsiness) will often help without producing hangovers or other untoward effects. If a sleeping medication is necessary, the dose and the type should be suited to the person taking it, and the mildest one that works will be the

best. Temporary recourse to a sedative to secure sleep may be extremely worthwhile during periods of great stress. One need not be afraid of becoming "addicted" to the drug. Generally, as the stress subsides and the tension diminishes, the capacity to sleep is restored.

Q-37. *Should I make a point of doing exercises?*

A. The contribution to health that exercise makes has been appreciated more and more in recent years. For example, some important studies have revealed that in persons who are physically active throughout their lifetime heart attacks seem to be less frequent, are more apt to occur later in life, if at all, and are less likely to be fatal. For this reason the prudent person might well consider some program of regular exercise. There are other values to regular exercising. These include the following:

• Some evidence exists that the tendency to grow fat may in large measure be due to a disproportion between output of energy, as represented by work and exercise, and intake of calories, as dictated by one's appetite. This has been demonstrated even with animals. Experiments have shown that when an animal is not allowed to exercise, it may grow fat, whereas when the animal is allowed perhaps an hour or so of exercise per day, it will maintain an even weight. Although at one time the value of exercise was downgraded in programs for reducing for overweight, there has been an increasing tendency to advocate moderate exercise, at least some walking daily, as part of the total program of keeping weight under control.

• Most doctors now agree that exercise tends to improve the performance and capability of the heart and lungs in the face of unexpected or strenuous effort. This is due to its toning or conditioning effect. Many aspects of this are not well understood, although it is known that the trained athlete's heart can pump much larger amounts of blood with greater ease than the heart of the former athlete who has lost his conditioning.

• In the absence of exercise, muscles do not merely remain what they were; they tend to shrink and lose their power. Flabbiness of the muscles may contribute to various kinds of stresses and strains which are not experienced by the physically well-conditioned person. One example is the low backache. This is more likely to occur in sedentary persons with poor musculature than in active ones with well-developed muscles. Indeed, there is a growing belief that for certain kinds of low backache, the best long-term answer may be a program of exercises.

• Exercise has a tonic and stimulating effect on the organism. Sedentary persons who constantly feel tired find that when they exercise, the tiredness disappears and they feel invigorated. They may also find that they have more "pep" and an improved sense of well-being.

The exercise problem is growing as the white-collar population increases, as labor-saving machinery is more widely adopted, and as cars and readily available public transportation lead to less walking. Housework and similar tasks are not the equivalent of exercise—there is considerable difference between standing in the kitchen washing dishes and taking a bracing walk out of doors.

A system of progressively graded exercises which, when followed by a sedentary person whose muscles have had very little use for many years, will produce muscle-toning and conditioning without the risk of harmful over-exertion at the beginning. In the absence of graded exercises, walking for a mile or more per day has much to recommend it. Some exercises for low backache are also good as toning-up exercises, and can be performed routinely by anyone in his or her own bedroom.

Q-38. _Since I turned sixty, I have noticed that my hearing seems poorer. What can I do for this?_
A. The hearing mechanism involves the external auditory canal, which runs from the opening in the outer ear to the eardrum; a series of small bones in the middle ear; the cochlea, or the hearing organ itself, in which sound impulses are changed into nerve impulses; the auditory nerve, which conducts the nerve impulses to the brain.

Disease processes at any point on this path can interfere with hearing. A plug of wax in the external canal, a bony engulfment of little bones in the middle ear by otosclerosis, or damage to the cochlea and auditory nerve are among the many conditions that can cause hearing impairment.

The diminished hearing that occurs in the elderly primarily involves the hearing organ and the auditory nerve. The exact cause of senescent hearing loss is unknown but may be regarded as a deteriorative process perhaps comparable to cataracts in the eyes. The diminished acuity of hearing is sometimes called presbycusis (presby- meaning old and -cusis, hearing). Hearing loss attributable to aging comes on very gradually and, in fact, some hearing loss may be demonstrable fairly early in life. Thus there are very few persons past the age of thirty who can hear the high-pitched squeak of the bat. Hearing loss severe enough to interfere with ordinary conversation is not likely to occur before the age of fifty or sixty, but thereafter tends to be somewhat progressive.

The loss is greater in the higher frequencies, so that a person may understand such words as "one" and "mother" better than higher pitched words such as "six" and "sister." A certain amount of "figuring out" goes on with a person who is hard-of-hearing. Sometimes he guesses wrong, with confusion and embarrassment for those concerned.

There seems to be no reliable treatment for presbycusis. Large doses of vitamin B complex occasionally help. The most practical solution is a hearing aid. A doctor should prescribe the type of hearing aid needed. As long as the auditory nerve functions reasonably well, the hearing aid will help the elderly in ordinary social situations. When the auditory nerve is too badly damaged, however, even a hearing aid may not be of any help. (See Presbycusis in the section Ear, Nose and Throat Conditions.)

Q-39. _Since reaching the age of seventy, I have noticed increasing dimness of vision. What could be doing this?_
A. This is most likely due to cataract formation, a fairly common condition in the eyes of the elderly.

As light passes through the eyeball it is focused on the retina at the back of the eye by a clear crystalline structure called the lens. Any opacity in the lens is referred to as a cataract. Some cataracts are present at birth (congenital cataracts); others are caused by injury (traumatic cataracts). By far the most frequent type is the one that appears in old age. Such cataracts are at first small, produce no significant impairment of vision, and often the person who has one is unaware of its existence. A small cataract produces no visual problem. However, any of a number of factors may cause a small cataract to progress slowly. It may become large enough to be clearly visible as a whitish area within the pupil.

Certain metabolic disorders, such as diabetes, thyroid disease, or disorders of the parathyroids (the glands regulating the calcium content of the body), may predispose to cataract formation. However, cataracts often occur in aged or aging persons who are apparently in sound general health.

There is no treatment for cataracts other than surgical removal when they reach a certain point of maturation ("ripe" cataracts). Until that point is reached, changes in prescriptions for glasses, good illumination, and magnifying devices may be helpful. Cataracts tend to appear in both eyes, but their rate of development is generally unequal, and only one cataract at a time will be operated upon. Surgery consists of removal of the lens, a procedure that is usually performed without complication thousands of times each day. To make up for the loss of the lens, an implant or compensating glasses must be worn. With such glasses, excellent restoration of vision can be expected to follow cataract removal. (*See* CATARACT in the section EYE AND VISION CONDITIONS.)

Q-40. *I have frequent colds. What can I do for this?*
A. The fact that solutions for the common cold are less than satisfactory is indicated by the numerous remedies and programs advocated. Colds vary, are undoubtedly caused by different viruses, and are far more severe in some epidemics than in others. These variations undoubtedly contribute to the belief in certain "cures" which people claim to have experienced.

Actually, shortening of the duration of the cold or lessening of symptoms after taking medication "X" may be due to the fact that the attacking virus is less vicious than usual, or that one's resistance and capacity to shake off the cold may be somewhat higher than previously, rather than to any value in medication "X" itself. Nevertheless, once medication "X" seems to have worked, its "beneficiaries" persist in taking it whenever they have a cold, however improbable it is that "X" could have any effect.

At the first sign of a cold, many people dose themselves with whisky. Others take a laxative. Nothing that we know about the tissue reactions to colds, or about the effect of agents like alcohol or laxatives on the body as a whole, or the body's resistance and defense mechanisms, indicates that either procedure can be of any value.

But even the skeptic will admit that there are some useful procedures and drugs:

• Cutting down on one's work and activities, even to the point of resting in bed for a day or so, may reduce the intensity of the symptoms and the feeling of wretchedness, and certainly may lower the fever (not generally high in most colds).

• Aspirin is likely to offer some relief for the headaches or vague muscular aches that accompany respiratory illnesses.

• In recent years there has been a boom in the use of drugs such as the antihistamines and other decongestant agents known as the sympathomimetic amines, very often in combination. These appear to decrease congestion and the amount of nasal secretion formed, results not to be shrugged off.

When nasal congestion is intolerable, the sparing use of nose drops may unblock the nasal passages sufficiently to permit a reasonably free nasal breathing. Infants with nasal congestion may experience a great deal of difficulty and be most uncomfortable when attempting to nurse. This results from an inability to take in air because of the stoppage of the nasal passages and the presence of the bottle or breast in the mouth. Sparing use of nose drops may make the baby a good deal more comfortable.

There has been considerable argument back and forth as to whether antibiotics or other germ-killing drugs should be used for the treatment of simple colds. The consensus, concurred in United States government statements, is that antibiotics are of no help in the therapy of the simple cold. In addition, quite a few studies, mostly based upon college students and similar groups, have indicated that the course of the cold is the same whether or not antibiotics are also given.

For the overwhelming majority of people the simple cold is a nuisance disease, not a threat. For the cough itself, there are innumerable preparations sold over-the-counter at any drug store. Among the classic cold and cough remedies are such familiar ones as elixir of terpinhydrate (ETH) and codeine, syrup of wild cherry, and syrup of coccilana. When the cough is more severe, the doctor may prescribe medications containing codeine and codeine-like drugs which have a cough-suppressant effect.

Expectorants which increase the amount of phlegm are common ingredients of cough syrups and mixtures. Sucking on cough drops is often of some help for a harassing cough, and so is the inhalation of steam and the maintenance of humidity in the sickroom by vaporizers. Finally, it may be noted that avoidance of colds is always better than treating them. While most people feel that there is no escape, here are several facts to be kept in mind:

• The common cold is a contagious disease, hence one should avoid undue exposure to individuals with colds who are coughing and sneezing.

• There is a resistance factor to colds. For many individuals, excessive fatigue seems to be a predisposing cause and should be avoided. The fatigue may be physical or emotional. Since it may be a long time before we have immunization against colds, it is wise to study the pattern which precedes the development of one's own colds and learn from such experiences. (*See* COMMON COLD in the section INFECTIOUS DISEASES.)

Q-41. *I have a definite pain in the throat when I try to swallow. What can I do for this?*
A. This is usually due to inflammation of the pharynx, producing pharyngitis or sore throat. It is of some importance to establish the type of sore throat that is causing the pain. For example, sore throats due to the streptococcus (strep throat) usually produce a beefy red throat with some white exudation. It is important that the patient with a strep infection be treated with penicillin or some other antibiotic. Statistically, however, the most frequent causes of sore throat are the

various viral respiratory illnesses. Whatever the other symptoms they may give rise to in the nose, sinuses, or bronchial tubes, they are very likely to produce a sore throat as well. Since there are no specific drugs for viruses, treatment should be directed toward allaying the discomfort and other symptoms they produce. Among treatments which have proved to be of value are the following:

• Heat, or alternatively, cold may relieve discomfort. Heat may be applied by means of a heating pad wrapped around the neck, or possibly an infrared lamp or ordinary light bulb directed toward the same area. (Precautions, of course, should be taken against possible burns.) Occasionally, when heat is not helpful and when congestion, swelling, and difficulty in swallowing persist, cold may be effective. Chips of ice may be slowly sucked and swallowed. Here the cold has a numbing effect. It tends to cut down congestion and so may help diminish the inflammation and swelling that goes with the infection.

• Various types of gargles have been prescribed at one time or another. One consists of a teaspoon of salt in a glass of hot water. The addition of ten to fifteen drops of tincture of iodine to a glass of warm salt water sometimes seems to increase effectiveness, but precautions must be taken not to swallow this gargle; its use therefore cannot be recommended for small children. Still another gargle consists of one or two aspirin tablets crushed in a glass of warm water.

• Pain-killing drugs ranging from aspirin to stronger compounds such as Darvon® and codeine or its derivatives may be necessary to relieve more painful sore throats.

• Lozenges containing a local anesthetic are sometimes used to relieve the discomfort of a sore throat. There are a few individuals, however, who have local allergic reactions to these anesthetics. Unless you are quite sure that you will not have this type of reaction, the anesthetic lozenges are best avoided.

• With certain kinds of infection, where swallowing is very painful, cortisone-type drugs are occasionally used under a doctor's guidance.

• Some of the liniments, rubs, and ointments used for sore muscles, which work by producing local heat (rubefacients), may occasionally be helpful with sore throats. Care must be taken, however, not to allow the fumes which some of these give off to get into the nostrils and eyes.

• If warmth seems to be helpful, it may be wise to wear a scarf around the neck not only outdoors but indoors as well. Hot drinks such as tea may also have a soothing effect. For children, milk as warm as they can tolerate it may be used. (*See* Sore Throat in the section Ear, Nose and Throat Conditions.)

Q-42. *I develop nasal stuffiness in the early fall of each year which lasts for weeks. What causes this?*
A. This is probably a form of hay fever. At least five million Americans suffer from hay fever, an allergic disease affecting the lining of the nose. The sensitivity generally is to pollens and hence is more likely to be noted around June (grasses) and August (ragweed). Depending on climatic conditions and the pollen count, the victim may have a variable amount of nasal stuffiness, sneezing, a watery nasal discharge, itching of the eyes, and tearing. One of the earliest fundamental treatments for this condition was to give increasing doses of pollen extracts, which bring about a sort of increased resistance or tolerance for the pollens. This process of desensitization is still fundamentally sound. When successful, it may effect a complete cure. Desensitization is particularly desirable if there is accompanying asthma, an allergic condition involving the bronchial tubes. For mild cases and as a supplementary aid, the antihistamine drugs have proved very useful. These are combined with sympathomimetic amines (neosynephrine, ephedrine, and isopropylarterenol, an adrenalin-like substance), which are often efficacious in diminishing nasal congestion, thereby permitting a reasonable degree of free breathing through the nose.

In addition, the sparing use of nose drops may be of value when the nasal blockage seems intolerable. For severe degrees of nasal blockage, drugs of the cortisone group may be helpful; their use in any but small doses over brief periods of time, however, is not usually recommended. One of the consequences of this form of nasal allergy is the formation of polyps—pale, grapelike growths within the nasal cavity. The polyps by themselves may be, if not entirely, at any rate significantly re-

sponsible for nasal blockage. They are not likely to respond to medication and may have to be removed, a minor surgical procedure which may be performed at a doctor's office.

A somewhat similar condition involving nasal obstruction, increased secretion, and even the formation of polyps may be found in individuals who have not been previously allergic. This condition may appear for the first time in adult life—unlike hay fever, which is likely to be manifested in the child or the teenager.

Probably some of the cases that occur in middle life represent unusual allergies. Others have been classified under the term vasomotor rhinitis. This is thought to be an irritable and overreactive state in the nasal lining and not a true allergy. Middle-aged individuals with vasomotor rhinitis may notice more nasal difficulty when they are tense, after they have been drinking, or when they undergo temperature and humidity changes. They complain of being unduly disturbed by various kinds of dust, smoke, and fumes. The treatment for this condition is similar to that advocated for hay fever, but injections are unnecessary since the condition is not a reaction to an offending external agent such as a pollen. Generally, antihistamines are of value, the amount taken depending upon the extent of the disability and the doctor's prescription. (*See* Hay Fever; Vasomotor Rhinitis in the section Allergic Conditions.)

Q-43. *I get aching in the cheek bones and over the eyes, especially with colds. What causes this symptom?*
A. This is doubtless due to involvement of the sinuses. The sinuses are cavities within the bones of the face, and communicate with the nasal cavity. They are lined by a mucus-secreting layer of cells, just like the nasal lining; they behave in general as the nasal lining does with respect to infections, allergic responses, dust, and other substances. Between the sinus and the nasal cavity is a small opening called the ostium. It is this anatomical construction that is likely to create difficulty since, if enough swelling of the lining occurs to close off the ostium, swelling and accumulated secretions within the sinus may cause increasing pain.

One or another set of sinuses may take part

in this process: the maxillary sinuses, which are in the cheek bones just below the eyes; the frontal sinuses, located in the bones just above the eyes; or the ethmoid sinuses, located in the nasal bones between the eyes. When this occurs, a painful headache may be noted. In addition, severe infection may be accompanied by fever.

When there is fever, antibiotics or other germ-killing drugs are generally prescribed. Antihistamines and nose drops may be of value in unblocking the openings of the sinuses to permit drainage. Once drainage has been established, pain is likely to diminish. Heat is often soothing, and can be given in the form of hot wet compresses or a heating pad applied to the face. Special narrow heating pads designed for use in sinusitis are available. Aspirin and other pain-killing drugs may also make a useful contribution.

Sinusitis may be intermittent, occurring several times during the winter, and not at all at other times of the year. However, for chronic sinusitis, surgical methods are sometimes employed. For the very common kind of chronic sinusitis in the maxillary sinuses, a useful procedure can be to establish surgically a new opening between the sinus and the nasal cavity to provide free drainage. The procedure may be compared to opening up a boil, for once the pus is discharged, relief of the pain, swelling, and inflammation generally occurs.

Since the introduction of antibiotics, severe sinusitis and chronic sinusitis have markedly diminished. Before trying surgical methods for severe forms of chronic sinusitis, these drugs or antihistamines, as well as similar medications, are generally tried first; they frequently produce satisfactory results. Another procedure that can be performed at the doctor's office is to puncture the sinus. It can then be irrigated or washed out. The treatment is designed to relieve the infection and with it the discomfort. Sometimes, several such treatments may lead to a marked improvement. (*See* SINUSITIS in the section EAR, NOSE AND THROAT CONDITIONS.)

Q-44. *Why do I sometimes feel mucus in the back of my throat?*

A. This is probably due to the condition sometimes referred to as postnasal drip. Postnasal drip refers to the dripping into the upper back part of the throat of mucus from the nasal cavity. It is a condition that occurs regularly with most colds and similar respiratory illnesses. A postnasal drip that is associated with a viral respiratory illness normally ceases as the illness abates. Where there is chronic infection of the nose and sinuses, however, postnasal drip may be present much of the time. Obviously, the treatment of such a condition would be directed toward clearing up the infection, as described in the discussion of sinusitis. Chronic irritation, in which cigarette smoking may be the leading offender, can also be responsible for postnasal drip. (*See* SINUSITIS in the section EAR, NOSE AND THROAT CONDITIONS.)

Q-45. *I have cough with phlegm for long periods of time. How can I clear this up?*

A. A cough of long duration is generally an indication of an irritation either in the larynx and trachea (the vocal cords and windpipe), or the bronchial tubes themselves.

It should always be possible to account for a chronic cough. A cough should not be allowed to go on indefinitely without being brought under close scrutiny and the reasons for it ascertained. There are dozens of possible causes for chronic cough, but in actual practice a few of the most common ones far exceed the others in incidence.

Perhaps the most common of all is chronic bronchitis, which is an infection of the bronchial tubes usually due to bacterial infection. Normally, because of good self-cleansing mechanisms, the bronchial tubes are virtually free of bacteria. If bacterial infection gains a foothold and lasts for any length of time, increased secretions (phlegm) and chronic cough may be the body's answer to the infection. Both of these are mechanisms for getting rid of the invading bacteria. The phlegm formed under these circumstances may have a yellow tinge and a thickened consistency.

Chronic bronchitis seems to be on the increase and may predispose to emphysema, another lung condition in which the sacs of the lung are overdistended and shortness of breath is experienced. It should not be disregarded, and efforts should be made to treat it rather than to put up with it. The single most important contributing factor to chronic bronchitis is undoubtedly cigarette smoking, and it is a waste of time to treat chronic bronchitis if the victim continues to smoke.

However, chronic bronchitis does exist in nonsmokers. Not infrequently it is secondary to an infection of the sinuses, with a chronic postnasal drip, and the condition is referred to as sinobronchitis. Antibiotics and germ-killing drugs are often useful in the treatment of sinobronchitis. Occasionally, special treatment may be necessary for the sinusitis before the bronchitis clears up.

Some cases of chronic bronchitis seem to follow the acute bronchitis set up by certain respiratory infections. Here again, antibiotics may be administered for a period of time. When large amounts of phlegm are produced, postural drainage by a physician is indicated. This involves the placement of the body into various positions, generally with the head lower than the waist. This facilitates the outward flow of the phlegm. By lying first on one side, than on the other, gravity may aid in bringing the phlegm from the smaller bronchial tubes out toward the larger ones. From there, the phlegm can easily be brought up by less strenuous coughing. Often the chronic cough itself will improve as a result of postural drainage. Inhalations of steam, sometimes mixed with other agents, and the use of various expectorant mixtures, may also be helpful.

No one should attempt self-diagnosis of a cough. Coughs may arise from such serious conditions as pulmonary tuberculosis and tumors of the lung. Also, they may occur in association with mild degrees of asthma, inflammation due to fungus and other organisms, not to mention certain forms of heart disease, emboli (or clots) in the lung, and other possibilities too numerous to mention here. Coughs, phlegm, and chest pains should never be lightly dismissed. All too frequently they are attributed to cigarette smoking and to other banal causes, with the result that serious underlying conditions are allowed to proceed undiagnosed and untreated. Anyone with a chronic cough who brings up phlegm or has frequent chest pains should avoid self-help measures and should instead seek professional advice at once. (*See* BRONCHITIS; COUGH in the section RESPIRATORY CONDITIONS.)

Q-46. *Why do I often feel "all out of breath"?*

A. A variety of heart, circulatory, and lung conditions may contribute to shortness of breath. We must remember, however, that shortness of breath can be experienced without any serious underlying disease. Sedentary persons, unaccustomed to physical effort, may experience shortness of breath when called on to exert themselves physically, even if the effort is nothing more than climbing a low hill or a few flights of stairs. The fact that this condition is due to a lack of conditioning, and is reversible, is indicated by the observation that performance improves following suitably graded exercises. Persons who are moderately or markedly overweight often complain of shortness of breath on exertion. Contributing factors here include not only the dead weight of the fat, but also the fact that the heavy deposits of fat on the chest and abdomen mechanically interfere with breathing.

Smokers often complain of shortness of breath. This is due to obstructive bronchiolitis, an inflammation of the lining of the tubes, with accumulation of mucus. This leads to partial clogging of the smaller bronchial tubes. Fortunately, this is usually cleared when smoking is discontinued, so that several weeks afterward the ex-smoker may find himself able to perform without shortness of breath, tasks that were formerly very trying. All of the factors just mentioned—lack of training, obesity, and cigarette smoking—are reversible.

Other conditions of the lung that impair ventilation and produce shortness of breath may not be so successfully reversed. This is true of certain kinds of chronic inflammation, for example, when there has been a good deal of scarring (fibrosis) which interferes with the ability of the lungs to expand and contract. Sometimes extensive scarring interferes with the exchange of oxygen around the innumerable small blood vessels of the lung, thus setting up a mechanical barrier to oxygenation.

A condition that seems to be on the increase, known as emphysema, may also contribute to shortness of breath. A form of this is seen in many aging people. The more severe grades of emphysema are a consequence of chronic bronchitis and are seen especially in persons who have smoked for long periods.

The basic trouble in emphysema is that the little air-containing sacs of the lungs are overdistended and have lost their elasticity. Hence they do not properly expand with inspiration and contract with expiration, and the total flow of air in and out of the lungs is considerably decreased.

In addition to lung factors, heart factors are also involved. Often, as people get older, the capacity of the heart to handle the increased demands produced by exercise diminishes. Hence shortness of breath is experienced as one attempts to run for a bus or train, climb several flights of stairs, shovel snow, or perform any other physical effort that taxes the heart muscle. The ability to face up to an unexpected or unusual demand on the heart's pumping function is sometimes referred to as the myocardial reserve (myocardium being equivalent to heart muscle). Various illnesses, past and present, may diminish the myocardial reserve. A heart attack that knocks out a portion of the heart muscle can do this; so can hardening of the coronary arteries that nourish the heart. Damage to the heart valves produced by rheumatic heart disease may lead to a considerable decrease of this reserve, as can various forms of congenital heart disease and such glandular disturbances as thyroid disease.

A variety of heart troubles may lead to congestive heart-failure. This is a condition produced when the heart's pumping function is inadequate, so that congestion in the lungs, the liver, or the lower extremities becomes apparent, and is manifested by accumulation of fluid in these sites. Pulmonary congestion or fluid in the lungs may be greatly improved by various prescribed programs. These may include instituting the use of such drugs as digitalis and the diuretic drugs, which pull water out of the body. These drugs may clear up pulmonary congestion and lead to marked relief from shortness of breath. Rest alone leads to temporary relief but the shortness of breath returns with exertion or other special effort. The patient may even experience spasm of the bronchial tubes with wheezing, quite like that seen in asthma. Obviously, shortness of breath is only a symptom, one that can arise in a variety of situations. The determination of the precise cause or causes will require examination by a physician. (*See* INDEX for specific entries.)

Q-47. *I sometimes develop wheezing and feel short of breath. What is the cause of this?*

A. One probable cause is a form of asthma. In asthma, the chief difficulty is due to an intense spasm of the bronchial tubes. When this is marked, the victim finds it difficult to breathe. Also, expiration, which is normally a passive process requiring no effort, becomes difficult and energy-consuming. In a severe case, the victim seems to gasp for air, and is obviously laboring hard to perform the act of breathing.

Most cases of asthma are due to some allergic reaction, most commonly to pollens, but occasionally to various other items including foods and drugs. If the reaction is to pollens, the discomfort is experienced at particular seasons. Desensitization is brought about by giving injections of the pollen extract. This may gradually build up the body's capacity to tolerate the offending agents and thereby result in cure. Often, however, there may be a multiplicity of substances to which the asthmatic patient is allergic. For these patients, desensitization may be a complicated and protracted process. Whatever the offending agent, drugs of various kinds may be necessary to relax the bronchial spasm. These drugs are known as bronchodilators. They include such agents as ephedrine, aminophylline, and certain related synthetic drugs. These are the drugs commonly found in various asthma remedies and may be given in pills or, occasionally, in suppositories, or in enema form. For very severe cases of asthma, steroid drugs (cortisone derivatives) may be helpful in tiding over a severe episode. Pocket inhalators, small enough to be carried around, are available. A few whiffs of these inhalators may give prompt relief in an asthma attack.

Asthmatoid bronchitis is a somewhat similar condition in which there is also bronchial spasm. This condition tends to appear in middle or later life, although occasionally it is found in some individuals in association with respiratory illnesses at any age. Patients with this condition do not have a history of allergic reactions to pollens, and their bronchospastic disorders are not limited to a particular season of the year. Instead, they seem to develop asthma in association with a bronchial infection—bronchitis—hence the term asthmatoid bronchitis.

Since it is often difficult to clear up bronchitis, the asthmatic tendency manifested by wheezing, coughing, and shortness of breath —particularly on exertion—may be present a considerable part of the year. Many of the drugs used for the treatment of asthma will help with asthmatoid bronchitis. Often combinations of drugs have to be used to achieve maximum control. In addition, since there is an infectious component to asthmatoid bronchitis, antibiotics may be prescribed. Antibiotics may be particularly useful when a person who is subject to asthmatoid bronchitis starts coming down with a cold or similar respiratory illness.

Antibiotics are seldom of value in the treatment of uncomplicated allergic asthma, except when the individual develops a superimposed infection, not infrequently a bronchopneumonia.

Mild forms of asthmatoid bronchitis frequently escape detection. They have all the qualities of a chest cold with cough, but may be more drawn out than usual. A wheeze and a long siege of a choking, hacking cough may well connote asthmatoid bronchitis. (*See* Asthma in the section Respiratory Conditions.)

Q-48. *How can I break the cigarette habit?*

A. Smokers are sometimes surprised to find that giving up cigarettes is far less of a struggle than they had supposed. This includes, to begin with, persons who have stopped smoking for several days during a bout with a cold, persons who light a cigarette and can forget it so that it burns itself out, and persons who, in places of employment that forbid smoking, manage to go for a substantial number of hours without lighting a cigarette. Unfortunately for the majority of individuals, a true habituation or addiction does seem to exist, so that for them to stop smoking does in fact produce tension and disagreeable symptoms. In addition to their preoccupation with the idea

of smoking, some people feel definitely under par during the withdrawal period, and they may experience trouble in concentrating on their work.

Other symptoms are a tendency to constipation during the first few days, some difficulty in falling asleep, marked feelings of hunger, and sensations of warmth in the extremities together with a noticeable slowing of the pulse rate. Withdrawal symptoms are most marked during the first few days, then tend to taper off over the next two weeks. Those abandoning the habit, however, should be advised that, from time to time during the early weeks following cessation of smoking, an intense though brief craving for smoking may reappear and must be firmly denied.

There is no doubt that considerable firmness or self-discipline is necessary for most hardened cigarette smokers who wish to give up the habit. A person seriously interested may wish to consult a doctor who will be in a position to prescribe mild stimulants, sedatives, or alternatives and substitutes that may partially compensate for the tobacco craving. Some people, those who feel truly wretched during the first few days, may be helped by a nicotine-containing chewing gum, while those who feel nervous may profit by small doses of sedatives. A drug of variable efficacy known as nicorette has been used to help relieve the symptoms. When an individual who wishes to stop makes a compact with another smoker, the knowledge that someone else is faced with the same problems is a barrier to falling back into the habit and a help in fighting temptation.

A cigarette smoker who stops should be good to himself and should seek other satisfactions. Since he often has an increased appetite, he should eat, suck on candy and mints, and be prepared to gain a few pounds—a temporary indulgence well worth the price. Women who hesitate to stop smoking due to a fear of gaining weight should be advised that a modest weight gain is no health hazard and that the increase can be reversed once the nonsmoking status has been achieved.

It is important for those giving up the smoking habit to realize that not only will they escape such statistical possibilities as lung cancer and heart attack, but that within a few weeks various kinds of pleasant improvements may be noted. Usually the wind is markedly improved, and shortness of breath disappears. The "cigarette cough" vanishes as the chronic bronchitis which afflicts most smokers generally clears. There is sometimes an enormous improvement in the sense of taste and smell, and the flavor of food seems to be doubled or tripled. In addition, many ex-smokers notice that their pep increases, and that sometimes sexual drives and capacities improve. The latter may represent an overall improvement in performance and health brought about by the discontinuance of smoking. (*See* Smoking in the section Miscellaneous Health Conditions.)

Q-49. *I seem to cough less on filter cigarettes. May I continue with them?*

A. There is no evidence that present-day filters will necessarily change the picture, as no one knows whether the particular agent responsible for some of these illnesses is held back or passes through the filters.

As early as 1938, it was demonstrated that heavy smokers live on an average four years less than nonsmokers. The American Cancer Society studies have repeatedly shown that the chances of developing lung cancer are multiplied a hundredfold when one compares the incidence of lung cancer in heavy smokers as against nonsmokers.

Even more perturbing was the American Cancer Society's finding that the incidence of coronary thrombosis (heart attacks) was definitely higher in heavy smokers than in nonsmokers. In addition, studies indicated that chronic bronchitis and emphysema, a condition which produces shortness of breath and which is most difficult to treat, was almost exclusively a disease of cigarette smokers, and so was cancer of the larynx (voice box), as well as cancer of the mouth and tongue.

The risk inherent in cigarette smoking is significant at the ten-cigarette-per-day level. The risk moves markedly upwards as the amount of cigarette smoking increases. For example, a man of sixty, smoking two packs per day, has one chance in ten of dying of lung cancer alone, not to mention the other smoking-related illnesses to which he may succumb.

All investigations point to the dramatic but inescapable fact that cigarette smoking is by far the most important single preventable agent contributing to illness and death on the American health scene today. It becomes the clear responsibility of every individual, therefore, with even a modest regard for the health of his own body, to desist from cigarette smoking. (*See* Smoking in the section Miscellaneous Health Conditions.)

Q-50. *Why do I often have dull pains in the lower back?*

A. Most chronic backaches arise in the musculoskeletal system, in this case the spinal column, the pelvis, and their associated muscles and ligaments. Various kinds of pulls, stresses, and strains on these structures will produce backaches. They are most commonly felt in the region of the lower back, the "small of the back," and will sometimes be more pronounced on one side than on the other. Back pains in this area may have a constant dull aching quality. Changes in posture or in the physical demands made on the low-back structure will have an effect on the pain. Such changes may be taken as a good indication that the ache does arise in the musculoskeletal system.

Quite often, sitting in certain positions, driving, or standing in one spot may make the backache worse. Bending so that the body goes into a partial stooping position may relieve the backache, as may supporting some of the body's weight on the outstretched hands. A backache which occurs mostly upon arising in the morning raises the possibility that a sagging mattress may be responsible. Backache of a similar quality may be experienced in the upper part of the back by individuals who have a curvature of the spinal column in this region. Here again special stress, which results in the ache, is being placed on muscles and ligaments.

Laymen tend to assume that aching in a particular region signifies some disorder in an organ nearby. Thus they assume incorrectly that an ache in the low back is due to something wrong with the underlying kidneys; or that, when it occurs higher up, it is due to pleurisy. But ninety-nine times out of a hundred the pain is in the muscle walls and ligaments rather than in a diseased organ underneath. This is not to deny that disease in the kidney is occasionally felt in the low back, or that a uterus which is tipped back (retroverted uterus) may produce a chronic low backache.

In addition, a physician will keep in mind other possible causes for backache, since various diseases of the musculoskeletal apparatus may be present. Such disorders include osteoarthritis; another form of arthritis known as spondylitis; osteoporosis, a condition in which the vertebrae become weak because of their loss of protein and calcium; herniated discs; tumors; neuritis or inflammation of nerves; and other rare possibilities. (*See* INDEX for specific entries.)

Q-51. *What should I do for frequent nagging aching in the back?*

A. If, after an examination by the doctor, it becomes clear that this is the usual postural type of chronic low backache, it should nevertheless be treated as a definitely individual problem. However, experience indicates that these backaches often have common features and that certain common approaches may be of value.

• A mild low backache may occasionally intensify rapidly after a sudden stress or pull on the back. In severe cases, the victim may be unable to straighten up, and every movement of the back may be agonizing. Sometimes chronic low backaches are ushered in by an acute, severe one. Generally, it is best that the individual get off his feet and go to bed. In bed, a slightly bent position of the back is usually the most comfortable. This can be achieved by elevating the knees and the lower extremities on several pillows, perhaps also raising the mattress at the head of the bed. Pain-killers, varying from aspirin to stronger combinations, may be necessary. Intermittent use of a heating pad placed on the lower back is often helpful. During this stage, a tight support such as a sacroiliac belt or a girdle may be of value.

• The victim of low backache should pay special attention to his bed and mattress. As mentioned earlier, if the backache is worse on arising in the morning, it is often found that a sagging mattress is to blame. A mattress should be quite firm and should provide good support under the hips and low back. A mattress that is too soft or has too much "give"

may be firmed by inserting boards between the mattress and spring. Sometimes placing newspapers, books, or a pillow under the center of the mattress helps give additional support in this region.

• Similar attention should be paid to seating. Pillows placed so as to support the small of the back may enable one to drive a car or work at a desk without getting backache.

• Supports for the back, such as sacroiliac belts, are often helpful. Women sometimes find that wearing a tight girdle is useful. A pad exerting moderate pressure against the small of the back may be of further value.

• Stresses and pulls on the back should be avoided. When one stoops to pick up a heavy object, this should be done by bending the knees, never by bending with the knees held stiffly. To keep the knees straight while lifting places all the strain on the low back.

• The best sitting posture for people with low backache is one which keeps the back slightly rounded. This is best achieved by ensuring that the knees are at a higher level than the hips. Thus a good chair for someone with low backache would slope downward from front to back. Another helpful arrangement is to have the feet elevated on a low hassock or stool.

• Finally, back-strengthening exercises should be seriously considered.

Q-52. *What sort of exercises are useful for chronic low backaches?*

A. Because low backaches may be a source of discomfort for months or years, and because they often suddenly give rise to episodes of aggravated or disabling pain, there have been increasing efforts to work out long-range solutions to the low-back problem.

In a few instances this may be easy, for example the disappearance of the low backache when the victim shifts from a sagging to a firm mattress. Not uncommonly, however, low backaches may persist, coming and going but never quite gone.

For many sufferers, exercises designed to strengthen the muscles of the low back may afford the best permanent relief. These not only strengthen the supporting muscles of the back, but are also sometimes intended to correct a tendency of the hollow in the small of the back to increase. Many authorities agree that the key to low backaches is a structural weakness in the lumbosacral region, or hollow, on which the weight of the trunk falls. Increasing strength in this region may therefore be of fundamental importance in dealing with low backache.

It has been clearly shown that daily exercise will cure, or significantly help, some low backaches. When, because of inertia or for other reasons, exercise is discontinued, the backache returns. Among the exercises that have been advocated are the following:

• Lying on the back, raise each leg alternately ten to fifteen times. Then repeat with both legs. The legs need not be returned to the resting position, and it is in fact preferable that they be lowered to from six to twelve inches above bed or floor level, from where the exercise is repeated.

• "Kissing the knees." While lying on the right side in the straight position, bring the left leg toward the chin, bending the knee. Repeat on the opposite side. While lying on the back, draw the legs upward, bending them at the knees. At the same time bend the trunk forward as far as it can go. With some practice it should be possible to bring the knees up to the face, first on one side, then on the other. This exercise should also be repeated ten to fifteen times.

• Knees-over-head exercise. In this exercise, the extended legs are brought up over the head as far back as they will go, then returned to a position in which the legs are six to ten inches off the floor. This can be repeated several times.

• The familiar touch-the-toes exercise should be modified. The knees should be kept slightly bent rather than rigidly straight. It is not necessary to touch the toes, nor should the back be completely straightened in the return sweep of the exercise.

• Squats. From a slightly stooped position, with knees slightly bent and arms hanging downward between the lower extremities, bend the knees until the knuckles touch the floor. Then straighten up to the partially erect position, and repeat.

These exercises should be started cautiously by sedentary individuals, and are best not done at all when the backache is acute. The number of repetitions can be slowly increased. If there is any increase in backache, the number of exercises may have to be decreased, and a physician should be consulted. The general aim of these exercises is to strengthen the back muscles, but in none of them should the hollow of the back be accentuated. This is the reason for not completely straightening out in some of them, and also the reason why the emphasis is placed on such others, as "kissing the knees," which have a tendency to straighten out the hollow. In addition, the back may be strengthened by exercises such as bowling, swimming, golfing, and pulling of weights.

Q-53. *I have noticed in recent years some thickening around my finger joints. What causes this?*
A. The thickening of the finger joints which appears in some people in their forties is a form of the disease called osteoarthritis. The thickening is due to an increased formation of bone around the joint. The condition is sometimes called Heberden's node. It seems to be more common in women, may run in some families, and may show some progression, but sometimes long periods will pass without any apparent further thickening. Very few people reach their sixties and seventies without some degree of osteoarthritis of the fingers. Occasionally, it may produce angulation so that the fingertip appears to be slightly crooked.

Mild degrees of this disorder may produce no discomfort. At times stiffness and slight aching in a joint may be noted. This may be more marked on arising in the morning, and may improve soon after a person gets up and starts using the hand. The condition is seen in sedentary individuals as well as those who work with their hands, so that work is not a primary cause. Women who are proud of their grooming and appearance will, of course, find the condition a little more annoying than those who are more philosophic about their appearance.

Unfortunately, nothing is known about the cause of this disease or how to alter its course. When pain or stiffness are present, soaking the hands in hot water usually limbers up the fingers and alleviates pain. Aspirin or similar drugs may be taken to decrease the ache. If exposure to cold seems to increase the discomfort, gloves should be worn. In most individuals, the condition is more of a nuisance than a disease process. It has no special relation to osteoarthritis elsewhere in the body, has nothing to do with rheumatoid arthritis, a far more crippling disorder, and is perfectly compatible with excellent health. (*See* ARTHRITIS, DEGENERATIVE in the section MUSCULO-SKELETAL CONDITIONS.)

Q-54. *Why do I have pains and difficulty in turning my head?*
A. This is sometimes referred to as a stiff neck and is usually due to a painful spasm in one of the major muscles at the back of the neck. The spasm produces pain, often increased by attempts to move the head about. Such movement generally is restricted to one side. The spasm may make the affected muscle appear to stand out more than the corresponding one on the opposite side of the neck. Stiff necks produce all degrees of incapacity, from slight discomfort to a severely painful spasm of the neck muscles which makes any motion impossible. Most such conditions are set up by a stress or unusual strain on the neck. Occasionally people wake up with such a stiff neck because the neck has been in an awkward position during sleep.

Occasionally, a stiff neck may occur after a twisting motion of the neck, just as a severe backache can result from an innocent maneuver such as reaching down to pick up a shoe. This is due to a slippage between the connections of the spinal vertebrae, setting up a reflex spasm in the muscles producing pain and then immobilization. Exposure to a cold wind or draft sometimes results in a stiff neck. It is thought that the cold produces some temporary change in the muscle, leading to the stiffness and pain. A variety of other neck pains are somewhat similar to the stiff neck. Arthritis in the neck area, degeneration of the discs between the vertebrae, pressures on the nerves where they exit through the vertebrae, and changes in the alignment of the vertebrae of the neck may all lead to uncomfortable and painful sensations in the neck region. These too are often aggravated on attempted motion.

Many of these conditions are treated by traction, in essence a stretching of the neck produced by a collar and weights. The collar is slung around the head and jaw and is connected to a rope passed over a pulley. The opposite side of the pulley is weighted, and produces a degree of tension that can be regulated and varied by a physician. The neck is stretched by this device for periods of five to fifteen minutes per day. Traction may relieve pain considerably. Aspirin and other painkillers are often useful in treatment. Also effective is massage.

Q-55. *My daughter has a breaking out of the face for some days before her period. What is this?*
A. This is probably acne (pimples) which is almost an inevitable part of every adolescent's development. Its appearance during adolescence is due to the fact that acne is related to sex hormone stimulation of the oil glands of the skin. Acne is a good deal more common in boys than in girls, but is found in both sexes. As a matter of fact, both male (androgen) and female (estrogen) sexual hormones are found in each sex. In girls, the flare-up of acne that occurs just prior to the menstrual period is related to the altered hormonal secretions at that time. Fortunately, in the great majority of adolescents acne is mild. It may consist of occasional crops of pimples on the face, forehead, or back which vary in number, and perhaps form whiteheads, but which leave little or no scarring. When the acne has run its course, as it generally does by the age of twenty, little in the way of significant skin blemishes can usually be noted. (*See* ACNE in the section SKIN CONDITIONS.)

Q-56. *What can I do for excessive perspiration?*
A. Excessive perspiration is an accompaniment of some diseases, such as overactivity of the thyroid, and episodes of excessive sweating are complained of by some women during the menopause. But many persons have this affliction without any obvious link with disease or organic condition. Hyperhidrosis, the medical term for it, is most often confined to a specific part of the body. A fairly common complaint is excessive perspiration from the palms of the hands. It occurs in moderate degree when people are nervous or tense, as the result of adjusting to a new business or social situation, or when they are experiencing anxiety or fear. Occasionally, excessive perspiration from the hands seems unrelated to the

emotions, and may reach the point of dripping. Excessive perspiration is also complained of in the armpits and on the feet.

There are, of course, innumerable antiperspirants for use in the armpits. Most of them contain an aluminum salt which inhibits the activity of the sweat glands. They generally also incorporate agents to reduce the odor of the sweat. Some seem to be a little more effective than others, and some individuals have to apply them more than once a day. Generally, however, washing the underarm region daily with an antibacterial soap such as Phisohex® or Dial®, and then using the antiperspirant, gives adequate relief. Even with antiperspirants, some women find dress shields necessary to protect their clothing. Similar measures will generally help excessive perspiration of the feet. Wearing sandals or open-toed shoes and porous cotton stockings, rather than synthetics, is of further help.

Excessive perspiration may sometimes be partially but not completely controlled. In the unusual cases in which the excessive perspiration reaches the point of large-scale dripping and is not controlled by the usual measures, surgical procedures may be effective. One of these is the severing of the sympathetic nerves which control the particular area. When they are cut, marked dryness in that part of the skin to which the nerves go will occur. The operation is by no means a minor one, however, and should be considered only when the degree of hyperhidrosis warrants it. Sweat glands have been removed to control excessive sweating from the armpits. The operation is simpler than cutting the nerve supply. Again this is for desperate cases. (*See* PERSPIRATION, EXCESSIVE in the section SKIN CONDITIONS.)

Q-57. *How much exposure to sun should I give my skin?*

A. In general, sun exposure and sun tanning are of medical value for only a limited number of people. Where there is excessive oiliness of the skin and acne formation, tanning the skin may have therapeutic value. However, many individuals, particularly sun-worshipers who toast themselves on the beach for prolonged periods, are only injuring their skin. The tanning reaction is the skin's and the body's attempt to protect against further injury.

Excessive exposure to the sun has been demonstrated to age the skin. Loss of elasticity and tone, and thinning and atrophy of the subcutaneous tissue (the tissue just under the skin) are all aging changes which are hastened by excessive, prolonged, or repeated exposure to sunlight. Thus, although a tan is prized as a sign of good health and, admittedly, gives that healthy outdoors look, overindulgence should be viewed with considerable restraint. This is not to say that getting an occasional brief sunning, or developing a tan during a summer vacation, is necessarily harmful. It is frequent and prolonged exposure to the sun that should be avoided. Application of sunscreen lotions before exposure is recommended.

A further factor to be considered is the fact that large doses of sunlight over long periods of time increase the rate of formation of skin cancers. Cancer of the skin is known to be more prevalent in people who work out of doors, with constant exposure to the elements, as do farmers and sailors. While slight tanning and exposure to the sun may be defended from the cosmetic point of view, and even, perhaps, from the medical point of view as giving rise to vitamin D formation, they should be indulged in with restraint. (*See* SUNSCREENS in the section SKIN CONDITIONS.)

Q-58. *Sometimes I feel as though I "itch all over." Yet when I look, I can't see anything wrong with my skin at the place that itches. What can be the reason for this?*

A. Many individuals suffering from nervous stress experience itchiness of the scalp or other parts of the body. The itching is essentially transient, and need not call for special measures. Some persons complain of itching as they lie in bed before falling asleep. They experience prickling, itching sensations in different parts of the body which respond to scratching; after a time, the sensations diminish, and the person falls asleep.

Other forms of nervous itching can be quite chronic, sometimes very stubborn, and present a variety of skin changes. Some patients undergoing particularly stressful periods experience diffuse itching sensations which are relieved by scratching. The scratching may produce a weltlike or reddish elevation of the skin, a condition technically called dermo-graphism—literally, skinwriting. Sometimes, however, there is a full-fledged skin eruption, which is very often symmetrical in shape. The eruption may be on both elbows, or on the backs of both knees, or it may be on various other parts of the body, such as the neck. The skin in these regions becomes reddened or purplish, appears slightly thickened, and the normal linear skin markings are somewhat more prominent than usual. Itching may be so intense as to lead to repeated scratching even to the point of drawing blood. (*See* ITCHING in the section SKIN CONDITIONS.)

Q-59. *What can be done for cracking and itching between the toes?*

A. The most common cause for these complaints is the condition termed athlete's foot. Athlete's foot is the popular term for a skin disease of the feet produced by a fungus organism. (A fungus organism differs somewhat from bacteria, one of the important distinctions being a greater hardiness and resistance to treatment.) (*See* ATHLETE'S FOOT in the section INFECTIOUS DISEASES.)

Q-60. *I have slight itching and flakiness of the scalp. What can be done for this?*

A. This is most often due to the disorder popularly termed dandruff. A wide range of scalp disorders, from light flakiness to extensive reddened and weeping, crusted patches, may be referred to as dandruff, or more properly as seborrheic dermatitis. Mild cases, which produce a little flakiness on one's collar, need not cause concern. Sometimes, particularly when the hair is not shampooed for a period, some itching may be noted. With any form of seborrhea, it is advisable not to let the hair grow too long, nor to use oily or greasy lotions and dressings. Thick hair and greasy lotions prevent proper aeration of the scalp and consequently promote dandruff. When considerable flaking, itching, and redness occur, a crew cut or a very short haircut may be advisable. (*See* SEBORRHEIC DERMATITIS in the section SKIN CONDITIONS.)

Q-61. *On waking up this morning, my father couldn't move his left arm and leg. What is happening?*

A. The most common cause for this is a stroke. In a stroke, a certain number of brain cells are damaged. The damage may occur because of a thrombosis or clot in the artery which supplies blood to these cells or, less commonly, a cerebral hemorrhage due to a leakage of blood from the blood vessel. Often the physician cannot be sure which has happened, and the event is referred to generally as a cerebral vascular accident, or CVA. A CVA can occur in any part of the brain, and multiple CVA's occur in which small groups of brain cells are damaged, sometimes with surprisingly little functional evidence of impairment. However, most people think of stroke-caused brain damage in terms of the control of voluntary motion. The brain cells involved are sometimes referred to as the motor cells, and are the ones that enable a person to move his arms or legs, speak, swallow, and smile, or perform other facial movements at will.

The motor cells which control each half of the body are located in the opposite half of the brain, that is, damage in the left side of the brain will produce paralysis on the right side of the body, and vice versa. There is but one speech center in the brain, the center that controls the complicated movements and acquired information that go into the process of talking. In right-handed persons, this center is located in the left half of the brain, in left-handed individuals, it is on the right side. As a result, impairment or loss of speech, known as aphasia, will not occur if a right-handed individual suffers a stroke affecting the left side of his body.

The extent of loss of function that occurs with a stroke varies from slight weakness affecting a limb, with or without speech difficulty, to full paralysis in which the entire affected half of the body appears to be knocked out. The latter condition is referred to as a hemiplegia. In the early stages of a hemiplegia the victim may be completely unable to move either the arm or the leg. Fortunately, however, it is generally found after the passage of some days that a degree of voluntary motion is coming back. Most often voluntary control returns first to the lower extremity, in which some motion can be achieved, even though requiring considerable effort.

As a rule, so long as some motion is evident

it is safe to predict that the victim will be able to walk after a period of rehabilitation. The degree to which control returns to the upper extremity is variable. Because of the complexity of human hand motion, and also because a very large number of motor cells are involved in controlling the arm, hand, and fingers, impairment of hand and finger motion is generally more apparent and also more distressing than loss of function in the leg. Particularly, of course, if the dominant side (the right side in a right-handed individual, and vice versa) is affected, difficulties and tribulations will be more marked. Characteristically, finely coordinated finger motions such as those involved in writing, picking up objects, or other everyday motions may be lost or severely impaired.

Various degrees of functional restoration usually take place during the days and weeks immediately following a stroke. This slow healing process may go on for months, at a rate that varies considerably from one person to another. Therefore, one cannot be certain of the permanent damage caused by a stroke for several months. Improvement may continue for as long as a year. Rehabilitation therapy is of great value following a stroke. If the stroke victim can raise his foot even slightly off the bed, the outlook for his eventually walking is quite good. However, before he walks again, a considerable program of effort, exercise, and persistence on his part and that of those caring for him may be necessary. Generally, the affected limb is quite stiff (the technical term for this is spasticity) and control over the spastic extremity is at first slow, weak, and distressingly inadequate. With practice, however, more and more control over the damaged extremity ordinarily returns.

The situation of the stroke victim can be likened to that experienced by the infant when he first attempts to walk. Before he can gain the necessary control and mastery of his muscles, many weeks of trying and of practice are necessary. The person who has suffered a stroke must go through a somewhat similar process of reeducation before he can walk again. A brace is of great help in this process. The brace may be a long one, which runs from the hip down to the foot, or a short one starting below the knee. Braces are designed to stabilize the spastic extremity. With the aid of a brace, and perhaps with the help of canes,

the use of a "walker," and manual support from an attendant, the patient eventually learns to walk again. Not uncommonly, his rehabilitation progresses from the use of a long leg brace to a short one, and he may even be able to discard all bracing after a period of time. As a rule, however, a cane or other support is useful in stabilizing the individual who has had a stroke.

The outlook for the hand and fingers is often less certain. It is not uncommon to see excellent restoration of function in the lower extremity, with only poor or partial restoration of function in the corresponding upper extremity. Again, only the passage of time, and earnest rehabilitation efforts, will enable one to judge what the residual disability is going to be.

The rehabilitation programs of the past thirty years have clearly shown that the outlook following a stroke is better than had previously been believed possible. Many stroke patients who once would have been consigned to a wheelchair or bed for life can be made independent again in the activities of daily living, so that they may be able to dress themselves, feed themselves, and take care of the bodily needs. The attainment of this level of competence, however, ordinarily requires the aid of certain specialists. The physiatrist is a doctor who specializes in rehabilitation. The physical therapist (physiotherapist) is a person trained in giving and supervising remedial and restorative exercises. (*See* STROKE in the section NERVOUS SYSTEM CONDITIONS.)

Q-62. *Some days I notice a forceful thumping in the left chest. What causes this?*
A. This is probably what many laymen refer to as palpitations. Most individuals look upon palpitations in terms of heart consciousness; they are aware of the beating of the heart, which is described as beating with greater force than usual. Often they describe a longer pause than usual between beats, or a series of rapid beats followed by a pause. The sequence of one or more strong beats followed by a slight pause is sometimes indicated on an electrocardiogram, or ECG. Not uncommonly, this condition is produced by a premature beat, one which comes a little ahead of schedule, followed by a compensatory pause, a rest

interval which is longer than usual. Other variations in the heart rate and beat may contribute to the sensation described as palpitation. This may be noted at irregular intervals during the day, sometimes in "bursts." At other times palpitations recur in fairly regular fashion, every minute or two.

Often, palpitations are not a sign of heart disease. They can occur in persons whose heart, blood pressure, and general status are perfectly normal. However surprising or upsetting the sensation may be, there is usually no legitimate cause for worry. Palpitations may sometimes occur as a result of known causes which can be identified. Among these are fatigue and stress, too much smoking, or too much coffee or other stimulants. Palpitations often occur after a period of illness and in convalescence, or following abdominal distention or other digestive upsets. Overindulgence in tobacco, particularly cigarette smoking, may regularly produce skipped beats and other transient disorders, and can be regarded as a warning to cut out smoking. Occasionally persons with this complaint are found to be suffering from some form of heart disease so the problem should not be dismissed without consulting a doctor. (*See* HEARTBEAT, IRREGULAR in the section CARDIO-VASCULAR CONDITIONS.)

Q-63. *I notice large bluish veins over the upper leg, especially after standing. What causes this?*
A. This is probably the condition termed varicose veins. The chief difficulty in varicose veins is that the usual flow of blood through them is reversed. Instead of conducting blood upward toward the heart, the varicose vein often carries it in a reversed direction. The blood is finally siphoned off into the deep veins, and through them it is carried back on up to the heart. Varicose veins have a hereditary aspect, for the condition is sometimes seen in several members of a family.

Mild degrees are not a cause for concern. Women, however, often regard varicose veins as objectionable enough to demand treatment. Elastic stockings, by compressing the varicose veins, may afford relief of pain and diminish the swelling of the legs associated with the varicosities. Very small varicose veins are sometimes injected with a scleros-

ing solution. This is a chemical agent that is injected into a segment of the vein. It produces inflammation and scarring, so that the vein is transformed into a scarred, little vessel.

Often, when the varicose vein is large and extensive, a stripping operation is performed. The segment of the vein is tied off at its upper portion, and through a series of small incisions the entire length of the varicose vein (it may extend from the groin down to the calf) is removed. The operation, of course, offers a total cure by virtue of total removal.

Q-64. *Why does my child throw himself on the floor and then kick and scream?*
A. These are doubtless temper tantrums. Temper tantrums may take various forms and be most disturbing to parents. One is breathholding, in which the child may hold his breath long enough so that he turns purple. More often, the temper tantrums consist of outbursts of stamping, kicking, and crying, with the child seemingly out of control and responding poorly to attempts to admonish or soothe him. Temper tantrums are by no means rare in children.

There are phases in the development of the child during which bouts of negativism are quite common. It is as though the child has sensed that he is an independent human being and is flaunting this fact by saying "no" to all requests, and by indulging in tantrums. Very often, the child is quite unresponsive to persuasion or discipline during the tantrum. One may have to stand by and wait for the tempest to blow itself out. Sometimes the child can be picked firmly off the floor, taken to his own room, and placed on his own bed. One may appropriately sit by the bedside and await the end of the tantrum. Some children will respond to a quiet talking-to, but with others this may be of no value.

Occasionally temper tantrums and breathholding are used as weapons to frighten or blackmail parents into certain kinds of indulgences. Here firmness and consistency are necessary. Once the child learns that the maneuver will not work, and once this fact is increasingly driven home to him, the episodes may end. Sometimes temper tantrums represent an outlet for a sense of dissatisfaction and discontent that has developed within the child. The rivalry with a new baby, jealousy of the attention being given to another child in the family, a feeling of neglect, and the desire to gain attention may be contributing factors. Frequent and prolonged or persistent use of the temper tantrum by the child should lead the thoughtful parent searching for causes and for ways and means of dealing with the problem to consultation with a specialist. (*See* TEMPER TANTRUMS in the section MENTAL HEALTH.)

Q-65. *I often have spells of jumpiness and irritability. What causes this?*
A. Symptoms of this sort are grouped into the category referred to as nervous tensions. By nervous tension most people mean a whole range of subjective sensations, including feeling of inner turmoil, jitters, and irritability. In some individuals the tension is manifested by a feeling of uneasiness, an anticipation that things may go badly. It may be associated with a sinking sensation in the abdomen, sometimes described as "butterflies in the stomach." This sensation, technically known as anxiety, is a fundamental aspect of nervous tension. Therefore, the fundamental question to be asked when someone describes such symptoms is: "What is the cause of the anxiety?"

In this age of physical violence, ranging from threats of worldwide atomic war to assassinations of presidents and all sorts of local acts of violence, many people experience tension caused by anxiety over the possibility of physical damage to themselves and their families. Many of us harbor anxieties generated by concern over the opinions of those about us, that is, fear of their disapproval or criticism. Sometimes our fears may be related to figures in authority, such as a parent, a boss, or a teacher. These examples show that sometimes the cause of tensions can be pinpointed fairly precisely while at other times, in the course of focusing on it and evaluating it, it may be seen by the patient as quite unjustified. Some reduction in anxiety and tension may then occur. What happens in psychotherapy is a prolonged investigation into the causes and origins of anxiety, and it is well established that this process does in fact free many people, to a considerable extent, from many of their nervous tensions.

The reality of many tensions is undeniable, and they may be experienced by many people. For immediate relief, medications are available which will allay the feelings of tension. Originally called sedatives, of which phenobarbital was a well-known early example, more recent drugs are referred to as tranquilizers. The presumed advantage of the tranquilizer is that it diminishes anxiety with relatively little effect on intellectual performance, so that feelings of sleepiness and difficulty in concentration need not be marked. The drugs meprobamate (Miltown®, Equanil®) and Librium® are some of the better-known tranquilizers that have been developed in recent years. Their advantage over old-fashioned phenobarbital is still being debated. Another group of drugs known as the phenothiazine drugs are sometimes referred to as major tranquilizers. They are prescribed for very disturbed states and have been effective in the control of various forms of psychosis, a major mental disturbance.

However, many people find ways and means of reducing their nervous tension without taking drugs. A warm bath or shower, a walk or some other physical activity, various kinds of diversion, all may have a tension-reducing effect. Certainly many people become overweight because they find that eating has a relaxing value for them. Anyone who experiences feelings of nervous tension frequently or repetitively should discuss this with a physician much as he would a fever or any other symptom, with the reasonable expectation that the doctor will be equally ready to treat emotional or psychic complaints. (*See* the section MENTAL HEALTH.)

Q-66. *My grandfather is forgetful and sometimes seems silly. What causes this?*
A. This is most likely the condition referred to as senility. With the markedly increased life span of the United States population in recent decades, more and more elderly individuals are showing an impairment of brain activity. There seems to be little question that most of this is due to changes and losses in brain cells often classed as Alzheimer's disease. The result is a progressive enfeeblement of brain function. It starts off at first with signs of increased forgetfulness, wavering attention, difficulty in concentration, poor

judgment in business and social dealings, negativism and irritability, and poor temper control. This sort of impairment can be somewhat trying on family and friends, but if it progresses no further than this, little difficulty in relations with the aging person is likely to occur.

In some individuals, however, further symptoms begin to appear. These include increased confusion, especially at night; insomnia, with a tendency to reverse the day-night cycle, so that the individual is up at night and drowses during the day; tendencies to wander and perhaps to level unjust accusations at other members of the household. Obviously, senility to this degree is difficult to live with; it also presents safety factors, since the individual may absentmindedly turn on the gas jet and not light it, or wandering off, may get lost.

Sometimes, a "total-push" program involving good nutrition, supplementary vitamins, pleasant stimulation, and encouragement to participate in activities at some level, may bring improvement. When it does not, and when the care of such a patient becomes very trying to the members of the family—as it often does because of the round-the-clock care that may be involved—custodial placement may be advised. This generally means a nursing home, where custodial nursing care and supervision are available. This solution is often difficult for families to face, and sometimes it is only a last resort when patience and strength have been exhausted. (*See* the section AGING.)

GUIDE TO PRESCRIPTION AND OVER THE COUNTER DRUGS

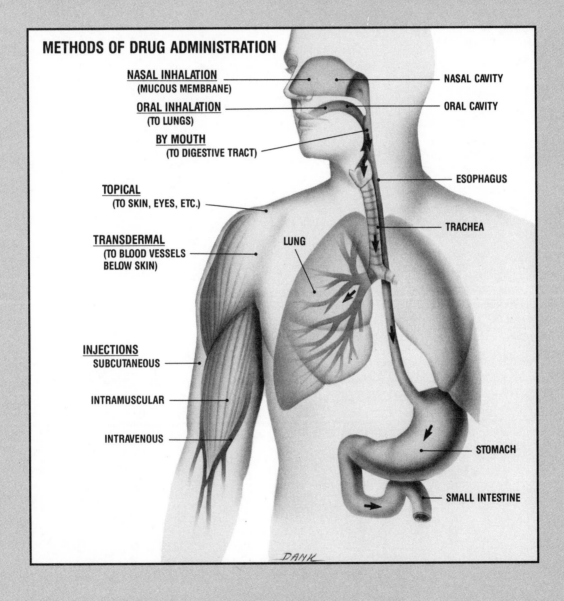

METHODS OF DRUG ADMINISTRATION

NASAL INHALATION (MUCOUS MEMBRANE)

ORAL INHALATION (TO LUNGS)

BY MOUTH (TO DIGESTIVE TRACT)

TOPICAL (TO SKIN, EYES, ETC.)

TRANSDERMAL (TO BLOOD VESSELS BELOW SKIN)

INJECTIONS
SUBCUTANEOUS

INTRAMUSCULAR

INTRAVENOUS

NASAL CAVITY

ORAL CAVITY

ESOPHAGUS

TRACHEA

LUNG

STOMACH

SMALL INTESTINE

DANK

Modern medical practice relies on the availability of drug preparations to provide relief from symptoms and to aid in effecting a cure. Research in various medical specialties has meant that newer, more effective products are constantly being introduced. Regulated by the Federal Drug Administration (FDA), drug products are available either by prescription only or over the counter without a prescription. Drugs that are habit-forming, toxic, or not safe for use except under a doctor's supervision can be dispensed only on prescription. Nonprescription, or over the counter (OTC) drugs, are primarily for symptom relief and can have the same potential for harmful side effects as prescription medications. Patients should ask their physicians and/or pharmacists any questions about the particular medication they are taking.

This section examines common medical conditions and the process for selecting medication. Certain drugs are more effective in treating certain conditions. A physician must weigh a patient's overall physical health in deciding which medicine to prescribe. The layman is often faced with the same choice when selecting over the counter medications for common ailments. This section will explain the drug choices, give some criteria for selection, and identify common side effects. Also discussed is the area of drug abuse, a problem that involves more than just illegal substances.

The following terms are identified in this section:

ABUSE OF DRUGS
ACQUIRED IMMUNE DEFICIENCY
  SYNDROME MEDICATIONS
ALLERGY AND COLD MEDICATIONS
ANALGESICS (PAIN MEDICATIONS)
ANTI-INFECTIVE MEDICATIONS
ARTHRITIS MEDICATIONS
CANCER MEDICATIONS
CARDIOVASCULAR MEDICATIONS

EPILEPSY MEDICATIONS
GASTROINTESTINAL MEDICATIONS
HORMONE REPLACEMENT
  MEDICATIONS
PARKINSON'S DISEASE MEDICATIONS
PSYCHIATRIC MEDICATIONS
RESPIRATORY MEDICATIONS
SUNSCREENS
VITAMINS

An Overview

What are drugs? Do we know how they work? Often when people talk about medications, they speak as though there is something magical or mystical about them. The answers to these questions may not always be firm, but for most medications, we do have a general understanding of how and why they work.

Drugs are chemicals that interact with other chemicals in our bodies. Pharmacologists often refer to some of these body chemicals as receptors. A receptor may be an enzyme, a component of body cells, or some other substance. Medications seem to bind temporarily to the receptor, stimulating or blocking its action.

Ideally a drug would have the desired effect without any undesired effects, or so called side effects; however, this usually is not the case. Side effects may occur because the medication interacts with many different enzymes or receptors or because the targeted receptor has more than one function. More specifically, the receptor functions differently depending on where it is located in the body. When choosing drug therapy the physician weighs the beneficial effects of the drug against the potential for adverse effects. Even medications with severe side effects may be used if the potential for benefit is great.

In the past most medicines were derived from plants or other naturally occurring substances. Often these products were very crude preparations and had varying degrees of potency. As technology improved, active ingredients were identified and isolated. Eventually, medicinal chemists began to alter natural substances or design completely new chemicals in an attempt to improve effectiveness or decrease side effects. Today pharmacologists continue to develop medications that have more specific actions. These extraneous chemicals can cause other side effects since until recently most drugs were foreign substances, not normally found in the body. Consequently, researchers have begun developing drugs which are identical to the body's own chemical regulators. It is likely that the trend toward this approach will continue.

Many factors affect how the body responds to a drug. How the drug is administered, the specific formulation (or drug product, which is the active chemical and other ingredients) used to produce the drug product, certain characteristics of the patient, and what other medications are also taken are important. When a patient takes a medication, many complex processes begin which may be modified by these factors. Drugs given orally, rectally, or intramuscularly must first be absorbed into the blood stream for effect. Once in the blood the drug is affected by the patient's metabolism, excretion, and sensitivity to the desired and undesired effects.

Medications active by mouth must be absorbed in the stomach or intestines for systematic effect. Absorption is affected by the product formulation, or the presence of gastrointestinal disease; with some drugs, the presence of food or other medications may interfere with absorption. The drug's formulation determines how much drug is released from the tablet or capsule and at what rate. Patients with diarrhea or other intestinal disorders may pass the drug before it is completely absorbed, while food or drugs may bind other drugs and thus prevent or hinder absorption. Some drugs are not absorbed by mouth and must be given by injection.

After a drug reaches the blood stream it must reach the site of action in sufficient amounts to attain the desired effect. The concentration of drug in the blood and the length of time the desired concentration is present is determined by the rate at which the patient metabolizes and excretes the drug. These processes can vary greatly between patients, accounting for variability in the drug's effect. Metabolism and excretion can also be modified by underlying medical problems. Drugs metabolized by the liver may be affected by liver disease, while those excreted by the kidney are affected by changes in kidney function. Interacting drugs can also affect metabolism and excretion.

Another important patient characteristic is sensitivity or responsiveness. Patient sensitivity to the actions of the drug may be determined by psychological factors and receptor site affinity for the drug. Some patients may be very sensitive and respond to low levels of the drug, while for other patients the opposite may be the case. Differences in patient sensitivity can also explain differences in occurrence of side effects. Other factors affecting response are the dosage amount, the interval between dosages, and how well the patient complies with the dosage schedule.

The primary difference between prescription and over the counter drugs is the potential for side effects and/or abuse. Some drugs are available both as prescription and over the counter products. When this occurs, the prescription product is usually available in a higher strength. For many common ailments such as uncomplicated colds, allergy symptoms, simple diarrhea, mild aches and pains, nausea and vomiting, and occasional insomnia, treatment with over the counter medication may be just as effective and less expensive.

It must be emphasized that all drugs have desired and undesired effects. It is important to keep this fact in mind when deciding to take any medication. Many side effects are dependent on the dose and can be predicted to occur if a drug is taken in an excessive dose or inappropriately. The following section is designed to explain the method physicians use in making drug selections. It is not intended to be a detailed description of each drug's effects and side effects. For more complete or specific information you should consult your physician, pharmacist, or product literature.

ABUSE OF DRUGS All drugs have some potential for abuse. Patients are known to abuse therapeutic agents such as diuretics, laxatives, pain medications, sedatives, medication for sleep, antibiotics, and steroids. In fact, nearly all of what are considered drugs of abuse have now or at one time had some therapeutic purpose. Problems arise when individuals develop physical or psychological dependence on the drugs or when their social and occupational functioning are impaired by drug use. Patients with physical dependence experience a characteristic set of symptoms when the drug is withheld; the symptoms of withdrawal may vary with different drugs. Some drugs produce no physical dependency but cause an uncontrollable desire for the drug to produce pleasure or avoid discomfort. Collectively, these conditions are referred to as addictive disease.

Drug abuse is found in all social, economic, and cultural groups; drug abuse is not limited to any particular personality type. What causes a person to develop an addiction to a drug is unknown although there is some evidence that a person can be genetically predisposed to addiction, particularly to alcohol.

The commonly abused drugs are hallucinogens, central nervous system stimulants, marijuana products, opioids, CNS depressants, and anticholinergic agents. Prescription, over the counter, recreational, and illicit drugs are included in these classes. In addition, compounds technically not drugs are often abused. Included in this group are solvents, glues, and various other chemicals which can be inhaled.

Abused substances.

Cocaine. The most publicized drug of abuse at this time is cocaine. A CNS stimulant extracted from cocoa leaves, it is available in several forms. Until recently, cocaine hydrochloride was sold as a white powder. Although some people inject the cocaine into a muscle or vein with a syringe, it is most often inhaled or "snorted" into the nose and carried to the bloodstream by the tiny blood vessels in the nose. Used in this way the drug limits its own absorption by shrinking the blood vessels. Slow absorption and dilution with other substances reduce the effect. Cocaine hydrochloride powder cannot be smoked because it decomposes when heated.

"Crack" is a form of cocaine which is more stable upon heating and can be smoked. This form of the drug is prepared by mixing cocaine hydrochloride with water and ammonia, with or without sodium bicarbonate, and heating it to remove the hydrochloride. The result is almost pure cocaine which, when smoked, produces an effect comparable to intravenous administration. Used this way an almost immediate intense effect occurs. However, this feeling of euphoria is short-lived, leading to frequent administration and rapid addiction in susceptible individuals. Other drugs may be abused in an attempt to overcome the cocaine "crash."

Cocaine can cause increased heart rate and blood pressure, seizures, ventricular arrhythmias, and elevated temperature. Anginal pectoris and myocardial infarction may also occur. Death may result from a number of factors, including seizure-induced low blood oxygen concentration. There appears to be great variation in individual response to the drug.

Hallucinogens. Hallucinogens, also called psychedelics, alter mood and perception. The most common of these is lysergic acid diethylamine (LSD). It is usually taken orally and the dosage necessary to produce a "trip" is small compared to other drugs. Flashbacks, recurrences of the LSD experience, may occur days or months later. Drugs in this category cause no true withdrawal syndrome, but patients may require treatment for anxiety and psychotic reactions.

Phencyclidine (PCP). A dissociative anesthetic, phencyclidine (PCP) crosses over a number of categories. According to dosage, it can have the effects of a stimulant, depressant, or hallucinogen. It is usually sprinkled on tobacco or marijuana cigarettes and inhaled.

CNS stimulants. Prescription, over the counter, and illicit drugs are represented in this class. Many of these drugs were once or are now used to manage obesity. Amphetamines, cocaine, methylphenidate, phenmetrazine, and phenylpropanolamine are frequently abused CNS stimulants. Phenylpropanolamine is the active ingredient in over the counter weight control and some cold and allergy products. These drugs cause adverse effects similar to cocaine. Withdrawal from these drugs can result in muscular pains, abdominal pain, chills, tremors, and other physical and psychological symptoms.

Marijuana products. Marijuana, hashish, hash oil, and THC (active ingredient in marijuana) can cause CNS changes. Withdrawal can result in various nonspecific symptoms such as loss of appetite, nausea, insomnia, restlessness, irritability, and anxiety.

Opioids. The most noted drug in this group is heroin, but similar prescription drug products are also abused. The narcotic analgesics morphine, codeine, meperidine, methadone, hydromorphone, opium, pentazocine, and propoxyphen (Darvon® and others) are routinely abused. Illicit drugs in this class may be contaminated with other drugs and unwanted material.

In overdose these drugs can cause respiratory depression, decreased blood pressure, coma, and death. Patients taking these agents will often have constricted pupils. Acute withdrawal may result in dilated pupils, rapid pulse, gooseflesh, abdominal cramps, muscle jerks, "flu" symptoms, vomiting, diarrhea, tremulousness, yawning, and anxiety.

CNS depressants. Alcohol is the oldest member of this group and is the nation's number one drug of abuse. Barbiturates, benzodiazepines (Valium®, Librium®, and others), and other sedative/hypnotic agents are abused CNS depressants. Acute intoxication can result in respiratory depression, drowsiness, coma, and death. Acute withdrawal can result in serious complications and may be life-threatening. Among reported withdrawal symptoms are tremulousness, insomnia, sweating, anxiety, cardiovascular collapse, agitation, delirium, hallucinations, convulsions, and shock. (*See also* ALCOHOLISM in the section MENTAL HEALTH.)

Inhalants. Nitrous oxide (laughing gas), amyl, and other nitrites are occasionally inhaled to attain a euphoric effect. Toluene, a solvent found in glue and paint, may also produce a similar effect along with hallucinations. The abuse of toluene is associated with numerous serious side effects. Other hydrocarbon solvents and gasoline have been used, and are very dangerous.

Signs of drug abuse. A person who is abusing drugs will usually exhibit certain behavior. Parents, spouses, friends, teachers, or employers might suspect a drug problem if the individual:

- changes moods or attitude abruptly
- is frequently late or absent from school or work
- withdraws from family or friends
- loses his or her temper frequently and for no apparent reason
- loses interest in activities which he or she previously enjoyed
- cares less about appearance and personal hygiene
- borrows or steals money from family, friends, school, or employer
- begins associating with a new group of friends, especially if they are known drug users
- becomes secretive about his or her actions and possessions
- has legal problems; for example, arrests for drunken driving, public misconduct.

Not all alcohol or drug abusers will exhibit all of these behaviors. Some behaviors depend on the type of drug that is being abused. However, if there is a pattern or enough indication that a problem exists, a physician or mental health counselor can evaluate the situation and help determine the best approach for confronting the individual about the problem and seeking treatment.

Treatment options. A number of alcohol and drug abuse recovery programs exist. The drug on which the individual is dependent may determine which program will be the most effective. Components of effective drug treatment programs include detoxification, individual counseling, group sessions, and aftercare.

Hospital-based detoxification. Before the drug abuser can begin recovery, use of the drug must cease. Because many drugs cause physical dependency, their withdrawal can have life-threatening effects. For that reason, a hospital setting, where the body's response to detoxification can be carefully monitored, is often required for abusers of alcohol, barbiturates, and other CNS depressants. In addition, some cases require the substitution of another drug that can gradually be withdrawn.

Hospitalization is often advised for those dependent on cocaine, amphetamines, and other stimulants as well. Although withdrawal from these substances is rarely life-threatening and involves less discomfort than many other drugs, users continue to crave the drug and often suffer from bouts of depression.

Detoxification usually lasts five to seven days. During this time patients may be prohibited from any external contact, either through telephone calls or visits.

Inpatient rehabilitation. Inpatient rehabilitation treatment takes about twenty-eight days, although in some cases it may last as long as six months. Patients undergo extensive individual counseling as well as group sessions. Family members may also be expected to spend several days or a week or more at the center. Special counseling sessions are designed to help relatives understand the disease and their role in the patient's recovery.

After rehabilitation, outpatient services may be offered to aid the transition to drug-free living. Counselors usually recommend the individual join Alcoholics Anonymous, Cocaine Anonymous, or Narcotics Anonymous and advise attending one meeting daily for the first ninety days. (*See also* ALCOHOL-ISM; GROUP THERAPY in the section MENTAL HEALTH.)

Outpatient detoxification. Detoxification can be accomplished through outpatient centers for certain drugs. For example, a narcotics user may be able to undergo detoxification on an outpatient basis because withdrawal from narcotics usually is not life-threatening, although it can cause great physical discomfort.

Therapeutic communities. Therapeutic communities offer a drug-free residential environment where the level of support is high and the atmosphere is designed to aid recovery. Detoxification is achieved without the use of any other drugs. Therapeutic communities usually offer long-term programs lasting up to one year.

Self-help programs. Some drug abusers have been able to overcome their problem through membership in Alcoholics Anonymous, Cocaine Anonymous, or Narcotics Anonymous. These organizations offer the recovering substance abusers fellowship and the opportunity to share their experiences. The programs offer twelve steps to recovery, which are recommended actions designed to lead to and maintain sobriety. The programs do not offer medical or psychiatric treatment. Many drug rehabilitation programs are based on the twelve steps created by Alcoholics Anonymous and adapted for Cocaine Anonymous and Narcotics Anonymous. (*See also* ADDICTION in the section MENTAL HEALTH.)

ACQUIRED IMMUNE DEFICIENCY SYNDROME (AIDS) MEDICATIONS

The drugs administered to patients with acquired immune deficiency syndrome (AIDS) are primarily for the treatment or prevention of parasitic, fungal, viral, or bacterial infections. Only one drug is currently marketed as an anti-HIV (Human Immunodeficiency Virus) drug, but several are under investigation. These patients often develop infections from organisms which are not commonly seen in patients with a normal immune system. Many of the drugs used to treat these infections have severe side effects which may interfere with the patient's therapy. Some drug side effects appear to occur more frequently and with greater severity in patients with AIDS than in others. Complications of AIDS may also influence how drugs may be given. Patients with decreased blood platelets may bruise easily if given intramuscular injections. A chronic diarrhea condition may affect drug absorption, and diarrhea may also cause dehydration which may favor the development of toxic blood concentration of drugs in the patient.

Parasitic infections. Pneumocystis carinii is an ameba-like parasite that can cause pneumonia in any patient with a defective immune system. However, Pneumocystis carinii pneumonia (PCP) appears to be more difficult to manage in patients with AIDS. Patients are usually treated with intravenous trimethoprim/sulfamethoxazole (Bactrim®, Septra®) for twenty-one days. Patients with AIDS appear to have a higher incidence and increased severity of side effects when taking this drug. An alternative agent is pentamidine (Pentam®). Pentamidine may be used intravenously to treat PCP or given by inhalation to prevent recurrence.

Infections from toxoplasma gondii (toxoplasmosis) are usually managed with sulfadiazine plus pyrimethamine. Sulfadiazine is an older sulfonamide antibiotic and requires good fluid intake to prevent kidney damage from crystalization in the urine. Patients may also develop cryptosporidium diarrheal infections. This organism does not respond well to anti-infective agents. Diarrhea is managed with fluids, electrolytes, and standard anti-diarrhea agents.

Fungal infections. Infections from Candida species, histoplasmosis, and coccidioidomycosis may respond to amphotericin B (Fungizone®) and/or ketoconazole (Nizoral®). Cryptococosis is usually treated with amphotericin B, but many patients may also receive flucytosine (Ancobon®).

Bacterial infections. Patients may become infected by any known bacteria, requiring the necessary antibiotic therapy. Some bacteria such as salmonella, streptococcus pneumoniae, and tuberculosis and tuberculosis-related organisms are commonly seen in AIDS patients. These infections are treated with standard antibiotics. Atypical tuberculosis-related infections may be difficult to treat, however. Ansamycin (investigational), clofazamine (Lamprene®), ethionamide (Trecator-SC®) and standard antituburcular drugs have been used to treat these organisms.

Viral infections. Infections with herpes zoster virus (shingles) and cytomegalovirus (CMV) are common. Herpes zoster responds to acyclovir (Zovirax®) and vidarabine (Vira-A®). Cytomegalovirus may be more difficult to treat. Combination therapy with vidarabine and acyclovir or other drugs have not altered the high mortality rate seen with this infection. Gancylovir (Cytovene®) has been recently approved by the FDA for the treatment of CMV infections of the retina. Its effectiveness has not been well established to date.

HIV infection. Zidovudine (Retrovir®), more commonly known as AZT, is currently the only drug marketed for the treatment of HIV infections. AZT is a semisynthetic thymidine analog which is used by the HIV virus instead of normal thymidine resulting in inhibition of viral DNA. The virus is more susceptible to the effects of AZT than are the cells in the patient's body. Patients taking AZT have an increase in the number of immune cells and improved function of the cells which have been affected by HIV. Studies comparing AZT to placebo (fake medicine) have shown a reduction in mortality rates.

AZT can cause serious side effects, however. Patients often develop anemia, reduced white blood cell counts, and decreased platelet counts. These effects are related to the dose and duration of treatment. Other side effects have also been reported. AZT is very expensive, a fact that has generated controversy. Other drugs similar to AZT are being investigated, as are drugs which modulate the immune response, as do interleukin-2 and alpha-interferon. To date no drug has been found to destroy the HIV virus.

ALLERGY AND COLD MEDICATIONS

There are literally hundreds of over the counter (OTC) medications which could be used to treat hay fever (allergic rhinitis) symptoms. The large number of products available, variously labeled indications for products with the same active ingredients, and the use of imprecise or misleading terminology by manufacturers can make product selection difficult. However, with just a little basic information, interpreting manufacturer's claims and list of ingredients can be made quite simple.

Products marketed for the treatment of hay fever and symptoms of the common cold can be very similar or even identical. Manufacturers may market identical products for either condition or for both conditions. A typical label may state that the product is beneficial for the treatment of hay fever, sinus headache, itchy eyes, and cold symptoms. Medication marketed for the treatment of symptoms of the common cold can be used to treat hay fever symptoms in most cases and may only differ by the addition of a cough suppressant, an ingredient often not required by hay fever sufferers. OTC medications marketed for the treatment of hay fever or other upper respiratory allergy symptoms usually contain an antihistamine, and/or a decongestant, and often an analgesic (pain reliever). These products are designed to treat the common symptoms of hay fever which include nasal discharge, itchy nose and eyes, watering and redness of eyes, nasal congestion, associated pain, and sneezing.

Antihistamines. Histamine is a substance released during allergic reactions and is responsible for many of the symptoms of hay fever. The FDA's OTC drug advisory panel has concluded that antihistamines are effective in treating runny nose, sneezing or itching of the nose or throat, and itchy, watery eyes. Any

LIST OF COMMON INGREDIENTS FOUND IN OTC
HAY FEVER REMEDIES

Antihistamines

Chemical Name	Brand Name	Ingredient In
Chlorpheniramine maleate	Chlor-Trimeton® and others	Various Products
Diphenhydramine HCL	Benadryl®	Benadryl® Complete Allergy and others
Triprolidine HCL	Actidil®	Actifed®
Pyrilamine maleate		Ursinus® inlay-tabs
Dexbrompheniramine maleate		Drixoral® and others
Brompheniramine maleate	Dimetane®	Dimetapp® Extentabs
Phenenindamine tartrate	Nolahist®	

Decongestants

Chemical Name	Brand Name	Ingredient In
Pseudoephedrine HCL	Sudafed®	Actifed® and others
Pseudoephedrine Sulfate	Afrinol Repetabs®	Chlor-Trimeton® decongestant and others
Phenylpropanolamine HCL		Comtrex® and others
Phenylephrine HCL	Neo-Synephrine®	Dristan® Advanced Formula and others

Analgesics

Chemical Name	Brand Name	Ingredient In
Aspirin	Vanquish® and others	Coricidin® Tablets and others
Acetaminophen	Tylenol® and others	Sinutab® Tablets and others

ANTIHISTAMINE CLASSIFICATION AND
SIDE EFFECT RATING

	Sedative Rating	Anticholinergic Rating
Class One		
Diphenhydramine HCL	+ + +	+ + +
Class Two		
Pyrilamine maleate	+	0
Class Three		
Triprolidine HCL	+	+ +
Chlorpheniramine maleate	+	+ +
Brompheniramine maleate	+	+ +
Dexbrompheniramine maleate	+	+ +
Miscellaneous		
Phenindamine tartrate	0	+ +

of these drugs are equally effective, but they may differ in side effects.

The most common side effect encountered with the use of antihistamines is drowsiness. In fact, antihistamines are often used as over the counter sleep aids. There is some variability in the severity of this effect from one class of antihistamine to another. (*See* Chart) Some experimenting with the various classes of antihistamines may identify the one which works best for you. Drowsiness may become less severe with continued use or if nonsedating products like Seldane® or Hismanal® are used. Products containing an antihistamine may be labeled "nighttime formula." These drugs can also cause blurred vision, urinary retention, and drying of the mucous membranes—side effects which also may vary between classes. (*See* Chart) These side effects are due to the anticholinergic action of antihistamine. As a result of their anticholinergic activity, patients with narrow angle glaucoma should not take antihistamines without the supervision of a physician.

Antihistamines are more effective if they are used chronically (steadily over a period of time) rather than sporadically (only an occasional dose) and if begun early in the hay fever season.

Decongestants. This group of drugs is used to reduce nasal congestion and may be sold separately or combined with an antihistamine. They are also sold for use in the nose as drops or sprays, and to be taken by mouth.

Oral decongestants, such as pseudoephedrine (Sudafed®) and phenylpropanolamine, are effective and are commonly sold combined with antihistamines. Side effects of decongestants include central nervous system stimulation and inability to sleep. For this reason products containing a decongestant without the addition of an antihistamine are often labeled "daytime formula." Patients with high blood pressure, heart disease, and diabetes should take these drugs only under the supervision of their physician.

Nose drops and nasal sprays are effective in reducing nasal congestion if used for a short period of time. However, if used more than three or four days these agents may cause rebound nasal congestion or a reverse of the desired effect. The longer acting products, such as oxymetazoline and xylometazoline hydro-

chloride, are less likely to cause this problem. If a nasal spray is used it is important for you to be in an upright position. Spray each nostril once. Wait three to five minutes; if you are still congested, blow your nose and spray each nostril once again. By waiting you allow your lower nasal passages to become less congested, thus allowing the second spray to reach the higher passages.

Analgesics. Some combination products contain an analgesic for the treatment of hay fever-associated headache or sinus pain. Either aspirin or acetaminophen (aspirin substitute) may be used, but acetaminophen is the analgesic most often found in combination products. While these two drugs are similar in their effectiveness, they differ in their side effects. Aspirin use is associated with more side effects, such as stomach irritation, than is acetaminophen. Nevertheless, acetaminophen should not be used chronically without consulting a physician, for long term use has been associated with liver damage, especially in alcoholic patients.

Manufacturers are limited by the number of decongestants, antihistamines, and analgesics available for use in OTC hay fever products. For this reason most products are very similar and may only differ in the presence or absence of one of the primary ingredients, either an antihistamine, a decongestant, or an analgesic. There may be some variation in side effects produced, based on the sufferer's sensitivities and the type of antihistamine or decongestant included in the product's formulation. You should refer to the product's label for more detailed list of side effects and restrictions. If you have any further questions, ask your physician or pharmacist for assistance.

Cough medications. There are many prescription and over the counter products available for the treatment of cough. Many of these products are combinations containing an antihistamine, a decongestant, and often an analgesic. They may also be combined with other cough-relieving drugs or available as a single drug.

Medications used to treat cough may be classified as antitussives (cough suppressants), expectorants (increase mucus excretion), hydrating medications (steam, vaporized products), and nonmedicated products. Cough drops, lozenges, rock candy, and horehound drops are commonly used nonmedicated medications.

A cough can result from various conditions involving the respiratory tract or other body systems. Most coughs are self limiting and often may not require any treatment beyond increased fluid intake. Nevertheless, most coughs are treated with some type of medication. Taking an antitussive usually does not result in any complications if the cough is nonproductive (does not result in expulsion of material) and due to mild respiratory infection or a cold. However, productive coughs generally should not be treated with antitussives, for they may interfere significantly with the resolution of the underlying disease. Additionally, narcotic cough suppressant drugs are rarely prescribed for infants, and used cautiously in children.

Available antitussive drugs may work through the central nervous system or the cough receptors in the respiratory tract. The most potent products are narcotics and usually require a prescription. However, codeine is available over the counter with certain restrictions. Several non-narcotic drugs are also available without prescription. The most commonly used non-narcotic antitussive agent is dextromethorphan. Products containing this drug are usually distinguished by the use of a "D" or "DM" as part of the trade name. Nonnarcotic medications are usually associated with few side effects when used as directed. All of these agents work through the central nervous system, while menthol and local anesthetics (Tessalon®, others) work locally within the respiratory tract.

The most commonly used expectorant is guaifenesin (Robitussin®, others), but others are available. These drugs enjoy widespread use, but their efficacy has not been well established. This is especially true of terpin hydrate, which is generally regarded to be ineffective.

When using any cough relieving medication, careful attention should be given to the manufacturer's instructions and cautions.

Eye drops. Various products are available by prescription or over the counter for the treatment of eye irritations and allergic reactions, such as allergies. Products available contain antihistamines, decongestants, as-

tringents (zinc sulfate), lubricants, or combinations of these medicines. Over the counter products, such as Visine® and Murine®, contain a decongestant which whitens the eye. A large number of lubricant products are available which are usually referred to as artificial tears (Liquifilm Tears®, Tearisol®, others). The product literature should be consulted for reported side effects and contraindications.

ANALGESICS (PAIN MEDICATIONS)

Analgesics are used to treat acute and chronic pain. The treatment of acute pain is usually easily prescribed, but the management of chronic pain may be difficult and perplexing.

All pain is a subjective response to a stimulus. It is modified by body chemicals, internalized social and cultural factors, physiological, and psychological factors. Acute pain is primarily associated with tissue injury and functions as a protective mechanism. Nevertheless, acute pain can actually be harmful, as may be the case after a heart attack, when the body's responses to pain may increase heart muscle damage.

Pain lasting for more than six months is considered by some physicians to be chronic pain. Chronic pain may also be defined as pain persisting after the disease has been cured or the injury healed. It is thought that patients with this problem continue to have the pain response because of psychological factors, such as depression and anxiety. For these patients, pain may not be a simple response to a stimulus, but more like hunger or thirst. A hunger disorder leads to obesity, while a pain disorder leads to chronic pain syndrome. Patients with chronic pain often do not respond to conventional therapy, such as analgesics. Seeking pain relief, they often confer with numerous physicians, undergo various surgical procedures, and try many strong analgesics, tranquilizers, and other agents.

The treatment of cancer pain also may be difficult. Unlike patients with chronic pain syndrome who respond poorly to increasing doses of analgesics, cancer patients often have analgesics inappropriately withheld because of the fear of addiction. Analgesics may be given in insufficient doses or at too long an interval between doses. Cancer patients often require large doses given at fixed intervals.

Administering these drugs only as needed often results in treatment failure.

Selection. Pain relieving medications can be classified in several ways. One of the most common ways is as prescription or non-prescription analgesics. Non-prescription pain relievers are mild analgesics with relatively few side effects and low potential for abuse. These drugs are preferred for treatment of common causes of mild to moderate pain. Prescription analgesics have greater side effects and/or potential for abuse and are reserved for patients with severe pain. While all analgesics may be abused to some degree, narcotic medications have the greatest potential for abuse.

When selecting an analgesic, the physician must consider the cause of the patient's pain, the patient's other medical problems, and the severity of the pain. Mild to moderate pain associated with inflammation may respond best to an analgesic with anti-inflammatory properties, such as aspirin or another non-steroidal anti-inflammatory drug (NSAID). Other types of mild pain, such as headache, may be treated with either aspirin or acetaminophen, an analgesic without anti-inflammation properties. However, acetaminophen may be preferred if the patient has a history of stomach ulcers or another condition worsened by NSAIDS. Severe pain associated with trauma, surgery, or cancer usually will require a narcotic analgesic for relief.

Additional factors considered in the selection of analgesic therapy are the onset and duration of drug effect, the patient's past response to drug therapy, and whether the pain is acute or chronic. Narcotic analgesics are avoided in patients with chronic pain syndrome because they are addicting and often not effective.

Recently new methods of administering oral and intravenous narcotics have been developed to increase the convenience and effectiveness. Morphine is now available in oral sustained release dosage forms, reducing the number of doses administered per day. Patient-controlled intravenous analgesia is now possible with programmable infusion pumps. These pumps allow the patient to administer his/her own intravenous medication in response to discomfort. This method of administration is very effective for relieving acute surgical pain. Portable infusion pumps are also available, allowing patients to become ambulatory earlier after surgery. These pumps can also be used to give constant infusions of narcotics to ambulatory cancer patients, those not confined to a bed.

Types of medications.

Non-steroidal anti-inflammatory agents (NSAIDS). Various NSAIDS are available as prescription and non-prescription analgesics. Aspirin and other drugs in this class are effective in treating mild to moderate pain, especially if there is inflammation. Aspirin may be combined with codeine or other narcotics for the treatment of moderate to severe pain. These drugs, when not combined with a narcotic, have a low potential for abuse. Nevertheless, NSAIDS can cause serious side effects, most commonly gastrointestinal conditions. NSAIDS may interact with other medications such as "blood thinners" and diuretics. Aspirin should not be administered to children, because of its association with Reye's syndrome.

Acetaminophen. Acetaminophen (Tylenol®, Datril® and others) is one of the most commonly used drugs for the treatment of mild pain. It too may be combined with a narcotic when a stronger analgesic effect is required. Acetaminophen is often touted as being safer than aspirin. While it does not commonly cause the gastrointestinal and bleeding side effects seen with aspirin, it is not necessarily safer. Acetaminophen is associated with severe liver damage when taken in overdose. Liver toxicity has also been reported in patients taking the drug in high doses for prolonged periods of time. This is especially true in alcoholic patients. Acetaminophen has no anti-inflammatory effects.

Propoxyphene (Darvon® and others). Propoxyphene hydrochloride and propoxyphene napsylate (Darvon-N®) are commonly prescribed alone or combined with aspirin or acetaminophen. These products may be no more effective than aspirin when taken in recommended doses.

Narcotic analgesics. Narcotic analgesics are thought to work in a manner similar to the body's own analgesics. Morphine and codeine were the earliest narcotic analgesics extracted from opium. Morphine is the most potent of these two agents and is used to treat severe pain associated with trauma, surgery, and cancer. Morphine is poorly absorbed when administered by mouth and is most effective when injected into a muscle or given intravenously. Codeine, while available as an injection, is most commonly administered by mouth combined with aspirin or acetaminophen. Both of these drugs are associated with constipation, nausea and vomiting, sedation, respiratory depression, and hypotension upon standing.

In an attempt to make more potent narcotic analgesics, manufacturers have modified the morphine and codeine molecules or developed synthetic derivatives. Fentanyl (Sublimase®), sufentanil (Sufenta®), and alfentanil (Alfenta®) are very potent agents used for surgical analgesia. Modifications have also resulted in better effectiveness when medication is taken by mouth. Hydromorphine (Dilaudid®), levorphanol (Levo-Dromoran®), oxymorphone (Numorphan®), and methadone (Dolophine®) are all potent narcotic analgesics effective orally. Oxycodone (various manufacturers) is usually prescribed combined with aspirin or acetaminophen for the treatment of moderate to moderately severe pain.

Meperidine (Demerol®) is a commonly used narcotic analgesic. However, it is not a very potent agent when taken by mouth and may lead to central nervous system toxicity when used for extended periods in patients with renal disease.

All narcotic analgesics can cause respiratory depression and dependence. Respiratory depression can be reversed with an injection of naloxone (Narcan®). While the potential for addiction is a limiting factor in the use of these agents, it should not prevent their use in patients with chronic cancer pain.

Narcotic agonist/antagonist. These drugs were developed to overcome some of the side effects encountered with narcotic agents. Pentazocine (Talwin®), butorphanol (Stadol®), nalbuphine (Nubain®) and buprenorphine (Buprenex®) cause less respiratory depression than narcotic drugs and have less potential for abuse. Unlike narcotic analgesics which cause a feeling of well being, these agents may cause behavior changes and unpleasant feelings. Narcotic agonist/antagonist can cause narcotic withdrawal when given to patients with narcotic dependence.

Anti-spasm medications. Although not technically analgesics, skeletal muscle relaxants are usually prescribed for relief of pain associated with involuntary contraction of a muscle group (spasm). Muscle spasm can result from many conditions, including muscle strains and minor injuries. Often these problems are selflimiting and respond to non-drug therapies such as rest and physical therapy. Carisoprodol (Rela®, Soma®), chlorphenesin (Maolate®), chlorzoxazone (Paraflex®), methocarbamol (Delaxin®, Robaxin®), orphenadrine (Norflex®), and cyclobenzaprine (Flexeril®) are frequently prescribed skeletal muscle relaxants. None of these agents has been shown to be any more effective than analgesic or anti-inflammatory medication.

These drugs are associated with various side effects, but the most commonly encountered adverse effect is sedation.

ANTI-INFECTIVE MEDICATIONS (ANTIBIOTICS, ANTIFUNGAL, AND OTHER AGENTS)

Anti-infective drugs are those drugs used to treat bacterial, fungal, viral, and parasitic infections. The development of effective antibacterial, antifungal, antiparasitic, and antiviral drugs with relatively few side effects is a continuing challenge to medical scientists. The use and abuse of penicillin and other older antibiotics has led to the emergence of antibiotic-resistant strains of organisms. Life support systems used to prolong life also have affected the types of organisms infecting hospitalized patients. The use of immunosuppressive drugs to treat cancer and/or prevent organ transplant rejection has resulted in infections from organisms previously unknown to cause or rarely cause infection. For these reasons the need for newer, more effective agents continues, as does the cost of treatment.

Selection. The selection of an appropriate anti-infective drug requires an in depth knowledge of the signs and symptoms of various infections, microbiology, and pharmacology.

If the patient has signs and symptoms of infection, the physician first must determine the site of the infection. This may be done with various diagnostic procedures, laboratory studies, and a physical examination. Once the site of the infection is determined, it is often possible to grow and identify the organism.

The identified organism's drug sensitivity may then be determined by the microbiology laboratory. It is not uncommon for two different organisms to be isolated from two separate sites or from the same site. Once the sensitivities of the organism(s) are known, the physician can develop a list of possible anti-infective choices. Final selection will be based on the patient's known drug allergies, the drug's potential for side effects, and the drug's ability to attain effective concentrations at the site of infection. If no organism can be isolated, the physician will select the single drug or drug combination most likely to be active against all the organisms generally known to infect the suspected site. This is referred to as a broad spectrum empiric therapy.

The usual infecting organisms will vary not only with site but also with the patient's clinical situation. Chronic pulmonary disease, diabetes, cystic fibrosis, alcoholism, cancer, and immunosuppression are among many medical problems predisposing patients to infection by certain organisms. Recent surgery, exposure history, and whether the infection was acquired at home or in the hospital are also factors considered in the selection of the appropriate drug.

The above principles apply more specifically to the selection of antibiotics than other anti-infective agents. Antiviral and antiparasitic agents are rarely administered empirically, nor are antifungal agents, with the exception of feverish patients with very low white blood cell counts not responding to empiric antibiotic therapy.

Decisions on the length of therapy, whether to give the drug by mouth or by injection, and whether to hospitalize the patient are dependent on the severity and location of the infection. Uncomplicated urinary tract infection, bronchitis, and other mild infections may be treated at home with oral antibiotics. Other more serious infections, such as pneumonia or meningitis, may require hospitalization. Most infections are treated for seven to ten days;

however, infections of the bones, brain, and heart valves require a longer treatment period. Hard to treat organisms may also require longer therapy.

Antibiotics are not only used to treat infections. Clinical studies have found that certain antibiotics prevent infections if given just prior to surgery. The drugs of choice for numerous surgeries are well established.

Antibiotics. The term antibiotic often is used to indicate any anti-bacterial agent, man-made or naturally occurring. Technically, antibiotics are compounds derived from microorganisms that suppress the growth of or kill other microorganisms. A large percentage of the antibiotic drugs used today are naturally occurring compounds produced by fungi. Penicillin is produced from a common mold found in every home. Some antibiotics are semisynthetic derivatives of natural compounds. Other drugs referred to as antibiotics, as are the so called sulpha drugs, are actually man-made chemicals.

Antibiotics can be grouped using various classifications, but for the purpose of this discussion the following general classes will be used: penicillins, cephalosporins, erythromycins, aminoglycosides, tetracyclines, sulphonamides, fluoroquinolones, and miscellaneous antibiotics. These drugs are used to treat infections caused by three types of organisms: gram positive, gram negative, and anaerobic bacteria. Gram (negative or positive) simply indicates whether or not the organism's cell wall is colored by a special laboratory stain. Anaerobic organisms are those that grow without oxygen. They may be either gram negative or gram positive.

Penicillins. There are four general types of penicillin antibiotics: natural penicillins, aminopenicillins, anti-staphylococcal, and extended spectrum penicillins. All drugs in this class interfere with bacterial cell wall synthesis. Natural penicillins, such as penicillin G, penicillin V and procaine penicillin G, are most active against gram positive organisms. Many staphylococcus and Neisseria gonorrhaeae, while once very sensitive to natural penicillins, have developed resistance to them. Resistance is usually due to the production of an enzyme (penicillinase) that destroys penicillin. Nevertheless, penicillin remains effective treatment for many streptococcal infections and syphilis. The major side effects encountered with natural and other penicillins are allergic or hypersensitivity reactions. These reactions on occasion may be life threatening. Patients with a history of true penicillin allergy should not receive penicillin. However, if it does become necessary to use one of these agents under this circumstance, it is possible to desensitize a patient.

Anti-staphylococcal penicillins, methicillin (Staphcillin®), nafcillin (Unipen®), dicloxacillin (Dynapen®), and oxicillin (Prostaphlin®) were developed to be more resistant to penicillinase. Methicillin was the first agent produced, but because of its more frequent association with kidney damage it is now rarely used. Only a few Staphylococcus aureus organisms remain sensitive to penicillin G. Nevertheless, resistance is now developing to anti-staph agents and may be a significant problem in some hospitals. Methicillin-resistant Staph. aureus (MRSA) infections are treated with vancomycin.

Semisynthetic aminopenicillins were developed to increase gram negative activity. Ampicillin (various manufacturers) and amoxicillin (Amoxil®, and others) are aminopenicillins with good activity against many gram-negative microorganisms. Amoxicillin is closely related to ampicillin, but it has several advantages which may make it the preferred agent of this class. It may be given less frequently and may cause less diarrhea.

Neither natural nor aminopenicillins are active against the clinically important organism Pseudomonas aeruginosa. Pursuit of an effective agent resulted in the development of extended spectrum penicillins. These drugs are highly active against many gram-positive, gram negative, and anaerobic bacteria, but they are ineffective against penicillinase-producing staphylococci and some gram negative organisms that produce penicillinase. Carbenicillin (Geopen®) was the first agent in this class, but it is less frequently used today to treat serious systemic infections. However, carbenicillin indanyl sodium, an oral form of carbenicillin, is used by some physicians to treat certain urinary tract infections. More commonly used, ticarcillin (Ticar®), mezlocillin (Mezlin®), and piperacillin (Pipracil®), are all effective in treating se-

rious P. aeruginosa infections when combined with an aminoglycoside antibiotic. Drugs in this class are associated with bleeding problems, low blood potassium, seizures in certain patients at risk, and those side effects seen with other penicillins.

Recently inhibitors of penicillinase have been developed. The products which are available are combinations of a penicillin and a penicillinase inhibitor. Ticarcillin plus clavulanate (Timentin®) and amoxicillin plus clavulanate (Augmentin®) are combinations of a penicillin with the penicillinase inhibitor potassium clavulanate. The addition of the inhibitor extends the activity of both penicillins. Ampicillin combined with the penicillinase inhibitor sulbactam (Unasyn®) is also available. It is anticipated that many of the antibiotic/penicillinase inhibitor combinations will be available in the future.

Cephalosporins. Cephalosporin antibiotics compose a large class of drugs which are highly marketed by drug manufacturers. These drugs inhibit bacteria cell wall synthesis as do all β-lactam antibiotics (penicillins, cephalosporins, cephamycins, carbapenems, and monobactams). These drugs are indicated for the treatment of various gram-positive, gram-negative and anaerobic infections and for the prevention of surgical infections. Unlike penicillins, cephalosporins are less likely to be associated with allergic reactions. Low side effect potential, broad spectrum activity, and increased marketing have made this the most highly used class of antibiotics. They are also among the most expensive. Development of new cephalosporins is targeted toward agents with an increased spectrum of activity and decreased dosing frequency..

Erythromycin. Various erythromycin salts are available. This drug is the drug of choice for the treatment of Mycoplasma pneumoniae (walking pneumonia) and Legionnaires disease. Erythromycin is commonly used to treat community acquired gram positive infections in patients allergic to penicillin. Gastrointestinal irritation is the most common side effect reported; diarrhea, abdominal pain and cramping, nausea and vomiting are common. Liver toxicity has been reported with its use, especially with the estolate salt. Erythromycin may interact with other drugs, such as theophylline and cyclosporine, resulting in increased side effects of these drugs.

Aminoglycosides. These drugs are very active against many gram-negative bacteria. They are primarily used to treat serious infections. Gentamicin (various manufacturers) was the first clinically useful agent for the treatment of Pseudomonas aeruginosa infections. Tobramycin (Nebcin®) and amikacin (Amikin®) are other agents commonly used. Other agents in this class (kanamycin, streptomycin, netilmicin) are less frequently used. Aminoglycosides are very effective agents, but they are also toxic. Safe use of gentamicin, tobramycin, and amikacin requires monitoring of blood concentration to avoid kidney and hearing damage.

Tetracyclines. Tetracycline (various manufacturers), oxytetracycline (Terramycin®), chlortetracycline (Aureomycin®), demeclocycline (Declomycin®), doxycycline (Vibramycin®), methacycline (Rondomycin®), and minocycline (Minocin®) are currently available tetracyclines. These drugs are useful in the treatment of many sexually transmitted diseases. They are also effective for treating brucellosis, Rocky Mountain spotted fever, tularemia (rabbit fever), Lyme disease, and cholera. Doxycycline is useful for the prevention of traveler's diarrhea. Tetracyclines commonly cause gastrointestinal irritation, which may be reduced if the medication is taken with food. However, these drugs should not be taken with milk or certain antacids. Tetracyclines should not be given to pregnant women or patients younger than eight years of age.

Sulfonamides. Sulfonamides are often referred to as sulfa drugs. Many agents in this class were commonly used in the past, but only a few continue to be used for systemic administration. The most common agent used is a combination of sulfamethoxazole and trimethoprim (Bactrim® and Septra®). When combined in the correct ratio, these two agents work together against many gram-positive and gram-negative bacteria. This combination is effective in treating many gastrointestinal, urinary, and respiratory tract infections. Trimethoprim-sulfamethoxazole (TMP-SMX) is useful in the treatment and prevention of Pneumocystis carinii pneumonia in AIDS and other immune deficient patients. This drug is, however, associated with allergic reactions and bone marrow suppression. TMP-SMX is contraindicated during pregnancy. All sulfonamide agents are known to interact with certain other drugs which may require that dosage adjustment be made.

Fluoroquinolones. Norfloxacin (Noroxin®) and ciprofloxacin (Cipro®) are members of this newer class of anti-infective agents. These drugs have a broad spectrum of activity and may be administered by mouth. They are active against many gram-positive and gram-negative organisms, including Pseudomonas aeruginosa.

Antituberculous agents. Isoniazid (various manufacturers), rifampin (Rifadin®, Rimactane®), streptomycin, ethambutol (Myambutol®), and pyrazinamide are the most commonly used antituberculous agents, although others are available. These agents may be used singularly or in combination depending on the clinical circumstances. Isoniazid, which may be used for treatment or prevention, is associated with many side effects.

Other antibiotics. Vancomycin (various manufacturers) is an agent which is being used more frequently. This increased use is primarily due to the emergence of methicillin resistant staphylococcal infections. It is also used as a substitute for penicillin in patients with penicillin allergy. Vancomycin is the drug of choice for the treatment of Clostridium difficile induced diarrhea. Older, more impure preparations of vancomycin were associated with kidney and hearing problems; however, newer products appear to be safer. Nevertheless, a unique problem called the "red man" syndrome persists. Patients develop itching and a rash involving the face, neck, and upper torso during vancomycin injections. This reaction can be avoided by slow infusion of the drug.

Chloramphenicol (various manufacturers) is less commonly used today because of its potential for causing serious bone marrow toxicity. However, it is still an important agent in the management of typhoid fever.

Clindamycin (Cleocin®) is primarily used to treat abdominal, pelvic, and pulmonary infections when anaerobic organisms are identified or suspected. It is often combined with an aminoglycoside.

Imipenem/cilastatin (Primaxin®) is the first carbapenem antibiotic available. This drug has the broadest spectrum of activity of any available antibiotic. It is effective against gram-positive, gram-negative (including P. aeruginosa), and anaerobic organisms. Cilastatin is combined with imipenem to prevent its degradation by the kidneys. This drug may cause seizures if given in high doses, especially in patients with a pre-existing seizure disorder.

Aztreonam (Azactam®) is the first monobactum antibiotic available. It is primarily active against gram-negative organisms. Presently this agent is felt to be useful in patients with unstable kidney function who are sensitive to all penicillins or cephalosporin-like antibiotics.

Antiviral and antifungal agents. Several antiviral agents are available for the treatment of influenza A, herpes simplex, herpes zoster, cytomegalovirus, HIV and other viruses. Products are available for systemic and local infections. Many of these agents are associated with severe side effects.

The most useful antifungal agent for systemic fungal infections is amphotericin B (Fungizone®). This drug is active against many fungal organisms. Intravenous administration of amphotericin B is associated with various side effects, including kidney damage. Other agents are available for systemic and topical use.

ARTHRITIS MEDICATIONS Rheumatoid arthritis, juvenile rheumatoid arthritis, and osteoarthritis are common medical problems. These chronic systemic inflammatory diseases can inflict severe pain, disability, and loss of time from work. Drug treatment is directed toward reducing the inflammatory process. The objective of therapy is to relieve the symptoms and improve quality of life. Drug treatment may delay, but will not prevent, the progression of the disease process.

Selection. A nonsteroidal anti-inflammatory agent (NSAID) is the drug of first choice for each of these conditions. NSAIDs are analgesics with anti-inflammatory properties. (*See also* ANALGESICS in this section.) The most commonly used NSAID is aspirin. Aspirin, a salicylate, is the drug to which all other NSAIDs are compared. It is the least expensive NSAID available. Some patients are not able to tolerate the high doses of aspirin

needed for treating arthritis. At these dose levels, patients may develop gastrointestinal side effects. Other salicylates used do not cause many of the adverse effects associated with aspirin. These agents also do not affect platelet function and are less likely to cause bleeding than is aspirin or newer NSAIDs. However, some physicians question their effectiveness.

Newer NSAIDs are as effective as aspirin and cause fewer gastrointestinal side effects. Consequently they may be selected as initial therapy by some physicians. Of the many NSAIDs available, no one has been shown to be more effective than another. Nonetheless, some patients may respond to one agent but not another. All of these agents can cause essentially the same side effects, and the choice for the safest agent may be a matter of opinion. Acetaminophen does not have anti-inflammatory properties, and theoretically, it should not relieve pain associated with the inflammatory process.

Patients with osteoarthritis not responding to a NSAID usually receive no further systemic treatment, but they may be given injections of glucocorticoids into the problem joint. Frequent use of steroid injections can lead to overuse of the joint and other problems, and should be avoided.

Patients with other forms of arthritis not responding to NSAIDs are given second-line drugs. All of these drugs have a potential to cause severe side effects. Although these agents do not cause immediate relief of pain, they may slow the progression of the disease. Selection of the second agent can depend on many factors. In general, drugs which are most likely to be tolerated are used initially. Depending on the patient's clinical response and development of side effects, therapy may be changed or other agents added to the regimen.

Types of medication.
Salicylates. Aspirin, sodium salicylate, salsalate (Disalcid® and others), magnesium salicylate (Magan®, Mobidin®), choline salicylate (Arthropan®), diflunisal (Dolobid®) and choline magnesium trisalicylate (Trilisate®; and others) are salicylates used to treat arthritis. Agents other than aspirin are considered nonacetylated salicylates. These drugs do not interfere with platelet function nor in-

crease the patient's bleeding time. Nonacety-lated salicylates may be safer to use than aspirin in some patients. At least one study has shown nonacetylated salicylates to be as effective as aspirin. Other available products which may reduce gastrointestinal side effects are enteric coated and sustained-release aspirin. These products may reduce or prevent aspirin release in the stomach. Another approach has been the use of combinations of aspirin and a buffering agent. While some patients may tolerate these products better than aspirin, there is no evidence that formulations like Ascriptin® and Bufferin® reduce gastrointestinal microbleeding. The use of products other than plain aspirin tablets may substantially increase the cost of therapy. Regardless of the product selected, therapy with a salicylate is usually adjusted using blood salicylate concentration measurements.

Other NSAIDs. Numerous other NSAIDs are available by prescription and one, ibuprofen, is available by prescription (Motrin®), and over the counter (Nuprin® and others). Many patients tolerate other NSAIDs better than high-dose aspirin. Even though they may cause fewer gastrointestinal side effects than aspirin, these and other side effects are common. The combination of gastrointestinal irritation and decreased platelet function often results in the development of gastric ulcers in certain patients at risk. Misoprostol (Cytotec®) is now available for the prevention of NSAID-induced gastric ulceration. Additionally, other NSAIDs are more expensive than aspirin. These drugs and aspirin can interact with other drugs and exacerbate certain medical problems. They can cause sodium and water retention, interfering with antihypertensive therapy. Other NSAIDs may cause asthmatic attacks in asthmatic patients sensitive to aspirin.

Hydroxychloroquine (Plaquenil®). This drug may be effective as a second-line agent. It is an antimalarial drug which can cause many serious side effects. However, serious irreversible side effects are rare with recommended doses and close monitoring of the patient. Close monitoring is especially important to prevent visual problems resulting from retinal toxicity.

Cloroquine (Aralen®) is another antimalarial agent used to treat arthritis.

Gold Salts. Gold sodium thiomalate (Myochrysine®) and aurothioglucose (Salganal®) are injectable gold products. Auranofin (Ridaura®) is the oral dosage form. These compounds are very effective and may prevent progression of some of the disease process. Dosage adjustment and clinical response may take many weeks to months to evolve. Like other second-line agents, gold therapy can cause many severe side effects. Oral gold may cause fewer mouth sores, bone marrow suppression, and kidney toxicity but more gastrointestinal side effects than the injectable forms.

Immunosuppressive agents. Azathioprine (Imuran®), chlorambucil (Leukeran®), cyclophosphamide (Cytoxan®), and methotrexate (Rheumatrex®) are immunosuppressive agents used to treat cancers and other disease processes. These drugs are all second-line agents. All of these agents are associated with severe side effects when used to treat other medical conditions, but they may be well tolerated in the dosages recommended for treatment of arthritis.

Sulfasalazine (Azulfidine® and others). This drug has been used for many years to treat inflammatory bowel disease. It has also been shown to be very effective for the treatment of arthritis. It may be more effective and better tolerated than some of the other second-line agents.

Penicillamine (Depen®, Cuprimine®). This is another second-line agent which may be effective in patients who do not respond well to other therapies. It may delay progression of some of the disease process, but its benefits must be weighed against the potential to cause severe toxicities.

Corticosteroids. Steroids may benefit patients during periods of active inflammation. They usually must be given daily, which can lead to many body changes, including loss of bone minerals. Methods to overcome these problems have not proven effective.

CANCER MEDICATIONS The treatment of cancer is very complex and beyond the scope of this discussion, as is a review of individual chemotherapeutic (anti-cancer) agents. More detailed information on these subjects is available from the American Cancer Society. However, even though the selection and use of these agents is complex, a few basic concepts do prevail.

Ideally, the goal of any chemotherapeutic regimen is to rid the body of all tumor cells. Some cancers can be cured, although this goal cannot always be attained. Chemotherapy may be administered to produce long term remissions or to relieve symptoms. To accomplish these goals, the physician may combine other treatment methods, such as surgery and/or radiation.

The function of chemotherapeutic agents. Until recently, most chemotherapeutic agents available worked by interfering with different phases of the cancer cell growth cycle. As a group these agents are referred to as cytotoxic drugs. Normal and cancer cells have the same growth cycle, but, with the exception of certain cell types, normal cells are less likely to be dividing. The normal cell cycle consists of a resting phase (G_0), a cell-division preparation phase (S-phase), a pre-division (G_2), and cell division (M-phase). Some cytotoxic drugs interfere with a specific phase. These drugs are called cell-cycle specific and are most effective when given continuously. Others may work throughout the cell cycle and are called cycle-nonspecific. Cell cycle-nonspecific drugs are more effective when administered intermittently. Intermittent drug administration also allows normal cells to recover, reducing complications, and also may help eradicate cells not affected by prior therapy.

Cytotoxic agents are not very active during the G_0 or resting phase. This is a very useful property, because most normal cells are in this phase and are less likely to be damaged. However, this is true also of a proportion of cells in large tumors. Consequently, cytotoxic agents are more effective when administered during early stages of the disease, when more cells are dividing. Knowing when an agent is active in the cycle is important in choosing drug combinations and timing administration.

The exact mechanism by which cytotoxic agents work is highly variable from one agent to the next, but they can be grouped into similar pharmacological classes. The earliest class of agents developed was the alkylating agents. The first drugs in this class were derived from nerve gasses. Alkylating agents are cell cycle-nonspecific. Other classes are antimetabolites, antitumor antibiotics, vinca alkaloids, podophyllotoxins, anthracenes, and protein inhibitors. Many of these agents are derived from naturally occurring yeast and plants.

Two other types of chemotherapeutic drugs used are hormones and biologic response modifiers. Certain cancers are responsive to the administration of hormones, while others are not. Biologic response modifiers have recently been intensely investigated. These agents are designed to help or modify the immune response. They may also be cytotoxic. Only one agent, interferon alpha, is currently marketed.

Drug side effects. Anti-cancer drugs are well recognized to be highly toxic to the patient. Toxicities can be so severe that some patients refuse to continue therapy. Cytotoxic agents are associated with the most severe toxicities. Most but not all normal body cells are in a resting phase, and less likely to be damaged by these drugs. Nevertheless, organs like the skin, hair follicles, nails, gastrointestinal tract, and bone marrow have large populations of cells in the growth phase. These organs have a high cell turnover rate and are at a greater risk of being damaged by cytotoxic agents; side effects commonly seen involve these organs. Nausea, vomiting, hair loss, skin ulceration, and bone marrow depression are routinely encountered. Bone marrow depression leads to many other complications, such as bleeding, anemia, and infection.

Other organ systems may be uniquely affected by a given drug within a pharmacological class. The anti-cancer antibiotic doxorubicin (Adriamycin®) is associated with congestive heart failure, while bleomycin (Blenoxane®), also an antibiotic, causes pulmonary (lung) toxicity. Cisplatin (Platinol®), an alkylating agent, commonly causes kidney damage if certain precautions are not taken. Many of these agents can cause severe pain and tissue injury if allowed to escape into tissue from intravenous catheters. Vinca alkaloids, such as vincristine and vinblastine, may cause neurotoxicity resulting in numbness and other nerve changes.

Selection. The selection of chemotherapeutic agents to treat a specific type of cancer is somewhat predetermined, but it may change regularly, reflecting new developments. Extensive clinical trials establish which combinations of agents are first line treatment. For some cancers the first line therapy is potentially curative and for others only palliative. If a patient fails to respond to first choice combination therapy, he or she may begin second-line therapy. For treatment of cancers with no known curative therapy, patients who desire it may be placed on investigative protocols, or experimental drugs. Many patients choose to do so, and this is a necessary means for the development of more effective drug treatments.

In addition to the type of cancer, treatment choice may be determined by staging. Staging is a procedure developed to determine how quickly the tumor is growing, if it has spread (metastasized), where it has spread to, and the prognosis of the disease. The criteria for staging are uniform for each tumor type and guide the physician in the selection of therapy.

CARDIOVASCULAR   MEDICATIONS

The types of heart conditions which respond best to cardiac medications are angina pectoris, arrhythmias (abnormal heartbeats), heart failure, and hypertension. Other therapies which relate to the heart and blood vessels are medications to lower blood cholesterol levels, blood thinners (or anticoagulants), and clot busters (thrombolytics).

Angina Pectoris

Angina pectoris (angina) can be described as a feeling of discomfort resulting from deficient blood flow to the heart muscle. Nevertheless, deficient blood flow can occur without the perception of pain. Angina may develop after strenuous physical exertion, or in advanced stages after little or no exertion. In addition to pain or discomfort, angina is accompanied by changes in the electrocardiogram. Most angina is associated with narrowing of major arteries in the heart, but it can be caused by spasms of otherwise normal heart arteries. The goal of therapy is to reduce the number of angina attacks, improve the patient's exercise tolerance, improve quality of life, and prevent myocardial infarction (heart attack). (See ANGINA PECTORIS in the section CARDIOVASCULAR CONDITIONS.)

Once atherosclerotic plaques obstruct 70 percent of the artery or more, angina usually develops; however, it can develop with less obstruction. Obstruction of the artery does not allow for an increase in blood flow as the heart increases its work. When the patient exercises, the heart muscle does not receive enough oxygen and pain occurs. Factors other than an imbalance in oxygen demand and supply may also be involved. These areas of atherosclerosis may be further obstructed by vessel spasm, platelet plugs, or thrombus (blood clots). Drug therapy is directed toward increasing oxygen supply, reducing oxygen demand, preventing platelet plugs, and occasionally preventing clots.

Types of medication.

Nitrates (Nitroglycerin). The mechanism of action of nitrates, like nitroglycerin (NTG), is not completely understood. However, it is felt that these drugs relax the muscles in the veins and arteries, resulting in dilatation. In usual dosages nitrates predominantly dilate veins, decreasing the amount of blood returned to the heart. This reduces the amount of work performed by the heart and decreases oxygen demand. NTG is also given intravenously to treat congestive heart failure for this reason. While arteries outside the heart may not be, heart arteries are dilated, thus increasing oxygen delivery to the heart muscle.

For many years NTG has been widely used under the tongue (sublingually). NTG is very effective administered in this manner in response to angina pain development. A rapid onset of action makes sublingual or lingual NTG the drug of choice for acute angina attacks. NTG is also effective in preventing pain if taken before heavy exertion. However, isosorbide dinitrate (Isordil®) given during the day is effective and more convenient to use. In an attempt to make NTG more convenient to use, other dosage forms have been developed. A topical ointment, slow release patch, and slow release capsule are available. NTG sublingual tablets require protection from heat and light and should be stored in their original container. Poor storage can result in lack of effectiveness. A NTG oral spray was developed to minimize this problem.

The major limiting side effect of all nitrates

is hypotension and headache. If signs and symptoms of hypotension occur the dosage must be adjusted. Tolerance to the development of headache may evolve after several weeks of therapy. Tolerance to the beneficial effects of nitrates can also occur. This is most common with long acting products, such as sustained release oral nitrates, patches, and ointment. Allowing nitrate free periods in the dosing regimen can minimize this problem.

Beta-adrenergic blocking agents (beta-blockers). These drugs reduce heart oxygen demand by blocking the beta receptor. It is possible that they have other beneficial effects not yet well described. The dose of beta-blocker may be calculated in relation to the heart rate; however, documentation of increased exercise tolerance is a more reliable method. Selection of a beta-blocker is dependent on the patient's other problems and/or previously encountered side effects. Beta-blocker therapy should not be abruptly withdrawn. This action could result in myocardial infarction. (*See also* HYPERTENSION in this section.)

Calcium channel blocking agents. These drugs block the movement of calcium into cells, decreasing cardiac and smooth muscle contraction. The resulting effects beneficial to the treatment of angina are vasodilation and reduced spasm of coronary arteries. In the United States two types of calcium channel blockers are available. Type 1 drugs, verapamil (Calan®, Isoptin®) and diltiazem (Cardiazem®) dilate coronary arteries more than other arteries, decrease heart contractions, and affect cardiac electrical signals. Type 2 drugs, nifedipine (Procardia®, Adalat®) and nicardipine (Cardene®), dilate coronary arteries less and other arteries more and have minimum effects on heart rhythm and contractions. The differences between the two types of calcium channel blockers are important to the physician in making a drug selection. The more potent effect of type 2 blockers on arteries outside the heart can result in increased heart rate and exacerbation of angina. If this occurs, a beta-blocker may be added to offset this effect. Type 1 drugs can increase conduction abnormalities in the heart.

Antiplatelet therapy. Platelets are small particles involved in the body's clotting mechanism. When an injury occurs in a blood vessel, blood platelets are exposed to substances which cause them to adhere to the surface. This action is the first step in clot formation and helps prevent excessive loss of blood. Platelets do not stick to normal uninjured blood vessel surfaces.

Platelets may also play an important role in the development of atherosclerosis, angina pectoris, and myocardial infarction. Three antiplatelet drugs—aspirin, dipyridamole (Persantine® and others), and sulfinpyrazone (Anturane®, and others)—have been studied in patients with angina. Only aspirin has been shown to reduce mortality and myocardial infarction in patients with unstable angina or previous myocardial infarction. Aspirin has two effects on platelet function; one effect is beneficial and the other is possibly harmful. The harmful effect may be reduced if aspirin is given in low doses. For this reason only one aspirin a day is usually prescribed.

Fish oil. Fish oil has recently been promoted to be effective in preventing heart disease. Eskimos have been reported to have a low incidence of coronary thrombosis, beneficial blood lipid changes, long bleeding times, and decreased platelet stickiness. Thus, it has been proposed that these changes are the result of eating large amounts of fish. It is known that cold water fish fats can affect platelet function, but the clinical importance of these findings is not known. Presently, there is no evidence that these products can prevent heart disease.

Arrhythmias (Abnormal Heartbeats)

The development of abnormal heart beats is commonly caused by heart attacks, abnormal heart valves, atherosclerosis, infections, caffeine and certain medications. The actual mechanism by which arrhythmias are produced is extremely complex and difficult to understand, even for persons working in medical fields. In the same manner, it is difficult to understand how antiarrhythmic agents work. The procedures used to select antiarrhythmic drug for a patient can also be very complex.

The chambers of the heart must be filled with blood and then contracted to force the blood out and into the arteries. In order for the heart to pump effectively it is important that its parts function in coordination with each other. In addition it must pump automatically, without conscious control by the brain. To accomplish this task, the heart tissue has a property called automaticity. This means that certain heart muscle cells can initiate the stimulus to contract on their own. Under normal circumstances impulses stimulating contraction are generated by the sinus node, located on the upper right side of the heart. This is the heart's normal pacemaker. It initiates the heart contraction. When the sinus node releases an electrical impulse, it is carried down the upper chambers of the heart to the lower chambers (ventricles) by special conducting tissue. Before the impulse passes into the ventricles, it must travel through the AV node which helps regulate the heart rate by regulating impulse passage. Once through the AV node the impulse is carried toward the ventricles by the bundle of His and then into the ventricles by its two major branches called the right and left bundle branch. These conductors can be thought of as electrical cables. Arrhythmias can arise when the SA node malfunctions, tissue other than the SA node becomes a pacemaker, the AV node is damaged, or conduction is abnormal.

Selection. Arrhythmias arising above the ventricles are called supraventricular arrhythmias. Those arising below the bundle of His are called ventricular. A third type, conduction blocks, can occur above or below the ventricles. Antiarrhythmic drugs are used in an attempt to correct one or more of these defects. Not all antiarrhythmic agents are equally effective in correcting all of these problems. Antiarrhythmic drug selection is dependent on the patient's arrhythmia type, other medical problems, and the likelihood that the drug selected will correct the cause of the arrhythmia. The physician must use many tools to help diagnose the arrhythmia, select the proper antiarrhythmic agent, and assess response to therapy.

Types of medication. The majority of antiarrhythmic drugs are arranged into six groups, according to how they affect electrical conduction in the heart. The groups are called Class IA, IB, IC, II, III, and IV. Digitalis has antiarrhythmic properties but does not fit into one of these classes.

Class IA drugs. The drugs in this class are quinidine (many manufacturers), procainamide (Pronestyl®, Procan SR®, and others), and disopyramide (Norpace® and others). These drugs may be useful in the treatment of atrial fibrillation and prophylaxis (prevention), abnormal atrial contractions, rapid ventricle rate, abnormal ventricular contractions (PVC's), and Wolff-Parkinson-White syndrome. When treating atrial fibrillation or flutter with either quinidine or procainamide, the patient must be first given digitalis to control heart rate.

Quinidine and procainamide are available in oral and intravenous dosage forms. Both are also marketed in a sustained release dosage form for more convenient administration. Procan SR®, a sustained release form of procainamide, may appear in the stool unchanged, which often causes concern by the patient. However, this is normal for this drug since it is a wax matrix formulation. The tablet may appear intact in the stool, but all the procainamide will have been released.

These drugs have similar adverse effects on the heart when taken in high doses. However, disopyramide may cause additional cardiac problems. This drug can induce or aggravate congestive heart failure. Each drug has other non-cardiac side effects not commonly shared by the others. Quinidine causes diarrhea, other gastrointestinal symptoms, fever, and decreased platelets. Procainamide is noted for causing a lupus-like syndrome that reverses upon discontinuing therapy. Disopyramide can cause urinary retention in men and women.

Class IB drugs. Lidocaine (Xylocaine®), phenytoin (Dilantin®), mexiletine (Mexitil®), and tocainide (Tonocard®) are included in this class. These drugs are used most often to treat ventricular arrhythmias, (PVC's), abnormal ventricle contractions, rapid ventricle rate, and ventricular fibrillation. Phenytoin is rarely used for treating arrhythmias and then only for a brief period of time. (*See also* ANTICONVULSANT DRUGS in this section.) Lidocaine must be given as an injection and therefore is used primarily in the hospital. Mexiletine and tocainide are newer drugs which can be given orally. The major side effects encountered with lidocaine, tocainide, and mexiletine involve the central nervous system. These effects are related to blood concentration. Patients may become drowsy, agitated, develop slurred speech, ringing in their ears, coma, and seizures.

Class IC drugs. Flecainide (Tambocor®) and encainide (Enkaid®) are Class IC drugs. These agents have only recently been made available and were initially felt to be the drugs of choice for PVC's. These drugs are also useful for treatment of supraventricular arrhythmias. Though once considered relatively safe agents, these drugs are now felt to have serious side effects. Flecainide and encainide can induce arrhythmias which can be hard to control. For this reason the FDA has required the manufacturers of these agents to change their approved indications. These drugs are now reserved for treatment of patients with life threatening arrhythmias unresponsive to less toxic compounds.

Class II drugs. Beta-adrenergic blocking drugs are considered class II antiarrhythmic agents. These drugs are useful for control of ventricular rate in patients with very rapid beating of the upper chambers of the heart and abnormal ventricle contractions. (*See also* BETA BLOCKING DRUGS in this section.)

Class III drugs. Amiodarone (Cordarone®) and bretylium (Bretylate®) are found in this class. Bretylium is available as an injection and amiodarone as a tablet. Bretylium is primarily used in the hospital for short-term treatment of rapid ventricle rate and ventricular fibrillation resistant to other treatment. Amiodarone is very effective orally for treating ventricular arrhythmias, but has many severe side effects. Amiodarone is reserved for the treatment of life-threatening arrhythmias which do not respond to other agents.

Class IV drugs. Calcium channel blockers are considered Class IV antiarrhythmic agents. Verapamil (Isoptin®; Calan®; and others) is the calcium channel blocker used as an antiarrhythmic agent. It is very effective for treatment and prevention of supraventricular tachycardias, such as atrial fibrillation. Verapamil can aggravate congestive heart failure and may interact with many drugs.

Digitalis drugs. Digoxin (Lanoxin®) and digitoxin (Crystodigin®) are commonly used to reduce the ventricular rate of patients with atrial fibrillation or flutter.

Heart Failure

Heart failure occurs when the heart is unable to effectively push the blood out of its chambers. Three factors contribute to this problem: the heart muscle's ability to contract, the amount of blood returning to the heart, and blood pressure (resistance). A failing heart is no longer able to pump blood against the blood pressure effectively. This causes blood to back up as it returns to the heart, creating more work for it to accomplish.

There are two primary types of heart failure. The least common type is called high output failure. This type of failure is due to some underlying medical problem, such as severe anemia or hypothyroid disease, that causes the heart to beat very rapidly to meet the metabolic requirements of the body. Treatment of high output failure requires correction of the underlying disease and will not be discussed here. The most common type of failure is low output failure. This is also called congestive heart failure (CHF). The causes of congestive heart failure are varied. Common causes are poorly managed high blood pressure, myocardial infarction (heart attack), and diseased heart valves. Surgery is usually required to correct diseased valves. Treatment of other causes of congestive heart failure is directed at improving the pumping action of the heart.

Heart pumping action can be improved by drugs that improve the heart muscle's ability to contract, reduce the resistance against which it is required to pump (blood pressure), and/or decrease the amount of blood returning to the right side of the heart. The goals of therapy are directed at decreasing the symptoms of CHF. Many of the symptoms are the result of excessive fluid accumulating in the tissues. In addition to administering cardiac drugs, the physician may restrict the patient's physical activity and salt intake. Bedrest reduces the effects of gravity on edema formation and increases blood flow to the kidneys assisting in fluid excretion. Salt restriction helps reduce the volume of blood.

Types of medication.

Diuretics. Diuretics are used to enhance the removal of water and sodium. Diuretics reduce blood volume, thus reducing the resistance to the heart's pumping action. Effective water removal also decreases edema (water accumulation in the tissue) and lung congestion. Thiazide diuretics may not be potent enough to effectively remove water in these patients. A loop diuretic, such as furosemide (Lasix®), is usually required. Diuretics usually cause a decrease in body potassium concentration. When treating hypertension, the physician may not always give the patient a potassium supplement. However, it is important to take potassium supplements whenever diuretics are used with digitalis drugs. (*See also* ANTIHYPERTENSION and POTASSIUM SUPPLEMENTS in this section.)

Digitalis. Digoxin (Lanoxin®) and digitoxin (Crystodigin®) are often referred to as digitalis glycosides. These drugs are derived from the foxglove plant. The leaf of this plant was once ground and used as a medicine. Eventually the active ingredients were identified and purified. Digoxin and digitoxin are not the only active compounds in digitalis leaf, but they are the only ones commonly used in this country. Both of these drugs have two major effects on the heart. They increase the force of contraction of the heart muscle and aid conduction of electrical signals. This latter effect is useful in treating certain abnormal heart beats. (*See* IRREGULAR HEARTBEATS in this section.) By increasing the force of contraction these drugs increase output of the heart. This results in better blood flow to body tissues and to the kidneys. The kidneys are able to excrete more water, reducing blood volume, edema, and lung congestion. As the heart does less work, its size returns toward normal. While the traditional role of digoxin and digitoxin in the treatment of CHF has recently been challenged, these drugs remain an important component of the drug treatment of CHF.

Selection. The selection of one of these drugs is, to a large extent, determined by physician preference. Digoxin is currently the drug most commonly prescribed. Its advantages are more theoretical than real. Digoxin is removed from the body more rapidly than digitoxin, which may be an advantage in a patient who has developed a toxic blood level. Digitoxin requires a longer time to be eliminated and would expose the patient to toxic levels for a longer period of time. However, digoxin is dependent on good kidney function for removal from the body, while digitoxin is not. Sudden decreases in kidney function can easily lead to excessive levels of digoxin but have no effect on digitoxin blood levels. Digoxin blood levels may also be increased by certain other drugs.

Digoxin and digitoxin can cause serious side effects when taken in excessive dosages. Therapy with either drug is assisted by measurement of blood concentrations. It may take several weeks to determine the proper dosage. The physician may give a large dose (starting dose) over the first twenty-four to forty-eight hours to shorten the period of time necessary to achieve the required blood concentration. Once the proper dosage of digitoxin is established, it is unlikely to cause toxic effects unless the patient develops severe liver failure or low blood potassium or magnesium levels. Conversely, the dosage requirement of digoxin is influenced by many factors. Decreased kidney function, addition of certain drugs, and low blood potassium and/or magnesium can increase the patient's response to an established maintenance dose. Common signs of digitalis toxicity are nausea and vomiting, loss of appetite, decreased heart rate, and abnormal heart beats.

Vasodilators. Vasodilators work by reducing pumping resistance (blood pressure) and/or the amount of blood returning to the heart. Some drugs dilate veins, reducing the amount of blood returning to the heart, while others dilate arteries, and increasing flow from the heart. Direct vasodilators, α-blocking agents, calcium channel blockers, and ACE inhibitors may be used for treatment of CHF. The use of ACE inhibitors has become common recently. These drugs are more effective than other vasodilators in producing long term dilation of veins.

Angiotensin converting enzyme (ACE) inhibitors. Angiotensin converting enzyme (ACE) inhibitors were first developed to treat hypertension (high blood pressure). Soon after ACE inhibitors were released for this use, it was discovered that they can help some patients with chronic congestive heart failure (heart failure). The standard treatment for this condition has consisted of oral diuretics and digitalis-related drugs. When this standard treatment fails to help the patient, the addition of an ACE inhibitor may be beneficial. In fact, some physicians feel that these drugs can be used as substitutes for digitalis drugs.

There are currently three ACE inhibitors marketed. Captopril (Capoten®) and enalapril (Vasotec®) are approved by the FDA for treatment of congestive heart failure in patients not responding to a diuretic and digitalis. Lisinopril (Prinivil®), the last drug released, is currently only approved for treatment of hypertension. Only captopril is approved for treatment of heart failure in patients who cannot tolerate digitalis. However, it must be noted that FDA approval for an indication does not necessarily mean that a drug is ineffective for other treatments, nor does it prohibit a physician from prescribing a drug for that use if in his judgment available alternatives are not desirable.

ACE inhibitors may also decrease some of the side effects caused by diuretics and digitalis. The addition of an ACE inhibitor may reduce the amount of potassium lost with diuretic use and thus reduce the potential to develop side effects from digitalis drugs. However, ACE inhibitors can cause other serious side effects in themselves. They can cause decline of kidney function in patients with certain underlying problems and low blood pressure. Some patients develop persistent cough which may interfere with continued use of the drugs.

Hypertension

Hypertension (high blood pressure) is a common medical problem. While the cause of some forms of hypertension may be known, most hypertension is caused by unidentifiable factors. This form of hypertension is called essential hypertension and usually requires long term management consisting of weight loss, sodium and fat restriction, exercise, cigarette and alcohol control, and often treatment with antihypertensive agents. Untreated, hypertension can result in serious damage to major organ systems. Effective hypertension management can reduce organ damage, but there has been some controversy concerning at what level of hypertension drug therapy should begin. Current discussion has centered on the fact that diuretics increase blood lipid and decrease blood potassium levels which

may offset the benefit gained by lowering the blood pressure in certain patients.

The function of antihypertension agents. To understand how antihypertensive agents work, the factors that determine the body's blood pressure must first be briefly reviewed. The body's circulation system, which determines blood pressure, consists of a pump (the heart) and a series of pipes (blood vessels). This system is filled with a fluid (blood) which is pumped to various parts of the body and back to the heart. Simply stated, pressure in this system can be increased by increasing the pumping force of the heart, increasing the amount of fluid in the blood vessels, decreasing the diameter of the blood vessels, or various combinations of these factors. The numerous drugs used to treat hypertension either decrease the heart's pumping force, reduce the amount of fluid in the vessels, or increase the diameter of the blood vessels. A few of the drugs affect more than one factor, but most affect only one. Initial therapy usually consists of one drug. Other drugs may be added as needed.

Selection. Until recently most physicians used a planned approach to drug treatment of hypertension called "stepped-care." Some scientists are now recommending movement away from this approach. The main incentive for this change in philosophy has been the development of new classes of drugs. Before the development of these new agents, it was important to initiate a diuretic first (step one). Diuretics cause patients to excrete water, thus reducing blood volume and blood pressure. It was important to use an agent that would increase water loss first, because the other available drugs that may subsequently be added cause water retention, making them less effective.

The second step, if required, consisted of the addition of a drug to decrease the pumping force of the heart or decrease blood vessel wall muscle tone. These drugs were called sympatholytic agents. The first sympatholytic agents worked in the brain (centrally), while later agents worked outside the brain (peripherally). Early step two drugs were reserpine and α-methyldopa (Aldomet®). These drugs could not be used alone, because they caused reflex salt and water retention which counteracted their effects.

The ability of these agents to reduce heart rate was important, because step three drugs, blood vessel dilating (vasodilating) agents usually induced a reflex increase in heart rate. When vasodilating agents dilate the blood vessels, the body responds by causing salt and water retention and increased heart rate. Use of a diuretic offsets salt and water retention, and a beta-blocker or centrally acting sympatholytic agent prevents an increase in heart rate. Thus the principle of "stepped care" was a very logical approach to hypertension management.

Nevertheless, introduction of beta-blocking agents and new drug classes, such as calcium channel blockers and angiotension converting enzyme (ACE) inhibitors, has made the principle of stepped care less necessary. These agents are effective when used alone. They do not cause salt and water retention and reflex increases in heart rate. Furthermore, these new drugs do not increase blood lipid levels nor decrease potassium levels which may lead to irregular heartbeats.

Also it is now known that response to a given type of agent is not the same for all patients. In other words, some patients may benefit from diuretic therapy, while others may respond more favorably to another class of agents. It is thought that response to a specific class of antihypertensive agent may be somewhat determined by the level of the enzyme renin present naturally in the blood. A complete description of the function of renin is beyond the scope of this discussion, but in simple terms, it plays a role in the normal maintenance of blood pressure. Renin can indirectly influence blood vessel constriction and sodium and water retention. Patients may be classed as high, normal or low renin hypertensives. Patients with low renin hypertension tend to respond better to diuretics. Conversely, others respond better to a beta-blocking agent. In response to these differences, current therapy of hypertension is more individualized to match the patient's characteristics and needs.

Types of Antihypertension Medications.

Diuretics. Diuretics work by causing excretion of salt and water, thus reducing blood volume. They can be grouped into three classes, thiazide, loop, and potassium sparing diuretics.

Thiazide and thiazide derivative diuretics comprise the largest group. The most commonly prescribed drug in this group is hydrochlorthiazide, available in generic form and usually relatively inexpensive. All agents in this class have similar effects and side effects. These agents generally are less effective in patients with poor kidney function except for metolazone (Zaroxolyn®) and indapamide (Lozol®). Thiazide diuretics are effective when used alone and add to the effectiveness of other antihypertensive agents when combined. They can cause low blood potassium levels, increased blood lipids, and other blood chemical abnormalities. However, these changes may be overcome by using low doses, taking potassium supplements, and altering diet. Once considered the drugs of first choice, their standing is now shared with beta-blocking agents, calcium channel blockers, and angiotensin converting enzyme (ACE) inhibitors.

Furosemide (Lasix®), bumetanide (Bumex®), and ethacrynic acid (Edecrin®) are loop diuretics. The term "loop" diuretic refers to the site in the kidney where these agents work. Although loop diuretics are more potent diuretics than thiazides, they are not as effective in reducing blood pressure. This is thought to be due to a lack of effect on blood vessel tone. These agents do have the advantage of inducing significant diuresis in patients with poor kidney function. Loop diuretics are usually reserved for use in patients not responding to thiazides or those who have poor renal function.

Three potassium-sparing diuretics are available, spironolactone (Aldactone®), amiloride (Midamor®), and triamterene (Dyrenium). These agents are poor diuretics but do not cause potassium loss. Potassium sparing diuretics are rarely used alone but are combined with a thiazide diuretic in an attempt to overcome thiazide induced low blood potassium. Patients on these agents generally should not take a potassium supplement, for a dangerously high potassium level may develop. High blood potassium levels can also occur in patients with chronic kidney dysfunction, diabetes mellitus, and a form of hypoaldosteronism. These agents may cause elevated potassium levels when taken with other drugs, such as angiotensin-converting enzyme inhibitors and pain medications such as aspirin and related compounds.

Centrally acting sympatholytic agents. Commonly known drugs in this group are clonidine (Catapres®) and methyldopa (Aldomet®), but others are available. These drugs stimulate an area in the brain that reduces blood vessel muscle contraction. They have other actions that may also be beneficial. These drugs are effective alone only in high doses, which may have many side effects. Therefore, they are combined with diuretics to increase their effectiveness and reduce side effects.

Even in lower doses these drugs are not without severe side effects. Sedation and lethargy can be severe. Clonidine can be associated with severe rebound hypertension if the medication is stopped abruptly under certain conditions.

Peripherally acting sympatholytic agents. These drugs work outside the brain to reduce blood pressure. Reserpine, an old drug, is probably the most useful in this group. It is very inexpensive, effective, and well tolerated in low doses. Other members of this class, guanadrel (Hylorel®) and guanethidine (Ismelin®), have severe side effects.

Beta adrenergic receptor antagonist (beta-blocking agents). These drugs may be used alone or in combination with other agents. If a physician is using stepped-care, a beta-blocker would most likely replace a centrally acting sympatholytic as a step-two agent, since, as previously noted, these agents do not cause the metabolic abnormalities seen with diuretics. In addition, they have beneficial cardiac effects and may benefit other medical problems which commonly occur in patients with hypertension. For these reasons beta-blocker use has increased greatly since propranolol was first approved by the FDA.

All agents in this class are effective in reducing blood pressure. They work by decreasing the pumping output of the heart. Beta-blocking agents are so named because they work by preventing the activation of the beta-adrenergic receptor in certain body tissues. There are two types of beta-adrenergic receptors responsible for many body activities. The receptor in heart tissue is called β_1; blocking this receptor results in the beneficial antihypertensive effects of beta-blockers. A second receptor (β_2) is found in the lungs and other tissues; blocking this receptor results in many of the unwanted effects. The first beta-blocker marketed, propranolol (Inderal®), blocked both receptors equally. Propranolol can cause problems when given to patients with lung disease, diabetes, and peripheral vascular disease. To overcome these problems, manufacturers developed drugs which block the β_1 receptor predominantly (cardioselective). Propranolol also has properties which allow it to cross into the central nervous system (CNS), causing headache, drowsiness, fatigue, and other problems. Manufacturers have created drugs such as nadolol (Corgard®) and others that do not cross into the CNS as well. All these products have different characteristics which may influence the doctor's selection of a particular one. If a patient fails to respond to one beta-blocking agent, he/she is not likely to respond to another.

A physician selects a beta-blocking agent based on the patient's underlying medical problems, previously encountered side effects, and convenience of drug administration. Patients with angina pectoris, certain heart rhythm problems, and record of previous heart attack may especially benefit from beta-blocker therapy. Conversely, patients with lung diseases, heart failure, diabetes, and peripheral vascular disease may be more at risk to developing adverse effects. The later patients may benefit from an agent more specific for blocking β_1 receptors. Also agents which are eliminated slowly by the body require less frequent dosing and may be more convenient for some patients to take.

Vasodilating agents.
• Direct acting vasodilating agents. Hydralazine (Apresoline®) was the first agent of this class introduced. The drugs in this class increase the diameter of the blood vessel reducing blood pressure. These drugs are usually combined with a diuretic and a sympatholytic agent to increase their effectiveness. Occasionally they may be given without the sympatholytic agent to patients

over 65, who are less prone to develop reflex increases in heart rate.

Minoxidil (Loniten®), another drug in this class, is very potent and must be given with a diuretic. Thiazide diuretics are usually not effective in preventing water retention when minoxidil is given, but loop diuretics are. Minoxidil is usually reserved for treatment of patients not responding to standard antihypertensive therapy.

Both drugs in this class have many side effects which limit their use. Hydralazine can cause a condition that resembles the disease systemic lupus erythamatosis (lupus). Minoxidil may cause hair growth on the face and body which may cause problems in women.

- α-Receptor blocking agents. These drugs cause vasodilation by blocking the α-receptor in the blood vessel wall. The body stimulates this receptor when vasoconstriction is needed. Blocking this receptor reduces vasoconstriction. Older drugs in this class are not useful for long term treatment of hypertension. However, newer class members, prazosin (Minipress®) and terazosin (Hytrin®), are more useful because they are more specific in decreasing vasoconstriction. These drugs do not cause reflex increases in heart rate as do the direct vasodilators, but both drugs can cause decreased blood pressure upon standing. This is especially a problem after the first dose. Giving a small first dose at bedtime can prevent this from occurring.
- α- and β-receptor blocking agents. Labetalol (Trandate®, Normodyne®) is the only drug in this class. This drug has side effects similar to drugs discussed above that block these two receptors singularly.

Angiotensin-converting enzyme (ACE) inhibitors. These drugs are also vasodilators but do not cause a reflex increase in heart rate or low blood pressure upon standing. They are very effective when used alone in certain patients. The addition of a diuretic enhances their effect. This class of drugs is also useful for the treatment of congestive heart failure.

ACE inhibitors work by blocking the action of angiotensin converting enzyme. This enzyme converts angiotensin I to angiotensin II, a naturally occurring vasoconstrictor. It is thought that the long term effects result from local blocking of angiotensin II production in tissue, rather than blood. Available products, captopril (Capoten®), enalapril (Vasotec®), and lisinopril (Prinivil®, Zestril®), appear to be equally effective and have similar side effects. The most common serious side effect is kidney failure, which can occur in patients with obstruction in the arteries going to the kidneys. Chronic cough, spasm of the tubes in the lungs, and high blood potassium levels may occur. The drugs enalapril and lisinopril may be given once a day.

Calcium channel blockers. Calcium channel blockers were first approved for the treatment of angina pectoris (heart pain). They are also useful in treating certain abnormal heart rhythms. These agents reduce blood pressure by causing blood vessel dilatation. Nifedipine (Procardia®) has the greatest vasodilating effect and least effect on heart rhythm; therefore, nifedipine may cause increased heart rate. In contrast, verapamil (Calan®, and others), nicardipine (Cardene), and diltiazem (Cardizem®) reduce blood pressure without an increase in heart rate. These drugs, like diuretics, may be more effective in certain patients.

Choice of a calcium channel blocker is determined by the patient's additional medical problems and ability of the drug to ease or aggravate that problem. All of the drugs in this class should be used cautiously in patients with congestive heart failure. Verapamil and diltiazem should be used with caution in patients receiving beta-blockers. These drugs may cause other side effects.

Other Therapies for Cardiovascular Conditions

Cholesterol-Lowering Drugs. Recently concern about blood cholesterol levels has resulted in many articles being published in newspapers, magazines, and scientific journals. Additionally, many products have been marketed to take advantage of this concern. Not only have drugs been developed to lower cholesterol, but also certain food products and diet programs. Products high in fiber or low in saturated fats are flaunted on television and in magazines.

Low-density lipoproteins (LDL) carry most of cholesterol in the blood. A high blood concentration of LDL is associated with an increased risk to developing coronary heart disease. Patients are first asked to change to a low fat diet and to lose weight. If these measures fail, then administration of cholesterol-lowering drugs may be considered.

Selection. The drugs available for lowering cholesterol are cholestyramine (Questran®), clofibrate (Atromid-S®), colestipol (Colestid®), gemfibrozil (Lopid®), lovastatin (Mevacor®), niacin (nicotinic acid), neomycin, and probucol (Lorelco®). The choice of drug used is primarily determined by demonstrated effectiveness, the patient's lipid problem, the patient's tolerance of the drug's side effects, and safety of long term use. Sometimes these drugs may be used in combination. None of these compounds will cure the problem, and cholesterol levels will return to pretreatment values when treatment is stopped.

Types of Medication. Cholestryramine (Questran®) and Colestipol (Colestid®) are resins which bind bile acids resulting in rapid cholesterol removal from the body. In high doses these drugs may decrease fat absorption which may also contribute to their effect. These drugs have similar side effects. The most common side effects involve the gastrointestinal (GI) tract. The most common side effect is constipation, especially with high doses. This effect is often controllable, but withdrawal of the drugs may be necessary. Abdominal pain, heartburn, nausea, bloating, flatulence (gas), and belching may also occur. These drugs may interfere with the absorption of fat soluble vitamins and other drugs.

Clofibrate (Atromid-S®) is more effective in lowering blood triglyceride concentrations than it does LDL cholesterol. This drug has been associated with the development of certain types of cancer and gastrointestinal problems. An increased incidence of gallstone development has been reported. It also may interact with anticoagulants (blood thinners). For these reasons this drug is usually reserved for treatment of patients with severe lipid problems that have not responded to other therapies and are a high risk of developing life-threatening complications.

Gemfibrozil (Lopid®) reduces triglycerides and LDL cholesterol. It has been shown to increase high density lipoproteins, which may have a protective effect. This drug, though chemically similar to clofibrate, does not cause as many severe side effects. However, it is also associated with gallstone formation and may interact with blood thinners.

Lovastatin (Mevacor®) inhibits the action of the enzyme that helps in the production of cholesterol. Lovastatin reduces total and LDL cholesterol and may be more effective than any other medication when used alone. At usual dosages this drug is usually better tolerated than other cholesterol-lowering drugs. However, several side effects involving muscle inflammation, kidney problems, and liver damage have been reported. Long-term safety has not been established, and some physicians are concerned that persistent reduction in the production of cholesterol may cause problems. Even though high blood levels of cholesterol are not desirable, a certain level is normal for it is a necessary component of body cell membranes. For this reason some physicians may reserve lovastatin for those patients who can not tolerate other possible choices.

Niacin (Nicolar®) is a vitamin and is available without a prescription. It is also available as a generic as well as a brand name product. It is not known how niacin works, but it is effective in lowering total and LDL-cholesterol, triglycerides and very low density lipoprotein (VLDL). It elevates HDL and has been shown in scientific studies to lower nonfatal heart attack and to affect the progression of atherosclerosis (hardening of the arteries). The most common complaint from patients taking this drug is severe flushing, itching, and gastrointestinal distress. This can often be prevented by starting treatment with a lower dose then gradually increasing it, taking the dosage on a full stomach, or dividing the dosage. If this does not work, then one aspirin taken 30 minutes before the niacin may be effective.

Neomycin is an antibiotic which can lower LDL cholesterol but also may decrease HDL. It is not approved by the FDA for this indication and can cause serious side effects in patients at risk.

Probucol (Lorelco®) lowers total cholesterol and LDL cholesterol and HDL cholesterol. When combined with colestipol, serum cholesterol is reported to be lowered to a great extent than when each is used alone. Probucol is cleared slowly from the body. It can cause loose stools and diarrhea and cause electrocardiogram changes in some patients.

Anticoagulant (Blood Thinner) Medications. Anticoagulant drugs are used to prevent blood from clotting, while thrombolytic agents dissolve existing blood clots. Even though these agents function differently, they may be used under the same circumstances. At present, however, thrombolytic agents are used predominantly to dissolve blood clots in the coronary arteries and certain intravascular devices.

Blood clots present a major problem when they develop in important vessels of the legs, lungs, brain, and heart. Clots developing in the large veins of the legs may cause some local damage. However, these clots are a greater threat to survival if a piece breaks away and travels to a major organ. If this occurs, the condition is called an embolism. Clots in the large veins of the legs (deep vein thrombosis) are a common source of emboli blocking arteries to the lungs (pulmonary embolism). In a similar manner, patients with atrial fibrillation can develop clots in the upper chambers of the heart. Fragments of these clots can travel to the brain causing stroke.

The formation of clots in atherosclerotic arteries of the heart plays a role in many heart attacks. Under certain circumstances, patients are thus at a greater risk for developing clots. When this is the case, the physician may use an anticoagulant to reduce the risk. Once a clot has developed, the physician may use an anticoagulant to prevent further growth and allow the body to dissolve the clot on its own. When it is important to rapidly remove the clot, the physician may choose a thrombolytic agent to dissolve the clot or in rare circumstances have it removed surgically.

The clotting mechanism of the body is important for survival. When a break occurs in a blood vessel, a set of reactions occurs resulting in clot formation, preventing major blood loss. These reactions are initiated by exposure of blood components to certain substances in the damaged tissue. Normal blood vessel walls do not cause blood to clot. If a clot does develop, it is eventually dissolved once it is no longer needed. The body removes clots with a naturally occurring thrombolytic agent called plasmin. However, there are circumstances when unwanted clots can develop. These circumstances are associated with blood stasis, vessel wall damage, and/or an overactive clotting mechanism (hypercoagulability). Any medical problem resulting in immobility can result in blood stasis in large vessels of the legs. Hypercoagulability may be precipitated by major surgery, trauma, genetic deficiency in natural clot preventers, bed rest, pregnancy, oral contraceptives, fractures of major bones, and other conditions.

Thus, anticoagulant agents are used to treat and/or prevent deep vein thrombosis, pulmonary embolism, and thrombotic stroke. Thrombolytic agents are used to treat deep vein thrombosis, pulmonary embolism, and myocardial infarction. Thrombolytic drugs are also useful for opening intravenous lines and other intravascular devices.

Types of anticoagulant drugs. The drugs in this class are often referred to as blood thinners. This term does not accurately describe the action of these agents. Anticoagulant drugs in no way increase the viscosity of blood or make it thin. They interfere with various steps in the body's coagulation mechanism, resulting in a decreased tendency to form a clot. While this effect may be necessary to treat the patient, it can result in unwanted bleeding.

There are two anticoagulant drugs commonly used in this country. These drugs are heparin (various manufacturers) and warfarin (Coumadin®). Heparin is always administered by injection, while warfarin is taken orally. These drugs are used for the same indications, but they are not necessarily interchangeable. Neither will dissolve a clot, but each will prevent the initiation or continuation of the clotting process. Both drugs may be used for various time periods; however, warfarin is more commonly used for long-term anticoagulation. This is primarily because it may be taken orally. Conversely, heparin is usually, but not always, administered for a short period of time. The major side effect of either drug is bleeding. Anticoagulant blood loss can be life-threatening. Patients taking anticoagulants should watch closely for signs of internal bleeding.

Selection. Most physicians follow a standard procedure for the use of these drugs.

Once the physician suspects the diagnosis of deep vein thrombosis or pulmonary embolism, heparin therapy is usually begun. Heparin produces immediate anticoagulation by enhancing the activity of an anticoagulant protein found in blood (antithrombin). Warfarin inhibits the production of vitamin K dependent clotting factors and may not cause adequate anticoagulation for several days. Immediate anticoagulation is necessary to prevent further clot formation.

Some physicians also begin warfarin along with heparin or within a few days. Heparin is continued until the anticoagulant effect of warfarin has reached adequate levels. Adequate anticoagulation is determined by blood clotting studies. Heparin is commonly monitored using the activated partial thromboplastin time (aPTT) and warfarin with the prothrombin time (PT).

The patient is usually continued on warfarin for six weeks to six months depending on his or her medical conditions. Patients with recurrent clots may be treated for even longer periods of time. After discharge from the hospital warfarin therapy will be followed with periodic measurement of the PT. Occasionally patients are unable to tolerate warfarin and will be instructed to give themselves small injections of heparin into the subcutaneous layer of the skin.

There are circumstances when heparin is given without additional warfarin therapy. Heparin is often given for short periods of time after myocardial infarction, during periods of unstable angina pectoris, and after procedures for opening blocked heart arteries (subcutaneous transluminal coronary angioplasty). It may also be given in small subcutaneous doses to prevent clots during periods of immobilization or before major surgery.

The doses required to anticoagulate a patient with either drug may be influenced by certain factors. Hereditary or temporary deficiencies in antithrombin may result in an increased heparin requirement. Families resistant to warfarin effects have also been discovered. Warfarin's effects may also be altered by the amount of vitamin K in the diet or the coadministration of drugs that affect vitamin K levels, such as antibiotics. Warfarin is especially susceptible to interactions with other drugs. Drugs which can affect the platelet function such as aspirin and non-steroidal anti-inflammatory agents (Motrin®, Indocin®, others) should be avoided. Drug interactions are most likely to cause a problem when a drug is begun or discontinued while taking warfarin.

Thrombolytic (clot buster) drugs. Thrombolytic drugs work by directly or indirectly increasing the breakdown of fibrin, a major protein component of a clot. The body normally dissolves fibrin with the enzyme plasmin, which is stored in an inactive form called plasminogen. Plasminogen is converted to plasmin by tissue plasminogen activator (rtPA, Alteplase, Activase®). Similarly, urokinase (Abbokinase®) directly stimulates the conversion of plasminogen to plasmin. Streptokinase (Kabikinase®, Streptase®) must first combine with plasminogen, forming a complex that enzymatically converts plasminogen to plasmin.

All three available thrombolytic agents are effective in dissolution of both arterial and venous clots. They have an advantage over anticoagulants because they enhance clot dissolution rather than preventing clot growth. Although indicated for deep vein thrombosis and pulmonary embolism, they are most commonly used to treat myocardial infarction. These agents are most effective in decreasing the extent of the infarction and preventing heart failure when used within a few hours of onset of a heart attack.

Selecting a thrombolytic agent. A physician's selection is influenced by cost, side effects, time after infarction, and physician preference. Streptokinase is the least expensive agent, but it has a greater potential to cause allergic side effects. Nevertheless, it is preferred by many physicians because of its effectiveness and low cost. Urokinase, while more expensive than streptokinase, remains less expensive than rtPA. It is the opinion of some experts that rtPA has not been demonstrated to have sufficient advantages over the other agents to justify its added cost.

EPILEPSY MEDICATIONS Chronic seizure disorders (epilepsy) must be managed with drug therapy. Anticonvulsant drugs, like some heart medications and intravenous antibiotics, have many serious side effects that may occur at normal doses. This occurs because the level of drug needed in the blood for the wanted effect (therapeutic concentration) is very close to the level that causes unwanted effects (toxic concentration). In fact there is some overlap in the two blood concentrations. In addition, the drug concentration produced by a given dose varies greatly from one patient to the next. This occurs because these drugs are metabolized in the body and their removal from the body is dependent on the patient's ability to metabolize the drug administered. The rate of metabolism is dependent on the patient's natural ability to metabolize the drug and the influence of certain underlying diseases and interfering drugs. To overcome this problem the physician measures the amount of drug in the patient's blood to determine proper dosage.

However, dosage is not solely based on blood concentration. The physician must also consider the patient's response to the drug. One of the drugs, phenytoin (Dilantin®), presents an additional dosing dilemma. This drug's metabolism is different from most other drugs. Usually when a physician increases the dose of a drug, the blood concentration increases proportionally; thus when the dose is doubled, the blood concentration will double. However, the body metabolizes phenytoin at a constant rate regardless of the dose. Therefore, doubling the dose may more than double the blood concentration.

Selection. Usually seizure disorders are initially managed with a single drug. The drug first chosen is determined by the type of seizure disorder diagnosed, but some of the drugs can be used for more than one type of disorder. The dose of the single agent is adjusted in response to seizure frequency, side effects, and measurement of drug concentrations in the blood. A change to a different single agent may occur in response to development of intolerable adverse effects. A second agent may be added if maximum doses of the single agent are not effective or if the patient has more than one seizure type.

It is no longer considered necessary to continue drug therapy for epilepsy on a lifelong basis for all patients. Medications can successfully be withdrawn from certain patients. The physician may decide to do this after the patient has been seizure free for two or more years. The presence of specific risk factors may predict those patients in which seizures are likely to recur.

Types of medications. Carbamazepine (Tegretol®) is indicated for the treatment of several seizure disorders. This drug has many side effects, but is considered by some clinicians to be the drug of choice for treatment of generalized tonic-clonic seizures. Carbamazepine may be better tolerated if it is begun at a low dose, and the dosage slowly increased. Some serious but rare side effects may not be dose-related.

Clonazepam (Klonopin®) is not considered to be the drug of first choice for any type of seizure. It is considered an alternative drug for the treatment of certain types of seizures. It may be effective when other drugs have failed but is generally less effective than other choices and tolerance may develop. This drug is a benzodiazepine and causes side effects common to this drug class.

Diazepam (Valium®) and lorazepam (Ativan®), two drugs used to treat anxiety and sedation, are effective intravenously for the acute treatment of sustained seizure activity (status epilepticus). Phenytoin is also useful but may not be given at first because it takes longer to begin working.

Ethosuximide (Zarontin®) is indicated for the treatment of uncomplicated absence seizures (petit mal). Toxic blood concentrations can cause mental changes. Allergic type reactions have been reported as well as other side effects.

Phenobarbital (various manufacturers) is considered an alternative drug for the treatment of generalized tonic-clonic and partial seizures. Phenobarbital may be the preferred drug when treating infants, but the mental side effects make it less useful in older children and adults. In fact many physicians avoid the long term use of this drug if at all possible.

Phenytoin is the most commonly prescribed antiseizure medication for adult epileptics. It is available in several dosage forms and may be prescribed for other indications. Phenytoin is indicated for the treatment of generalized tonic-clonic, and partial seizures. It has many side effects but is selected over carbamazepine by some physicians because of the latter's serious, but rare, blood cell toxicities. However, phenytoin more commonly interferes with thought processes in a learning situation. The physician must closely monitor patients taking phenytoin. To do this, certain physical signs of toxicity must be watched and blood concentrations of phenytoin periodically measured. Adjusting the dosage of phenytoin is not an easy task since phenytoin is not metabolized in the same manner as other drugs. It may take many weeks to determine the required dosage. The side effects associated with high blood concentrations are irregular movement of the eyes (nystagmus), unsteadiness (ataxia), and other mental changes. Many non-dosage related unwanted effects have also been associated with phenytoin.

Primidone (Mysoline®) is indicated for the same types of seizures as phenobarbital. In fact, some of the activity of primidone is due to its conversion in the body to phenobarbital. To overcome many of the side effects seen with this drug, primidone dosages should be gradually increased. Like phenobarbital, primidone is considered an alternative agent.

Valproate (Depakene®; Depakote®) is used for the treatment of generalized tonic-clonic, absence, and myoclonic seizures. It is also effective for treatment of mixed forms of seizures, but valproate is FDA-approved only for treatment of absence seizures. Valproate does not cause serious mental side effects, and other serious side effects are not common.

GASTROINTESTINAL MEDICATIONS
Upper gastrointestinal (GI) diseases, including peptic ulcer disease (PUD) and gastroesophageal reflux, are common in our society. The most common sites for the development of PUD are the duodenum and the stomach (gastric or "stomach" ulcers). The development of gastric ulcers is associated with the use of aspirin and similar antiarthritis medications, while duodenal ulcers are not. Use of alcohol, coffee and smoking may delay healing of gastric and duodenal ulcers. Another gastrointestinal problem, gastroesophageal reflux, is often referred to as heartburn. This too may be affected by life style and medications.

Peptic ulcer disease. When food is consumed, the body is stimulated by various substances and processes to release acid and pepsinogen into the stomach. In the presence of acid, pepsinogen is converted to pepsin. The acid-pepsin complex formed is essential in the digestion of food. Under normal conditions, the stomach is protected from self digestion by several mechanisms. The body reduces acid secretion when it senses an excessive amount. The intestinal tract secretes mucus, which acts as a protective barrier. Prostaglandins and bicarbonate are secreted which are also protective, as are other activities. When there is a defect in one or more of these defenses or an excess in acid, pepsin, or other digestive substances, a peptic ulcer may develop. While there is great variability, in general, duodenal ulcers are associated more with excessive acid secretion and gastric ulcers with defective protective barriers.

The goals of medical treatment are to heal the ulcer, relieve pain, prevent serious complications, and prevent recurrences. This is not always accomplished by medical treatment alone. Patients who continue to smoke will most certainly experience a relapse. Some patients will develop more than two recurrences per year, in spite of maintenance therapy. Unfortunately, no drug therapy has been shown to alter the long-term natural history of the PUD. These patients may require permanent reduction of acid secretion by surgery.

Selection. Antacids, H$_2$-antagonist, and sucralfate are equally effective in treating PUD when given in a sufficient dose. Drug selection is primarily based on patient acceptance, convenience, and potential for side effects.

Antacids must be taken frequently and in large doses. The taste of these agents may not be acceptable to some patients, and they frequently cause diarrhea. They have the potential for other adverse reactions and may interact with other medications. For these reasons, many practitioners may prescribe antacids only as needed for relief of pain.

H$_2$-antagonists may be given in large single doses at bedtime, thus making them easier to take. These drugs are relatively free of side effects, and newer agents are less likely to interact with other drugs. However, it is not known what the long term effects of continuous acid suppression are.

Sucralfate does not affect acid secretion or neutralization, nor is it absorbed in a significant amount. It may cause minor side effects, such as constipation. It must be given more frequently than H_2-antagonists, but not as often as antacids.

The physician will consider the above factors in selecting an agent. Occasionally, two agents will be used together, but there is no evidence that the combination of two agents is any more effective than either used alone; however, this practice has been shown to increase cost. The combined use of antacids as needed for pain and therapeutic doses of either of the other two agents is rational.

Treatment is usually continued for six to eight weeks. Long term maintenance therapy must be initiated if recurrence takes place within three months of the end of acute therapy, or if more than two times within one year.

Types of medications.

Antacids. There are many antacids available over the counter. Antacids work by neutralizing the acid found in the stomach. These products vary in the amount of acid neutralizing capacity, flavor, chemical composition, side effects, and added ingredients. Many products contain simethicone (anti-gas agent) which probably does not benefit the PUD patient. Products with high acid neutralizing capacity (Mylanta®II) may be more palatable due to the smaller volume required per dose. Antacids containing magnesium are more likely to cause diarrhea, while aluminum-containing products may cause constipation. Alternating a magnesium product with an aluminum product may counteract the side effects of each. Some products are a mixture of aluminum and magnesium salts. In the past, the majority of products were high in sodium content and could cause problems in patients on sodium restricted diets. However, most antacids have been reformulated so that this is no longer a problem.

H_2-antagonist. Histamine is involved in many activities within the body. Cold and allergy medicines contain antihistamines to block the allergic processes caused by the presence of histamine. The receptor responsible for allergic responses is called the H_1-receptor. H_2-receptors are found in the stomach and other organs. In the stomach these receptors cause acid secretion when stimulated. H_2-antagonist bind to these receptors, reducing acid release. All H_2-antagonists work by this mechanism. They differ mainly in potency, type and potential for side effects,

duration of action, and potential to interact with other drugs.

Cimetidine (Tagamet®) was the first H_2-antagonist marketed in this country. This product was accepted quickly as effective and convenient therapy of PUD. Cimetidine is the least potent of the available agents. It has more potential to cause side effects and to interact with other drugs than does ranitidine (Zantac®), famotidine (Pepcid®), and nizatidine (Axid®). When given in a single bedtime dose for the treatment of PUD, the differences between these agents may be very small.

Sucralfate. Sucralfate (Carafate®) binds to protein in the gastric and intestinal linings. It favors binding to diseased tissue, but it will bind to normal lining. This drug forms a barrier which inhibits the local action of the acid-pepsin complex. It has other activities which may be beneficial as well. Sucralfate is as effective as antacids and H_2-antagonists and has fewer side effects. It is normally given one gram four times a day, but studies of two grams given twice a day have had promising results.

Anticholinergic Agents. Anticholinergic drugs inhibit gastric secretion mediated by the vagus nerve. These drugs must be given in large doses to be effective, resulting in numerous side effects. Therefore, they are primarily used as supplemental therapy. The addition of an anticholinergic agent may benefit patients with nocturnal pain unresponsive to conventional therapy.

Misoprostol (Cytotec®). Approximately one-third of gastric ulcers are associated with the use of aspirin and other nonsteroidal anti-inflammatory agents (NSAIDs). Neither antacids, H_2-antagonists, nor sucralfate has been shown to prevent NSAID-associated gastric ulcers. Misoprostol is a synthetic analog of prostaglandin E_1 that is approved for the prevention of gastric ulcers in high-risk patients taking NSAIDs. Prostaglandins are substances secreted by the stomach lining and other body organs that facilitate many body functions. The E class prostaglandins inhibit gastric acid secretion, dilate blood vessels, increase movement of the GI tract, and cause contractions of the uterus in women. They also stimulate the stomach lining to secrete other substances that protect against ulcer formation. This agent has the potential for many side effects, especially in women. It is contraindicated in pregnancy and may cause other gynecological disturbances. The long term effects of this agent are not known.

Gastroesophageal reflux. Patients with this condition are unable to prevent the movement of stomach contents back into the esophagus. The resulting irritation and pain are often referred to as heartburn. Reflux occurs when the sphincter at the junction between the esophagus and stomach is not functioning properly. It is most likely to occur when the volume of stomach contents is high, stomach emptying is delayed, and/or the patient is lying down. Antacids or H_2-antagonists may be administered to neutralize stomach acid and thus reduce tissue irritation. Sucralfate has been used to protect the damaged tissue. Bethanechol (Urecholine®) increases the tone of the esophageal sphincter, while metoclopramide (Reglan®) increased sphincter tone and decreased stomach emptying time, helping reduce reflux. The last two drugs may cause severe side effects and may be reserved for patients with uncontrolled symptoms.

Laxatives. Laxatives help the passage of feces through the large intestines. Most laxatives are available without a prescription and are often overused, resulting in laxative dependence, habituation, and decreased response to their action. Healthy individuals eating adequate amounts of natural laxative foods and drinking adequate amounts of fluid should have no problems with bowel function. However, constipation can develop if a balanced diet is not maintained, the urge to defecate is ignored, or the patient has a medical condition resulting in decreased movement of the intestines. These medications are not always used to treat constipation, but they may be used to assist defecation under certain circumstances. Laxatives are indicated to relieve pain, reduce straining and intra-abdominal pressure, and to relieve constipation associated with certain conditions.

Drugs in this class may also be referred to as cathartics. Cathartics produce rapid results, while laxatives are slower acting. In general most types of laxatives/cathartics promote defecation by increasing the amount of water in the intestines. The additional water can lead to reflex evacuation, softened stools, or enhanced movement of the stool through the intestines. These drugs may be classed as stimulant (Dulcolax®, cascara sagrada, castor oil, others), saline (milk of magnesia, Phospho-Soda®, others), lubricant (mineral oil, glycerine suppositories), stool softening (Colace®, Surfak®, others), or bulk-forming (Metamucil®) laxatives, indicating the method of action. The selection of an agent is primarily determined by patient preference. Under certain conditions, the use of these medications can result in serious side effects such as precipitation of congestive heart failure, body fluid and mineral abnormalities, abdominal cramping, and other problems.

Nausea and Vomiting. Vertigo (dizziness), nausea, and vomiting are symptoms of underlying problems. Correction of these problems is the most effective remedy for these troublesome symptoms, but certain drugs may be indicated for persistent difficulties.

Effective medications include anticholinergic drugs (scopolamine patches), antihistamines (Dramamine®, Benadryl®, Antivert®, others), metoclopramide (Reglan®), certain tranquilizers (Compazine®, others), and miscellaneous drugs (Pepto-Bismol®, Emetrol®, others). These drugs are more effective for the prevention of vomiting than the treatment. The most common side effect encountered with this group of drugs is sedation.

Most over the counter products are used to treat motion sickness or vomiting associated with acute gastroenteritis. Caution should be taken when using these products for they may mask the symptoms of underlying medical problems. Additionally, self medication may delay contacting a physician. Since persistent vomiting can lead to serious depletion of body fluids and minerals, this delay could lead to serious consequence, especially in children.

Antidiarrheal medications. Acute severe or mild chronic diarrhea can cause dehydration and loss of body minerals, resulting in weakness and feebleness. Additionally, frequent defecation can produce discomfort and local irritation. The use of antidiarrheal drugs can ease these problems but may prolong infectious diarrhea. In addition to antidiarrhea agents, patients with mild uncomplicated diarrhea should drink plenty of clear liquids to replace lost fluid. Children and patients with severe diarrhea should be seen by a physician.

The most effective antidiarrheal drugs slow the movement of the gastrointestinal tract and prolong the time it takes for substances to move through the intestines. Effective drugs include codeine, loperamide (Imodium®), and diphenoxylate with atropine (Lomotil®). Paregoric is also widely used, either alone or combined with kaolin (Parepectolin®). These drugs are not associated with significant side effects when taken in recommended antidiarrheal doses.

Bismuth subsalicylate (Pepto-Bismol®) is effective for the treatment of diarrhea associated with a certain bacteria and as a non-specific antidiarrheal medication. Other commonly used medications are water absorbent substances, such as psyllium seed derivatives (Metamucil®, others), and kaolin (Kaopectate®). Live cultures of lactobacillus (Bacid®, Lactinex®) are reported to be useful in managing antibiotic associated diarrhea, but it is thought that most of the organism should be killed by stomach acid.

HORMONE REPLACEMENT MEDICATION Hormone replacement agents are used to treat various gynecologic and endocrine disorders, as well as other medical problems. Commonly used agents are male and female sex hormones, corticosteroids, thyroid hormone, parathyroid hormone, pituitary hormones, and insulin.

Corticosteroids. Corticosteroids are produced by the adrenal cortex, and are responsible for many important body activities under normal conditions and in times of stress. The body is capable of regulating corticosteroid levels by a complex system involving the brain and pituitary glands. The amount of drug equivalent to the amount of natural corticosteroid released by the body daily is called the physiologic dose. Doses greater than the physiologic dose are called pharmacologic doses.

These agents are usually classified as mineralocorticoids or glucocorticoids based on their main pharmacological activity. However, agents can have a significant amount of each activity. Aldosterone is a naturally occurring mineralocorticoid, while hydrocortisone and cortisone are naturally occurring glucocorticoids. Mineralocorticoids alter electrolyte and fluid balance by increasing the kidney's retention of sodium and potassium and hydrogen excretion. Glucocorticoids aid the body's breakdown of protein, production of glucose, and redistribution of fat from peripheral to central areas of the body. They also affect the immune response and certain blood cells.

When given in pharmacological doses, these agents affect many body functions and suppress the hypothalamic-pituitary-adrenal axis and the release of adrenocorticotropic hormone, ACTH, from the pituitary. If the corticosteroid is suddenly withdrawn, the patient may develop secondary adrenocortical insufficiency, which can be life threatening during periods of stress. The physician overcomes this problem by tapering the dose over a long period of time.

Long term use of pharmacological doses also produces hypercorticism. These patients are said to be cushingoid and have many identifiable physical changes. They may develop a rounded face (moon face) and fat build-up on the upper back (buffalo hump), as well as other body changes.

Glucocorticoids and mineralocorticoids are used for replacement therapy in patients with primary adrenal insufficiency (Addison's disease). Other indications include certain dermatologic, allergic, ocular, respiratory, hematologic, gastrointestinal, rheumatological, and neoplastic (cancer) disorders. High dose parenteral glucocorticoids may also be useful for treatment of brain edema associated with head injury. Mineralocorticoids may be useful in the management of certain types of low blood pressure.

Corticosteroids currently available may be given by mouth, injection, enema, inhalation, or topically. These drugs are associated with increased susceptibility to infection, fluid and electrolyte disturbances, weight gain, edema, ocular damage, peptic ulcers, mental disturbances, increased blood sugar, and many other side effects.

Contraceptives. Use of an oral contraceptive (birth control pill) is the most common form of contraception in the United States. Other drugs or chemical forms of contraception are available but are less commonly used because of higher reported failure rates, lack of FDA approval, and/or inconvenience. Another method, medroxyprogesterone acetate

(Depo-Provera®) administered intramuscularly every three months, may be as effective as tubal sterilization. It is commonly used in other countries but is not approved for this indication in the U.S. Chemical spermacides are also available in different forms of delivery. This method of contraception is not convenient and has a higher reported failure rate than the use of medroxyprogesterone acetate or oral contraceptives. On the other hand, chemical spermacides combined with condoms may offer the best protection against sexually transmitted diseases.

Selection. There are two types of oral contraceptives available. A small number of products contain the hormone progestin only (An intrauterine device that releases progesterone is also available.) The most commonly marketed oral contraceptives are combination products. Combination products contain variable amounts of estrogens and progestins. Not only do products differ in the estrogen and/or progestin combination used, but they also may differ in the dosage of these two drugs. The most popular oral contraceptives vary the dosage of progestin and occasionally estrogen in two or three phases. In theory, these drugs better mimic the normal body fluctuation in the amount of these hormones during the menstrual cycle. It was surmised that mimicking the body's release of hormones would less likely disrupt the body's normal metabolic patterns. However, no studies have documented occurrence of these theoretical advantages. Nevertheless, a physician may consider these theoretical differences when making a selection.

When taken as directed, both classes of oral contraceptives are effective, but there is a small difference in their reported failure rate. Progestin-only products have a slightly greater failure rate. This class is primarily indicated for nursing mothers, since estrogen found in the combination type products may decrease lactation and therefore is contraindicated. Additionally, these products may be used in women with estrogen-dependent breast cancer.

Safety. The potential risk of taking oral contraceptives has received much media attention. Most of the concern arose because of serious side effects documented to occur with older formulas. Use of older, high dose estrogen products is associated with an increased risk of cardiovascular disease and breast cancer. Consequently, manufacturers reduced the amount of estrogen and progestin used. Studies in women using newer combination products have not shown a relationship to these unwanted consequences. Nevertheless, it is possible that oral contraceptives may increase the risk of breast cancer in some groups of women. However, oral contraceptives may protect against endometrial and ovarian cancer.

Estrogens. Estrogens are naturally occurring hormones secreted mainly by the ovaries, and to a lesser extent other female and male organs. Natural and manmade estrogens are used to treat various gynecological disorders associated with a deficiency of these substances. They may also be effective in retarding further bone loss and the progression of osteoporosis associated with menopause. They may also be useful as palliative treatment of various inoperable male and female cancers. In high doses these drugs are associated with increased risk of blood clots, stroke, heart attack, hypertension and other problems.

Androgens. Androgens are male sex hormones. Testosterone is the principal naturally occurring androgen. Testosterone is responsible for normal growth and development of male sex organs and for secondary male sex characteristics. All drugs in this class are anabolic hormones and increase protein production. Androgens may enhance the release of the hormone that stimulates red blood cell production and may be used to treat certain anemias. The administration of androgens results in the inhibition of testosterone release by the body. Testosterone and other androgens are used as replacement therapy in male patients with congenital or acquired deficiencies in testosterone secretion. They are also used in the management of certain cancers and anemias. Androgens are also used for certain unapproved indications. These are the agents abused by athletes seeking to enhance muscle strength training. These drugs are associated with many severe side effects, such as hypertension, liver toxicity, cancer, and sterility. Female patients may experience development of virilization.

Thyroid hormones. Various natural and synthetic thyroid hormones are available as replacement therapy. These drugs are primarily used as replacement therapy in patients with hypothyroidism of various causes. Levothyroxine sodium is considered the thyroid agent of choice for the control of symptoms secondary to hypothyroidism. The use of thyroid hormones for the management of obesity is considered unjustified.

Overdosage of thyroid hormone results in weight loss, increased appetite, palpitations, nervousness, diarrhea, abdominal cramps, sweating, increased heart rate, elevated blood pressure, cardiac arrhythmias, and other abnormalities.

Insulin. Insulin is a hormone produced and released by the pancreas. Insulin stimulates carbohydrate metabolism by assisting transport of glucose into the body cells. Insulin replacement in patients with diabetes mellitus restores the ability to maintain reasonable blood glucose concentrations. Insulin is available from human and animal sources. Animal source insulin is obtained from beef and pork pancreases and is available as single and mixed source products. Pork insulin most closely approximates human insulin. Presently available products are designated "purified" for they contain less contaminates than earlier products. Human insulin is also commercially available. It is manufactured by special strains of bacteria using recombinant DNA technology or by modifying pork insulin.

The various forms of insulin available differ in time of onset, peak, and duration. The physician chooses the appropriate form based on close monitoring of the patient's blood glucose measurement. The most serious side effect of insulin therapy is hypoglycemia.

Topical Steroid Products. Topical corticosteroids are available for the treatment of various dermatological conditions. These drugs reduce redness, itching, and other troublesome symptoms. Topical corticosteroids are available as lotions, creams, and ointments in a variety of potencies and strengths. Drug selection is dependent upon many considerations including drug potency, drug concentration, product formulation, site of problem, and expense. Products requiring a prescription are generally more potent and more expensive. Hydrocortisone is available over the counter in a 0.5 percent strength for relief of minor skin problems.

PARKINSON'S DISEASE MEDICATIONS Parkinson's disease can be described as a problem with one of the electrical systems of the brain, the extrapyramidal nervous system. The brain uses several substances to help send messages along its different systems. Some of the messages sent are inhibitory (stop activities), while others are excitatory (start activities). Patients with Parkinson's disease have a decrease in dopamine, a substance which helps transmit inhibitory signals, and a relative increase in acetylcholine, a substance responsible for excitatory signals. The imbalance in the inhibitory and excitatory helping substances results in the symptoms observed in patients with this disease. At present Parkinson's disease is not curable. Therefore, treatment is primarily targeted toward reduction in the symptoms. Drug treatment plays an important role in the attempt to correct this imbalance. There are five types of drugs currently being used to treat this disease. These drugs are anticholinergic agents (which block effects of excitatory system), amantadine (which may help the release of dopamine), levodopa (which enters the brain and is converted to dopamine), dopamine agonists (which mimic dopamine), and monoamine oxidase (MAO)-type B inhibitors (which prevent breakdown of dopamine).

Selection. Selection of initial therapy may be influenced by the type and severity of symptoms. In the early stage of the disease anticholinergics, or more commonly amantadine, may be used alone. As the disease progresses levodopa is added. As the effectiveness of levodopa dwindles with time, the addition of other medications may be considered.

Anticholinergics. These drugs were once used alone to treat Parkinson's disease. With the introduction of levodopa their role in the management of this disease has diminished. Anticholinergic agents may be used for their additive effects at any point in the progression of the disease. Examples of this class of drugs are trihexylphenidyl (Artane®), biperiden (Akeneton®), benztropine (Cogentin®), procyclidine (Kemadrin®), and ethopropazine (Parsidol®). Antihistamines with anticholinergic activity may also be prescribed. Common adverse effects are dry mouth, constipation, and urinary retention.

Amantadine. Amantadine (Symmetrel®; and others), an antiviral agent, was accidentally discovered to reduce symptoms of Parkinson's disease. The mechanism of action of this drug is not completely understood, but it is thought that it enhances release of dopamine. Amantadine is effective in reducing the symptoms of this disease in about half the patients, but many will develop a decrease in response within one to three months. As with levodopa, this drug may regain some of its effectiveness when temporarily withdrawn and then reinstituted. This situation is called a drug holiday.

Amantadine is relatively free of severe side effects. The side effects commonly seen involve mainly the gastrointestinal, cardiovascular, and central nervous systems. The most common side effects involve the central nervous system. Patients may develop confusion, dizziness, disorientation, depression, nervousness, and hallucinations. Amantadine has some anticholinergic effect which may result in an increased incidence of CNS effects when combined with an anticholinergic drug. Ankle edema is also commonly reported. A benign reversible condition called livedo reticularis can occur in up to 80 percent of the patients. This adverse effect is noted by rose colored mottling of the skin, usually involving the lower extremities.

Levodopa and carbidopa. Levodopa is rapidly degraded outside the brain requiring the administration of large doses when not combined with an inhibitor of degradation. Carbidopa is an enzyme inhibitor combined with levodopa in the product Sinemet®. The presence of carbidopa reduces the amount of levodopa required for the desired effect. In addition, many of the side effects seen when levodopa is used alone in high doses are prevented with the levodopa/carbidopa combination. This combination is the most effective treatment of Parkinson's disease available in this country.

The time to add levodopa therapy during the progression of the disease has been somewhat controversial. Levodopa does not alter the course of the disease and its effects diminish with time. Some physicians believe that the effectiveness of levodopa may have a time limit. These physicians would recommend re-serving this drug for severe forms of the disease. Conversely, others believe that the effectiveness of levodopa is dependent on the duration of the disease and recommend early use. When a decrease in effectiveness does occur the physician may withdraw levodopa for a period of time (drug holiday). This has been shown to improve response and reduce side effect in some, but not all studies. A drug holiday can produce serious psychological and physical problems, and its use probably should not be routinely employed.

Side effects. The dosage of levodopa/carbidopa is adjusted to get maximum benefit with minimum side effects. As the dosage increases the patient is more likely to develop involuntary movements (dyskinesias, dystonias). This requires careful monitoring of the patient and periodic changes in dosage. Other problems associated with this drug are unpleasant dreams, hallucinations, excitement, agitation, and depression. Mental changes are most often seen in patients with underlying mental conditions or are receiving high doses.

Unwanted response fluctuations such as the "on/off" and "wearing off" effects may be partially explained by fluctuation in the amount of drug found in the blood stream. Improvement of these problems may be managed by shortening the interval between doses or adding a supplemental agent as a dopamine agonist. Sustained release formulations of levodopa are being investigated in an attempt to alleviate these problems.

Dopamine agonist (mimic dopamine). Bromocriptine (Parlodel®) is a dopamine agonist. It mimics the effects of dopamine and may reduce symptoms.

PSYCHIATRIC MEDICATIONS

Benzodiazepines. One of the most common class of drugs dispensed in this country is the benzodiazepines. These drugs are used to treat several problems but their most common use is to treat anxiety (nervousness) and insomnia (inability to fall asleep). The two oldest examples of benzodiazepines are Librium® (chlordiazepoxide) and Valium® (diazepam). These two drugs have been widely dispensed for many years and are now available in the generic form.

Selection. All benzodiazepines are effective in treating anxiety and insomnia and can be used interchangeably for these purposes. However, different manufacturers of benzodiazepines have chosen to market their products differently. The majority of products are marketed to treat anxiety. A smaller number is marketed to treat insomnia, and one drug, clonazepam (Klonopin®), is marketed only for the treatment of seizures. Midazolam, (Versed®) is marketed to relieve anxiety, induce light anesthesia, and produce amnesia for certain surgeries and uncomfortable diagnostic procedures. To some degree the selection of a benzodiazepine may be influenced by the targeted use chosen by the manufacturer.

How the drug is absorbed and metabolized (pharmacological properties) can also play an important role in product selection. While most benzodiazepines are similar in their effectiveness in treating the same indications, they may differ greatly in their pharmacological properties. Some have a rapid onset of action, while others may be slow in onset. Some have a short duration of action, while others may have a long duration of action. These differences may be very important. It would seem logical that a drug with a short onset of action would have an advantage over one with a slow onset, when treating insomnia. Additionally, a drug with a long duration of action may cause unwanted sedation and interfere with normal daily activities. A physician must consider these factors in determining medication for a patient.

Common uses. This class of drugs may be used to treat anxiety, insomnia, muscle spasms, seizures, and alcohol withdrawal.

Anxiety and insomnia. Benzodiazepines are generally preferred over other classes of medications to treat these indications. This preference is due to the effectiveness and relative safety of benzodiazepines when compared to other possible choices such as barbiturates (phenobarbital and others) or meprobamate (Equanil® and others).

Diazepam (Valium®), lorazepam (Ativan®), and midazolam (Versed®) can be given intravenously before certain surgeries and diagnostic studies to relieve anxiety. These drugs will also cause the patient to forget the events of the surgery or procedure. The ability to cause the patient to forget the events surrounding the surgery or study can be a very useful property, especially when given before cancer drug therapy. Many cancer drugs cause such severe nausea and vomiting that, once a patient has experienced this side effect, it may be induced subsequently upon seeing the medication or the nurse or doctor that administered the drug. When benzodiazepines are given before cancer therapy, beginning with the first treatment, patients will often tolerate the anti-cancer drugs better.

Alprazolam (Xanax®) may be useful for the treatment of depression and prevention of panic attacks.

Alcohol withdrawal. Benzodiazepines are used to manage agitation and tremor associated with acute alcohol withdrawal. They may prevent or relieve symptoms of delirium tremens (DT's) and hallucinations.

Seizure disorders. Diazepam (Valium®) has been used intravenously for many years to treat a condition called status epilepticus and seizures associated with drug overdoses and poisons. However, it is not used for treatment of chronic seizure disorders such as epilepsy. Clonazepam (Klonopin®) is the only drug in this class used orally to treat chronic seizure problems. It may be used alone or in combination with other anticonvulsants (seizure-preventing medications).

Treatment of muscle spasms. The effectiveness of these drugs to relieve pain associated with acute skeletal muscle conditions, such as that produced by strains and physical injury, is not well established. Published studies have produced conflicting results. Benzodiazepines are effective in the short and long term management of skeletal muscle spasm caused by local trauma and inflammation, cerebral palsy, paraplegia, and other disorders such as tetanus.

Adverse effects. Some of the effects which may make benzodiazepines useful when treating one type of condition can become unwanted effects when treating another condition. All drugs in this class can cause sedation, interfere with normal daily function, and impair memory. Older patients may be especially susceptible to these unwanted effects. These drugs may become habit forming after extended periods of use. They can cause a since of well being under certain conditions which may explain why they are often abused. In some elderly patients, benzodiazepines may produce unexpected excitement instead of sedation.

Sedation and impaired function. Benzodiazepines with a long duration of action (slowly removed from the body by metabolism and excretion) can accumulate producing unwanted sedation and impair daily mental and physical function. Some patients may not be aware of this effect.

Memory loss. This effect is highly variable depending on the drug used, the dose, and how it is given. Two drugs, triazolam (Halcion®) and lorazepam (Ativan®) have been implicated more often than other benzodiazepines.

Problems with chronic use. Tolerance (decrease in effectiveness) and dependence can occur. Tolerance can compound the potential for psychological and physical dependence. Sudden cessation of benzodiazepine therapy may produce severe withdrawal symptoms similar to those seen with barbiturates and alcohol dependence. Symptoms may not occur for days in patients taking benzodiazepines which are slowly removed from the body. Mild forms of withdrawal resulting after discontinuance of these drugs for insomnia may be mistaken to be a reoccurrence of the patient's sleeping problems and result in reinstitution of the drug.

Antidepressants. A tricyclic antidepressant (Elavil®, Norpramin®, Sinequan®, and others) is usually the drug of first choice for treatment of major depression. Several tricyclic antidepressants are available in the generic form and may be less expensive than newer classes of antidepressants.

Even though TCA's are considered by many physicians as the drugs of choice for treatment of this disorder, they do have several drawbacks. These drugs can cause serious life threatening side effects when taken in an overdose. Additionally, they may interact with other drugs taken by the patient and can cause annoying side effects in standard doses. Adverse effects on the heart have been a major concern in some patients with underlying heart disease.

For these reasons drug manufacturers have developed newer antidepressants in an attempt to overcome these concerns. Newer drugs may have fewer side effects, but none have been shown to be decidedly more effective than the older TCA agents.

Patients may be diagnosed to have depression in conjunction with some other psychiatric diagnosis. These patients may receive an antidepressant in conjunction with another type of drug such as a neuroleptic (drug for psychotic behavior).

Tricylic antidepressants (TCAs). The precise cause of depression is not known, but several theories have been proposed. Neither is the mechanism by which TCAs help ease depression known. Nonetheless, it is felt by scientists that these drugs, as well as other antidepressants, affect levels of chemicals in the brain and/or the brain's sensitivity to chemicals responsible for mood. TCAs may be used alone or in conjunction with other methods of treatment such as psychotherapy and electroconvulsive (shock) therapy, depending on the degree and type of depression diagnosed by the physician. Depression can be induced by some diseases and by certain medications. If this is the case, the physician may treat the patients with a TCA until these problems are resolved. Establishment of the proper TCA dosage takes close monitoring of the patient. The adjustment of the dosage of TCAs may also be aided by monitoring drug blood concentrations. Dosage adjustment may take several weeks to accomplish.

Selecting a tricyclic antidepressant. The selection of a TCA is dependent on many factors. If, on one hand, the patient has been newly diagnosed to have major depression, then selection may be determined by the patient's current medical problems, attitude, and the symptoms of depression present. These drugs, as a class, have effects on the heart, urinary bladder, the brain, as well as other organs. Fortunately, not all of the TCAs have the same degree of effect on these body systems. The doctor tries to select the drug which would most likely have the least effect on the patient's other health problems. In the same manner, if agitation or inability to sleep is a major symptom of the patient's depression, the physician will choose a drug which will most likely help the troublesome symptom. On the other hand, if the patient has been treated previously for depression, the choice of TCA will be based on past response to drug therapy and/or side effects encountered with past therapy.

Side effects. These drugs, as a class, cause

certain characteristic side effects, but the seriousness of each side effect varies from one TCA to another. Common side effects are dry mouth, dilated pupils, urinary retention, increased heart rate, drowsiness, and weight gain.

OTHER ANTIDEPRESSANTS

Second generation antidepressants. Two members of this group, amoxapine (Asendin®) and maprotiline (Ludiomil®), offer no real advantages over the TCAs. However, two others, fluoxetine (Prozac®) and trazodone (Desyrel®), may cause fewer side effects and fewer problems after overdose.

Monoamine oxidase inhibitors (MAOIs). MAOIs are used as alternatives to TCAs in patients who do not respond or do not tolerate their side effects. MAOIs may be more effective in patients with atypical depression or phobic disorders (unrealistic fear or avoidance of certain things or situations). These drugs also have many side effects. The most common ones are decreased blood pressure upon standing, weight gain, sexual dysfunction, and water retention. In addition these drugs interact with many drugs and certain foods. MAOIs inhibit an enxyme in the body responsible for breaking down chemicals which can increase blood pressure. Tyramine is a chemical which when ingested can increase these chemicals. Tyramine is found in foods like cheese, chocolate, red wines, and others. If a patient is taking a MAOI and ingests a food containing tyramine, a very harmful increase in blood pressure may occur. When a doctor places a patient on one of these agents, he will give the patient a list of drugs and foods to avoid.

Lithium. Lithium is a drug used to treat manic depressive illness. It has been used to treat other conditions, and at one time it was used as a salt substitute. The latter use resulted in severe lithium poisoning in some patients, leading to it being labeled a poison. It is not known how lithium works in this disorder. Its long term use prevents both the depressive and manic episodes of bipolar affective disorders. Lithium's effects may take two to three weeks to occur requiring temporary treatment with other medications. Lithium dosage is adjusted using close monitoring for side effects and measurement of blood concentrations. Many medical conditions, age,

drugs, and salt intake can effect lithium blood concentrations. For this reason the physician will carefully instruct the patient on how to take medication and what things to avoid.

ANTIPSYCHOTIC DRUGS (TRANQUILIZERS) Major tranquilizers may be referred to by several names. Commonly they are called antipsychotic agents or neuroleptics. This class of drugs may be used for various mental disorders but are most often used to treat schizophrenia. Like other drugs used to manage mental disorders, neuroleptics are fraught with many side effects. Furthermore, it is not known exactly how these drugs work. Nevertheless, it is felt that they block the site of action of a brain signal transmitting chemical (dopamine). Most of the neuroleptic agents block the site of action of dopamine. Not only is blocking of dopamine activity felt to be responsible for the antipsychotic activity of these drugs, but also they prevent nausea and vomiting. These wanted effects are counterbalanced by unwanted effects of dopamine blocking activity. The most notable unwanted effects are a collection of body movement disorders which can be very troublesome. Along with this problem, chronic dopamine blocking can lead to tardive dyskinesia, a movement disorder caused by an oversensitivity to dopamine stimulation. Another serious side effect relatively unique to this group of drugs is neuroleptic malignant syndrome. This adverse effect occurs more with the most potent agents with highest dopamine blocking activity. Neuroleptic malignant syndrome is similar in some ways to heat stroke. Patients develop a high temperature, mental changes, and signs of muscle damage.

Neuroleptic drugs can be classified in many ways. Scientists commonly use their chemical classification, but they may grouped by potency or extent and type of side effects.

The goal of therapy with neuroleptic agents is reduction is the symptoms of schizophrenia with minimum adverse effects.

Selection. Studies evaluating neuroleptic agents suggest that they are equally effective when given in ample dosages. In a specific individual this may not be the case. The failure of a patient to respond to one agent does not indicate that he or she will fail to respond to another. Why this occurs is not known, but it may be related to differences in how individuals metabolize the drugs or possible differences in the cause of schizophrenia. The side effect profile of various agents also plays an important role in drug selection. As with TCAs there are differences in intensity of each side effect between various agents in the class. Again the physician attempts to match the drug with the patient's needs and accompanying medical problems.

SEDATIVES (DRUGS THAT INDUCE SLEEP) Sedative/hypnotic drugs are the class of drugs commonly used to treat difficulties in initiating or maintaining sleep. There are multiple causes of insomnia, but a large proportion of patients with chronic insomnia have underlying psychiatric disorders. Other patients may have a psychological, physiological, or drug induced cause. The underlying condition must be diagnosed for successful management of insomnia. The long term use of sedatives or hypnotics for the management of insomnia cannot be recommended. In fact, it is generally recommended that these drugs be used for no longer than six weeks.

Selection. Several factors are important in selecting a sedative or hypnotic. The drug should have minimal effect on normal sleep patterns, not cause hangover, and have minimal effects upon withdrawal. The class of drugs which most closely meets this criteria are the benzodiazepines. Barbiturates, such as phenobarbital, are no longer considered to be indicated for this problem by many physicians. Additionally other classes of sedative or hypnotics have fallen into relative disuse. Short acting benzodiazepines are currently the drugs of first choice for the treatment of insomnia. Nevertheless, these agents should only be used for short periods of time. It should be kept in mind that these agents do interrupt normal sleep patterns may cause hangover and withdrawal side effects.

Over the counter sleep aids. All over the counter sleep aids primarily contain antihistamines. Some products contain diphenydramine (also referred to as Benadryl®). A sleep aid promoted in health food stores contains L-tryptophan, a naturally occurring aminoacid. There is some evidence that both these agents will reduce the time it takes to

fall asleep in study patients. Conflicting studies of L-tryptophan, however, have found it to be no more effective than a placebo (sugar pill).

RESPIRATORY MEDICATIONS In general there are two types of lung disease. The first, restrictive lung disease, is characterized by a decrease in the ability to breathe in air. Lung fibrosis and pneumonia are examples of restrictive lung disease. The second, obstructive lung disease, is distinguished by a decrease in the ability to breathe out air. Asthma and bronchitis are examples of this type. Drug treatment may benefit either of these types of lung diseases but is most beneficial if the problem is reversible. Reversible lung disease is associated with spasm of the lung passageways (bronchospasm). The physician can determine the type of lung disease and its reversibility by performing a lung function test.

The drugs used for the treatment of intermittent and chronic asthma, emphysema, and chronic bronchitis are essentially the same. However, they may be used in slightly different ways and one medication, cromolyn sodium (Intal®), is used only for asthma prevention. Drug treatment is directed at dilatation of the breathing passageways (bronchodilatation), reducing inflammation, and prevention of acute attacks. Drugs used to treat precipitating factors, such as infection, will not be discussed.

Selection. The following discussion will be in general terms. There are five classes of drugs used to treat these problems. They are beta-agonist, theophylline, steroids, anticholinergic agents, and cromolyn sodium. Cromolyn sodium is used to prevent certain asthmatic attacks. The manner in which the other drugs are used is dependent on the type and severity of the problem, and to some extent, physician opinion.

Patients may have either intermittent or chronic asthma. Patients with intermittent asthma are usually treated only during an attack. These patients appear to benefit most from inhalation of a beta-agonist for bronchodilatation. The use of theophylline has not been shown to be as effective as parenteral or inhaled beta-agonist for initial therapy of acute attacks of asthma. Furthermore, it is the opinion of some physicians that the addition of theophylline in this situation may increase side effects without added benefit.

Patients not responding completely to inhaled beta-agonist may benefit some from the addition of an inhaled anticholinergic agent. The timing of the addition of corticosteroids (steroids) to initial therapy is somewhat controversial. Early use of steroids may prevent hospitalization. However, many patients will respond adequately to bronchodilator therapy alone. Patients requiring hospitalization will usually receive a short course of intravenous steroids, after which oral steroid therapy is begun. Length of the oral therapy is dependent on the patient's clinical condition.

Patients with chronic asthma may be treated similarly during acute attacks. However, these patients require maintenance therapy to reduce the number of attacks. To accomplish this, the patient may be treated with theophylline or cromolyn sodium. Patients not controlled on the combination of theophylline, inhaled cromolyn, and inhaled beta-agonist may benefit from steroid therapy. Short courses of oral steroids may be beneficial, but chronic administration can lead to serious side effects. The administration of inhaled corticosteroids may be prescribed to overcome this problem.

Chronic bronchitis and emphysema are referred to as chronic obstructive pulmonary disease (COPD). Patients with COPD are treated in a manner comparable to patients with chronic asthma. Theophylline may have additional beneficial effects other than bronchodilatation in this group of patients. It may improve contraction and reduce fatiguing of the breathing muscle (diaphragm). Patients with COPD may benefit more from inhaled anticholinergic agents than patients with asthma. Acute worsening of COPD is managed in a similar manner as acute asthma.

Types of medication.
Adrenergic Drugs. These drugs cause bronchodilation by stimulating lung receptors. These drugs may be given by mouth, injection, or inhalation. Their effectiveness and adverse effects are dependent on the route of administration. When given by the oral route, beta-agonists are slow in onset and erratically absorbed. The parenteral route appears to be no more effective than inhalation and may cause more side effects. Clinical studies have shown the inhaled route to be effective and relatively free of side effects. Several methods of administration are available for inhalation therapy. Recent studies have shown the use of metered-dose aerosols to be the most cost effective method. Nevertheless, certain handicapped adults and young children may have difficulty using an aerosol canister. These patients may benefit from the use of a tube-spacer device. If this does not help, the drug may be delivered using compressed air nebulization.

Theophylline. Theophylline produces bronchodilatation by enhancing β_2 stimulation. It may also have other beneficial effects when used in patients with COPD. Theophylline has limited usefulness for the acute treatment of asthma attacks. However, its use does benefit patients with chronic asthma and COPD by decreasing the frequency and severity of attacks.

Theophylline is manufactured in intravenous, rectal, and oral dosage forms. The intravenous route is no more effective than oral, but it may be used when the patient is unable to take medications by mouth. The rectal route may be used in the rare occasion when neither oral or intravenous routes are preferable. Nevertheless, it must be noted that rectal suppositories are erratically absorbed, and their use is avoided when possible. Many oral products are available, making product selection confusing.

There are several products that are theophylline derivatives or theophylline salts. One product, dyphylline (Dilor®, Lufyllin®, and others) is of questionable effectiveness, cannot be monitored by blood concentration measurement, and should be avoided. Theophylline salts, aminophylline, oxtriphylline (Choledyl®), theophylline sodium glycinate (Synophylate®), and others, have no proven advantage over theophylline. Aminophylline, a complex of theophylline and ethylenediamine, is becoming less frequently used. Fixed-dose combination products, such as Tedral® and Marax®, are often not rational and are avoided by most clinicians. Products containing theophylline alone are preferred. They are sold as a liquid, regular tablets, and sustained release tablets and capsules. The sustained release products are preferred, because they can be given less frequently and produce more consistent blood concentrations. Nevertheless, not all products are alike. It is not easy to manufacture a product that evenly and consistently releases the drug over a long period of time (twelve hours or more). The best products produce blood theophylline concentrations that fluctuate only slightly over a twelve hour period. Only two or three manufacturers produce products that do this. These products are preferred by most practitioners.

Theophylline can cause many adverse effects. The occurrence of these effects may be affected by changes in metabolism, taking the product with or without food, and interactions with other drugs. The physician will attempt to avoid side effects by carefully monitoring the patient for toxic symptoms and measuring blood theophylline concentrations.

Cromolyn Sodium. This drug prevents the release of histamine from certain body cells, but its precise mechanism of action is still unknown. Histamine release is known to play a role in hyperreactivity of lung passageways. Cromolyn sodium is not a bronchodilator and is only effective for the prevention of symptoms. This drug is available as a powder for inhalation through a spinhaler, a nebulized solution and a metered-dose aerosol. Cromolyn has very few side effects.

Anticholinergic agents. Anticholinergic agents in the form of "asthma cigarettes" and other products have been available for many years. Until recently, the use of these agents had declined, but lately interest in these agents has been revived. Anticholinergic agents cause bronchodilatation by a mechanism separate from β_2 stimulation. Ipratropium bromide (Atrovent®) is a new agent available for inhalation. It has additive effects when combined with other bronchodilators.

Corticosteroids. Steroids reduce inflammation which can influence the severity of pulmonary symptoms. They are associated with many side effects and are reserved for the treatment of acute or chronic symptoms unresponsive to bronchodilators. Serious side effects are rare with short term use of oral or parenteral products or the use of inhaled products.

Over the counter asthma products. Epinephrine (Primatene Mist®) is available for inha-

lation. It is much shorter acting and less β_2-selective than newer prescription products.

SUNSCREENS   The shelves of most drug, grocery, and department stores are lined with a plethora of over the counter sunscreens. These products vary greatly in the type of vehicle (medium in which active ingredient is delivered), active ingredient, and degree of sun protection provided. This large selection of products has been brought about by the demand created by a health conscious consumer.

Selecting a sunscreen. The selection of a vehicle (alcohol, cream, gel, lotion, or oil) in which the active ingredient is delivered is somewhat a personal choice and will not be discussed here. These products may contain one of two types of active ingredients, a chemical or physical blocker. Physical sunblockers, such as products containing titanium dioxide, talc, or zinc oxide should be limited to use on small areas of skin, such as the ear tips, lips, and/or nose. These products are opaque and scatter light, thus preventing harmful rays from reaching the skin.

The most effective sunscreens contain chemical sun blockers. These products will contain either aminobenzoic acid esters, anthranilates, benzophenones, cinnamates, or salicylates. All of these substances are effective when used properly. The type of chemical used is of primary importance to those individuals with a known sensitivity to one of the active ingredients. These individuals should avoid products containing the offending ingredient.

Chemical sunscreens absorb ultraviolet-light. This is a type of light energy which normally can not be seen. This light energy is responsible for causing the damage known as sunburn. It is also responsible for skin aging and certain types of skin cancers. There are two types of ultraviolet energy, UVA and UVB. UVA levels are constant throughout the day. UVA exposure is not a major cause of sunburn in temperate areas of the world, but it can cause chronic skin damage, aging, and cancer. Most chemical sunscreens do not block this form of ultraviolet light effectively. They are most effective in blocking UVB which is the major cause of sunburn in temperate areas.

The major consideration when choosing one

of these products is the amount of sunburn protection needed. The amount of protection required is dependent on the individual's sensitivity, time of day and altitude at which the exposure will occur, and the amount of reflected light present. Levels of UVB are greatest between the hours of 10:00 AM and 3:00 PM. The degree of exposure is increased by 4 percent with each 1000-foot increase in altitude. Snow, sand, white painted surfaces, and, to a small degree, water, reflect UVB-causing additive damage.

Chemical sunscreens are rated by "Sun Protection Factor" or SPF value. Commercially available products range in rating from a value of two to fifty. These ratings are determined in a laboratory and may not truly predict the protection provided outdoors. A product with a SPF 2 value will double the time of development of sunburn redness in an individual. An exposure which would cause redness in one hour without the sunscreen would not cause redness until after two hours of exposure with the SPF 2 value sunscreen. It is important to realize that the degree of protection does not change with reapplication. Reapplying a SPF 2 value sunscreen in two hours does not delay the onset of sunburn redness beyond two hours. Rarely is a SPF value greater than 15 needed for maximum benefit.

Application. The effectiveness of a sunscreen is dependent on the amount applied and reapplication after swimming and sweating. Products labeled "water-proof" may be removed by toweling dry and sweating and should be reapplied as necessary.

Adverse effects. Allergic skin reactions have been reported with active ingredients and inactive substances found in sunscreen vehicles. UVB energy is required for the body to make vitamin D. Vitamin D deficiency could occur in elderly individuals using sunscreens regularly.

VITAMINS AND MINERALS In this country there are few sound reasons for taking vitamin and mineral supplements. Nevertheless, a large proportion of the population does. Healthy individuals who consume a balanced diet will not benefit from these products and could potentially encounter adverse effects. Patients that may benefit from supplementation include strict vegeterians (B_{12}, vitamin D), patients on low-calorie diets (multivitamins with minerals), nursing infants (vitamins K and D), certain children (fluoride), pregnant and lactating women (iron, and folic acid), and patients on an artificial kidney machine (folic acid, pyridoxine, vitamin C, and possible vitamin E). Elderly patients usually do not need vitamin supplementation unless their diet is not adequate, in which case a multivitamin with minerals is often prescribed. Any condition which results in malabsorption of fat will result in a deficiency in the fat soluble vitamins (A, D, E, and K).

The indiscriminate use of vitamin and mineral supplements results in unnecessary expense and possible toxic effects. Toxicity can result from excessive dosages of vitamins A and D. Vitamin A toxicity can result in many severe symptoms and liver damage. Excessive dosages of vitamin D can also result in severe complications. Prolonged overdosage can cause mental and physical retardation, certain physical changes, kidney failure and death. In normal children and adults excessive dosages of vitamin D result in high blood levels of calcium and its associated symptoms. Prolonged use of high doses can result in permanent kidney damage and death.

INDEX OF BLACK AND WHITE ANATOMICAL AND MEDICAL ILLUSTRATIONS

INDEX

Boldface Indicates Chapter Titles

THE RESPIRATORY AND DIGESTIVE SYSTEMS

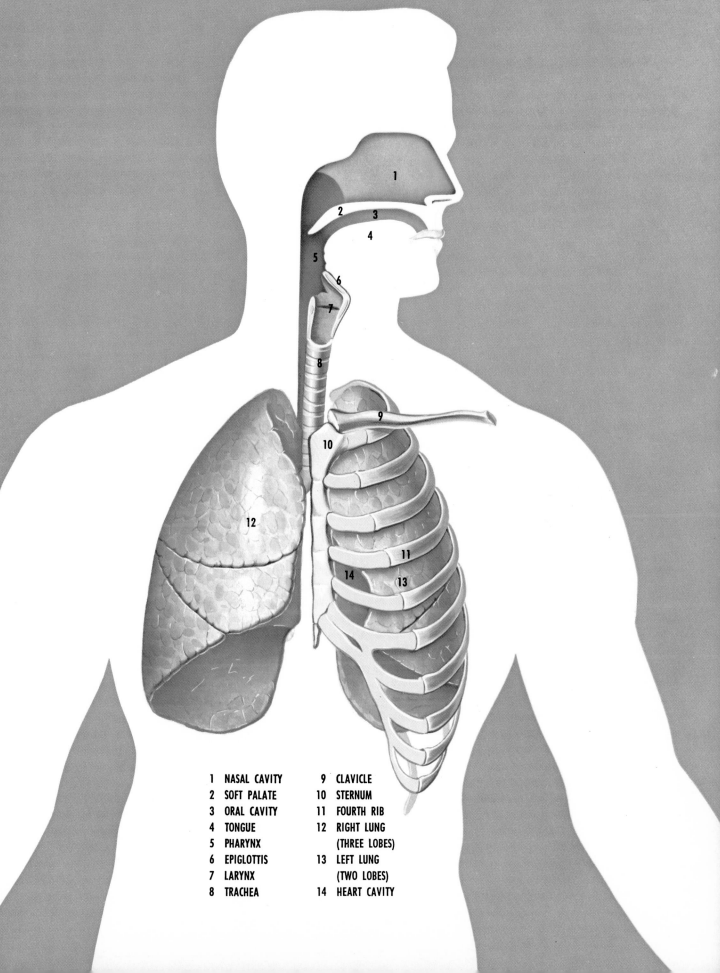

1	NASAL CAVITY	9	CLAVICLE
2	SOFT PALATE	10	STERNUM
3	ORAL CAVITY	11	FOURTH RIB
4	TONGUE	12	RIGHT LUNG
5	PHARYNX		(THREE LOBES)
6	EPIGLOTTIS	13	LEFT LUNG
7	LARYNX		(TWO LOBES)
8	TRACHEA	14	HEART CAVITY

RESPIRATORY MOVEMENTS

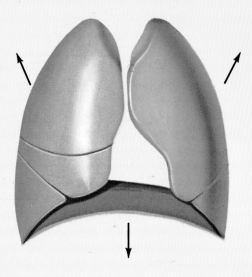

INSPIRATION

As the rib cage rises and the diaphragm falls, the lung area enlarges.

EXPIRATION

As the rib cage falls and the diaphragm rises, the lung area is decreased.

THE BRONCHIAL TREE

1 TRACHEA
2 LEFT BRONCHUS
3 SMALLER BRONCHUS
4 BRONCHIOLE
5 ALVEOLI

FUNCTION OF BRONCHIAL TREE

The bronchial tree is a system of branching hollow tubes whose function is to convey air to and from the alveoli (small hollows). Not shown are the companion arteries and veins which follow the branchings of the tree. At the level of the alveoli, these blood vessels become a capillary network embedded in the alveolar wall.

THE ALVEOLI
(IN CROSS SECTION)

Plate A3

1 ARTERIAL CAPILLARY
2 ALVEOLAR WALL CUT
3 CO₂
4 O₂
5 VENOUS CAPILLARY
6 ALVEOLAR WALL
7 BRONCHIOLE

Blood within the arterial capillary coming from the heart is laden with carbon dioxide. The latter passes through the capillary wall into the hollow alveoli and is exhaled during the next expiration. Each inspiration brings in air rich in oxygen which passes through the venous capillary wall, is absorbed by the blood, and returns to the heart for distribution throughout the body. Only at the microscopic level of the alveoli are the tissues thin enough to permit this gaseous exchange.

THE DIGESTIVE SYSTEM

Plate A4

1 NASAL CAVITY
2 SOFT PALATE
3 ORAL CAVITY
4 TONGUE
5 PHARYNX
6 ESOPHAGUS
7 CLAVICLE
8 STERNUM
9 FOURTH RIB
10 LIVER
11 STOMACH
12 SMALL INTESTINE
13 LARGE INTESTINE
14 PELVIC BONES

THE MECHANICS OF DIGESTION ▶

Digestion involves three simultaneous processes: mechanical passage of food through the continuous, hollow tube called the digestive tract; the chemical breakdown of the food; and absorption of the food.

To propel food forward, the muscular walls of the various portions of the tract undergo rhythmic contractions called peristalsis.

After being masticated by the teeth, the tongue pushes the food down the esophagus into the stomach. Successive waves of contraction beginning at mid-stomach travel down its muscular walls, churning the food. In the small intestine, two types of peristalsis occur: nonmoving, segmental contractions that occur 10 to 30 times a minute and mix the food with secretions from the liver and pancreas; and waves of peristalsis that propel the food forward. The large intestine has infrequent waves which move the undigested waste into the rectum where it is stored until elimination.

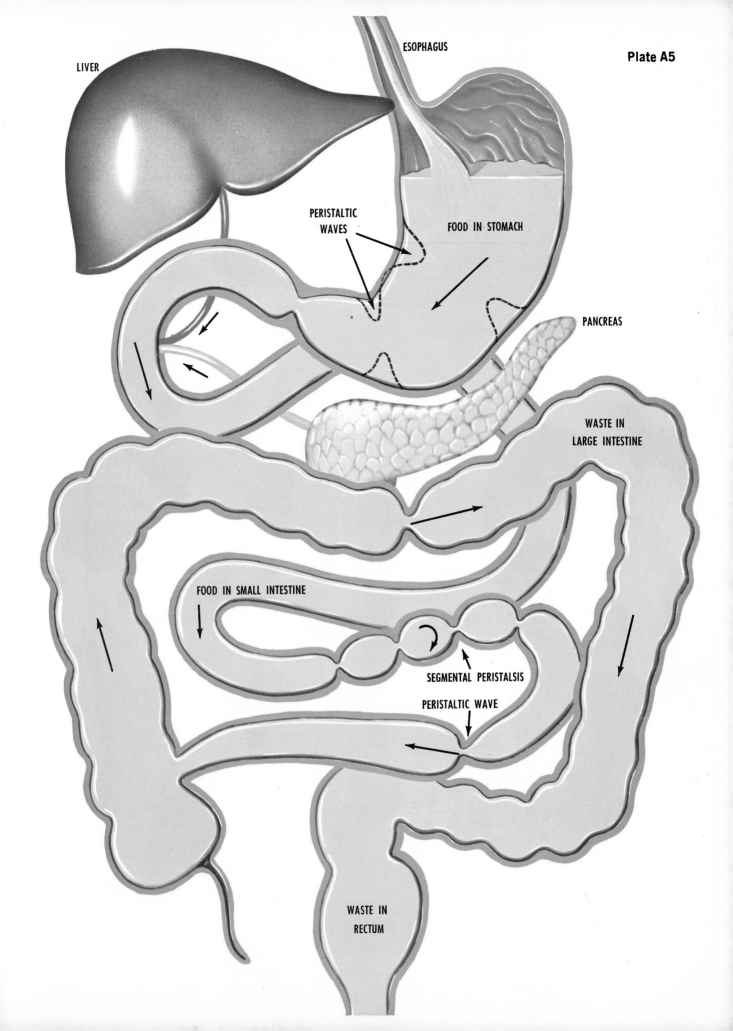

LIVER

ESOPHAGUS

Plate A5

PERISTALTIC WAVES

FOOD IN STOMACH

PANCREAS

WASTE IN LARGE INTESTINE

FOOD IN SMALL INTESTINE

SEGMENTAL PERISTALSIS

PERISTALTIC WAVE

WASTE IN RECTUM

THE CHEMISTRY OF DIGESTION

During their passage — through the composite digestive tract shown on these two pages, —foods are broken down by the action of enzymes secreted by the digestive glands. Each enzyme breaks down a specific food type: sugar, fat, or protein.

PROTEIN CHAINS

FATS

STARCHES

TWO-SUGAR UNITS

MUCUS CELLS

HCL

PEPSIN

MUCUS CELLS

PTYALIN

MUCUS CELLS

MOUTH AND ESOPHAGUS

Three salivary glands in the mouth secrete mucus to moisten food, and ptyalin which splits off two-sugar units from the starch chain. Fats and proteins are not affected. The esophagus has a few isolated mucus-producing glands.

STOMACH

The stomach has two types of glands; the gastric glands and the pyloric glands. The gastric glands secrete mucus, pepsin, and hydrochloric acid (HCl). The latter two break protein chains into shorter segments. Fats and sugars are unaffected. The pyloric glands produce mucus only.

PANCREAS

LIVER

SUGARS

PROTEINS

FATS

VILLUS

MUCUS
CELLS

MALTASE AND PEPTIDASE

LYMPH VESSEL

BLOOD VESSELS

SMALL INTESTINE

LARGE INTESTINE

The pancreatic secretions emptying into the small intestine contain three powerful enzymes: amylase, trypsin, and lipase. Amylase splits off two-sugar units. Trypsin splits proteins into shorter chains. Lipase, in conjunction with liver bile, decomposes fats into their simplest units. The intestinal glands located between villi produce mucus and two enzymes: maltase and pepitidase which complete the breakdown of sugar and protein, respectively. All absorption takes place in the lower small intestine. Fats are absorbed into the lymph vessels, sugars and proteins by the blood vessels. The large intestinal glands secrete mucus to lubricate the undigested food in its passage to the rectum.

NERVOUS CONTROL OF DIGESTION

BRAIN · **VAGUS NERVE** · **STOMACH**

PERISTALTIC WAVE

THE EMPTY STOMACH

At the individual's sight, smell, and taste of food, the brain sends impulses over the vagus nerve to the stomach, causing peristalsis and gland secretion.

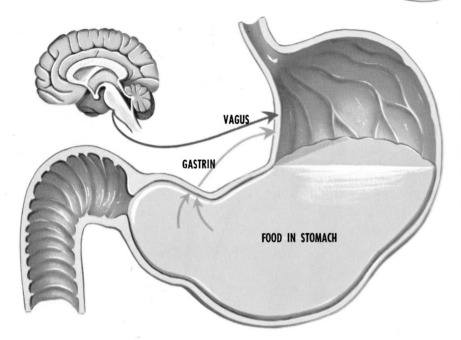

VAGUS · **GASTRIN** · **FOOD IN STOMACH**

FOOD IN THE STOMACH

During filling, peristalsis decreases. The stomach walls relax to accommodate the food. When filled, stomach peristalsis increases via vagus nerve control. The food itself stimulates the release of gastrin which travels to the gastric glands, increasing the secretion of gastric juices.

FOOD IN THE INTESTINES

If too great a food bulk reaches the duodenum, stomach peristalsis (still under vagus control) is slowed down. Food itself stimulates the release of gastrin (to stomach) and secretin which stimulates pancreatic secretions.

Food in the small intestine causes the secretion of enterogastrone which travels to the stomach and inhibits gastric gland secretion.

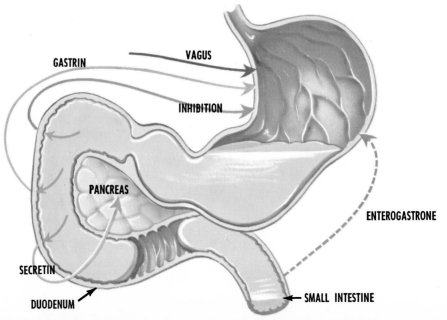

GASTRIN · **VAGUS** · **INHIBITION** · **PANCREAS** · **ENTEROGASTRONE** · **SECRETIN** · **DUODENUM** · **SMALL INTESTINE**

THE CIRCULATORY SYSTEM

ANTERIOR VIEW OF HEART

THE HEART

1 ARCH OF AORTA
2 SUPERIOR VENA CAVA
3 PULMONARY ARTERY
4 RIGHT AURICLE
5 LEFT AURICLE
6 RIGHT VENTRICLE
7 LEFT VENTRICLE
8 INTERVENTRICULAR
  ARTERY AND VEIN

VENTRICLE WALL

CROSS SECTION OF HEART

1 AORTIC VALVE
2 SUPERIOR VENA CAVA
3 PULMONARY VALVE
4 RIGHT AURICLE
5 LEFT AURICLE
6 RIGHT VENTRICLE
7 TRICUSPID VALVE
8 BICUSPID VALVE
9 PAPILLARY MUSCLE
10 LEFT VENTRICLE

ILLUSTRATED BY

LEONARD D. DANK

ST. LUKE'S HOSPITAL
NEW YORK CITY

CARDIAC CYCLE

HEART SOUNDS

Both auricles fill with blood and contract. Blood flows through the open atrioventricular valves into the ventricles.

As the ventricles begin to contract, the atrioventricular valves snap shut.

As the ventricles continue to contract, the semilunar valves are forced open. Blood is pushed into the aorta and pulmonary artery.

When all the blood is gone, the ventricles relax. Blood is prevented from returning to the heart by the semilunar valves.

Sounds produced by the valves enable the doctor to form an impression of the cardiac cycle. The typical lub-dub sounds are produced by the closing of the atrioventricular and semilunar valves. If any valve does not close properly, a murmuring after-sound results.

CONTROL OF THE CIRCULATORY SYSTEM

Four regulatory centers in the medulla of the brain control the circulatory system. Their action can best be explained by three conditions described below.

1. A RISE IN BLOOD PRESSURE (Red Arrows)

The carotid sinus is stimulated by the rise in pressure. It sends warning impulses to the cardioinhibitor and vasodilator centers. These centers send impulses to the heart causing it to slow down, and to the arterioles of the stomach causing them to enlarge. Both actions rapidly lower the blood pressure.

2. A FALL IN OXYGEN WITHIN THE BLOOD (Blue Arrows)

A node of tissue in the aorta, stimulated by low oxygen levels sends impulses to the cardio-accelerator and to the vasoconstrictor centers. The centers send impulses to the heart causing it to speed up, and to the stomach arterioles causing them to constrict. Both actions raise the blood pressure, thus insuring an adequate supply of oxygen to vital organs.

3. DURING SUSTAINED EXERCISE (Dotted Blue Arrow)

The right auricle is stimulated by a high venous pressure. It sends impulses to the cardioaccelerator and vasoconstrictor centers. Together with impulses from the aorta due to low oxygen, the carotid sinus protective mechanism (see above RISE IN BLOOD PRESSURE) is blocked. Thus a necessary sustained high blood pressure can be maintained.

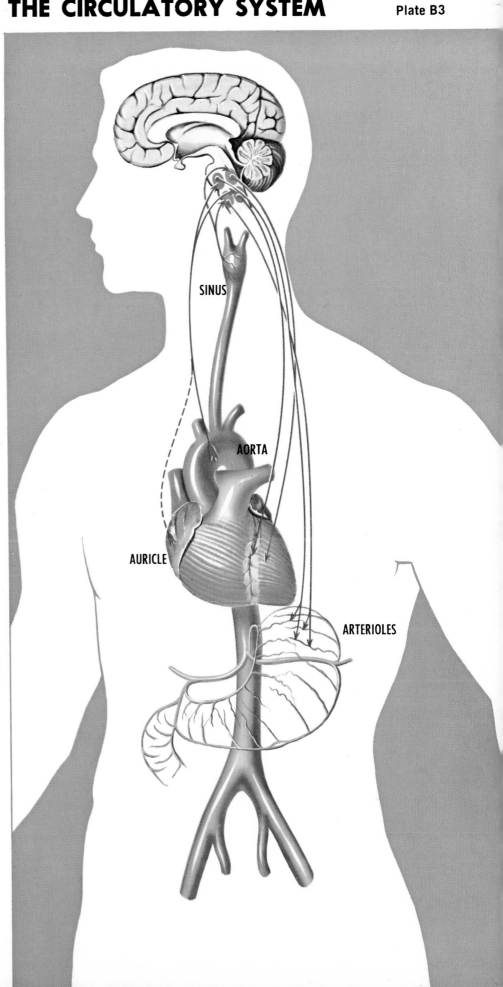

SINUS

AORTA

AURICLE

ARTERIOLES

THE BLOOD VESSELS

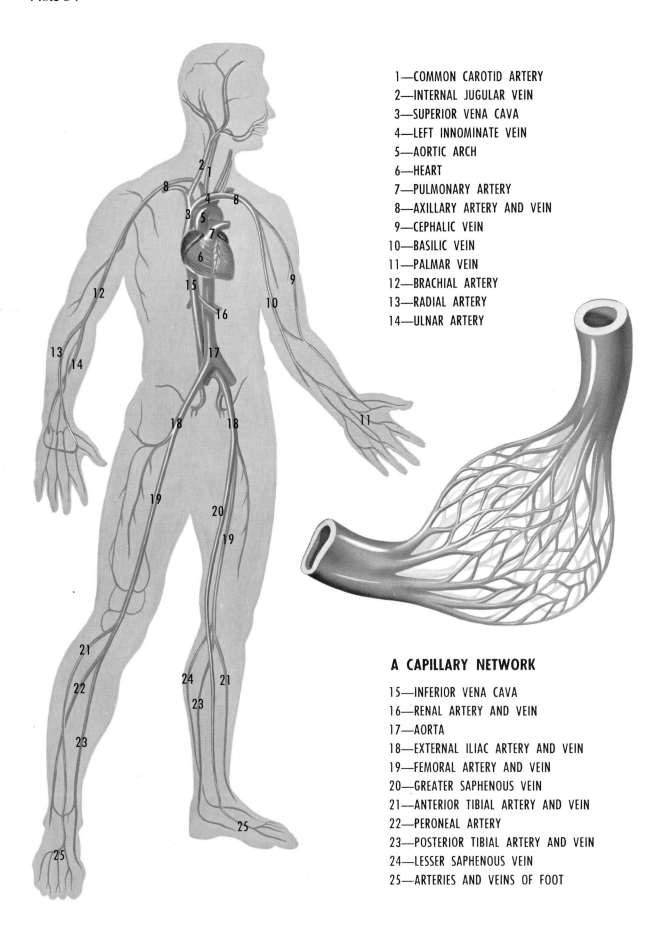

1—COMMON CAROTID ARTERY
2—INTERNAL JUGULAR VEIN
3—SUPERIOR VENA CAVA
4—LEFT INNOMINATE VEIN
5—AORTIC ARCH
6—HEART
7—PULMONARY ARTERY
8—AXILLARY ARTERY AND VEIN
9—CEPHALIC VEIN
10—BASILIC VEIN
11—PALMAR VEIN
12—BRACHIAL ARTERY
13—RADIAL ARTERY
14—ULNAR ARTERY

A CAPILLARY NETWORK

15—INFERIOR VENA CAVA
16—RENAL ARTERY AND VEIN
17—AORTA
18—EXTERNAL ILIAC ARTERY AND VEIN
19—FEMORAL ARTERY AND VEIN
20—GREATER SAPHENOUS VEIN
21—ANTERIOR TIBIAL ARTERY AND VEIN
22—PERONEAL ARTERY
23—POSTERIOR TIBIAL ARTERY AND VEIN
24—LESSER SAPHENOUS VEIN
25—ARTERIES AND VEINS OF FOOT

THE COMPONENTS OF BLOOD

ERYTHROCYTES
(5 Million per cu. mm)

CARRY OXYGEN
AND CARBON DIOXIDE

LYMPHOCYTES
(1200-2300 per cu. mm)

IMPORTANT IN COMBATING
INFLAMMATION

NEUTROPHILS
(3000-6000 per cu. mm)

IMPORTANT IN RIDDING THE
TISSUES OF BACTERIA

PLATELETS
(250,000 per cu. mm)

IMPORTANT IN THE
CLOTTING MECHANISM

PLASMA PROTEINS
(7 per cent of plasma)

ALBUMIN REGULATES THE FLUID
LEVEL OF BLOOD

FIBRINOGEN IS IMPORTANT
IN CLOTTING MECHANISM

GLOBULINS CONTAIN ANTIBODIES

BACTERIA

GLOBULIN

GAMMA GLOBULIN
(2.3 per cent of plasma)

CONTAINS ANTIBODIES WHICH
CAUSE BACTERIA TO AGGLUTINATE

THE ANCIENT CONCEPT OF CIRCULATION

ACCORDING TO GALEN (129-200 A.D.)

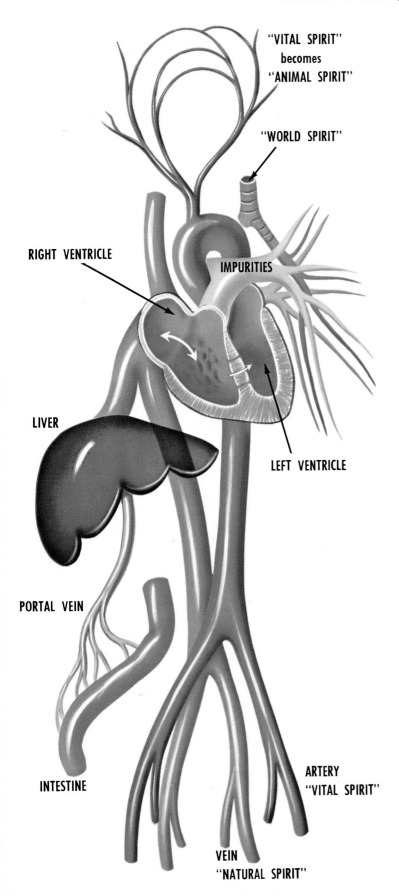

"VITAL SPIRIT"
becomes
"ANIMAL SPIRIT"

"WORLD SPIRIT"

RIGHT VENTRICLE

IMPURITIES

LIVER

LEFT VENTRICLE

PORTAL VEIN

INTESTINE

ARTERY
"VITAL SPIRIT"

VEIN
"NATURAL SPIRIT"

GALEN'S THEORY

Galen's theory of circulation dominated men's minds and actions for 1,400 years. He believed that dissolved food, transported from the intestines to the liver by the portal vein, was transformed into venous blood to which was added "Natural Spirit." The liver distributed this venous blood throughout the veins in which it ebbed and flowed.

When the venous blood reached the right ventricle, impurities flowed out of the pulmonary artery to the lungs and then these impurities somehow found their way into the bronchi and were exhaled.

"World Spirit" was inhaled, traveled to the bronchi and found its way via the pulmonary vein into the left ventricle. Here "World Spirit" encountered some venous blood that had seeped through the interventricular septum. "World Spirit" mixed with venous blood and became "Vital Spirit" which was distributed throughout the arteries.

"Vital Spirit" upon reaching the brain became charged with "Animal Spirit" which flowed out through the supposedly hollow nerves.

"Natural, Vital, and Animal Spirits" were the cornerstone of physiology until the seventeenth century.

THE MODERN CONCEPT OF CIRCULATION

RIGHT VENTRICLE

THE PULMONARY CIRCULATION

The right ventricle pumps carbon dioxide- (CO_2) saturated venous blood into the pulmonary artery which branches repeatedly, finally becoming a capillary network surrounding the alveoli of the lungs. The carbon dioxide is exchanged for oxygen (O_2). The oxygen-saturated arterial blood returns to the heart for distribution to the body.

LUNG TISSUE

CO_2 O_2

ARTERY

VEIN

SYSTEMIC CIRCULATION

The left ventricle pumps the oxygen-saturated blood to all parts of the body. In the body tissues, the arteries (red) branch repeatedly until they become a capillary network surrounding the cells. Oxygen is exchanged for carbon dioxide. The carbon dioxide-saturated veins (blue) return the blood back to the heart to go through the pulmonary circulation.

BODY TISSUE

O_2 CO_2

THE PORTAL CIRCULATION

Venous blood carrying dissolved foods from the intestines takes a special route: the portal vein, to the liver. In the liver, the portal vein again becomes a capillary network. Excess dissolved food is stored. The veins regroup again to join the main veins just before they enter the heart.

BLOOD TYPES

Gamma globulin antibodies agglutinate foreign red cells just as they do with bacteria. Red cells also have chemicals (antigens) which react with antibodies.

TYPE O

TYPE O CELLS CONTAIN NO ANTIGENS
TYPE O GLOBULIN CONTAIN A & B ANTIBODIES

TYPE A

TYPE A CELLS CONTAIN A ANTIGEN
TYPE A GLOBULIN CONTAIN B ANTIBODIES

TYPE B

TYPE B CELLS CONTAIN B ANTIGEN
TYPE B GLOBULIN CONTAIN A ANTIBODIES

TYPE AB

TYPE AB CELLS CONTAIN A & B ANTIGENS
TYPE AB GLOBULIN CONTAIN NO ANTIBODIES

If type B blood is transfused into type A blood, the cells of both types will agglutinate. The clumps of red cells may block small capillaries, leading to shock and possible death.

CHILD GROWTH AND BEHAVIOR

Parents should always be aware that statistics, behavior patterns, growth charts and norms for all growing children generally represent averages or medians. Parents should expect some variations from such printed data in their own children's development. Development norms are influenced by heredity, environment, nutrition, and a variety of other factors. An observable marked retardation from so-called norms should be brought to the attention of a physician.

FOUR WEEKS

Baby does not really see yet or focus the eyes but does follow a moving light. Sleep takes up on an average of twenty hours of the infant's day. Body temperature is steady and not as subject to fluctuations as it was the first weeks after birth. Baby gains about six ounces a week and has grown about one inch since birth.

EIGHT WEEKS

Baby is able to recognize familiar people and objects. Sleep has been cut to about eighteen hours a day. Weight increases at about three ounces a week. Height is still increasing at about one inch a month.

SIXTEEN WEEKS

Baby sees objects very well now and reaches for them. Length of sleep is about the same as at eight weeks. Weight is increasing at a steady rate and will be doubled at about twenty weeks. Objects now are grasped and held. Baby laughs.

SIX MONTHS

Baby still sleeps about sixteen hours a day and may sleep through the night. Weight may be increasing by two to three ounces a month. Baby probably is about six inches taller than at birth. Hearing is showing a marked development and there is a definite response to sound. Of the twenty temporary teeth baby is to get, the first two, the lower center incisors, may now appear. Baby may try to sit up without help, and may attemp to pick up and grasp small objects, and shift them from hand to hand. Baby turns over but may have started to do so even at five months.

TEN MONTHS

Baby may now be sleeping only fifteen hours a day. Gets around by crawling, and can sit unsupported and also change from a sitting to a prone position. Baby generally can pull himself up to a standing position and may be able to imitate simple syllables such as "da da."

TWELVE MONTHS

The baby can now distinguish colors in this order: yellow, red, blue. Some babies now sleep about fourteen hours a day but there are some who still need sixteen full hours. The scale will show that baby's weight has tripled since birth. Height is still increasing at about three inches a year. To the two lower central incisors will have been added four upper incisors. Baby crawls and can walk by holding on to chairs and other objects nearby and some may be able to walk without support.

FIFTEEN MONTHS

In addition to the previous temporary teeth, baby has added two lower lateral incisors. Baby can walk and attempts to climb stairs. Toys and dolls are hugged and just as readily thrown away. Although baby is not talking yet, demands are made known by pointing and shouting. Some babies are now trying to feed themselves by attempting to drink from a glass or cup and by using a spoon.

EIGHTEEN MONTHS

Baby has added the four canines to the temporary teeth already in, and is growing at the rate of about three inches a year. This is the age when being "contrary" is the normal way to be. Baby is able to climb and run and does so at every opportunity.

Plate C4

TWO YEARS

Baby is now sleeping twelve to fourteen hours and may skip the daytime nap more often than parents would like. The balance of the temporary teeth (four posterior molars) are coming in now. Motor control has improved. He points to his eyes, nose, and ears and may be toilet-trained. He understands more and makes himself understood.

TWO AND ONE-HALF YEARS

Baby's weight has quadrupled since birth, and he probably is about thirty-five inches tall and all the temporary teeth are in. Speech has progressed to the point where the child is talking in three-word sentences. Play is very vigorous and from the parents' point of view, hazardous. Climbing instinct may show itself and the child may even grasp small trees as if about to climb them. There will be genuine attempts to dress and undress, with undressing preceding the attempt to dress. Some children actually succeed in pulling on socks and slipping a foot into a shoe.

THREE YEARS

Child feeds himself, talks in short sentences, and generally is toilet-trained by this age. Motor control is improving — he can now build and keep from tumbling a large number of blocks. He can manage physical activities that were beyond his capacity only a few months ago. Emotionally he is temporarily becoming a conformer and will follow suggestions and orders from elders. He is more cooperative and will share toys with friends.

THREE AND ONE-HALF YEARS

Sudden changes occur. Child seems to temporarily slip back in motor coordination, despite the fact that for several months already he has been riding a tricycle, is now feeding himself with a minimum of spilling, and is able to put on his shoes quite well. Temporary regression shows itself in fear of heights. Stuttering may appear and temporary crossing of the eyes is also symtomatic of this strange age. The child seems to need greater expressions of affection and is constantly accusing parents of not loving him. Fortunately this "retardation" is temporary and will disappear as quickly as it came.

FOUR YEARS

The four-year-old can dress and undress himself and even lace his shoes. He can skip on one foot and can wash and dry himself and brush his teeth. Generally, he plays cooperatively with his friends.

FIVE YEARS

By the time the child is five years old, he is interested in looking at pictures in books and magazines and actually can draw pictures and print some letters. He can recognize and name some coins. Socially he is very cooperative and is described as being a "good child."

SIX YEARS

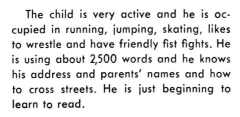

The child is very active and he is occupied in running, jumping, skating, likes to wrestle and have friendly fist fights. He is using about 2,500 words and he knows his address and parents' names and how to cross streets. He is just beginning to learn to read.

SEVEN YEARS

The child seems to suddenly develop nervous habits such as nail-biting and tongue-sucking. He has begun to be keenly competitive in play and dresses like his friends. He is becoming aware of the social and economic differences between himself and his classmates. He is beginning to understand addition and subtraction concepts and is able to tell time and may know what month it is. Child may now show great curiosity about the sexes and how babies are born.

EIGHT YEARS

The eight-year-old can swim and ride a bicycle. He begins to respect the property rights of others and he is becoming more "choosy" in selecting his friends. He is beginning to read the comics and the funnies in the newspapers and attempts to spend more time watching television. This is merely an expression of a greater interest in the world about him.

NINE YEARS

The nine-year-old can bathe, comb his hair and take care of other physical needs. He is beginning to be able to use tools very well. Boys and girls are beginning to play separately now and there is a greater variety in their play activities. There is a greater interest in visiting friends and sleeping away from home. In school work he is now able to do some multiplication and division. Generally he is interested in how things are made. There is curiosity about science, nature, and the world around him.

TEN YEARS

The ten-year-old is showing a greater involvement in hazardous games and activities. There is a greater interest in organized games and teamwork spirit is developing. In school, numbers beyond 100 are being used and examples and problems involving simple fractions are now understood. There is a growing interest in other people and their ideas.

MUSCULAR
AND
SKELETAL
SYSTEMS

THE MUSCLES

1 STERNOCLEIDOMASTOID
2 TRAPEZIUS
3 PECTORALIS MAJOR
4 DELTOID
5 BICEPS
6 TRICEPS
7 BRACHIALIS
8 BRACHIORADIALIS
9 FOREARM FLEXORS
10 EXTERNAL OBLIQUE
11 RECTUS ABDOMINIS
12 TENSOR FASCIA LATA
13 ILIOPSOAS
14 PECTINEUS
15 ADDUCTOR LONGUS
16 GRACILIS
17 SARTORIUS
18 RECTUS FEMORIS
19 VASTUS LATERALIS
20 VASTUS MEDIALIS
21 PATELLA
22 TIBIALIS ANTERIOR
23 TIBIA
24 GASTROCNEMIUS
25 SOLEUS
26 EXTENSOR TENDONS OF FOOT

ILLUSTRATED BY

LEONARD D. DANK

ST. LUKE'S HOSPITAL
NEW YORK CITY

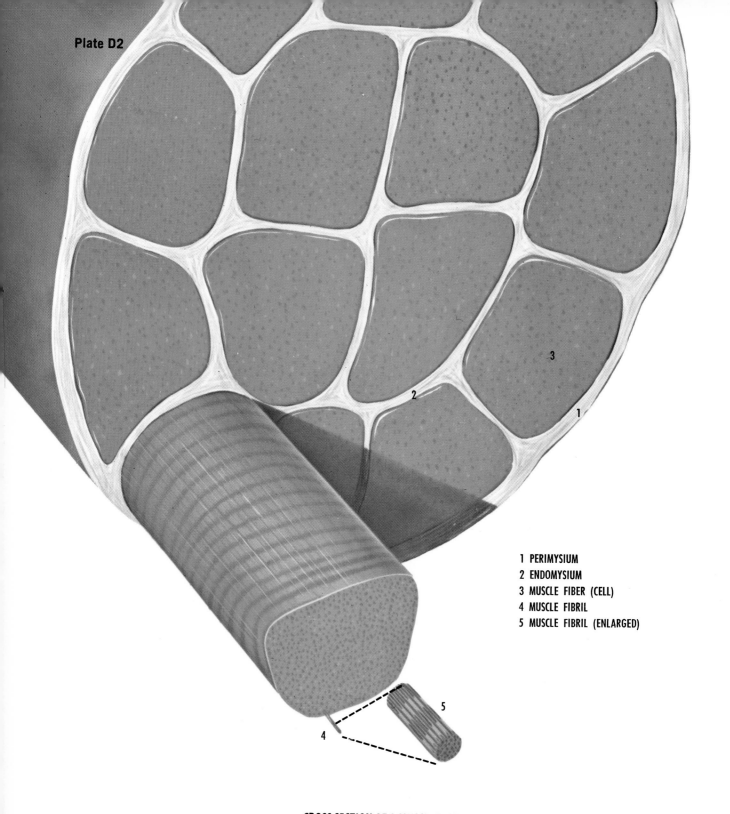

1 PERIMYSIUM
2 ENDOMYSIUM
3 MUSCLE FIBER (CELL)
4 MUSCLE FIBRIL
5 MUSCLE FIBRIL (ENLARGED)

CROSS SECTION OF A MUSCLE BUNDLE

A voluntary muscle is composed of numerous muscle bundles. Each bundle, surrounded by an outer covering (perimysium) contains many muscle fibers (cells). Each fiber, ensheathed in the endomysium, contains thousands of longitudinal fibrils. Each fibril is composed of long and short filaments (5) which impart a cross-striated appearance. Since the striations of all the fibrils are in register, the fiber as a whole seems to be cross-striated. The actual mechanism of contraction is thought to involve the sliding of the short over the long filaments.

CONTROL OF THE MUSCLES

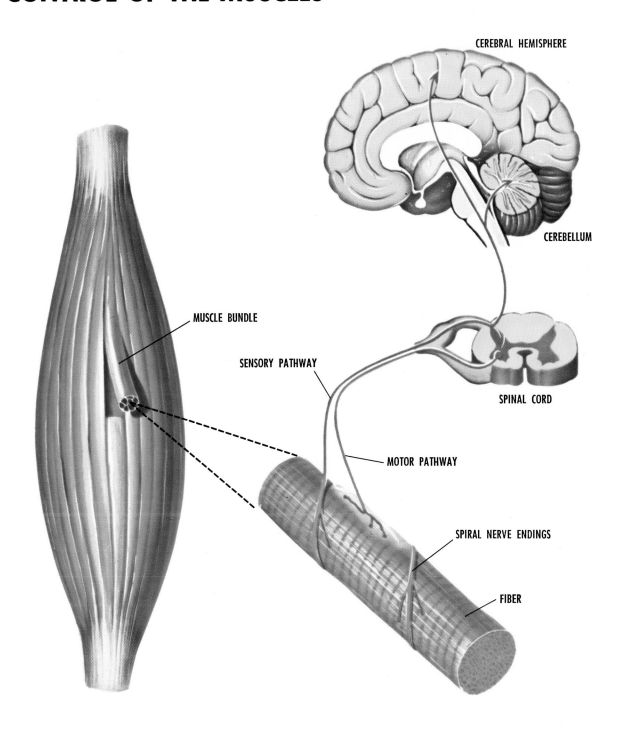

CEREBRAL HEMISPHERE

CEREBELLUM

MUSCLE BUNDLE

SENSORY PATHWAY

SPINAL CORD

MOTOR PATHWAY

SPIRAL NERVE ENDINGS

FIBER

Where fibers stretch or relax, they stimulate spiral nerve endings which send sensory impulses to the spinal cord. Motor impulses are activated and return to the fiber causing it to contract. This unconscious "stretch reflex" maintains the muscles in a state of balanced partial contraction called "tonus." If many muscles are involved, sensory impulses are sent to the cerebellum, the chief unconscious muscle coordination center. Impulses may also go to the cerebral hemispheres, to inform the conscious mind of the state of the muscles.

MUSCLE ACTION

1 SCAPULA
2 HUMERUS
3 TRICEPS
4 BICEPS
5 ULNA
6 RADIUS

In order to produce movement, a muscle must be attached to at least two bones. When the triceps, attached to the scapula, humerus, and ulna, contracts, it extends the ulna. Muscles occur in antagonistic pairs: the triceps extends, the biceps flexes the forearm.

As the biceps contracts, the triceps relaxes.

The fully contracted biceps has flexed the forearm. The triceps is fully relaxed.

ANATOMY OF BONE

1 ARTICULAR CARTILAGE
2 NECK OF FEMUR
3 GREATER TROCHANTER
4 LESSER TROCHANTER
5 MUSCLE ATTACHMENT
6 SHAFT
7 ARTICULAR CARTILAGE

CROSS SECTION OF HEAD AND NECK OF FEMUR

Cancellous bone forms a light-weight system of struts for efficient weight-bearing.

POSTERIOR VIEW OF FEMUR

CROSS SECTION OF SHAFT

Bone is hollow to reduce weight.

SKELETON IN INFANCY

Most bones are preformed as cartilage which bone tissue gradually replaces. Some bones are not fully replaced until the late teens; the articular cartilage is never replaced.

Bone tissue replaces dying cartilage, causing an increase in bone length at ends only.

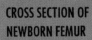

CROSS SECTION OF NEWBORN FEMUR

yellow = bone
blue = cartilage

Pins inserted in femur at birth will be same distance apart in adult. Only circular growth occurs in the shaft.

SKELETON IN ADULT

Some cartilage persists in the adult. This cartilage lines the joints, and forms part of the rib cage.

GROWTH OF A BONE (Femur)

INFANT

10 YEARS

ADULT

Bones elongate and increase in width. They are also remodeled to reach final conformation.

ARTICULATION OF BONE AT A JOINT

1 ILIUM
2 PUBIS
3 ISCHIUM
4 FEMUR
5 ARTICULAR CARTILAGE
6 LIGAMENTS
7 SYNOVIAL CAVITY

CROSS SECTION OF FEMERO-PELVIC JOINT

Most of the freely movable joints are of the synovial type. Both bones are covered with a thin layer of articular cartilage to reduce friction. The inside of the joint contains a mucous lubricant called synovial fluid. Various ligaments hold the joint together.

PHYSICAL FITNESS AND REDUCING EXERCISES

The exercises illustrated in this eight-page full-color insert are useful for general body conditioning and for reducing flabbiness and girth in specific parts of the body. If, for example, the goal is to reduce the size or flabbiness of the hips, spending a few extra minutes each day on the hip exercises will produce the desired results. Success both in body conditioning and weight control will be yours if you spend about thirty minutes a day on the exercises. The United States government publication Adult Physical Fitness, on which some of the exercises in this insert are based, cites a study by the Harvard School of Public Health for the claim that "one-half an hour of proper exercise each day can keep off or take off as much as twenty-six pounds a year."

TRUNK MUSCLES

This exercise is designed to condition and strengthen the trunk muscles. Stand with the feet shoulder-width apart. Turn the trunk to right and bend forward and touch the fingertips to the floor outside that right foot. Return to the starting position by sweeping the trunk and arm upward. Repeat the exercise to the left side. About fifteen repetitions on each side are recommended.

TRUNK AND WAIST

At the start stand erect with hands on waist and hips. Twist the trunk to the right but not the hips and head — they remain to the front. Return to the starting position. Repeat the exercise to the left side. About thirty daily repetitions on each side are suggested.

ABDOMINAL MUSCLES AND SHOULDER GIRDLE

This exercise is designed to strengthen the abdominal muscles and the shoulder girdle. Assume a squatting position with the hands touching the ground inside the knees. Thrust the legs to the rear with toes and heels together. Return to the squatting position and then to the starting position. Repeat about ten times but only if you can do so without strain.

START

LEG MUSCLES

This exercise builds leg muscles. It is quite strenuous and should be attempted only after considerable conditioning has been achieved. In the starting position, the knees are bent and the feet are set about eight inches apart. One foot is forward toe-to-heel distance. The back is erect. The fingers are joined on top of the head and the elbows are well back.

Now jump into the air, locking the knees and reversing the leg position. The feet come to rest but reversed from the starting position. Repeat up to four times, reversing the starting position from one leg to the other.

THIGH-TO-SHOULDER CONDITIONING

This is a good exercise for the thigh, abdomen, back and shoulder muscles. In the starting position spread the feet more than shoulder-width apart, arms straight overhead, palms facing. Now bend at the knees and waist, swing the arms down and reach between the legs as far as possible. Return to the starting position with a sharp and quick movement. Repeat, but without exertion or strain.

START

START

PUSH UPS—SHOULDER MUSCLES

This exercise will help to build the muscles of the shoulder. To assume the starting position lie on the floor, face down, legs together, hands on floor under shoulders with fingers pointing straight ahead. Now push the body off the floor so that the weight rests on the hands, and the legs and arms are kept straight. Then lower the body until the chest touches the floor. Repeat up to ten times and more if you can do so without strain.

HIPS

This is a good exercise for strengthening the hip muscles and reducing their flabbiness and girth. At the start kneel on the floor with the arms out in front. Now sit down, moving hips to one side as shown. Next, return to the kneeling position and repeat the exercise to the other side.

THIGHS

This exercise, although designed for thigh conditioning, is also effective for the back, neck, and other parts of the body. The exercise should not be attempted until the body has been conditioned by other milder exercises. Lie on the back and place the feet on a chair as in the starting position illustrated. Now raise the hips until the knees, thighs, and trunk are in line. Return to the the starting position. Repeat as often as comfortable without exertion.

ARMS

This exercise is designed to strengthen and condition the arm muscles. Stand in the straddle position (feet spread shoulder-width apart). Take a rubber ball, sponge, or any squeezable object in each hand. Now lean forward and bend the elbows. Next, bring the arms all the way back, at the same time squeezing the objects held in the hands. Repeat a few times until you can do about twenty exercises without exertion.

BUTTOCKS EXERCISE

This exercise is designed to reduce the flabbiness and girth of the buttocks. Rest one hand on a chair and then lift the opposite leg and swing it from front to back. Repeat the action five times and then change to the other leg. Repeat a few times but without exertion.

LEGS

This exercise is effective for strengthening and conditioning the leg muscles. Lie on your back, legs straight out. Bring one leg up as far as comfortable; now as you bring the leg down start the other leg upwards getting into a smooth scissors action. Repeat several times until you can do about twenty exercises without exertion.

ABDOMINAL EXERCISE

This abdominal exercise is designed to reduce the flabbiness and girth of the abdomen and to strengthen the abdominal muscles. Stretch out on your back, arms stretched sideways, legs together. Now bend the knees and bring them as close to the chest as possible. Now return the legs to the floor, first to the left side, and then to the right side. Bring the knees back to the chest. On the finish, straighten the legs to the starting position. Repeat several times.

WAIST AND BODY

At the start assume a straddle position (feet about shoulder-length apart). Raise the left arm up, keeping the right arm down. Bend and stretch far to the right with raised left arm following. Return to the starting position. Repeat to the other side.

HEAD AND NECK MUSCLES

This exercise will strengthen the neck muscles and reduce the girth and flabbiness of the chin and neck. The exercise may be done in a standing or in the illustrated sitting position. Hold the back straight and stretch the head as far back as possible. Now turn the head from side to side attempting to make a complete circle. Repeat as many times as you can manage without exertion.

Plate E6

BACK AND CHEST

This exercise will improve the posture by strengthening the back and chest muscles. Start the exercise by getting down on all fours. The first action is to stretch your right arm out straight. Then move it along the floor and under the left arm so that the right shoulder is resting on the floor. Now move your right arm out and back to the "first action" position. Now return to starting position. Repeat the exercise with the left arm. Do the exercise about four times. Do not strain.

SHOULDERS

This is a useful exercise for straightening the shoulders. Lie on the stomach in a prone outstretched position. Bend the knees back and grasp the feet as shown. Rock back and forth.

GENERAL CONDITIONING

This is a good exercise for putting many of the body muscles into action. To start, assume a straddle position (feet shoulder-width apart). Place the right hand on the hip and left arm straight out sideways. Bend the body forward and swing the left arm across body to the right as shown in the picture. Next, return to the starting position. Repeat several times and then reverse to the other direction.

POSTURE

While posture must necessarily vary from person to person due to inheritance and different growth and development characteristics, there is a generally accepted standard followed by physical fitness experts. For example, the United States Army Conditioning Manual describes this standard as follows:

"Good posture is characterized by true vertical aline-ment, in which certain body segments are alined, one above the other, so that they support each other along the line of the pull of gravity."

The publication Adult Physical Fitness, prepared by the President's Council on Physical Fitness, states:

"Good posture acts to avoid cramping of internal organs, permits better circulation, prevents undue tensing of some muscles and undue lengthening of others. It thus contributes to fitness.

"In turn, physical conditioning, by developing muscle tone, helps to make good posture more readily maintainable — and will help, too, if you have any bad postural habits you need to break.

"For good posture, the centers of gravity of many body parts — feet, legs, hips, trunk, shoulders, and head — must be in a vertical line. As viewed from the side when you are standing, the line should run through ear lobe, tip of shoulder, middle of hips, just back of kneecap, just in front of outer ankle bone."

The posture illustrations and texts shown on these pages are based upon material from these two publications.

STANDING

The ideal standing position is illustrated by the large figures of the man and the woman on the top left and right. Unfortunately, most people are quite careless about their standing postures and the most common postures with their faults are illustrated below.

FAIR

Head forward. Abdomen
 prominent.
Exaggerated curve in upper
 back.
Slight hollow back.

POOR

Relaxed posture.
Head forward.
Abdomen relaxed.
Shoulder blades prominent.
Hollow back.

VERY POOR

Head forward badly.
Very exaggerated curve
 upper back.
Abdomen relaxed.
Chest flat — sloping.
Hollow back.

WALK TALL

1. Knees and ankles limber, toes pointed straight ahead. 2. Head and chest high. 3. Swing legs directly forward from hip joints. 4. Push feet off the ground — don't shuffle. 5. Swing shoulders and arms freely and easily.

PLUMB-LINE TEST

Hang a plumb bob or any weight from the top of a mirror as shown. Stand in front of the mirror and position your body so that the string lines up with the lobe of your ear, the tip of the shoulder, the middle of the hip, the middle of the knee, and the front of the ankle bone. Practice keeping this position for a few minutes each day. Soon it will become so natural that you will not have to strain to maintain the position.

SIT TALL

1. Sit tall and back, with hips touching the back of the chair, feet flat on floor. 2. Chest out, back of neck nearly in line with upper back.

THE BACK-TO-THE-WALL TEST

Stand with your back against the wall. If your figure is as shown on the left illustration (or variations of it), then your posture does not conform to what is considered healthful and physically desirable. To correct this wrong posture, push your back against the wall as shown on the right illustration. Automatically you will stand in a position which more closely conforms to the plumb-line ideal.

WRONG

RIGHT

YOGA EXERCISES FOR HEALTH

Yoga has increasingly become popular in this country as an exercise procedure for achieving and maintaining good physical and mental health. Some of the basic positions are described in the succeeding pages.

THE LOTUS POSTURE

Practitioners of the Lotus Posture claim that it is the ideal position to practice meditation. The Lotus Position should be achieved by stages.

STAGE 1

As demonstrated in the picture, bring the right foot on to the left thigh with the heel touching the root of the left thigh with the sole upturned.

STAGE 2

Bring the other leg over the right leg and thigh so that the heel is close to the root of the thigh. Study the picture carefully, and maintain the position as closely as possible, initially for a brief time. Increase the time as you become more expert at assuming the Lotus Position.

HIP CONTROL

This is a very good exercise to achieve balance. It is also good for controlling the hips.

STAGE 1

Place one foot against the opposite thigh, as shown.

STAGE 2

Raise both hands and join the palms together.

STAGE 3

Conclude the position by bringing the palms in front of the chest. Maintain that position for a few seconds and change to the other side.

THE TREE POSTURE

STAGE 1

Assume the position shown in the illustration. Breathe deeply and bend the body laterally from the hips to the left until it is almost horizontal. Maintain the legs straight but extend the hips outward. Remain in the position a few seconds and then return to the upright position as you breathe out.

STAGE 2

Do procedure to the other side and repeat several times.

PLOW POSTURE

This is considered a good exercise for strengthening the abdominal muscles.

STAGE 1

Stretch out on your back with arms along the sides and palms down. Elevate the legs from the hip.

STAGE 2

Bring the legs over your head gradually lowering the toes to the floor.

STAGE 3

Bend the knees. Bring them close to your head. Maintain the position for a few seconds and then roll forward until your body has returned to the starting position.

FIRST AID AND LIFE SAVING

The object of first aid is to give emergency care to people who are injured or ill, to save life, to prevent death, to relieve pain, until such time as professional medical aid arrives.

The United States government publication **First Aid** describes the value of properly administered help in emergencies as follows:

"First aid, rendered correctly, in many instances can restore natural breathing, usually check loss of blood, prevent or moderate shock, protect wounds and burns from infection, immobilize fractures and dislocations, lessen pain, and conserve the patient's strength; and when medical aid can be obtained, his chance of recovery is greatly enhanced.

"The principal objects of first aid are:

(1) Prevention of further injury.
(2) Checking conditions known to be endangering life.
(3) Protecting injuries from infection and complications.
(4) Making the patient as comfortable as possible to conserve his strength.
(5) Transporting the patient to medical assistance, where required, in such a manner as not to complicate the injury or subject him to any more discomfort than is absolutely necessary."

CHOKING (Dislodging Objects From Throat or Mouth)

Very often an obstructing object can be dislodged by inserting the fingers into the child's mouth and removing the object. If this is not successful, turn the child upside down as shown in the illustration. Slap him on the back between the shoulder blades. This may dislodge the obstructing object. Of course, get medical aid immediately if you have not removed the object, and the choking continues.

In the case of a lightweight adult, the same procedure may be followed. If the patient is a large adult, stretch him across a bed face down with the face hanging over the side. Slap the patient on the back between the shoulder blades. In the absence of a bed or table, sit the patient on a chair and bend his head as far downward as possible and slap his back until the object is dislodged.

LIFE SAVING — DROWNING

If you cannot swim and the drowning person is near a dock or shore, there are many ways that you can help. The simplest and most effective is to reach out to him with a pole as illustrated. If a line or ring buoy is available, throw it to him. You can also extend your shirt and even tie the shirt and other part of your apparel together to make a longer line. Another way is to grab hold of part of the dock and extend your body to the drowning person; he may be able to grab your feet, and you can then pull him in.

Of course, if you are in a boat, row to the victim and help him grasp part of the boat. If you can pull him into the boat without risking capsizing it, then do so. If you can't safely help him into the boat, then row in with him and if that isn't possible, help him hold on to the boat and keep calling for more help. The American National Red Cross cautions against swimming rescues except by persons trained in life saving.

DROWNING

If there is no way to reach the drowning person by boat or line or other means, and you are a good swimmer and you must swim to him, then the cross-chest carry method of life saving is suggested. Follow this procedure:

Reach over the victim's shoulder and across his chest with your free arm and grasp his side just below the armpit as shown. Hold him so that your hip is directly under the small of his back, and the junction of his chest and head is under your armpit. Swim on your side using the scissors kick and the side arm pull. The side arm pull is executed by pulling the arm outward in a shallow sweep rather than in deep water. The strokes should be short and rapid.

RESCUE BREATHING

The instant you can touch bottom and stand with your own head outside the water, tilt the victim's head back and open his mouth. Place your mouth over his mouth and blow. Make sure to seal his nostrils shut with two of your fingers as shown in the illustration. The first series of breaths should be given as quickly as possible. Continue carrying the victim to shore but blow into his mouth at least once every ten seconds.

MOUTH - TO - MOUTH RESUSCITATION

Many people are under the mistaken impression that the restoration of breathing is applicable only in cases of drowning. Actually, there are many reasons for loss of breathing besides drowning. These are: choking, electric shock, gas poisoning, overdose of medicines, and many other causes. A knowledge of the four-step method described on these two pages may enable you to save somebody's life. It will only take a few minutes for you to master this knowledge. Once you know it, you will never forget it. It might even be a good idea to practice on someone now so that when an emergency arises, you will actually have some experience with this method.

1. Lay the victim on his back and turn the head to one side and remove with your fingers any foreign objects that may be in the victim's mouth. Now straighten the victim's head as shown in the illustration.

Put one hand under the victim's neck and tilt the head back by holding the head with the other hand.

2. Pull the chin upward until the head is tilted back fully.

3. Put your mouth tightly over the victim's mouth. Seal the nostrils shut with two fingers of your other hand. Now blow into the victim's mouth in order to make the chest rise.

4. Lift your mouth away from the victim and listen for the sound of returning air. If you don't hear the air, breathe again. If there is still no returning air, then there is a possibility that there is still some obstructing matter in the mouth or throat. Turn the victim's head to the side and attempt to dislodge such obstructing object. Then proceed to breathe into the victim's mouth as before. Always lift your own mouth away each time to permit the escape of air from the victim.

In the case of infants or young children, it is quite possible to obtain an airtight enclosure by covering both nose and mouth of the child with your own mouth. Continue breathing into the victim's mouth — don't give up. For a child, take short breaths, about twenty per minute; for an adult, breathe much more vigorously at the rate of about twelve times a minute. Get professional medical help without delay.

ELECTRIC SHOCK

Never touch a person directly with your own hands if he has made contact with a live electric wire or cable and is under a state of electric shock. Of course, if possible, cut off the current immediately, but if this is not feasible or instantly practical, break the contact of the person and the wire by using a long, dry stick as shown in the illustration. Make sure that your hands are dry and you are standing on a dry surface. Other devices that can be used are dry ropes or dry cloth. Once you have succeeded in breaking the contact with the current, and if the victim is not breathing, proceed to give mouth-to-mouth resuscitation.

TRIANGULAR-BANDAGE SLING

Sometimes it is important to know how to prepare a temporary sling; a very useful one is the triangular bandage sling which is illustrated. It is useful for supporting the arm, elbow, forearm, wrist, hand, or fingers.

Slings may be improvised with any one of objects such as belts, neckties, handkerchiefs and similar materials, but regular bandages are preferable. The illustration shows the triangular bandage sling. Put one end of an open triangular bandage over the shoulder of the injured side and allow the bandage to hang down in front of the chest as shown. Bend the arm at the elbow and bring the injured arm across the chest over the bandage. Now bring the end of the bandage over the shoulder of the injured side and tie as illustrated. Tuck the other end of the bandage in at the elbow, pinning it with a safety pin. Keep the fingertips exposed to detect the appearance of any interference with blood circulation.

MOVING VICTIM FROM DANGER ZONES

Sometimes it is important to move a victim away from a place of danger such as a fire or automobile accident. This action may even be necessary in the face of the possibility of additional injury but this is the only alternative to saving the victim's life. One quick method of moving the victim to safety is to place him on a blanket as shown and then to pull him away from the danger area. He should be pulled in the direction of the axis of his body, not sideways.

THE THREE-MAN CARRY

Sometimes it is necessary to lift a patient from the floor to carry him either to an ambulance or some other place for emergency medical help. The three-man carry is illustrated below.

In this carrying position two men kneel on one side of the victim and the third carrier faces them as shown. The carriers slide their hands under the victim's back as shown in step 1. The victim is then raised to the carriers' knees and rested on the knees. The carriers then slide their hands farther inwards under the victim and interlock their hands as shown in step

2. Notice that the hands of the carrier on the left are interlocked with the right hand of the front carrier and the left hand of the rear carrier. When the hands are interlocked, all carriers rise and stand erect as shown in step 3 — and carry the victim to the desired location and then lower him by reversing the lifting procedure.

1

2

3

PRESSURE POINTS

Often it is necessary to stop bleeding because of a wound or cut of an artery. Applying pressure at the nearest available pressure point between the heart and the cut may result in stopping or controlling the bleeding. There are actually twenty-two pressure points in the body, eleven on each side. Illustrated on this page are a number of the more important and accessible ones. The principle of the pressure points is somewhat similar to compressing a rubber tube to stop the flow of water through such tube. In some instances finger pressure may be sufficient to stop the bleeding, or it may be the only way to control bleeding. In other cases a tourniquet may be required. When a tourniquet is necessary, finger pressure should be applied first to stem the loss of blood while the tourniquet is being prepared and applied.

Illustrated at the top are various points to apply pressure to stop or control bleeding in shoulder, neck, and head. The application of the pressure should always be between the cut and the heart.

THE TOURNIQUET

The tourniquet can be made from a strap, belt, suspenders, handkerchief, necktie, rubber tubing, towel, or similar material. Do not use wire, cord, or anything that will cut the flesh. Place a hard pad or object over the artery so that when the tourniquet is tightened, it will press the pad or object against the artery. Sometimes a stick is placed through one of the knots as shown in the illustration. This is so that the tourniquet can be twisted and by twisting the stick, extra constricting force can be obtained in order to control the bleeding. Usually after a tourniquet is applied and remains on for several minutes the skin below the tourniquet turns white and then bluish. After the tourniquet is applied, the patient should be rushed to a physician and the physician should be the one to release or remove the tourniquet. United States Armed Forces experience indicates that a tourniquet can remain on for several hours without causing damage. This procedure of permitting the tourniquet to stay on is contrary to the old procedure which required release of the tourniquet after ten minutes and then its reapplication if necessary.

EARLY WARNING SIGNS OF A HEART ATTACK

Many lives might be saved, including your own, if the public learned to recognize early warning signs of a heart attack. A heart attack generally does not occur suddenly; the body gives some warning signs first. Knowing these signs might save your life.

1. One of the first signs is pressure or pain in the middle of the chest. Your heart is in the middle of your chest, not on the left as many believe.

2. The pain might get worse and also spread through the whole chest and down the left arm.

3. The pain might also spread to both arms, shoulders, neck or jaw. The sensation of pressure or fullness that often accompanies the pain is often mistaken for indigestion.

4. Pain may occur in any one or a combination of these areas at the same time. Pain might be intermittent—come and go. Often sweating, nausea, loss of breath and vomiting is accompanied with the pain.

WHAT TO DO IF YOU EXPERIENCE ANY OF THE ABOVE FOUR SIGNS

Call your doctor at once, or if he or any other doctor is not available, immediately go to the nearest hospital emergency room and ask for immediate treatment.

**IN CASE OF AN ACTUAL HEART ATTACK
FIRST AID SHOULD BE ADMINISTERED IMMEDIATELY— SEE PLATE F8D**

NEW LIFE SAVING TECHNIQUE TO HELP VICTIMS OF FOOD CHOKING "THE HEIMLICH MANEUVER"

A victim of food choking, unless helped immediately, will not be able to speak or breathe, usually turns blue, collapses and in most instances dies in about four minutes. Quick help is of the utmost importance. The procedure described below was developed by Dr. Henry Heimlich of the Jewish Hospital, Cincinnati, Ohio.

Place your arms around the victim's waist. Grasp your fist with your other hand. Place it against victim's abdomen above the navel and below the rib cage. Push fist into the abdomen with a quick upward thrust. If the food is not dislodged, repeat the procedure. A doctor should examine the victim after the food is dislodged. The Heimlich Maneuver can be self-administered.

If victim has collapsed and is lying down, kneel astride the victim's hips. Now place one hand on top of the other, as is shown in the picture. Place heel of bottom hand on victim's abdomen above the navel and below the rib cage. Push into the abdomen with a quick upward thrust. If food is not dislodged, repeat the procedure. As soon as the food is dislodged, the victim should be examined by a doctor.

LIFE SAVING TECHNIQUE FOR A HEART ATTACK

CARDIOPULMONARY RESUSCITATION

A heart attack victim may collapse, show no pulse and usually rapidly turns blue from lack of oxygen. The heart may have stopped beating. Often the heart can be restarted by a sharp rap with a clenched fist on the chest area above the heart. However, in most cases, it will be necessary to keep the circulation going and get air into the lungs. The instructions given below were written by Dr. Isadore Rossman, coauthor of *Medical Aid Encyclopedia for the Home* and appeared originally in *Health Digest,* a health newsletter published by *Parents' Magazine.*

This is the procedure called cardiopulmonary resuscitation and is most effective when performed by a two person team; one to compress the heart and another to blow air into the lungs.

1. *Cardiac massage.* Locate the rib margin and follow it to the middle of the body, to the breastbone. At the tip of the breastbone is a flexible, cartilaginous portion which confirms the central location. Three finger breadths above its tip (about 1 ½ inches) is the site for massage. The heel of the one hand is pushed downwards by the other hand. The intent is to depress this part of the lower breastbone by 2 inches, which in turn compresses the heart and ejects some of its blood into the arteries. Pressure is released and reapplied at a rather rapid rate, approximately 60 cycles per minute. Some rescuers count ''one thousand and one, one thousand and two, etc.,'' each count corresponding to one cycle of pressure and release and lasting about one second. There is a pause after the one-thousand-and-five count and then the cycle is repeated.

2. *Artificial respiration.* The other rescuer hyperextends the victim's head. (This is the head thrown back position one would assume to look at the top of a skyscraper.) With the thumb in the victim's mouth and the fingers under the chin, the rescuer takes the victim's jaw and brings it forcibly forward. The rescuer takes a deep breath and when the partner's count reaches one thousand and five, blows air into the victim's mouth by tightly sealing his mouth to the victim's. The rescuer should also hold the victim's nose to prevent air loss. There should be an obvious rise in the chest as air is blown into the lungs and a corresponding lowering of the chest as the air is subsequently released. This process (artificial respiration) is repeated once for every five depressions the other rescuer makes on the heart, ideally providing around 12 lung fulls of air every minute.

If only one person is available, he must perform both rescue operations, which is possible but not easy. The steps are the same with the rescuer shifting from pressing on the breastbone to artificial respiration after each fifth count. The maneuver should be kept up until an ambulance crew or medical help arrives. Individuals interested in learning more about cardiopulmonary resuscitation will find that many local communities and Red Cross chapters offer courses in the subject.

THE GLANDS

TYPES OF GLANDS

There are two classes of glands: exocrine (with ducts) and endocrine (ductless).

SIMPLE EXOCRINE

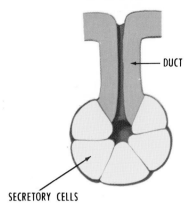

DUCT

SECRETORY CELLS

COMPOUND EXOCRINE

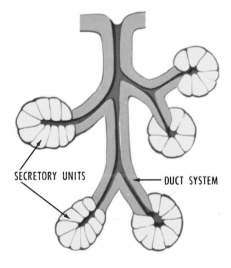

SECRETORY UNITS

DUCT SYSTEM

CAPILLARY

SECRETORY CELLS

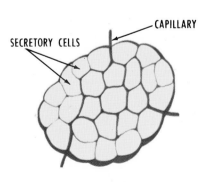

ENDOCRINE

THE MAJOR GLANDS

1 PITUITARY
2 PAROTID
3 SALIVARY
4 THYROID and PARATHYROIDS
5 LIVER
6 ADRENAL
7 GASTRIC
8 PANCREAS
9 INTESTINAL
10 TESTES
11 SKIN GLANDS

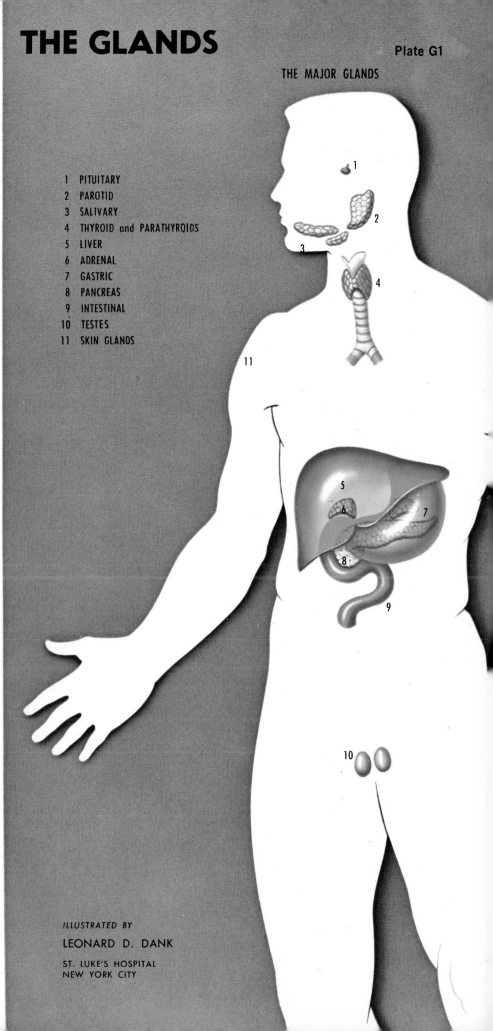

ILLUSTRATED BY

LEONARD D. DANK

ST. LUKE'S HOSPITAL
NEW YORK CITY

THE DEVELOPMENT OF GLANDS

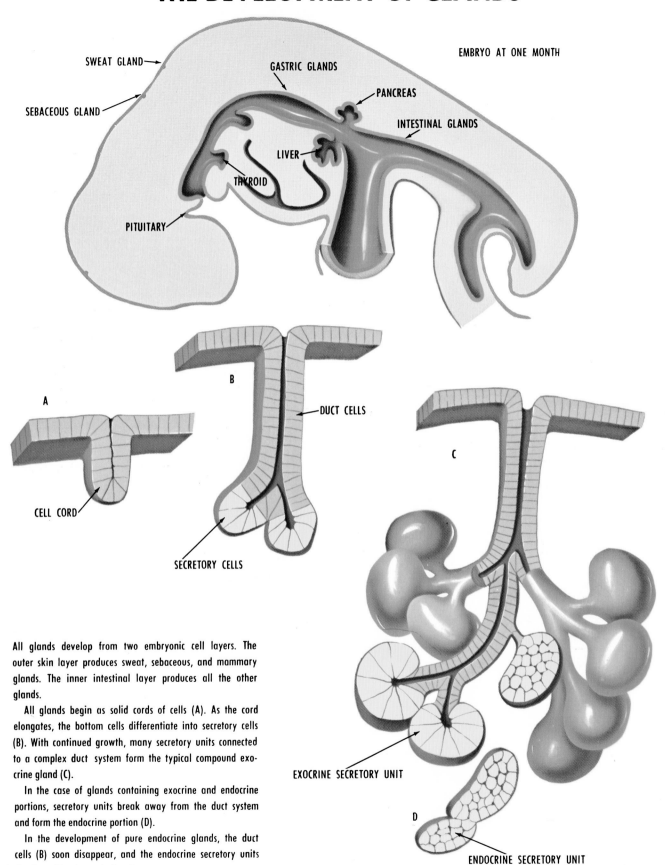

EMBRYO AT ONE MONTH

SWEAT GLAND

SEBACEOUS GLAND

GASTRIC GLANDS

PANCREAS

INTESTINAL GLANDS

LIVER

THYROID

PITUITARY

A

B

DUCT CELLS

CELL CORD

SECRETORY CELLS

C

EXOCRINE SECRETORY UNIT

D

ENDOCRINE SECRETORY UNIT

All glands develop from two embryonic cell layers. The outer skin layer produces sweat, sebaceous, and mammary glands. The inner intestinal layer produces all the other glands.

All glands begin as solid cords of cells (A). As the cord elongates, the bottom cells differentiate into secretory cells (B). With continued growth, many secretory units connected to a complex duct system form the typical compound exocrine gland (C).

In the case of glands containing exocrine and endocrine portions, secretory units break away from the duct system and form the endocrine portion (D).

In the development of pure endocrine glands, the duct cells (B) soon disappear, and the endocrine secretory units develop without any duct system.

THE EXOCRINE GLANDS

The sweat and sebaceous (oil) glands are distributed throughout the skin.

SWEAT GLAND

Numerous small glands located in the lips, tongue, palate, cheek plus the salivary glands empty into the oral cavity. All produce a complex liquid called saliva.

The esophagus has isolated mucus glands.

SALIVARY GLAND

The liver in addition to other functions produces bile, a digestive juice. Bile is stored in the gallbladder until needed.

The stomach contains an estimated 35 million gastric glands which produce digestive enzymes.

The exocrine portion of the pancreas produces the three most potent digestive enzymes.

The small intestine contains millions of glands producing digestive enzymes.

CONTROL OF EXOCRINE GLANDS

The exocrine glands are under involuntary nervous control. Sweat, sebaceous, and salivary glands, in response to local stimuli, adjust their secretory activity. For example, a temperature rise causes increased sweating.

The gastric and intestinal glands, the liver and pancreas are under both nervous and chemical hormonal control. The sequence of action and reaction between nerve and chemicals is described here in a simplified manner.

1   The sight, smell, taste of food stimulates a "hunger center" to send impulses to the hypothalamus.

2   The hypothalamus sends impulses over the vagus nerve to the gastric glands.

3   The vagus nerve stimulates the gastric gland cells and initiates secretion.

6   Food in the duodenum also causes the production of gastrin.

4   Gastric juice mixes with food.

5   Chemicals contained in all food cause the stomach lining to secrete the hormone gastrin. Gastrin travels to the gastric gland increasing the flow of gastric juice.

7   The interaction of hormones continues in the duodenum and small intestine. In brief, the duodenum produces the hormone secretin which causes the pancreas to secrete digestive juices. These juices cause the duodenum to secrete its own digestive juices.

THE ENDOCRINE GLANDS

The endocrine system is composed of widely scattered ductless glands which manufacture complex chemicals called hormones. The hormones empty directly into the blood stream, travel to their site of action and exert a powerful, long-sustained control over the body and each other.

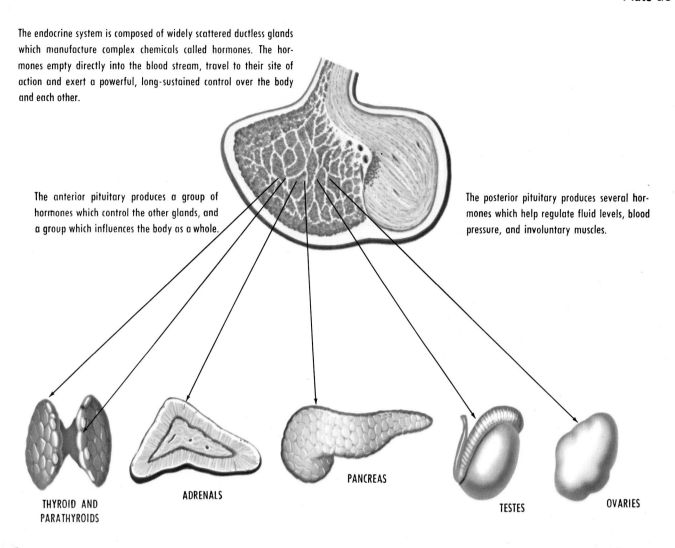

The anterior pituitary produces a group of hormones which control the other glands, and a group which influences the body as a whole.

The posterior pituitary produces several hormones which help regulate fluid levels, **blood** pressure, and involuntary muscles.

THYROID AND PARATHYROIDS

ADRENALS

PANCREAS

TESTES

OVARIES

BODY ACTIVITIES REGULATED BY THE ENDOCRINE GLANDS

ENERGY   CHEMISTRY   GROWTH   SEXUAL GROWTH   EMERGENCY

THE ADRENAL GLAND

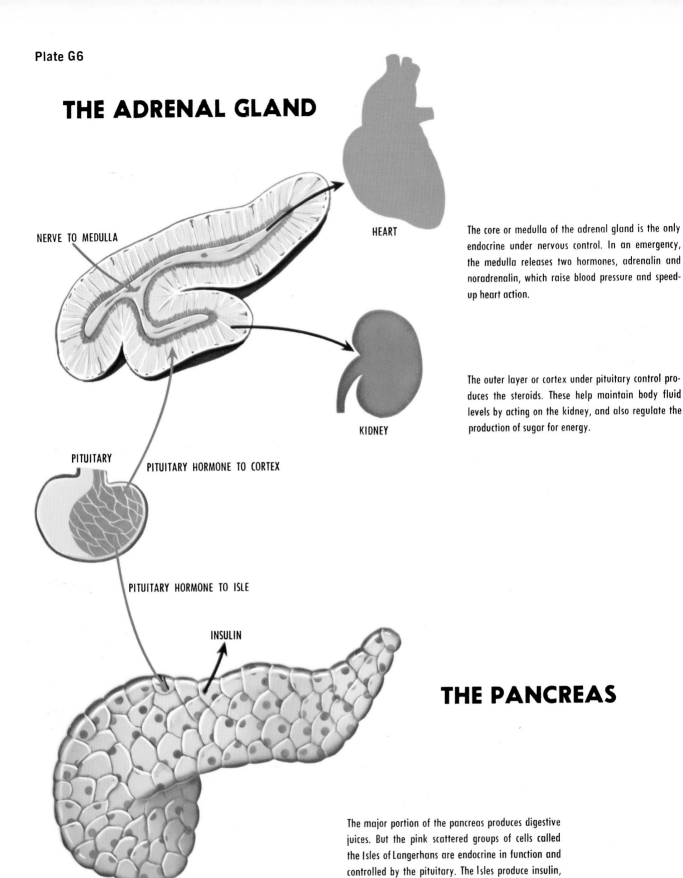

NERVE TO MEDULLA

HEART

The core or medulla of the adrenal gland is the only endocrine under nervous control. In an emergency, the medulla releases two hormones, adrenalin and noradrenalin, which raise blood pressure and speed-up heart action.

KIDNEY

The outer layer or cortex under pituitary control produces the steroids. These help maintain body fluid levels by acting on the kidney, and also regulate the production of sugar for energy.

PITUITARY

PITUITARY HORMONE TO CORTEX

PITUITARY HORMONE TO ISLE

INSULIN

THE PANCREAS

The major portion of the pancreas produces digestive juices. But the pink scattered groups of cells called the Isles of Langerhans are endocrine in function and controlled by the pituitary. The Isles produce insulin, a hormone essential to the storage and use of sugars by the body.

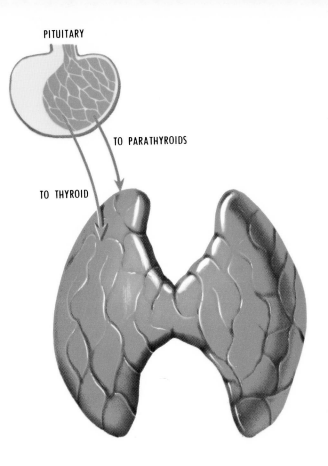

PITUITARY

TO PARATHYROIDS

TO THYROID

THE THYROID

The thyroid produces one hormone, thyroxin. Thyroxin regulates the metabolism (rate of energy consumption) and the physical and mental growth rate. The thyroid and parathyroids are under pituitary control.

THE PARATHYROIDS

The four yellow nodes located on the back of the thyroid constitute the parathyroids. They produce one hormone, parathormone, which has the sole function of regulating the calcium balance between blood and bone.

THE TESTIS

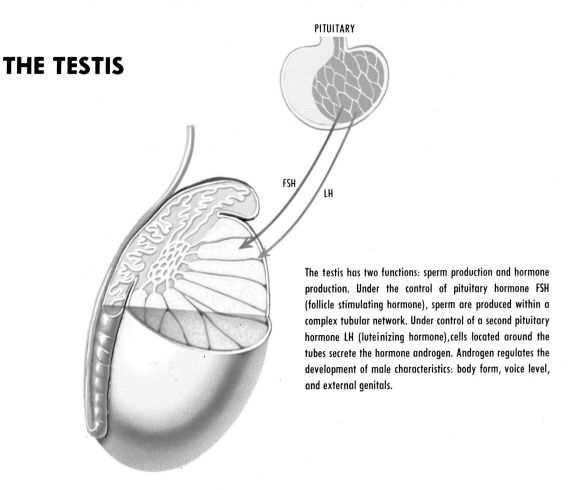

PITUITARY

FSH

LH

The testis has two functions: sperm production and hormone production. Under the control of pituitary hormone FSH (follicle stimulating hormone), sperm are produced within a complex tubular network. Under control of a second pituitary hormone LH (luteinizing hormone), cells located around the tubes secrete the hormone androgen. Androgen regulates the development of male characteristics: body form, voice level, and external genitals.

THE OVARY

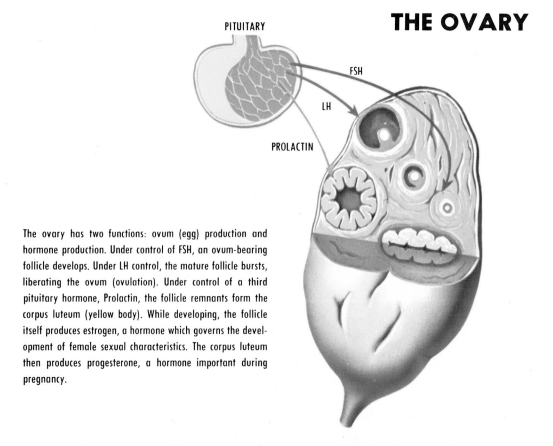

PITUITARY

FSH

LH

PROLACTIN

The ovary has two functions: ovum (egg) production and hormone production. Under control of FSH, an ovum-bearing follicle develops. Under LH control, the mature follicle bursts, liberating the ovum (ovulation). Under control of a third pituitary hormone, Prolactin, the follicle remnants form the corpus luteum (yellow body). While developing, the follicle itself produces estrogen, a hormone which governs the development of female sexual characteristics. The corpus luteum then produces progesterone, a hormone important during pregnancy.

THE NERVOUS SYSTEM

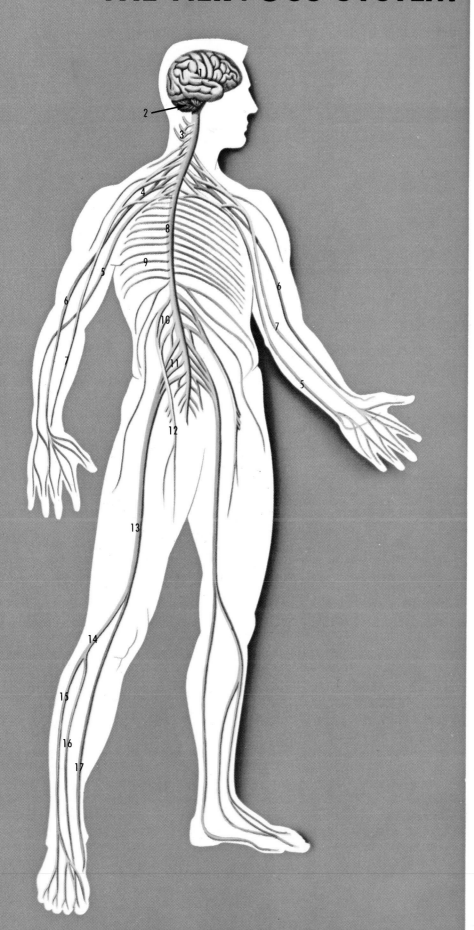

THE MAJOR NERVES

1 CEREBRUM
2 CEREBELLUM
3 CERVICAL PLEXUS
4 BRACHIAL PLEXUS
5 ULNAR
6 RADIAL
7 MEDIAN
8 SPINAL CORD
9 INTERCOSTAL
10 LUMBAR PLEXUS
11 LUMBO-SACRAL PLEXUS
12 FEMORAL
13 SCIATIC
14 COMMON PERONEAL
15 SUPERFICIAL PERONEAL
16 DEEP PERONEAL
17 TIBIAL

ILLUSTRATED BY

LEONARD D. DANK

ST. LUKE'S HOSPITAL
NEW YORK CITY

PARTS OF THE NERVOUS SYSTEM

BRAIN

GANGLION

SPINAL NERVE

SPINAL CORD

The central nervous system consists of the brain and spinal cord (yellow).

The peripheral nervous system consists of a series of 31 spinal nerves on each side which connect the central nervous system with the rest of the body (blue).

The autonomic nervous system has two subdivisions:

The sympathetic division consists of a series of 25 nodes (ganglia) on each side, connected to the spinal nerves and to each other. Sympathetic nerves leave the ganglia, travel to larger ganglia, and are distributed to the internal organs (black).

The parasympathetic division consists of 7 nerves (4 cranial and 3 sacral nerves) which are distributed to the internal organs (light grey).

ANATOMY OF THE CENTRAL NERVOUS SYSTEM

SENSORY CORTEX

THALAMUS

WHITE MATTER

GREY MATTER

CEREBELLUM

CROSS SECTION OF BRAIN

Nervous tissue is composed of grey and white matter. In the spinal cord, grey matter is within white matter. In the brain, grey matter is both over and within white matter. In general, white matter is for transportation of impulses, grey matter either relays or integrates these impulses.

White matter is arranged into fiber bundles. Sensory bundles ascend the cord, traverse the brain white matter, and end in brain grey matter. These bundles and their terminations in the brain are in tones of red and numbered 1-4. Motor bundles begin in brain grey matter, travel down brain white matter, and descend the cord. These bundles and their brain origins are in tones of blue and numbered 5-9. Not only does each bundle occupy a specific location in both brain and cord, it also carries a specific type of impulse. For example, pain-sensation impulses from most of the body ascend the lateral spinothalamic bundle, travel to the thalamus, and are relayed to the sensory cortex. Note that the right cord bundles are linked with the left side of the brain.

LATERAL SPINOTHALAMIC BUNDLE

CROSS SECTION OF SPINAL CORD

SPINAL CORD

DORSAL ROOT

DORSAL ROOT GANGLION

VENTRAL ROOT

SPINAL NERVE

SPINAL NERVE AND GANGLION CONNECTION

SYMPATHETIC GANGLION

SYMPATHETIC NERVE

RELATIONSHIP BETWEEN CENTRAL, PERIPHERAL, AND AUTONOMIC SYSTEMS

THE NEURON—LOCATION AND ANATOMY

TO AND
FROM BODY

TO INTERNAL
ORGANS

The neuron is the basic impulse-carrying cell of all parts of the
nervous system. Excluding specialized brain neurons, there are two
types. Sensory neurons (red) bring sensation impulses to the spinal
cord grey matter. They synapse with motor neurons carrying command or action impulses to the muscles and glands of the body and
internal organs.

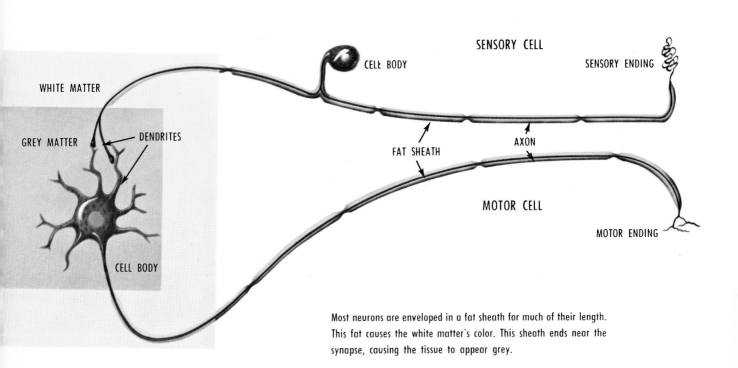

WHITE MATTER

GREY MATTER

DENDRITES

CELL BODY

CELL BODY

SENSORY CELL

SENSORY ENDING

FAT SHEATH

AXON

MOTOR CELL

MOTOR ENDING

Most neurons are enveloped in a fat sheath for much of their length.
This fat causes the white matter's color. This sheath ends near the
synapse, causing the tissue to appear grey.

SENSATION—CONTACT WITH THE ENVIRONMENT

PAIN

COLD

HEAT

TOUCH

TOUCH

PRESSURE

Through specialized sensory-neuron endings in the skin, the brain becomes aware of temperature, touch, pressure, taste, and pain. These sensory impulses ascend separate spinal cord bundles, ending in the brain sensory cortex. In the illustration on this page they are grouped into a common pathway. Sensory endings in muscles report to the cerebellum on muscular condition. Part of the inner ear informs the brain of body position and balance. The special senses of sight, smell, and hearing report directly to various sections of brain cortex.

MUSCLE SENSORY ENDING

CONTACT WITH THE MUSCLES

In response to the vast amount of information collected by the body, the brain directs innumerable movements. Motor impulses originating either in the brain grey motor cortex, or in other muscle coordinating brain centers, descend the spinal cord. The impulses travel out a spinal nerve to the muscle. A complicated voluntary movement may involve several hundred motor neurons.

CONTACT WITH THE INTERNAL ORGANS

The autonomic nervous system controls the internal activities. Each organ (the stomach is used as an example) receives a nerve supply from the parasympathetic division (light blue) which takes a direct route independent of the spinal cord. Each organ also receives a sympathetic nerve supply (dark blue) which descends the spinal cord, exits into a ganglion, and travels a sympathetic nerve to the organ. Sensory nerves (black) travel to the lower, nonconscious portions of the brain, where autonomic regulatory centers are located. In response to sensory information regarding the stomach's muscle and gland activity, a speed-up impulse is sent via the parasympathetic nerve, or a slow-down impulse via the sympathetic nerve. Thus each organ is maintained in delicate balance. Occasionally, unusual pain or discomfort will cause sensory impulses (dotted black) to register in the conscious mind.

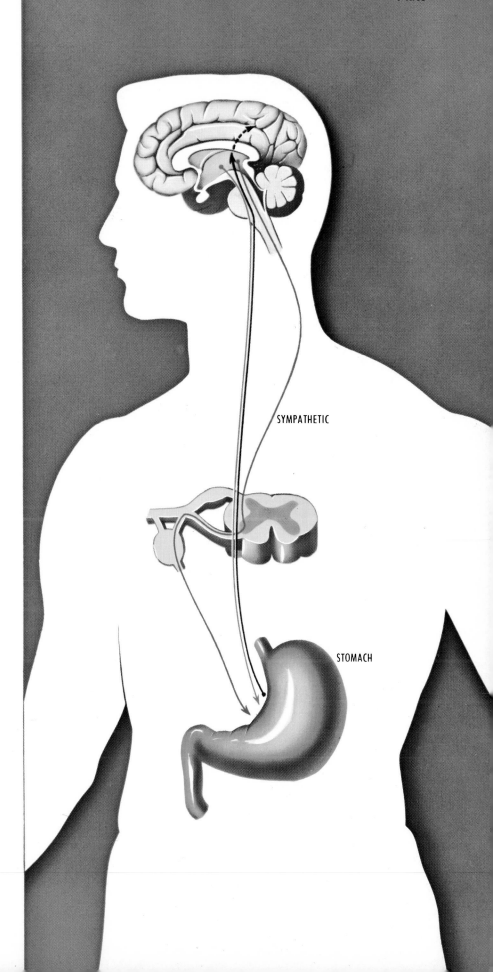

SYMPATHETIC

STOMACH

REFLEX ACTIVITIES OF SPINAL CORD

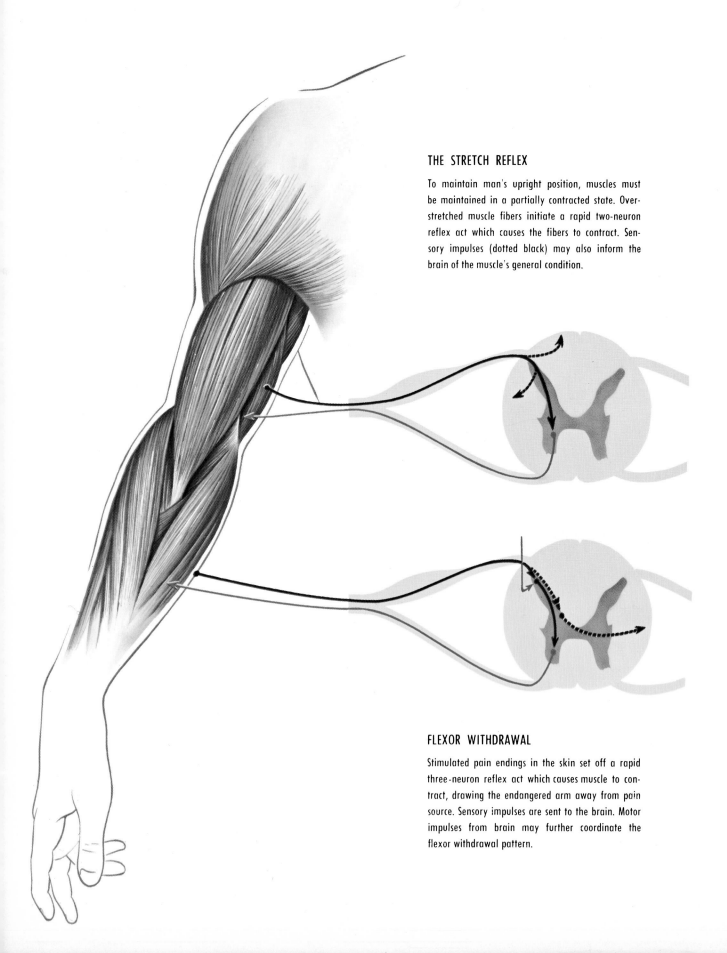

THE STRETCH REFLEX

To maintain man's upright position, muscles must be maintained in a partially contracted state. Over-stretched muscle fibers initiate a rapid two-neuron reflex act which causes the fibers to contract. Sensory impulses (dotted black) may also inform the brain of the muscle's general condition.

FLEXOR WITHDRAWAL

Stimulated pain endings in the skin set off a rapid three-neuron reflex act which causes muscle to contract, drawing the endangered arm away from pain source. Sensory impulses are sent to the brain. Motor impulses from brain may further coordinate the flexor withdrawal pattern.

REPRODUCTION AND FETAL DEVELOPMENT

THE FEMALE REPRODUCTIVE ORGANS

ON THE LEFT, THE ORGANS ARE SHOWN FROM BEHIND IN NATURAL
POSITION;   ON THE RIGHT THE ORGANS ARE IN CROSS SECTION.

Each month the ovary produces an ovum
(egg) which develops within a hollow follicle.
When ripe, the ovum bursts out of (ovulates)
the follicle, enters the mouth of the tube, and
is fertilized by male sperm. The follicle remnants form the corpus luteum. The fertilized
ovum, developing as it travels, takes 10
days to traverse the tube and implant in
uterine lining.

1   UTERINE MUSCLE
2   UTERINE CAVITY
3   IMPLANTATION SITE
4   FALLOPIAN TUBE
5   OVARY
6   OVUM WITHIN FOLLICLE
7   CORPUS LUTEUM
8   CERVIX
9   VAGINA
10 BROAD LIGAMENT
11 BLADDER

SIDE VIEW IN CROSS SECTION

ILLUSTRATED BY

LEONARD D. DANK

ST. LUKE'S HOSPITAL
NEW YORK CITY

THE MENSTRUAL CYCLE

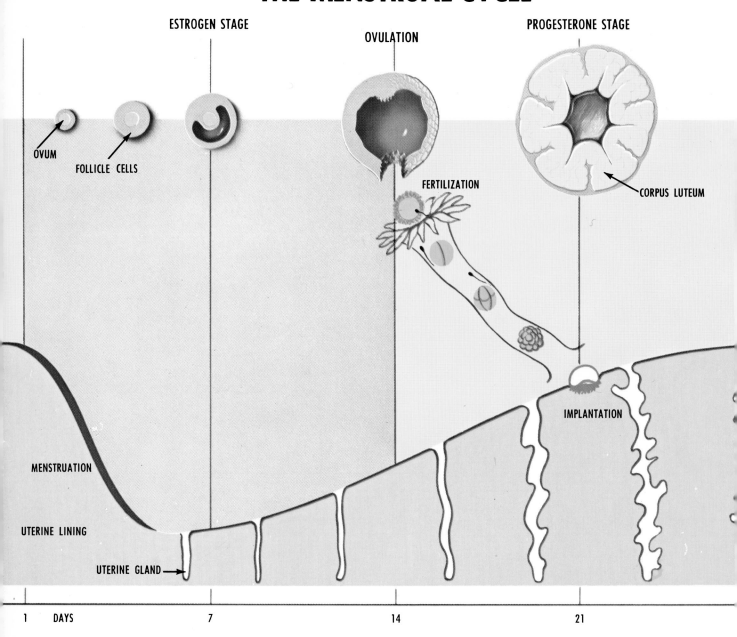

ESTROGEN STAGE

OVULATION

PROGESTERONE STAGE

OVUM

FOLLICLE CELLS

FERTILIZATION

CORPUS LUTEUM

IMPLANTATION

MENSTRUATION

UTERINE LINING

UTERINE GLAND →

1 DAYS   7   14   21

The 28-day cycle involves the simultaneous growth of an ovum
within the ovary, and the thickening of the uterine lining in preparation for receiving the ovum. The cycle can be divided into 2
equal stages.

ESTROGEN STAGE, DAYS 1 TO 14

As the ovum develops, the follicle cells secrete the hormone, estrogen,
which travels via the blood stream to the uterine lining. After the
cessation of menstrual flow, estrogen causes the lining to thicken.
The glands are straight tubes during this stage.

PROGESTERONE STAGE, DAYS 14 TO 28

When the ripe ovum is shed, it enters the fallopian tube, is fertilized, and travels down the tube to become implanted in the uterine
lining. After ovulation, the follicle cells form a new structure, the
corpus luteum, whose yellowish cells secrete the hormone, progesterone. Progesterone continues the uterine lining build-up in preparation for implantion, and persists until late in pregnancy.

PREGNANCY

(FIRST WEEK)

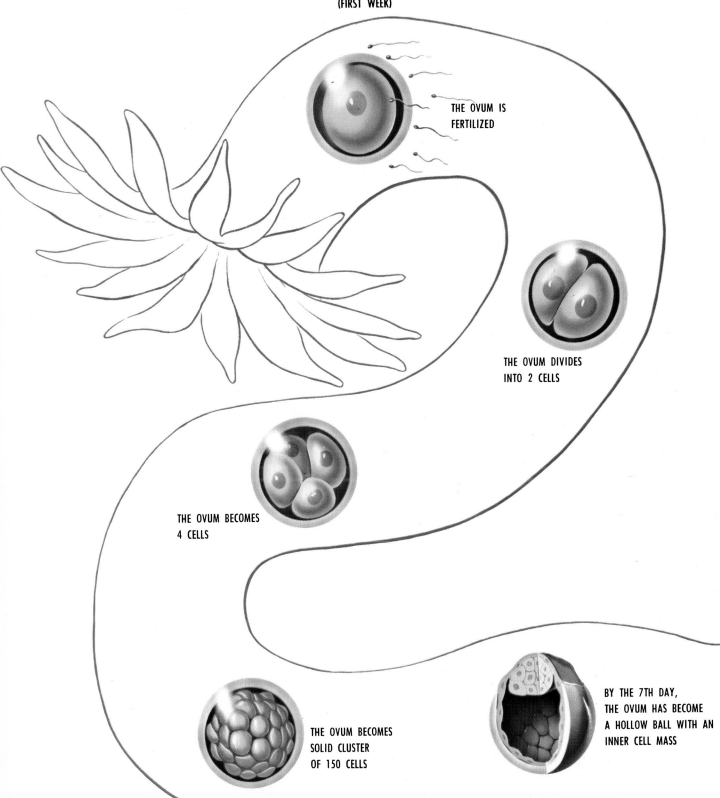

THE OVUM IS
FERTILIZED

THE OVUM DIVIDES
INTO 2 CELLS

THE OVUM BECOMES
4 CELLS

THE OVUM BECOMES
SOLID CLUSTER
OF 150 CELLS

BY THE 7TH DAY,
THE OVUM HAS BECOME
A HOLLOW BALL WITH AN
INNER CELL MASS

Plate J4

IMPLANTATION

PREGNANCY
(SECOND WEEK)

Pink — Maternal uterine lining
Red — Permanent placenta
Yellow — Embryonic temporary placenta
Blue — Embryo
Grey — Endoderm
Orange — Mesoderm

8TH DAY
The hollow ball of embryonic tissues pierces the uterine lining. A new cell layer, the endoderm, is formed by the embryo. Magnified 300 times.

9TH DAY
The embryonic tissues are completely implanted. The temporary placenta has established a blood supply for all the embryonic tissues. Magnified 230 times.

11TH DAY
The permanent placenta grows and forms a new tissue, the mesoderm. The embryo enlarges, and is now roofed over by the amnion. The endoderm develops a cavity, the yolk sac. Magnified 150 times.

14TH DAY
The permanent placenta lined by mesoderm is forming the villi. The amnionic and yolk sac cavities are well developed. Magnified 50 times.

PREGNANCY

(THIRD AND FOURTH WEEKS)

ONLY THE EMBRYO AND A PORTION OF THE PLACENTA ARE SHOWN IN THIS SERIES OF CROSS SECTIONS

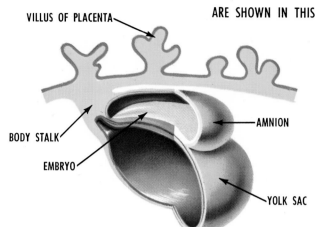

VILLUS OF PLACENTA

BODY STALK

EMBRYO

AMNION

YOLK SAC

16TH DAY

The flat embryo is roofed over by the amnion, and attached to the endoderm which forms the yolk sac. The mesodermic body stalk connects these tissues with the developing placenta. The embryo is 1/20 of an inch long.

19TH DAY

The embryo is beginning to curve. The mesoderm is pushing between the embryo and the endoderm.

22ND DAY

The mesoderm has pushed between the curved embryo and the endoderm. Head, tail, heart, and gut regions are defined. The yolk sac opening to the gut is narrowing.

GUT

HEART

HEAD

28TH DAY

By the end of the first month, the embyo is 1/5 inch long. The head, heart, and gut are more advanced.

THE SECOND MONTH

EXTERNAL APPEARANCE
OF 35–DAY–OLD EMBRYO.
SIZE IS 1/3 INCH.

1   BRAIN
2   HEART
3   LIVER
4   SPINE
5   YOLK SAC
6   BODY STALK

EXTERNAL APPEARANCE
OF 45–DAY–OLD EMBRYO.
SIZE 4/5 INCH.

COMPARATIVE SIZES
IN 3-12 WEEK EMBRYOS

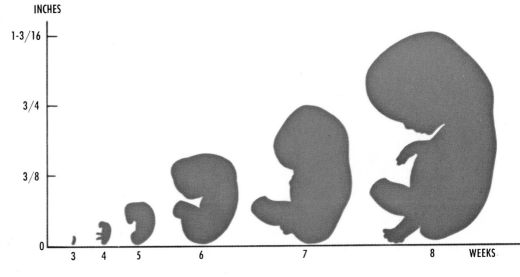

INCHES

1-3/16

3/4

3/8

0

3   4   5   6   7   8   WEEKS

INCHES   OUNCES

PERIOD OF THE FETUS

After the end of 8th week, the embryo, complete in external form, with all organs in place is called a fetus.

LENGTH

WEIGHT

LENGTH   WEIGHT

0   1   2   3   4   5   6   7   8   9   10

LUNAR MONTHS

Comparison of length and weight of embryo and fetus. For example: In 5th month fetus is 7-7/8 inches long and 61 ounces in weight.

9 WEEKS (1-3/4 in.)

12 WEEKS (3-3/16 in.)

THE TENTH MONTH

FETUS WITHIN AMNION
IN 38TH WEEK

FETUS ENTERING BIRTH
CANAL DURING LABOR

CLASSIFICATION OF FRACTURES

DIRECTION OF FRACTURE

OBLIQUE

SPIRAL

TRANSVERSE

A fracture is classified according to direction, extent, and displacement, i.e., a simple, spiral complete fracture, etc.

EXTENT OF FRACTURE

COMPLETE Bone is broken entirely across.

INCOMPLETE   (Linear or Greenstick)
A fracture which does not destroy
the continuity of the bone.

EXTENT OF DISPLACEMENT

COMPOUND
Bone penetrates overlying structures, causing
external wound. A simple fracture does not penetrate.

INJURIES PRODUCED BY A FALL

POSSIBLE INJURY SITES FOLLOWING A FALL

CLAVICLE

SHOULDER

ELBOW

PELVIS

FEMUR

WRIST

FINGERS

ANKLE

HEEL

KNEE

FRACTURE OF THE ELBOW

POSTERIOR DISLOCATION OF ELBOW

POSTERIOR DISLOCATION OF KNEE

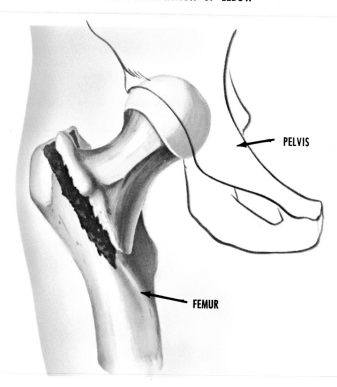

FRACTURE OF FEMUR

Curvature of spine (scoliosis) lateral displacement of vertebrae commonly due to poliomyelitis.

Traumatic torticollis is a scoliosis of the neck vertébrae due to an injury (blow on head). Congenital torticollis is due to an injury to the neck muscles. Both produce an outwardly similar deformity.

Ankylosis is the fusion of bones at a joint, due to an injury. Here the jaw and skull have fused, causing immobility.

Knock-knees in which the leg bones angle outward is generally due to rickets.

Clubfoot is any congenital turning of the bones of the foot. The foot may turn in, out, up, or down. The heel is also misplaced.

Congenital dislocation of hips. (Due to displacement of femoral head before birth). Pronounced lordosis and difficulty in walking become progressively worse without treatment.

BIRTHMARKS AND WARTS

Moles can be flat, raised, rough or smooth, hairless or hairy. Their color varies from brown to black. Hairy moles are apt to be congenital.

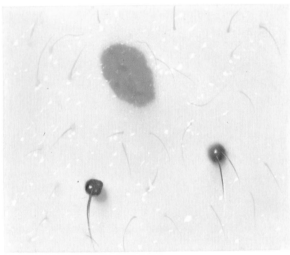

Port-wine stains are flat red discolorations located chiefly on the face and neck.

A wart is a virus-caused infection of the skin. Round, pea-sized, rough or smooth, yellow or brownish elevations occur singly or in groups, commonly on the hand.

SKIN RASHES

Contact dermatitis is an inflammation due to contact with irritant material. Poison ivy is an example.

Lupus erythematosus is a chronic skin disease. Patches with raised red edges, and depressed scaly centers commonly are found on the face.

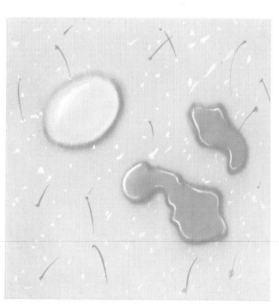

Urticaria (Hives) an inflammation characterized by the sudden appearance of pale, or reddish flat, smooth elevated patches or wheals. Severe itching and stinging is experienced. The wheals last minutes or hours, but disappear suddenly without a trace.

COMMON NASAL DEFORMITIES

Typical s-shaped nasal fracture causes a deviated septum, with resultant breathing difficulties.

Typical saddle-nose is result of depressed fracture of nasal bones

Typical nasal hump is produced by outward displaced fracture of nasal bones.

ILLUSTRATED BY LEONARD D. DAI

EMERGENCY SURVIVAL GUIDE continued

Rescue Breathing

1. Clear the airway.

A. Hold the victim's mouth open with one hand using your thumb to depress the tongue . . .
B. Make a hook with the pointer finger of your other hand, and in a gentle sweeping motion reach into the victim's throat and feel for a swallowed foreign object which may be blocking the air passage.
C. If you need to, reach all the way down to the voice box (larynx) and if there is a foreign object remove it.

2. Give mouth-to-mouth rescue breathing.

A. Put your hand on the victim's forehead, pinching the nose shut with your fingers, while holding the forehead back.
B. Your other hand is under the victim's neck supporting and lifting up slightly to maintain an open airway.
C. Take a deep breath. Open your mouth wide. Place it over the victim's mouth. Blow air into the victim until you see his or her chest rise . . .

D. Remove your mouth from the victim's. Turn your head to the side and watch the chest for a falling movement while you listen for air escaping from the victim's mouth as he or she exhales.
E. If you hear air escaping and see the chest fall you know that rescue breathing is working. Continue until help arrives.
F. Repeat the cycle every 5 seconds, 12 breaths per minute.

3. Mouth-to-mouth rescue breathing for a small child.

A. Be careful tilting a small child's head back to clear the airway. It cannot tilt as far back as an adult's.
B. Cover the child's mouth and nose with your mouth.
C. Blow air in with less pressure than for an adult. Give small puffs. A child needs less.
D. Feel the chest inflate as you blow . . .
E. Listen for exhales.
F. Repeat once every 3 seconds, 20 breaths per minute.

Note: It may take several hours to revive someone. Keep up rescue breathing until help arrives to relieve you. Remember you are doing the breathing for the victim. If you stop—in about 5 minutes—he or she could be dead!

Unconscious Person

Be careful approaching an unconscious person. He or she may be in contact with electrical current. If that is the case, turn off the electricity before you touch the victim.

There are hundreds of other possible causes of unconsciousness, but the first thing you must check for is breathing.

1. Try to awaken the person: Shake the victim's shoulder vigorously. Shout: "Are you all right?"
2. If there is no response check for signs of breathing.
   A. Be sure the victim is lying flat on his or her back. If you have to roll the victim over, move his or her entire body at one time.
   B. Loosen tight clothing around the neck and chest.
3. Open the airway:

A. Lift up the neck gently with one hand.
B. Push down and back on the forehead with the other hand.
C. Place your ear close to the victim's mouth. Listen for breath sounds. Watch his or her chest and stomach for movement.
D. If there is any question in your mind, or if breathing is so faint that you are unsure . . . assume the worst!
E. Give rescue breathing immediately. Have someone else summon professional help.